Maternal/Newborn
Plans of Care
Guidelines for Individualizing Care

Maternal/Newborn Plans of Care Guidelines for Individualizing Care
Third Edition

Marilynn E. Doenges, RN, BSN, MA, CS, APN

Clinical Specialist
Adult Psychiatric/Mental Health Nursing
Adjunct Faculty
Beth-El College of Nursing and Health Sciences
University of Colorado at Colorado Springs
Colorado Springs, Colorado

Mary Frances Moorhouse, RN, CRRN, CLNC

Nurse Consultant
TNT-RN Enterprises
Colorado Springs, Colorado

F. A. DAVIS COMPANY • Philadelphia

F. A. Davis Company
1915 Arch Street
Philadelphia, PA 19103

Printed in the United States of America

Last digit indicates print number: 10 9 8 7 6 5 4 3

Publisher, Nursing: Robert G. Martone
Production Editor: Elena Coler
Cover Designer: Alicia Boronsky

As new scientific information becomes available through basic and clinical research, recommended treatments and drug therapies undergo changes. The authors and publisher have done everything possible to make this book accurate, up to date, and in accord with accepted standards at the time of publication. The authors, editors, and publisher are not responsible for errors or omissions or for consequences from application of the book, and make no warranty, expressed or implied, in regard to the contents of the book. Any practice described in this book should be applied by the reader in accordance with professional standards of care used in regard to the unique circumstances that may apply in each situation. The reader is advised always to check product information (package inserts) for changes and new information regarding dose and contraindications before administering any drug. Caution is especially urged when using new or infrequently ordered drugs.

Library of Congress Cataloging in Publication Data

Doenges, Marilynn E., 1922–
        Maternal/newborn plans of care: guidelines for individualizing
    care / Marilynn E. Doenges, Mary Frances Moorhouse.—3rd ed.
            p. cm.
        Includes bibliographical references and index.
        ISBN 0-8036-0320-7
        1. Maternity nursing. 2. Pediatric nursing. 3. Perinatology.
        4. Nursing care plans. I. Moorehouse, Mary Frances. 1947–.
    II. Title.
            [DNLM: 1. Maternal-Child Nursing. 2. Patient Care Planning.
        3. Nursing Diagnosis. WY 157.3 D651m 1999]
    RG951.D64   1999
    610.73′678—dc21
    DNLM/DLC
    for Library of Congress   98-31646
                                                                    CIP

This book is dedicated:

To our husbands, the late Dean Doenges, who supported Marilynn and took great pride in her accomplishments; and Jan Moorhouse, who supports and cheers Mary when the going is rough.

To our children: Nancy (Jim) Daigle, David (Monita), Jim, Barbara (Bob Lanza), and John (Holly) Doenges: and Paul and Jason (Ellaina) Moorhouse, and grandchildren, Jennifer and Jonathan Daigle, Matthew and Tyler Doenges, Nicole and Kelsey Doenges; and Alexa and Mary Isabella Moorhouse, who provided us with first-hand knowledge about this subject.

To our mothers and fathers, who encouraged us to dream.

To our many friends, who discussed various concerns we had about differing viewpoints and ethical issues. Thanks!

To the FAD family for their support and friendship and for making us a part of the family, our great appreciation.

Special thanks to our editor, Robert Martone; production director, Bob Butler; production manager, Sam Rondinelli; production editor, Elena Coler, and the rest of the Production Department who survived our changes; and to Ruth de George, who relayed messages so well.

Thanks also to the staff of the Memorial Hospital Library, who so promptly provided us with articles we requested.

and

Finally, this book is dedicated to the student and practitioner who daily face the challenge of caring for the maternity client and her newborn and family in a rapidly changing healthcare environment.

Consultants and Contributors for the Third Edition

SANDRA CONANT, RN, MSN, CAS
Certified Addiction Specialist for Maternal/Infant
  Addictions
Topsfield, Massachusetts

SUSAN M. MOBERLY, RN, BSN, ICCE
Labor and Delivery Staff Nurse
ICEA Certified Childbirth Educator
Centura Health/Penrose Community Hospital
Colorado Springs, Colorado

CELESTE PHILLIPS, RN, EDD
President
Phillips and Fenwick a Women's Healthcare
Consulting & Management Company
Santa Cruz, California

Key to Essential Terminology

CLIENT ASSESSMENT DATA BASE

Provides an overview of the more commonly occurring etiology and coexisting factors associated with a specific maternal/newborn diagnosis as well as the signs/symptoms and corresponding diagnostic findings.

NURSING PRIORITIES

Establishes a general ranking of needs/concerns on which the Nursing Diagnoses are ordered in constructing the plan of care. This ranking would be altered according to the individual client situation.

DISCHARGE GOALS

Identifies generalized statements that could be developed into short-term and intermediate goals to be achieved by the client before being "discharged" from nursing care. They may also provide guidance for creating long-term goals for the client to work on after discharge.

NURSING DIAGNOSES

The general problem/concern (Diagnosis) is stated without the distinct cause and signs/symptoms, which would be added to create a diagnostic statement when specific client information is available. For example, when a client displays increased tension, apprehension, quivering voice, and focus on self, the nursing diagnosis of Anxiety could be stated: Anxiety, severe, related to threat to self-concept as evidenced by statements of increased tension, apprehension; observations of quivering voice, and feelings of inadequacy.

In addition, diagnoses identified within these guides for planning care as *actual* or *risk for* can be changed or deleted and new diagnoses added, depending entirely on the specific client information.

MAY BE RELATED TO/POSSIBLY EVIDENCED BY

These lists provide the usual/common reasons (etiology) why a particular problem may occur with probable signs/symptoms, which would be used to create the "related to" and "evidenced by" portions of the *client diagnostic statement* when the client situation is known.

When a risk for (formerly "potential") diagnosis has been identified, signs/symptoms have not yet developed and therefore are not included in the nursing diagnosis statement. However, interventions are provided to prevent progression to an *actual* problem.

DESIRED OUTCOMES/EVALUATION CRITERIA—CLIENT WILL

These give direction to client care as they identify what the client or nurse hopes to achieve. They are stated in general terms to permit the practitioner to modify/individualize them by adding time lines and individual client criteria so they become "measurable." For example, "Client will appear relaxed and will discuss feelings within 24 hours."

ACTIONS/INTERVENTIONS

Activities are divided into dependent and collaborative and are ranked in this book from most to least common. When creating the individual plan of care, interventions would normally be ranked to reflect the client's specific needs/situation. In addition, the division of independent/collaborative is arbitrary and is actually dependent on the individual nurse's capabilities and hospital/community standards.

RATIONALE

Although not commonly appearing in client plans of care, rationale has been included here to provide a pathophysiologic/psychosocial basis to assist the nurse in deciding about the relevance of a specific intervention for an individual client situation.

Contents

Introduction

One of the most significant achievements in the healthcare field during the past 20 years has been the emergence of the nurse as an active coordinator and initiator of client care. Although the transition from helpmate to healthcare professional has been painfully slow and is not yet complete, the importance of the nurse within the system can no longer be denied or ignored. Today, the nurse designs care interventions that move the whole client/family toward a positive outcome and optimal health.

The current state of the theory of nursing process, diagnosis, and intervention has been brought to the clinical setting to be implemented by the nurse. This book gives definition and direction to the development and use of individualized nursing care for women during the childbearing years, and their families. Therefore, this book is not an end in itself, but a beginning for the future growth and development of the profession.

Professional care standards, along with physicians and clients, will continue to increase expectations for nurses' performance as each day brings advances in the struggle to understand the mysteries of normal body function and human response to actual and potential health problems. With this increased knowledge comes greater responsibility for the nurse. To meet these challenges competently, the nurse must have up-to-date physical assessment skills and a working knowledge of pathophysiological concepts concerning the common changes occurring during pregnancy and birth and the conditions or diseases that may have an impact on the outcome. This book is a tool, a means of attaining that competency.

In the past, plans of care were viewed principally as learning tools for students and seemed to have little relevance after graduation. However, the need for a written format to communicate and document individualized client care has been recognized in all care settings. In addition, governmental regulations and third-party payer requirements have created the need to validate the appropriateness of the care provided, as well as the need to justify staffing patterns and monetary charges for client care. Documenting the expected and achieved outcomes serves this purpose. Thus, although the student's "case studies" were too cumbersome to be practical in the clinical setting, the client plan of care meets the above identified needs. The practicing nurse, as well as the nursing student, will welcome this text as a ready reference in clinical practice.

The primary focus of this book is on wellness, with inclusion of common health problems that impact on the maternity client and her newborn as well as plans of care identifying general considerations for the high-risk maternity client who presents with less common health problems. This book is designed for use in the maternal/newborn setting, serving as a guide for nurses who plan and promote healthcare for the maternity client and her family. The plans are organized by stages of pregnancy and address specific conditions and diseases in each stage for easy reference. Rationales (which not only state why an intervention is important but also provide related pathophysiological/psychosocial information, when applicable) enhance the reader's understanding of the intervention. This information also serves as a catalyst for thought in planning and evaluating the care being rendered.

Chapter 1 examines current issues and trends with their implications for the nurse caring for the client/family in the childbearing and early newborn phases. Trends in healthcare such as cost containment, shortened hospital stays, home care, and increased use of freestanding birth centers are examined in light of possible effects on the delivery of maternity care. An overview of cultural, community, sociologic, and ethical concepts impacting on the maternity nurse in a variety of healthcare settings is included. The importance of the nurse's role in collaboration and coordination with other healthcare professionals is integrated throughout the plans of care. Chapter 2 reviews the historical use of the nursing process in formulating plans of care and discusses the nurse's role in the delivery of that care. Nursing diagnosis is discussed to assist the nurse in understanding its role in the nursing process.

In Chapter 3, a nursing-based assessment tool is provided to aid the nurse in identifying appropriate nursing diagnoses. A sample client situation with individual data base and corresponding plan of care are included to demonstrate how critical thinking is used to adapt the nursing process theory to practice. Finally, evaluation and documentation are addressed to complete the nursing process cycle.

Chapters 4 though 6 provide plans of care that include information from multiple disciplines to assist the nurse in providing holistic care for the client/family during the prenatal, intrapartal, and postpartal phases within the community or acute care setting. Chapter 7 addresses the care of the newborn. Assessment guides incorporating the pertinent and customary questions to be asked of the client are included for each phase. Each plan includes a client assessment data base (presented in a nursing format) and associated diagnostic studies. After the data base is collected, nursing priorities are sifted from the information to help focus and structure the care provided. Discharge goals are listed to identify which general goals should be accomplished in situations in which care is expected to be terminated (e.g., prenatal infection) and not simply to progress to another stage (e.g., second trimester). The nursing diagnoses contain "related to" and "evidenced by" statements that provide an explanation of client problems or needs. Desired client outcomes are stated in behavioral terms that can be measured to evaluate the client's progress and the effectiveness of care provided. The interventions are designed to promote problem resolution.

The nurse acting independently or collaboratively within the health team uses a decision-making model to organize and prioritize nursing interventions. No attempt is made to indicate whether independent or collaborative actions come first, because this must be dictated by the individual situation. Inclusion of rationales for the nursing actions will assist the nurse in deciding whether the interventions are appropriate for an individual client. A bibliography follows the text to allow for further reference and research, as desired.

This book is designed for students who will find the plans of care helpful as they learn and develop skills in applying the nursing process and using nursing diagnoses in the maternal/newborn setting. It will complement their classroom work and support the critical thinking process. This book remains a ready reference for the practicing nurse as well as a catalyst for thought in planning, evaluating, and documenting care.

As a final note, this book is not intended to be a procedures manual, and efforts have been made to avoid detailed descriptions of techniques or protocols that might be viewed as individual or regional in nature. Instead, the reader is referred to an actual procedures manual or a book covering standards of care if detailed direction is desired.

INTRODUCTION

During the past 20 years, one of the most significant achievements in the healthcare field has been the emergence of the nurse as an active coordinator and initiator of client care. Although the transition from helpmate to healthcare professional has been painfully slow and is not yet complete, the importance of the nurse within the system can no longer be denied or ignored. Today the nurse designs care interventions that move the whole client/family toward a positive outcome and optimal health.

The current state of the theory of nursing process, diagnosis, and intervention has been brought to the clinical setting to be implemented by the nurse. This book gives definition and direction to the development and use of individualized nursing care for women and their families during the childbearing years. Therefore, this book is not an end in itself, but a beginning for the future growth and development of the profession.

Professional care standards, along with physicians and clients, will continue to increase the expectations for nurses' performances as each day brings advances in the struggle to understand the mysteries of normal body function and human response to actual and potential health problems. With this increased knowledge comes greater responsibility for the nurse. To meet these challenges competently, the nurse must have up-to-date physical assessment skills and a working knowledge of pathophysiologic concepts concerning the common changes occurring during pregnancy and birth and the conditions or diseases that may have an impact on the outcome. This book is a tool, a means of attaining that competency.

In the past, plans of care were viewed principally as learning tools for students and seemed to have little relevance after graduation. However, the need for a written format to communicate and document individualized client care has been recognized in all care settings. In addition, governmental regulations and third-party payor requirements have created the need to validate the appropriateness of the care provided, as well as the need to justify staffing patterns and monetary charges for client care. Documenting the expected and achieved outcomes serves this purpose. Thus, although the student's "case studies" were too cumber-some to be practical in the clinical setting, the client plan of care meets the above identified needs. Practicing nurses, as well as nursing students, will welcome this text as a ready reference in clinical practice.

The primary focus of this book is on wellness, with the inclusion of common health problems that affect the maternity client and her newborn as well as plans of care identifying general considerations for the high-risk maternity client who presents with less common health problems. This book is designed for use in the maternal/newborn setting, serving as a guide for nurses who plan and promote healthcare for the maternity client and her family. For easy reference, the plans are organized by stages of pregnancy and address specific conditions and diseases relevant at each stage. Rationales (which not only state why an intervention is important, but also provide related pathophysiologic information when applicable) enhance the reader's understanding of the intervention. This information also serves as a catalyst for thought in planning and evaluating the care being rendered.

Chapter 1 examines current issues and trends and their implications for the nurse caring for the client/family in the childbearing and early newborn phases. Healthcare trends, such as cost containment, shortened hospitals stays, home care, and the increased use of freestanding birth centers, are examined in light of possible effects on the delivery of maternity care. An overview of cultural, community, sociologic, and ethical concepts affecting the maternity nurse in a variety of healthcare settings is included. The importance of the nurse's role in collaboration and coordination with other healthcare professionals is integrated throughout the plans of care. Chapter 2 reviews the historical use of the nursing process in formulating plans of care and discusses the nurse's role in the delivery of that care. Nursing diagnosis is discussed to assist the nurse in understanding its role in the nursing process.

In Chapter 3, a nursing-based assessment tool is provided to aid the nurse in identifying appropriate nursing diagnoses. A sample client situation with individual data base and corresponding plan of care is included to demonstrate how critical thinking is used to adapt the nursing process theory to practice. Finally, evaluation and documentation are addressed, completing the nursing process cycle.

Chapters 4 through 6 provide plans of care that include information from multiple disciplines to assist the nurse in providing holistic care for the client/family during the prenatal, intrapartal, and postpartal phases within the community or acute care setting. Chapter 7 addresses the care of the newborn. Assessment guides incorporating the pertinent and customary questions to be asked of the client are included for each phase. Each plan includes a client assessment data base (presented in a nursing format) and associated diagnostic studies. After the data base is collected, nursing priorities are sifted from the information to help focus and structure the care provided. Discharge goals are listed to identify the general goals that should be accomplished in situations in which care is expected to be terminated (e.g., prenatal infection) and not simply to progress to another stage (e.g., second trimester). The nursing diagnoses contain "related to" and "evidenced by" statements that provide an explanation of client problems or needs. Desired client outcomes are stated in behavioral terms that can be measured to evaluate the client's progress and the effectiveness of care provided. The interventions are designed to promote problem resolution.

The nurse acting independently or collaboratively within the health team uses a decision-making model to organize and prioritize nursing interventions. No attempt is made to indicate whether independent or collaborative actions come first because this must be dictated by the individual situation. Inclusion of rationales for the nursing actions will assist the nurse in deciding whether the interventions are appropriate for an individual client. A bibliography follows the text to allow further reference and research, as desired.

This book is designed for students, who will find the plans of care helpful as they learn and develop skills in applying the nursing process and using nursing diagnoses in the maternal/newborn setting. It will complement their classroom work and support the critical thinking process. This book remains a ready reference for the practicing nurse as well as a catalyst for thought in planning, evaluating, and documenting care.

As a final note, this book is not intended to be a procedures manual, and efforts have been made to avoid detailed descriptions of techniques or protocols that might be viewed as individual or regional in nature. Instead, the reader is referred to a procedures manual or book covering standards of care if detailed direction is desired.

CHAPTER 1

TRENDS AND ISSUES IN MATERNAL/ NEWBORN CARE

In considering trends and current issues in maternal/newborn nursing care, one must look at the overall trends and restructuring within the healthcare industry. The impetus to restructure healthcare is partly a result of the rapidly rising cost of healthcare delivery, the increasing numbers of uninsured or underinsured consumers, and the need for allocation of resources. In addition, technological advances, the needs of special populations, changing roles for healthcare providers, ethical issues, and liability concerns will all affect the way in which maternity care is provided in the future. Nurses must be aware of these influences and be actively involved in formulating policies and standards of practice so that care continues to be provided at a high level of quality and client satisfaction is ensured.

THE CHANGING HEALTHCARE ENVIRONMENT

Healthcare Costs and the Allocation of Resources

Healthcare expenditures continue to rise. Public Law No. 98-21 changed the method of payment for federally subsidized healthcare for inpatient services from a cost-based retrospective payment system to a prospective payment system based on 467 diagnoses or diagnostically related groups (DRGs). Most states are considering (and some have enacted) options to similarly curb Medicaid reimbursement. Both government and private payors of healthcare are pursuing various methods of cost containment, including managed care and special incentives for the consumer and/or provider. Most insurance plans include precertification, early hospital discharge, outpatient care, and some home care services, with third-party payors negotiating with healthcare providers, agencies, and facilities to lower reimbursement rates or even to capitate fees based on both the numbers and on specific demographics of the insured population.

Cost-containment programs are having a significant impact on maternity care. For example, although new federal and state legislation requires private insurers to cover hospital stays of 48 hours for vaginal delivery and 96 hours for cesarean delivery, most women are discharged within 24 to 36 hours or 48 to 72 hours, respectively. Data are still being gathered regarding the impact that prospective payment systems are having on hospital costs for high-risk mothers and infants. Although some states have modified payment structures for high-risk services in certain perinatal centers not under the DRG reimbursement system, a national restructuring may be necessary for equitable treatment. Based on predetermined guidelines, such as gestational age and/or birth weight, this rationing of healthcare dollars or allocation of resources may mandate limiting the services and therapy modalities provided to preterm infants. Studies by the Division of Maternal and Child Health of the U.S. Department of Health and Human Services may provide the data for such a restructuring to help ensure that perinatal programs designed for the high-risk client are not unduly compromised.

In addition, within the current healthcare delivery system, there is a significant population of underserved and uninsured individuals. Some of these are uninsured by choice, such as young adults who may choose to budget their healthcare dollars elsewhere, believing that at this stage of their lives they will not need these services. Others may not have access to group coverage because they are self-employed, are not offered healthcare insurance by their employers, or cannot afford the cost of monthly premiums even if insurance is available. Even those with insurance may find that their policy does not provide maternity benefits.

3

Inadequate preventive and primary care for infants and for women of childbearing age has contributed to the lack of a decline in fetal mortality rates and to the increased cost of care for infants with special needs. Preconception counseling and prenatal and perinatal care for all women are necessary to effect change in these areas. Nurses can play a primary role in this change by providing leadership, client education, counseling, and screening. In 1991, the American Nurses Association (ANA), with the support of other nursing organizations, presented an Agenda for Health Care Reform, in which they proposed "delivering primary healthcare in community-based settings," "consumer responsibility for personal health, self-care, and informed decision making," and "utilization of the most cost-effective providers to include certified nurse midwives and nurse practitioners," among other proposals. This agenda continues to define the ANA's philosophy and to guide its public policy and legislative action for the way in which care should be delivered to all clients, and most certainly to maternal/newborn clients.

Managed Care— Restructuring Healthcare

With its changes in reimbursement, the shift to managed care has forced hospitals to restructure following methods borrowed from industry, such as re-engineering and work redesign, or according to methods developed specifically for the healthcare arena (e.g., accelerated clinical improvement) to achieve the goal of reduced cost without jeopardizing quality and customer satisfaction.

Restructuring the work force and patient care system was initially accomplished through downsizing and layoffs, with shifting of care from registered nurses (RNs) to licensed practical nurses (LPNs) and unlicensed providers, as well as through mergers and consolidations of services. Great concern has been raised by professionals regarding the quality of care provided as well as the perceived decline in customer satisfaction. In response to these concerns, some hospitals have formed collaborative practice teams whose goal is to totally revise the patient care system by the following means: reducing redundancy and eliminating nonproductive activities; relocating ancillary services, such as laboratory and x-ray services, to the client care areas; implementing cross-training of staff to enhance careprovider qualifications; implementing computerization; streamlining documentation; and developing structured care methodologies.

Using collaborative practice teams (including administrative and financial representatives) helps to ensure the quality and cost-effectiveness of client care through the inclusion of clinical research findings and sound fiscal policy. These activities have reaffirmed the client-focused care approach already taking hold in many obstetrical departments. Low-intervention, "family-centered" care is being encouraged through the use of labor, delivery, and recovery rooms (LDRs)

or labor, delivery, recovery, and postpartum rooms (LDRPs), which replace the need for three or four different rooms. This setup provides the same level of care, but allows relaxation of visitation policies both intrapartally and postpartally; the incorporation of birth plans developed by the client/couple, which can further individualize the birth experience; and a conscious effort by some providers to reduce the use of "technology." Cross-training of staff members to provide mother *and* infant care from admission through discharge and beyond helps promote continuity of care and enhances educational follow-through. A cross-trained/multiskilled staff allows flexible staffing to address fluctuations in client admissions and acuity. In addition, case managers are being added to the team to coordinate prenatal and postnatal care needs of special populations, helping to reduce the untoward effects of complications and to maximize outcomes while minimizing costs.

The reduction in the number of individuals providing direct client care has necessitated problem-solving activities to help nurses "work smarter." The use of computers has advanced beyond billing and order entry functions. Bedside terminals (or hand-held units) allow immediate data entry and file review/data retrieval. Other technological developments such as beepers/cordless phones facilitate communication between client/nurse, reducing response time. Documentation time is reduced through streamlining, such as using detailed flow sheets, charting "by exception," developing clinical pathways, and using computers to generate plans of care.

Clinical pathways identify specific outcomes and corresponding activities for a given population (such as Uncomplicated Pregnancy or Intrapartal Care for Spontaneous Vaginal Delivery), which aids in organizing, sequencing, and standardizing care. The use of clinical pathways provides the opportunity for healthcare providers to modify or incorporate care to reflect clinical innovations and research findings. (However, there is the possibility that the clinical pathway's philosophy of "one size fits all" may be at odds with the client's personal birth plans/preferences.) Finally, clinical pathways may be useful for identification of actual/potential "outlyers," allowing reallocation of resources to maximize mother/infant outcomes in a timely manner while controlling costs.

Other structured care methodologies allowing standardization of the care process include the use of algorithms, guidelines, protocols, and standing orders, which stabilize care practices, and system processes, which are designed to improve outcomes. In addition, shifting some care activities from the nurse to the client/family permits better use of nursing time and efforts. Promotion of self-care through participation in planning care, self-administration of nonnarcotic medications as indicated, self-guided tutorials/education modules, and rooming-in provide opportunities for the client to maximize the hospital experience and demonstrate newly learned skills.

Advances in Technology

Complex technological advances and scientific discoveries continue to alter the scope of maternity care. For instance, genetic research and engineering have expanded the scope of prenatal testing to encompass an ever-increasing number of diagnoses and interventions. Management of infertility problems now includes in vitro fertilization, gamete intrafallopian transfer (GIFT), and other procedures, as well as surrogate parenting. New pharmaceuticals have frequently been successful in controlling premature labor. Clients with high-risk pregnancies can often be monitored at home rather than in the hospital, using sophisticated communication systems linked to central computers or laboratories in large medical centers. Some women with long-standing severe health problems are successfully conceiving and delivering viable infants. Increasingly sophisticated methods for assessing fetoplacental well-being are available to detect problems during a high-risk pregnancy. Advances in ultrasonography have enabled surgeons to operate on the developing fetus for select problems. Neonatal intensive care units are equipped and staffed to provide life support to premature infants who previously would not have survived. With these advances come additional concerns, ethical dilemmas, and higher costs.

Special Populations

The mobility and displacement of people worldwide and the trend of immigrants to locate in specific urban areas and to retain their ethnic and cultural identity have created large numbers of clients and families with diverse backgrounds and needs. Furthermore, the shift from acute care to community-based care necessitates delivery of culturally congruent care to specific communities, integrating folk and lay care with professional services. In these populations, problems related to healthcare include language barriers, lack of knowledge or understanding, and unique health beliefs or practices that influence behaviors adopted during the prenatal, intrapartal, and postpartal periods. In addition, owing to a lack of immunizations, exposure to communicable diseases, the carrier status of diseases, poor health and hygiene habits, and variations in immune systems, there has been an increase in health-related problems among immigrant populations. These concerns are magnified in the illegal immigrant population, who receive no health screening before entry into this country and who are often reluctant to seek professional healthcare for fear of being deported. Nurses need to enhance their own cultural awareness and be adaptable, creative, and knowledgeable in dealing with the needs of these clients, their family members, and communities as a whole, in order to maximize healthcare outcomes, and to prevent cultural clashes or impositions.

Increasingly, women are electing to postpone childbearing until after they complete certain educational, personal, or professional goals, thereby entering childbearing as "older" primigravidas. These women may have some increased risk for complications during the prenatal, intrapartal, and postpartal periods. With shorter hospital stays, such clients may have a difficult time adapting to new mothering roles. For these women, who thus far have been able to control the events in their lives, hormonal fluctuations, medical restrictions, a crying baby, breastfeeding issues, and infant care tasks, in combination with other responsibilities, can be overwhelming. Unfortunately, these clients may not be recipients of the agency referral or support services afforded to many other high-risk groups. However, they often have problem-solving skills related to their work and life experience that can help them to adjust to this new situation. By creating and/or implementing a comprehensive plan of care, including home visits and/or timely telephone calls, the nurse can be instrumental in helping these clients cope positively. In addition, the nurse may be involved in establishing or teaching community-based parenting/postpartal classes to meet the needs of the family.

Not only are nurses caring for greater numbers of older maternity clients, but nurses also continue to care for large numbers of adolescents. With its identifiable physical and emotional risks, adolescent pregnancy affects approximately 1 million teenagers, their families, and their significant others annually. In creating and implementing a plan of care for the adolescent, the nurse must recognize that this client's developmental needs may interfere with her cooperation, necessitating alternative approaches to achieve the goal of optimal maternal and fetal well-being. Whether the adolescent chooses to terminate the pregnancy or carry it to term, either keeping the baby or relinquishing it for adoption, an educational program must include information about family planning methods, sexually transmitted diseases (STDs), and infant care/parenting, as applicable. The incidence of STDs tends to remain high, particularly among adolescents aged 15 to 19 years, and is related to a lack of treatment, drug use, multiple sex partners, and unsafe sex practices. As new and more virulent strains of STDs are identified, the incidence of chlamydia and gonorrhea infections remains high, and cases of syphilis and HIV/AIDS are reaching epidemic proportions. Such infections can have a negative impact on the outcome of a pregnancy and/or future childbearing capabilities. A new technique for locating the AIDs virus in the blood may help doctors predict if a baby born to an HIV-infected mother will eventually develop the disease, and ongoing research may lead to the establishment of new vaccines to protect the fetus from such threats as herpes, cytomegalovirus (CMV), and AIDS.

Current mortality trends indicate that HIV/AIDS is now one of the five leading causes of death in women of reproductive age. Because women infected with HIV are the major source of infection for infants, these trends in AIDS mortality in women forecast the impact of AIDS mortality in children as well. In addition, by the end of 1995, approximately 50,000 children/adolescents were left motherless. In meeting the physical and emotional needs of affected mothers, infants, and families, such statistics have tremendous economic implications for the healthcare delivery system. Primary prevention through health education programs aimed at the primary and secondary school level may be the most effective means to reduce the impact of this health problem.

The same approaches are being used to deal with the problem of substance abuse, which continues to have a significant effect on the prenatal well-being of the mother and her offspring. Cigarette smoking, alcohol, and prescription/street drug use have far-reaching short- and long-term effects. The National Institute on Drug Abuse estimates that 15% of American women between the ages of 15 and 44 years (or 8 million women) are currently substance abusers, and this number is increasing. The National Association for Perinatal Addiction Research and Education predicts that as many as 375,000 infants may be affected each year by their mothers' drug abuse during pregnancy. Cocaine use and abuse, particularly among women between the ages of 15 and 25 years, has increased dramatically in recent years, with a significant impact on women during the childbearing years, increasing perinatal morbidity and mortality rates. Researchers are now examining both the short- and long-term effects of maternal cocaine use on the pediatric population and the potential impact on the education system.

It is imperative that the healthcare system continue to develop methodologies to identify substance abuse in the prenatal client and to establish protocols for primary, secondary, and tertiary treatment. Using the media to educate the public about the dangers of substance use, particularly during pregnancy, is critically important. Prenatal programs must focus on educating the at-risk client about the dangers of substance abuse during pregnancy and must establish therapeutic networks between identified abusers and prenatal healthcare providers. Social policy must address who should pay for the healthcare and education required by the substance-abusing mother and her infant.

Consumer Participation

The self-care focus that began in the 1960s and 1970s is being sustained by the push to contain healthcare costs. Obstetric care is being redefined as providers move from a medical (or illness) model, where the focus was on the childbearing woman and her unborn baby with the "patient" in a passive role, to a family-centered model, where the "client" takes an active role and a collaborative team provides care to the woman and her family throughout her childbearing years. This approach requires the client to be assertive, to seek the necessary information to make informed decisions, and even to assume some primary care functions, including monitoring physiological status and the performance of diagnostic tests. This may be in direct conflict with the individual's personal, cultural, or religious beliefs, expectations, and practices. It is the

nurse's responsibility to be attuned to the client's needs in general and to recognize and incorporate these specific issues into the plan of care. The consumer must actively participate in the planning of care and in writing the plan of care or clinical pathway in lay terms to assist the client/family in anticipating care and accepting specific interventions to achieve agreed-on goals.

As consumers become increasingly sophisticated in their approach to maternity care, they have some expectations for specific labor, delivery, and postpartal experiences, such as a family-centered approach to childbirth with reduced medical intervention. These expectations are reflected in the consumer's choice of a care provider (e.g., certified nurse midwife [CNM] versus physician), delivery setting (e.g., homelike versus "hospital"), and individually written birth plan. Such sophistication, together with strong economic incentives to provide lower-cost alternatives to hospital care, has promoted the development of single-room maternity care (SRMC) and freestanding birth centers throughout the country. The focus is on "normalizing" the birth experience by allowing women with low-risk, uncomplicated pregnancies to give birth in a homelike setting without the need to rely on complex technology to monitor the progress of labor and fetal well-being. The nurse working in this setting needs to philosophically accept the mission, goals, and objectives of this decreased reliance on technology and to possess a broad base of clinical experience in prenatal care as well as labor and delivery.

Shortened maternity stays require nurses to provide a thorough assessment of needs and to create a comprehensive plan fostering self-care. Preparing the client and family for discharge within 12 to 36 hours after delivery also requires the nurse to demonstrate comprehensive skills in assessment of needs and health education for the postpartal family as well. Parenting and infant care classes and health-promotion programs are anticipated components of the nurse's role in providing support to the client and her family after discharge. An integral component of such a program involves outpatient or home follow-up assessments of both mother and infant at specific intervals during the early postpartal period. Because many new mothers experience some degree of anxiety and ambivalence in the first few days at home alone, these women can benefit from the additional teaching and assistance provided by a qualified nurse provider. Roadblocks to outpatient participation in care, including finances, transportation, child care, and cultural expectations, need to be identified and the consumer included in the problem-solving process if home follow-up programs are not available.

Expanding Roles for the Healthcare Professional

In an effort to contain costs and avoid the duplication of services, hospitals are regionalizing obstetric/perinatal units and defining the responsibilities of each agency based on its categorization as a Level I, II, or III/IV (primary, secondary, or tertiary) facility. Such regionalization may force the separation of families when a high-risk situation requires the hospitalization of the prenatal client and/or the birth of a preterm infant. Such a crisis presents unique challenges to the nurse, who may function as an information link between the larger medical center and the absent family.

The complexity of new technology and of new approaches to maternity care places enormous demands on the nurse providing care. Nurses are actively involved not only in the technological aspects of care, but also in the educational process of the client and family members. The rapidly changing knowledge base requires constant update of information. The continuation of education through formal classwork, workshops, seminars, and professional reading is essential. As nurses continue to assume the link between the client/family and the physician, the improvement of clinical practice skills for the advanced care of mothers and infants (particularly those in a high-risk category) must be ongoing.

A trend that causes concern is the public's increasing reliance on house or lay midwives. This is partly a result of the consumer's desire for providers who will respond to requests for a more personal, neutral, and nonintervening approach. By virtue of their educational background, scope of practice, standards of care, and access to resources (such as medical consultation), CNMs are better qualified to provide individualized, safe client care than lay midwives. However, without the support of physicians, legislators, and third-party payors, the acceptance of CNMs will be delayed, limiting the client's options and forcing clients to continue to choose between licensed physicians and lay midwives.

As managed care grows and the U.S. healthcare system shifts its focus from illness to wellness and healthcare promotion, new roles and broadened scopes of practice are being developed. Clinical studies and research have helped quantify the value and worth of primary care provided by nurse practitioners and CNMs. In addition to CNMs, advanced practice roles for nurses include family, maternal/child, perinatal, and neonatal practitioners (generally referred to as APNs). Together, APNs are being used in all settings from home care to office/clinics and acute care facilities. Some hospitals are using APNs to augment, or even replace, medical house staff as the number of medical residencies is reduced in response to changes in the marketplace and recommendations by the Pew Commission. (This Commission is a "think tank" group privately funded by the Pew Foundation to investigate social policy issues such as healthcare delivery and to make recommendations.)

Furthermore, the trend toward shorter hospital stays and the movement toward community-based care increases the need for nurses with advanced skills to coordinate care and to lead collaborative care teams for delivery of need-based, family-oriented care. The current stumbling blocks to independent practice and the use of APNs (as identified by the Pew Commission) include the lack of a common definition of the APN role among the 50 states, widely varying educational standards in regulatory language, the lack of required certification in some states, and the lack of consistency regarding requirements for licensure. These problems add to questions regarding entry-into-practice standards, prescriptive authority, freedom from physician supervision, and direct reimbursement.

The clarification of roles and progressive improvement in practice environments will encourage more nurses to take on the challenge of advanced practice roles/independent practice within a collaborative framework.

The strategies of early risk identification and timely intervention have made the United States the most effective country in the world at saving high-risk neonates. Now these same strategies are being applied to prenatal care (beginning even before conception) through an integration of home/community-based and acute care services under the auspices of an interdisciplinary team, often coordinated by APNs.

Nursing can increase the emphasis on health promotion and disease prevention by providing education and by developing family support programs with resources for caregivers to empower families to be more responsible for their own health and general well-being. Areas of focus should encompass high-concern needs such as effective parenting, family violence, substance use/abuse, and teenage sexual responsibilities (including issues of STD prevention and birth control). To accomplish these goals, nurses need to enhance their skills to deal with more serious health/family problems, increase their knowledge about and use of complimentary (alternative) therapies, engage in research to increase empirically based family nursing knowledge, encourage the use of APNs, and refer for case management, when appropriate.

Case managers may be hired by physician/CNM group practices, acute-care facilities (especially when payment is capitated), insurance companies, or even self-insured employers. Using medical case managers (generally nurses) to handle "outlyers" or high-risk clients can reduce/prevent the untoward effects of complications and minimize costs through timely intervention, coordination of care, and negotiation for payment of services not usually covered by the payor source but which are more cost effective than alternatives (e.g., home monitoring/IV therapy versus hospitalization, or homemaker/child care support for clients on bedrest to prevent preterm labor).

Home Care

Antepartum nursing care is provided to pregnant women before the onset of labor. Because of complications such as placenta previa, preterm labor, premature rupture of membranes, pregnancy-induced hypertension (PIH), and insulin-dependent diabetes, high-risk mothers-to-be may require antepartum care. Postpartum home care includes performing mother/

newborn physical, psychosocial, and environmental assessments, breastfeeding assistance, blood drawing, and referrals to community and medical resources.

Depending on a variety of reasons, including presumed availability of home care, cost-containment issues, low morbidity rates for mothers/infants after discharge, and consumer demand, discharge from the hospital typically occurs within 24 to 36 hours after vaginal birth, or 48 to 72 hours after cesarean delivery. Although early postpartum discharge (EPD) has become a common occurrence, many women report feeling rushed to discharge within a specific time frame (sometimes occurring during the night). New mothers also tend to feel more tired and uncomfortable than they expected, and the availability/usefulness of support may be less than anticipated. Thus, EPD needs to include timely follow-up care. The American Academy of Pediatrics recommends a follow-up office or home visit at 2 to 4 days of age for a newborn discharged before 48 hours of age. However, client barriers to a follow-up clinic or office visit include transportation, weather, child care for siblings, and client fatigue.

Home visits can facilitate the transition from hospital to home with home health nurses monitoring the recovery process, addressing potential parental fears/anxieties, identifying risk situations, and using client/family strengths to promote problem-solving. In addition, follow-up home care may help ensure patient satisfaction with the entire postpartal recovery process and alleviate potential parental fears and anxieties. Many communities are providing programs (e.g., First Visitor, Bright Beginnings) in which a trained volunteer visits the home to help the new mother learn skills of infant care and management.

Moral/Ethical Concerns

Advances in technology have created many moral and ethical dilemmas for the maternity nurse. Many more infants with low birth weights are now surviving, raising issues of quality of life versus sanctity of life for the offspring and parents. Depending on the degree of prematurity and the presence of birth defects/complications, the outcome may include the decision to withhold or withdraw treatment/support, or deal with long-term, severe, lifelong physical and mental disabilities. The physical, emotional, and financial burdens on the family can result in increased family discord, divorce, and child abuse, as well as physical and psychological illnesses. In addition, the ability to monitor fetal development, diagnose some life-threatening situations, and perform surgical procedures in utero can place the client at odds with the healthcare system if she chooses to refuse diagnostic/corrective interventions.

Unhealthy family interactions leading to physical and emotional abuse are not restricted to families with premature infants. Official U.S. government statistics indicate that 1 of every 10 women is abused by the man with whom she lives. Often, abusive episodes increase or occur for the first time during pregnancy, particularly if the male partner has an immature personality

and a weak ego identity. The nurse can play a major role in assessing the adequacy of available support systems and identifying and intervening with families in crisis.

The expanding field of genetics, comprised of research, screening, engineering, and counseling, raises many moral, legal, and ethical concerns for the individual and society. Society may eventually mandate genetic screening before marriage, as has been done in some other countries. Serum measurement of alpha-fetoprotein levels (AFP) and amniotic fluid analysis or chorionic villa sampling (CVS) for the detection of specific genetic or congenital disorders may be voluntary, or may be state- or federally mandated, as is phenylketonuria (PKU) screening. Nurses in expanded roles are becoming increasingly involved in genetic counseling and education and are dealing with more sophisticated consumers, who are aware of the effects of teratogens and hereditary disorders. Unresolved issues need to be addressed regarding the rights of the fetus, gene manipulation, artificial insemination, in vitro fertilization, gamete intrafallopian transfer (GIFT), embryo transfer, and even surrogate parenting. Dilemmas surrounding the artificial insemination of a surrogate include the possibility of a child with a birth defect, with all parties refusing to accept responsibility for this child, or the birth mother deciding not to relinquish the child. Furthermore, questions persist regarding the appropriateness of abortion, including its use when fertility drugs result in multiple fetuses, necessitating a decision whether or not to use "selective reduction" (the abortion of some fetuses to improve the outcome for the remaining fetuses).

Women of childbearing age now have more options related to family planning. The Food and Drug Administration (FDA) has approved the simple, effective implant contraceptive, levonorgestrel (Norplant), which effectively prevents pregnancy for up to 5 years. The National Institutes of Health report success with a long-acting contraceptive vaccine for women developed through animal studies using genetic engineering. Such a vaccine prevents the fertilization of eggs rather than interfering with the development of a fetus after conception. The issues of women's reproductive rights related to abortion will continue to create intense conflict. In Europe, women have access to RU486, an oral drug that safely accomplishes a first-trimester abortion without the need for surgical intervention. As yet, this controversial drug has been released for clinical trials but has not received FDA approval in the United States.

Of equal or even greater concern is the alarming trend among some healthcare providers to refuse care to individuals with communicable diseases, particularly those who are HIV-positive. Nurses are increasingly concerned about protecting themselves from contamination from certain communicable diseases (such as herpes, AIDS, hepatitis B and C, and syphilis), all of which are transmitted via blood products and body fluids. When appropriately implemented, Occupational Safety and Health Administration (OSHA) standards and universal precautions do provide adequate safeguards. The nurse has a primary role in educating the public—including clients, family members, peers, and the community—about preventive measures and modes of transmission to correct misconceptions and reduce inappropriate fears.

Finally, cultural conflicts, such as a client's request for repair of perineal tissues to maintain infibulation after delivery, raise ethical and legal concerns. Although laws are being enacted to prevent this procedure from being performed, if the repair is not made, the husband/family of the woman may cast her aside, leaving her with no family or means of support.

It is essential for healthcare providers to have objective support through peer support groups or counselors to help in dealing with moral/ethical issues and potential conflicts. In many cases the answers are not clear-cut, but discussion provides an opportunity to share feelings and approaches in coping with such dilemmas.

Liability Concerns

The increasing frequency of litigation is affecting the way in which maternity care is practiced. The heightened concern for fetal safety during labor has increased the use of invasive fetal monitoring, diagnostic testing, and even cesarean deliveries. These practices may create a conflict between healthcare providers and cost-conscious third-party payors as well as the client's desire for a "natural" birthing experience. Although the need for services and providers has increased, the crisis in liability insurance has caused a decline in the availability of general practitioners and specialists, who are choosing to discontinue obstetric services because of the high cost and difficulties of carrying liability insurance. The demand for healthcare providers in obstetrics will continue in the future. Where practice acts permit, CNMs can fill a vital role in providing the professional comprehensive care that mothers and infants deserve in a rapidly changing healthcare environment. In addition, plans to restructure healthcare are also recommending tort reform. Currently, some providers require clients to agree to mediation in the event of an untoward outcome. This may help control insurance costs, and these savings can then be passed on to the consumer.

A new area of liability concern revolves around the use of cross-trained nurses and the delegation of client care to unlicensed personnel. Cross-trained nurses require opportunities to perform tasks frequently enough to ensure and maintain competency in mother/infant dyad care, including education to support lactation and infant care. Finally, to assist nurses in addressing the complex issues associated with the delegation process, guidelines to help determine which tasks can be safely *and* legally delegated have been developed by the national council of State Boards of Nursing, Inc. (1995). The Five Rights of Delegation are:

Right task: One that can be delegated for a specific patient.
Right person: Right person is delegating the right task to the right person to be performed on the right person.
Right direction/communication: Clear, concise description of the task, including its objective, limits, and expectations.
Right supervision: Appropriate monitoring, evaluation, intervention, as needed, and feedback.

CONCLUSION

Nurses electing to care for the maternity client and her family face many exciting challenges created by the changing healthcare scene. Increased technological advances, expanded nursing roles and responsibilities, increased consumer participation in decisions, and an increased awareness of moral/ethical issues (often brought about by improved technology) impact the maternity arena. Professional nurses take individual responsibility for ensuring that their clinical skills and theoretical framework keep pace with these changes to meet the needs of individuals, families, and society as a whole.

CHAPTER 2

NURSING PROCESS: PLANNING CARE WITH NURSING DIAGNOSES

Nursing care is a key factor in achieving positive client outcomes, including the maintenance, rehabilitative, and preventive aspects of healthcare. To this end, the nursing profession has identified a problem-solving process that "combine[s] the most desirable elements of the art of nursing with the most relevant elements of systems theory, using the scientific method" (Shore, 1988).

The publication of the American Nurses Association (ANA) *Social Policy Statement* (1980), which defined nursing as the diagnosis and treatment of human responses to actual and potential health problems, in combination with the ANA *Standards of Clinical Nursing Practice* (1991), provided impetus and support for the use of nursing diagnosis in the practice setting. The prospective payment plans, the movement from acute care (hospital) to community settings, freestanding birth centers, home health services, the development and revision of specialty standards of care, (e.g., the Association of Women's Health, Obstetrics and Neonatal Nursing [AWHONN]: Nursing Standards for the Nursing Care of Women and Newborns [1991]), and other changes in the healthcare system have given rise to the need for a common framework of communication and documentation. The linkage of nursing diagnoses to specific nursing interventions and client outcomes (nursing intervention classification [NIC]/nursing outcomes classification [NOC]) has resulted in a standardized nursing language that can help ensure quality nursing care and continuity of care for the client who moves from one area of the healthcare system to another. Evaluating and documenting care helps to ensure that the care is appropriate and is available when the client/family receives care in different settings.

The concept of nursing process was introduced in the 1950s as a three-step process of assessment, planning, and evaluation based on the scientific method of observing, measuring, gathering data, and analyzing the findings. Years of study, use, and refinement have led nurses to the expansion of the nursing process into five steps: (1) assessment, including focus assessments (systematic collection of data relating to clients and their problems/needs); (2) problem identification (analysis and interpretation of data); (3) planning (choice of solutions, prioritizing, and goal setting); (4) implementation (putting the plan into action); and (5) evaluation (assessing the effectiveness of the plan and changing the plan as indicated by current needs). These five steps are central to nursing actions and the delivery of higher quality, individualized care in any setting. Although nurses use these terms separately, they are actually interrelated and form a continuous circle of thought and action, which, when combined with critical thinking skills, provide an efficient method of organizing thought processes for clinical decision making and active problem solving. The nursing process is included in the conceptual framework of all nursing curricula and is accepted as part of the legal definition of nursing in the Nurse Practice Acts of most states. To use this process, the nurse must demonstrate fundamental abilities of knowledge, intelligence, and creativity, as well as expertise in interpersonal and technical skills. The following are some critical assumptions for the nurse to consider in the decision-making process:

- The client is a human being with worth and dignity.
- There are basic human needs that must be met. When they are not met, problems arise requiring interventions by another person until the individual can resume self-care/independence.
- The client has a right to quality health and nursing care delivered with concern, compassion, and competence with the focus on wellness, prevention, and restoration.
- The therapeutic nurse-client relationship is a critical element in this process.

The important element for providing effective planned nursing care is its relevance as identified in assessments. According to the ANA *Standards of Clinical Nursing Practice*, client assessment is required in the following areas: physical, psychological, sociocultural, spiritual, cognitive, functional abilities, developmental, economic, and lifestyle. These assessments, combined with the results of medical findings and diagnostic studies, are documented in the client data base

10

and form a strong basis for developing the client's plan of care. In addition, hospitals accredited by the Joint Commission on Accreditation of Healthcare Organizations (JCAHO) must meet standards that further specify the parameters of obstetric and newborn assessment and documentation of care.

PLANNING CARE

Medicine and nursing, as well as other health disciplines, are interrelated and, therefore, have implications for each other. This interrelationship should allow exchange of data, sharing of ideas and thoughts, and development of plans of care that include all data pertinent to the individual client and/or family.

The plan of care contains not only the actions initiated by medical and nursing orders, but also the written coordination of care given by all related healthcare disciplines. The nurse becomes the person responsible for coordinating these different activities into a functional plan, which is necessary to provide holistic care for the client. Although independent nursing actions are an integral part of this process, collaborative actions are also included, based on the medical regimen as well as on suggestions or orders from other disciplines involved with the care of the client. In this book, collaborative actions in conjunction with other disciplines are identified to assist the nurse in choosing appropriate interventions for the individual client and setting. The educational background and expertise of the nurse, the standing protocols, the delegation of skills, the use of care partners, and the area of practice (rural or urban, acute care or community care settings) can influence whether an individual intervention is actually an independent nursing function or requires collaboration.

The written plan of care communicates the past and present health status and needs of the client to all members of the healthcare team. It identifies problems solved and those yet to be solved, approaches that have been successful, and patterns of client responses. The plan of care documents client care in areas of liability, accountability, and quality improvement. It provides a mechanism to help ensure continuity of care.

COMPONENTS OF THE PLAN OF CARE

For each plan of care presented in this book, a client assessment data base is established from information obtained from the history, physical examination, and diagnostic studies. Nursing priorities are then determined and ranked. The priorities included in this book represent a general ranking system for the nursing diagnoses in the plan of care and may be reworded and reorganized with time lines, according to the individual client and situation, to create short- and long-term goals. The nursing diagnosis then follows with possible related factors (etiology) and corresponding signs

and symptoms (cues), when present. Desired client outcomes for each problem/need area are followed by appropriate independent and collaborative interventions with accompanying rationales.

Client Data Base

Construction of the plan of care begins with the collection of data (through the history-taking interview, physical assessment, diagnostic studies, and review of other records). The data base consists of subjective and objective information encompassing the various nursing concerns identified in the 1996 list of nursing diagnoses developed by The North American Nursing Diagnosis Association (NANDA) (Table 2–1).

Interviewing

Interviewing provides data that the nurse obtains from the client and significant others through conversation and observation. This information includes the individual's perceptions; that is, what the person wants to share. It is important to accept what is reported because the client/significant other is the "expert" in this regard. However, the nurse needs to note incongruencies or dissonances, which may indicate the presence of other factors such as lack of knowledge, myths, misconceptions, or fear.

Physical Assessment

During this aspect of information gathering, the nurse exercises perceptual and observational skills, using the senses of sight, hearing, touch, and smell. The duration and depth of any physical assessment depend on the current condition of the client and the urgency of the situation but usually include inspection, palpation, percussion, and auscultation.

Diagnostic Studies

Laboratory and other diagnostic studies are included as part of the data-gathering process. The nurse needs to be aware of significant test results that require reporting to the physician and/or initiation of specific nursing interventions. Some tests are used to diagnose disease, whereas others are useful in following the course of a disease or in adjusting therapies. In many cases, the relationship of the test to the pathological physiology is clear, but in other cases it is not. This is the result of the interrelationship between various organs and body systems. Interpretation of diagnostic test results should be integrated with the history and physical findings.

Nursing Diagnosis (Problem/Need Identification)

Nursing diagnoses are a uniform way of identifying, focusing on, and dealing with specific client needs and

TABLE 2–1. NANDA Nursing Diagnoses Accepted for Use and Research Through 1998*

Activity Intolerance [specify level]†
Activity Intolerance, risk for
Adaptive Capacity: Intracranial, decreased
*Adult Failure to Thrive
Adjustment, impaired
Airway Clearance, ineffective
*Altered Dentition
*Altered Development, risk for
*Altered Growth, risk for
Anxiety [specify level]†
Aspiration, risk for
*Autonomic Dysreflexia, risk for

*Bed Mobility, impaired
Body Image disturbance
Body Temperature, risk for altered
Bowel Incontinence
Breastfeeding, effective
Breastfeeding, ineffective
Breastfeeding, interrupted
Breathing Pattern, ineffective

Cardiac Output, decreased
Caregiver Role Strain
Caregiver Role Strain, risk for
*Chronic Sorrow
Communication, impaired verbal
Community Coping, potential for enhanced
Community Coping, ineffective
Confusion, acute
Confusion, chronic
Constipation
Constipation, colonic
Constipation, perceived
*Constipation, risk for
Coping, defensive
Coping, Individual, ineffective

*Death Anxiety
Decisional Conflict (specify)
*Delayed Surgical Recovery
Denial, ineffective
Diarrhea
Disuse Syndrome, risk for
Diversional Activity deficit
Dysreflexia

Energy Field disturbance
Environmental Interpretation Syndrome,
    impaired

Family Coping: ineffective, compromised
Family Coping: ineffective, disabling
Family Coping: potential for growth
Family Process, altered: alcoholism
Family Processes, altered
Fatigue
Fear
[Fluid Volume deficit, hyper/hypotonic dehydration]†
Fluid Volume deficit [Isotonic dehydration]†
Fluid Volume risk for deficit
Fluid Volume excess
*Fluid Volume Imbalance, risk for

Gas Exchange, impaired
Grieving, anticipatory
Grieving, dysfunctional
Growth & Development, altered

Health Maintenance, altered
Health-Seeking Behaviors (specify)
Home Maintenance Management, impaired
Hopelessness
Hyperthermia
Hypothermia

Incontinence, functional
Incontinence, reflex
Incontinence, stress
Incontinence, total
Incontinence, urge
Infant Behavior, disorganized
Infant Behavior, risk for disorganized
Infant Behavior, organized, potential for enhanced
Infant Feeding Pattern, ineffective
Infection, risk for
Injury, risk for

Knowledge deficit [Learning Need]† (specify)

*Latex Allergy
*Latex Allergy, risk for
Loneliness, risk for

Memory, impaired

*Nausea
Noncompliance, [Compliance, altered]† specify
Nutrition: altered, less than body requirements
Nutrition: altered, more than body requirements
Nutrition: altered, risk for more than body
    requirements

(continued)

Source: North American Nursing Diagnosis Association: Definitions and Classifications, 1999–2000. NANDA, Philadelphia, 1999, with permission.
*New diagnoses accepted in 1998.
†Entries in brackets are author recommendations.

12

TABLE 2–1. NANDA Nursing Diagnoses Accepted for Use and Research Through 1998* (continued)

Oral Mucous Membrane, altered	Skin Integrity, impaired
	Skin Integrity, risk for impaired
Pain [acute]†	Sleep Pattern disturbance
Pain, chronic	Social Interaction, impaired
Parental Role conflict	Social Isolation
Parent/Infant/Child Attachment, risk for altered	Spiritual Distress (distress of the human spirit)
Parenting, altered	Spiritual Well-Being, potential for enhanced
Parenting, risk for altered	Spontaneous Ventilation, inability to sustain
Perioperative Positioning Injury, risk for	Suffocation, risk for
Peripheral Neurovascular dysfunction, risk for	Swallowing, impaired
Personal Identity disturbance	
Physical Mobility, impaired	Therapeutic Regimen: Community, ineffective management
Poisoning, risk for	Therapeutic Regimen: Families, ineffective management
Post-Trauma Response	Therapeutic Regimen: Individual, effective management
*Post-Trauma Syndrome	Therapeutic Regimen: (Individuals) ineffective management
Powerlessness	
Protection, altered	Thermoregulation, ineffective
	Thought Processes, altered
Rape-Trauma Syndrome	Tissue Integrity, impaired
Rape-Trauma Syndrome: compound reaction	Tissue Perfusion, altered (specify): cerebral, cardiopulmonary, renal, gastrointestinal, peripheral
Rape-Trauma Syndrome: silent reaction	
Relocation Stress Syndrome	
Role Performance, altered	Trauma, risk for
Self Care deficit [specify level]†: feeding, bathing/hygiene, dressing/grooming, toileting	Unilateral Neglect
Self Esteem, chronic low	Urinary Elimination, altered
Self Esteem disturbance	Urinary Retention [acute/chronic]†
Self Esteem, situational low	
Self-Mutilation, risk for	Ventilatory Weaning Response, dysfunctional (DVWR)
Sensory/Perceptual alterations (specify): visual, auditory, kinesthetic, gustatory, tactile, olfactory	Violence [actual/]† risk for, directed at self
Sexual dysfunction	Violence [actual/]† risk for, directed at others
Sexuality Patterns, altered	

Source: North American Nursing Diagnosis Association: Definitions and Classifications, 1999–2000. NANDA, Philadelphia, 1999, with permission.
*New diagnoses accepted in 1998.
†Entries in brackets are author recommendations.

responses to actual and high-risk problems. Nursing diagnosis labels provide a format for expressing the problem identification portion of the nursing process. NANDA has accepted the following working definition:

Nursing diagnosis is a clinical judgment about individual, family, or community responses to actual and potential health problems/life processes. Nursing diagnoses provide the basis for selection of nursing interventions to achieve outcomes for which the nurse is accountable.

The nursing diagnosis is as precise as the data will allow because it is supported by the immediate data collected. It communicates the client's present situation and reflects changes as they occur. It is necessary to seek, incorporate, and synthesize all the relevant data and make the diagnosis statement meaningful to provide direction for nursing care. The nurse needs to be aware of biases that may interfere with reaching an accurate diagnosis. Keeping an open mind to numerous possibilities and not becoming preoccupied with a single symp-

tom or thought facilitates this process. For example, when identifying a cue of restlessness in a client, the nurse may infer that the client is anxious. The nurse may believe that the restlessness is only psychologically based, overlooking the possibility that it could be a physiological response.

Analysis of the data involves examining assessment findings, grouping related findings, and comparing the findings against established normal parameters. The key, then, to accurate nursing diagnosis is problem/ need identification, which focuses attention on a current or high-risk physical or behavioral response that interferes with the quality of life that the client desires or which she is accustomed to. The nursing diagnosis addresses the client's, significant others', and/or nurse's concerns that require nursing intervention and management. In this text, the choice of an individual nursing diagnosis is validated by the related/risk factors and signs and symptoms most consistently associated with a specific situation or medical condition.

Nurses may feel at risk in committing themselves to documenting a nursing diagnosis; however, many references are currently available to aid in identifying and formulating the diagnostic statement. In addition, unlike medical diagnoses, nursing diagnoses change as the client progresses through various stages of illness or maladaptation to problem resolution. From the specific information obtained in the client assessment data base, the related factors, signs, and symptoms can be identified, and an individual statement of the client's problem/need or diagnosis can be formulated. For example, a client may report fatigue and inability to rest adequately while caring for children. These data, along with other cues, lead to a choice of the nursing diagnosis: Fatigue related to increased energy requirements, altered body chemistry, inadequate support system as evidenced by client reports of lack of energy, inability to maintain usual routines, and emotional irritability.

Nursing diagnosis, as the crux of the client's plan of care, focuses attention on certain areas and is the prime determinant of the style of nursing care to be delivered. Nursing actions have often been based on such variables as signs and symptoms, test results, and medical diagnosis. Nursing diagnosis is a uniform way of identifying, focusing on, and dealing with specific client problems and responses. The affective tone of the nursing diagnosis can shape expectations of the client's response and influence the nurse's behavior toward the client. For instance, if the nurse sees the client as noncompliant, the nurse's attitudes and behavior may reflect anger and mistrust, and judgmental decisions may be made that do not accurately treat the client's problem. However, accurate diagnosis of a client's problem (e.g., Ineffective Management of Individual Therapeutic Regimen related to medication side effects) can become a standard for nursing practice, understood by all who are using the plan of care, and thus can lead to improved delivery of care.

Planning (Goals and Actions/Interventions)

Goals are established, and outcome statements are formulated, to give direction to nursing care. Desired client outcomes emerge from the diagnostic statement and are defined as the results of nursing interventions and responses that are achievable, desired by the client and/or nurse, and attainable within a defined period, given the present situation and resources. They are used to evaluate the client's response to nursing intervention, which is the fifth step of the nursing process and is addressed in the sample client situation in Chapter 3. The terminology must be concise, realistic, measurable, and stated in words that the client can understand. Beginning the outcome statement with an action verb provides direction that is measurable (e.g., "client will: Verbalize"). It is important that multidisciplinary goals do not conflict. The Desired Outcomes in this book have been stated in general terms to permit the practitioner to individualize them by adding time lines, considerations of client circumstances and needs, and other specific qualifiers.

Interventions are prescriptions for specific behaviors expected from the client and carried out, or facilitated by, nurses to achieve desired client outcomes. The rationale for interventions needs to be sound and feasible and needs to reflect individualized client data. Actions may be independent or collaborative and encompass orders from nursing, medicine, and other disciplines. Again, using an action verb (e.g., "Instruct," "Demonstrate") provides direction for the nurse and client. These interventions have the intent of individualizing care by meeting a specific client need and should incorporate identified client strengths.

Finally, the nurse needs to formulate the plan of care with the client because both individuals are accountable for that care and for achieving the desired outcomes. The written interventions that guide client care need to be dated and signed to identify the person who is initiating and coordinating the care.

Rationales

Although rationales do not appear on agency plans of care, they are included in this book to assist the student and practicing nurse in associating the pathophysiological and/or psychological principles with the selected nursing intervention.

DOCUMENTING THE NURSING PROCESS

In general, the goals of the documentation system are to:

- Facilitate the quality of client care.
- Ensure documentation of progress with regard to client-focused outcomes.
- Facilitate interdisciplinary consistency and the communication of treatment goals and progress.

Two recent publications provide the nurse with guidelines for documenting the nursing process and for supporting the need for a written (or computer-generated) plan of care. The ANA *Standards of Clinical Nursing Practice* "delineate care that is provided to all clients of nursing services," and each standard includes a measurement criterion addressing documentation. In addition, the *Nursing Care Standards* (JCAHO, 1997) also focus attention on documentation, as presented in Table 2–2. These revised standards delineate the professional responsibilities of all registered nurses and provide criteria to assist in measuring the achievement of identified standards.

From a nursing perspective, documentation provides a record of the use of the nursing process for the delivery of individualized client care. The initial *assessment* is recorded in the client history or data base. The *diagnosis* of client problems/needs and the *planning* of client care are recorded in the plan of care. The *implementation* of the plan is recorded in progress notes and/or flow sheets. Finally, the *evaluation* of care is documented in progress notes, flow sheets, and/or the plan of care/clinical pathway.

The maintenance of a medical record is one of the most essential requirements for accreditation of healthcare facilities by JCAHO and/or other credentialing and licensing agencies. JCAHO standards state that the medical record must be documented accurately and in a timely manner. Therefore, the importance of completing notes on schedule and in a manner that facilitates retrieval of data should be emphasized.

Documentation is not only a requirement for accreditation, but it also provides a permanent record of what happens with each client. It is a legal requirement in any healthcare setting. In our society, with its many lawsuits and aggressive malpractice emphasis, all aspects of the medical record may be important for legal documentation. The plan of care that has been developed for a particular client serves as a framework or outline for charting administered care. Progress notes and flow sheets, therefore, reflect implementation of the treatment plan by documenting that appropriate actions have been carried out, precautions have been taken, and so forth. These notes need to be written in a clear and objective fashion and in a manner that reflects progress toward the stated outcomes with the implementation of planned staff interventions. These notations also need to be date- and time-specific and need to be signed by the person making the entry. Any error in the document must be crossed out with one line so that it is still legible, identified by the author as "error," and then initialed. "White-outs" or "cross-outs," which make the information unreadable, are not acceptable because they could be construed to mean that the individual or facility is trying to alter facts.

The medical record is always the primary source of providing proof of services, which is necessary to maintain revenues. Third-party payors insist that the why, when, where, how, what, and who of services be clearly documented. Absence of such documentation, may result in denial of authorization or termination of funding for individual clients, possibly delaying or ending their treatment. Therefore, progress notes must document what is happening to the client during all phases of pregnancy, intervention, and recovery. It is important to record information and observations that will assist the oncoming nurse and other healthcare providers to maintain continuity of planned care. Table 2–3 provides examples of information to be documented in the client record.

Whether charting is handwritten or electronically generated, a number of formats are currently used for documentation (e.g., block notes; problem-oriented medical record [POMR]; FOCUS® Charting). Regardless of the form used, to avoid confusion and to comply with existing agency policies and procedures, entries should be concise and consistent in style and format. Examples of documentation formats are included in Chapter 3.

TABLE 2–2. A Sample Portion of One Nursing Care Standard from the Joint Commission on Accreditation of Healthcare Organizations

NC.1.	Patients receive nursing care based on a documented assessment of their needs.
NC.1.3.4.	The patient's medical record includes documentation of:
NC.1.3.4.1	The initial assessments and reassessments
NC.1.3.4.2	The nursing diagnosis and/or patient care needs
NC.1.3.4.3	The interventions identified to meet the patient's nursing care needs
NC.1.3.4.4	The nursing care provided
NC.1.3.4.5	The patient's response to, and the outcomes of, the care provided
NC.1.3.4.6	The abilities of the patient and/or, as appropriate, his/her significant other(s) to manage continuing care needs after discharge

TABLE 2–3. **Contents of a Progress Note**

Unsettled or unclear problems or issues that need to be dealt with, including attempts to contact other client care providers

Noteworthy incidents or interviews involving the client that would benefit from a more detailed recording

Other pertinent data, such as notes on phone calls, home visits, and family interactions

Additional critical incident data, such as seemingly significant or revealing statements made by the client, an insight the nurse has into a client's patterns of behavior, client injuries, the use of any special treatment procedure, or other major events such as episodes of pain, changes in uterine contractile pattern, changes in fetal heart rate, exaggerated emotional responses, medication reactions, or suicidal/homicidal comments

Administered care, activities, or observations if not recorded elsewhere on flow sheets (physician/healthcare provider visits, completion of ordered tests, required medications)

Evaluation of care provided, client response to interventions

SUMMARY

This book is intended to facilitate the application of the nursing process and the use of nursing diagnosis for the maternity client, newborn, and family. Each plan of care is intended to be an informational guide, designed to provide generalized information on the associated medical condition. The guides can be modified by either using portions of the information provided or adding additional client-care information to the existing guides. The plan-of-care guidelines were developed using NANDA recommendations, except in a few examples in which we felt more clarification and enhancement were required. The ongoing controversy regarding the validity of the NANDA-approved nursing diagnosis Knowledge deficit is one example in which further clarification is provided through the addition of the term "Learning Need." For example, for the client with severe hypertension, a nursing diagnosis was developed with the following label: Knowledge deficit [Learning Need] regarding condition, prognosis, and treatment plan. Some diagnoses have been combined for convenience, e.g., Anxiety/Fear, indicating that two or more factors may be involved.

We recognize that not all of the NANDA-approved nursing diagnoses have been used in these plan-of-care guides, but we hope that these guides will assist you in determining the client's needs, outcomes, and nursing interventions.

Chapter 3 will assist you in the critical thinking process as you apply and adapt theory to practice.

CHAPTER 3

CRITICAL THINKING: ADAPTATION OF THEORY TO PRACTICE

Critical thinking is defined as "the intellectually disciplined process of actively and skillfully conceptualizing, applying, analyzing, synthesizing, and evaluating of information gathered from or generated by observation, experience, reflection, reasoning, or communication, as a guide to belief and action" (National Council for Excellence in Critical Thinking, 1992). Critical thinking requires cognitive, psychomotor, and affective skills to use the tools of a comprehensive knowledge base, the nursing process, and established standards of care, as well as nursing research to analyze data and plan a course of action based on new insights and conclusions. Although critical-thinking skills are used in all aspects of nursing practice, they are most evident when assessment data are analyzed to identify relevant information, make decisions about client needs, and develop an individualized plan of care. Therefore client assessment is the foundation on which identification of individual needs, responses, and problems is based.

To facilitate the steps of assessment and diagnosis in the nursing process and aid in the critical thinking process, assessment data bases have been constructed using a nursing focus instead of the traditional medical approach of "review of systems." To achieve this nursing focus, we have grouped the North American Nursing Diagnosis Association (NANDA) nursing diagnoses into related categories titled "Diagnostic Divisions" (Table 3–1), which reflect a blending of theories, primarily Maslow's hierarchy of needs and a self-care philosophy. These divisions serve as the framework or outline for the collection of data, directing the nurse to the appropriate corresponding nursing diagnoses as the client's information is recorded in the client's assessment data base (Table 3–2).

Because the divisions are based on human responses and needs and not on specific "systems," information may be recorded in more than one area. For this reason, the nurse is encouraged to keep an open mind, to pursue all leads, and to collect as much data as possible before choosing the nursing diagnosis label that best reflects the client's situation.

From the specific data recorded in the data base, the related/risk factors (etiology) and signs and symptoms can be identified, and an individualized client diagnostic statement can be formulated using the problem, etiology, signs/symptoms (PES) format to accurately represent the client's situation. For example, the diagnostic statement may read: "Knowledge deficit [Learning Need], regarding preterm labor, related to lack of information/misinterpretation, evidenced by questions and expression of concerns."

Desired client outcomes are identified to facilitate choosing appropriate interventions and to serve as evaluators of both nursing care and client response. These outcomes also form the framework for documentation.

Interventions are designed to specify the action of the nurse, the client, and/or significant other(s). Interventions need to promote movement toward independence, in addition to achieving physiological stability. This requires involvement of the client in her own care, including participation in decisions about the care and projected outcomes. In addition, although the pregnant woman is the primary client, significant other(s)/family members will also need consideration and inclusion in care.

To assist in visualizing this critical thinking process, a sample client situation and sample plan of care (Preterm Labor/Prevention of Delivery) provide an example of data collection and construction of the plan of care. As the client assessment data base is reviewed, the nurse can identify the related or risk factors and defining characteristics (signs/symptoms) that were used to formulate the client diagnostic statements. The addition of timelines to specific client outcomes and goals reflects the anticipated length of stay and individual client and nurse expectations. Interventions have been chosen based on concerns/ needs identified by the client/family, and nurse during data collection, as well as physician orders. Although not normally included in a plan of care, rationales are included in this sample for the purpose of explaining or clarifying the choice of interventions and enhancing the nurse's learning. Finally, to complete the learning experience, samples of documentation based on the client situation are presented.

TABLE 3–1. Nursing Diagnoses Organized According to Diagnostic Divisions*

ACTIVITY/REST—Ability to engage in necessary/ desired activities of life (work and leisure), and to obtain adequate sleep/rest
  Activity Intolerance
  Activity Intolerance, risk for
  Bed Mobility, impaired†
  Disuse Syndrome, risk for
  Diversional Activity deficit
  Fatigue
  Sleep Deprivation†
  Sleep Pattern disturbance
  Walking, impaired†
  Wheelchair Mobility, impaired†
  Wheelchair Transfer Ability, impaired†

CIRCULATION—Ability to transport oxygen and nutrients necessary to meet cellular needs
  Adaptive Capacity: Intracranial, decreased
  Autonomic Dysreflexia, risk for†
  Cardiac Output, decreased
  Dysreflexia
  Tissue Perfusion, altered (specify type): renal cerebral, cardiopulmonary, gastrointestinal, peripheral

EGO INTEGRITY—Ability to develop and use skills and behaviors to integrate and manage life experiences
  Adjustment, impaired
  Anxiety [specify level]
  Body Image disturbance
  Chronic Sorrow†
  Coping, defensive
  Coping, Individual, ineffective
  Death Anxiety†
  Decisional Conflict (specify)
  Denial, ineffective
  Energy Field disturbance
  Fear
  Grieving, anticipatory
  Grieving, dysfunctional
  Hopelessness
  Personal Identity disturbance
  Post-Trauma Response
  Post-Trauma Syndrome, risk for†
  Powerlessness
  Rape-Trauma Syndrome
  Rape-Trauma Syndrome: compound reaction
  Rape-Trauma Syndrome: silent reaction

  Relocation Stress Syndrome
  Self Esteem, chronic low
  Self Esteem disturbance
  Self Esteem, situational low
  Spiritual Distress (distress of the human spirit)
  Spiritual Distress, risk for†
  Spiritual Well-Being, potential for enhanced

ELIMINATION—Ability to excrete waste products
  Bowel Incontinence
  Constipation
  Constipation, colonic
  Constipation, perceived
  Constipation, risk for†
  Diarrhea
  Incontinence, functional
  Incontinence, reflex
  Incontinence, stress
  Incontinence, total
  Incontinence, urge
  Urinary Elimination, altered
  Urinary Retention [acute/chronic]
  Urinary Urge Incontinence, risk for†

FOOD/FLUID—Ability to maintain intake of and utilize nutrients and liquids to meet physiological needs
  Adult Failure to Thrive†
  Breastfeeding, effective
  Breastfeeding, ineffective
  Breastfeeding, interrupted
  Dentition, altered†
  Fluid Volume deficit [hypo/hypertonic dehydration]
  Fluid Volume deficit [isotonic dehydration]
  Fluid Volume excess
  Fluid Volume Imbalance, risk for†
  Fluid Volume risk for deficit
  Infant Feeding Pattern, ineffective
  Nausea†
  Nutrition: altered, less than body requirements
  Nutrition: altered, more than body requirements
  Nutrition: altered, risk for more than body requirements
  Oral Mucous Membrane, altered
  Swallowing, impaired

HYGIENE—Ability to perform activities of daily living
  Self Care deficit: feeding, bathing/hygiene, dressing/grooming, toileting

(continued)

TABLE 3–1. Nursing Diagnoses Organized According to Diagnostic Divisions* (continued)

NEUROSENSORY—Ability to perceive, integrate, and respond to internal and external cues
   Confusion, acute
   Confusion, chronic
   Infant Behavior, disorganized
   Infant Behavior, risk for disorganized
   Infant Behavior, organized, potential for
      enhanced
   Memory, impaired
   Peripheral Neurovascular dysfunction, risk for
   Sensory/Perceptual alterations (specify): visual,
      auditory, kinesthetic, gustatory, tactile, olfactory
   Thought Processes, altered
   Unilateral Neglect

PAIN/DISCOMFORT—Ability to control internal/external environment to maintain comfort
   Pain [acute]
   Pain, chronic

RESPIRATION—Ability to provide and use oxygen to meet physiological needs
   Airway Clearance, ineffective
   Aspiration, risk for
   Breathing Pattern, ineffective
   Gas Exchange, impaired
   Spontaneous Ventilation, inability to sustain
   Ventilatory Weaning Response, dysfunctional
      (DVWR)

SAFETY—Ability to provide safe, growth-promoting environment
   Body Temperature, risk for altered
   Environmental Interpretation Syndrome, impaired
   Health Maintenance, altered
   Home Maintenance Management, impaired
   Hyperthermia
   Hypothermia
   Infection, risk for
   Injury, risk for
   Latex Allergy†
   Latex Allergy, risk for†
   Perioperative Positioning Injury, risk for
   Physical Mobility, impaired
   Poisoning, risk for
   Protection, altered
   Self-Mutilation, risk for
   Skin Integrity, impaired
   Skin Integrity, risk for impaired
   Suffocation, risk for

   Surgical Recovery, delayed†
   Thermoregulation, ineffective
   Tissue Integrity, impaired
   Trauma, risk for
   Violence, risk for directed at others
   Violence, risk for self-directed

SEXUALITY [Component of Ego Integrity and Social Interaction]—Ability to meet requirements/characteristics of male/female role
   Sexual dysfunction
   Sexuality Patterns, altered

SOCIAL INTERACTION—Ability to establish and maintain relationships
   Caregiver Role Strain
   Caregiver Role Strain, risk for
   Communication, impaired verbal
   Community Coping, ineffective
   Community Coping, potential for enhanced
   Family Coping: ineffective, compromised
   Family Coping: ineffective, disabling
   Family Coping: potential for growth
   Family Process, altered: alcoholism
   Family Processes, altered
   Loneliness, risk for
   Parent/Infant/Child Attachment, risk for altered
   Parental Role conflict
   Parenting, altered
   Parenting, risk for altered
   Role Performance, altered
   Social Interaction, impaired
   Social Isolation

TEACHING/LEARNING—Ability to incorporate and use information to achieve healthy lifestyle/optimal wellness
   Development, risk for altered†
   Growth, risk for altered†
   Growth & Development, altered
   Health-Seeking Behaviors (specify)
   Knowledge deficit [Learning need] (specify)
   Noncompliance [Compliance, altered] (specify)
   Therapeutic Regimen: Community, ineffective
      management
   Therapeutic Regimen: Families, ineffective
      management
   Therapeutic Regimen: Individual, effective
      management
   Therapeutic Regimen: Individual, ineffective
      management

*After data are collected and areas of concern/need identified, the nurse is directed to the diagnostic divisions to review the list of nursing diagnoses that fall within the individual categories. This will assist the nurse in choosing the specific diagnostic label to accurately describe the data. Then, with the addition of etiology or related/risk factors (when known) and signs and symptoms, or cues (defining characteristics), the client diagnostic statement emerges.
†New NANDA diagnoses accepted for use and research from the 13th Conference, 1999–2000.

TABLE 3–2. **Prenatal Assessment Tool**

General information:
Name: _____ Age: _____ DOB: _____ Race: _____ Visit/Admission date: _____
Healthcare provider: Maternal: _____ Infant: _____
Father of child: Name: _____ Age: _____ Race: _____
Source of information: _____ Reliability: _____ (1–4 with 4 very reliable)

ACTIVITY/REST:

Subjective:

Occupation: _____
Usual activities/hobbies: _____
Leisure time activities: _____
Usual exercise: _____
Limitations imposed by pregnancy/condition: ____
Physical requirements of:
   Employment: _____ Home: _____
Sleep: Number of hours: _____
   Naps: _____ Aids: _____
   Insomnia: _____ Reason: _____

Objective:

Observed response to activity:
   Cardiovascular: _____ Respiratory: _____
Mental status (e.g., withdrawn/lethargic): _____
Neuromuscular assessment:
   Muscle mass/tone: _____ Posture: _____
   Tremors: _____ ROM: _____
   Strength: _____ Deformity: _____
   Other: _____

CIRCULATION:

Subjective:

History of elevated BP: _____
   Heart trouble: _____ Rheumatic fever: _____
   Ankle/leg edema: _____
   Phlebitis: _____ Slow healing: _____
Extremities: Numbness: _____ Tingling: _____
Cough/hemoptysis: _____
Change in frequency/amount of urine: _____

Objective:

BP: R and L: Standing: _____ Sitting: _____
   Lying: _____
Peripheral pulses: Radial: _____
   Dorsalis pedis: _____
   Jugular vein distention: _____
Heart sounds: Rate: _____ Rhythm: _____
   Quality: _____ Rub/murmur: _____
Breath sounds: _____
Extremities: Temperature: _____ Color: _____
   Capillary refill: _____ Homans' sign: _____
   Varicosities: _____ Nails (abnormalities): _____
Color/cyanosis: Overall _____
   Mucous membranes: _____ Lips: _____
   Nailbeds: _____ Conjunctiva: _____
   Sclera: _____
Diaphoresis: _____

EGO INTEGRITY:

Subjective:

Pregnancy planned (Y/N): _____
Client's/father's feelings about pregnancy: _____
Relationship status: _____
Report of stress factors: _____
   Financial concern: _____ Lifestyle: _____
   Recent changes: _____
Ways of handling stress: _____
Religion: _____ Practicing: _____
Cultural factors: _____
Feelings of: Helplessness: _____
   Hopelessness: _____ Powerlessness: _____
History of emotional problems: _____
   Psychological abuse/neglect: _____

Objective:

Emotional status: _____
Observed physiological response(s): _____

20

(continued)

TABLE 3–2. **Prenatal Assessment Tool** (continued)

ELIMINATION:

Subjective:

Usual bowel pattern: _____ Laxative use: _____
Character of stool: _____
   Bleeding: _____ Hemorrhoids: _____
   Diarrhea: _____ Constipation: _____
Usual voiding pattern: _____
Incontinence/when: _____ Urgency: _____
   Frequency: _____ Retention: _____
   Character of urine: _____
Pain/burning/difficulty voiding: _____
History of kidney/bladder disease: _____
Diuretic use: _____

Objective:

Abdomen tender: _____ Soft/firm: _____
Palpable mass: _____ Size/girth: _____
Bowel sounds: _____ Hemorrhoids: _____
Bladder palpable: _____
Overflow voiding: _____
Urinalysis: _____ Albuminuria: _____
   Glycosuria: _____ Occult blood: _____
Stool for occult blood: _____

FOOD/FLUID:

Subjective:

Usual diet (type): _____
   Number of meals daily: _____
   Last meal/intake: _____
Dietary pattern: _____
Loss of appetite: _____ Nausea/vomiting: _____
Heartburn/indigestion: _____
   Related to/relieved by: _____
Allergy/food intolerance: _____
Mastication/swallowing problems: _____
   Dentures: _____
Average nonpregnant weight: _____
   Pattern of weight gain/loss: _____
Diuretic use: _____

Objective:

Current weight: _____ Height: _____
Body build: _____ Skin turgor: _____
Mucous membranes moist/dry: _____
Hernia/masses: _____
Edema: _____ General: _____ Dependent: _____
   Periorbital: _____ Sacral: _____
   Digital: _____
Jugular vein distension: _____
Thyroid enlarged: _____
Halitosis: _____ Condition of teeth/gums: _____
Appearance of tongue: _____;
   Mucous membranes: _____
Bowel sounds: _____
Breath sounds: _____
Diabetic screening: GTT: _____
Thyroid studies: _____
Hb/Hct (anemia): _____

HYGIENE:

Subjective:

Activities of daily living:
   Independent/dependent (specify): _____
Equipment/prosthetic devices required: _____
   Assistance provided by: _____

Objective:

General appearance: _____ Manner of dress: _____
Personal habits: _____ Body odor: _____
Condition of scalp: _____
Presence of vermin: _____

NEUROSENSORY:

Subjective:

Fainting spells/dizziness: _____
Headaches: _____ Location: _____
   Frequency: _____ Tingling/numbness/
   weakness (location): _____
Stroke (residual effects): _____
Seizures: _____ Aura: _____
   How controlled: _____
Eyes: Vision loss: _____
   Last examination: _____
   Glaucoma: _____ Cataract: _____
Ears: Hearing loss: _____
   Last examination: _____
Epistaxis: _____ Sense of smell: _____

Objective:

Mental status: Oriented/disoriented
   (specify): _____
Glasses: _____ Contacts: _____ Hearing aids: _____
Usual speech pattern/impairment: _____

(continued)

TABLE 3–2. **Prenatal Assessment Tool** (continued)

PAIN/DISCOMFORT:

Subjective:

Location: _____ Intensity (0–10 with 10
    most severe): _____ Frequency: _____
    Quality: _____ Duration: _____
Precipitating factors: _____
    How relieved: _____
Associated symptoms: _____

Objective:

Facial grimacing: _____ Guarding affected
    area: _____ Emotional response: _____
Narrowed focus: _____

RESPIRATION:

Subjective:

Dyspnea (related to): _____
Cough/sputum: _____
History of: Bronchitis: _____ Asthma: _____
    Tuberculosis: _____ Emphysema: _____
Recurrent pneumonia: _____
Smoker: _____ Packs/day: _____
    Number of pack-years: _____
Use of respiratory aids: _____ Oxygen: _____

Objective:

Respiratory: Rate: _____ Depth: _____
    Quality: _____
Breath sounds: _____
Sputum characteristics: _____
Chest x-ray results: _____

SAFETY:

Subjective:

Allergies/Sensitivity: _____
    Reaction: _____
Previous alteration of immune system: _____
    Cause: _____
History of STDs/gynecologic infections
    (date/type): _____
High-risk behaviors: _____ Testing: _____
    Blood transfusion/number: _____
    When: _____ Reaction: _____ Describe: _____
Childhood diseases: _____
    Immunization history: _____
Recent exposure to German measles: _____
    Other viral infections: _____
    X-ray/radiation: _____ House pets: _____
Previous ob/gyn problems: Pregnancy-
    induced hypertension (PIH): _____
    Kidney: _____ Hemorrhage: _____
    Cardiac: _____ Diabetes: _____
    Infection/UTI: _____
        ABO/Rh sensitivity: _____
        Uterine surgery: _____ Anemia: _____
Length of time since last pregnancy: _____
    Type of previous deliveries: _____

Objective:

Temperature: _____ Diaphoresis: _____
Skin integrity: _____ Scars: _____
    Rashes: _____ Sores: _____
Ecchymosis: _____ Vaginal warts/lesions: _____
General strength: _____ Muscle tone: _____
    Gait: _____ ROM: _____
    Paresthesia/paralysis: _____
Fetal status: Heart rate: _____ Location: _____
    Method of auscultation: _____
    Fundal height: _____ Estimated gestation: _____
    Activity/movement: _____ Ballottement: _____
Fetal assessment testing: Date: _____
    Test: _____ Results: _____
Results of cultures, cervical/rectal: _____
Immune system testing: _____
Blood type: Maternal: _____ Paternal: _____
Screenings: Serology: _____ Syphilis: _____
    Sickle cell: _____ Rubella: _____
    Hepatitis: _____ HIV: _____ TB: _____
AFP: _____
    Health status of living children: _____
    History of accidental injuries:
        Fractures/dislocations: _____
        Physical abuse: _____
    Arthritis/unstable joints: _____ Back problems: _____
    Changes in moles: _____ Enlarged nodes: _____
    Impaired vision: _____ Hearing: _____
    Prosthesis: _____ Ambulatory devices: _____

(continued)

TABLE 3–2. **Prenatal Assessment Tool** (continued)

SEXUALITY (Component of Social Interactions)

Subjective:

Sexual concerns: _____
Menarche: _____ Length of cycle: _____
  Duration: _____
First day of LMP: _____
  Amount: _____ Bleeding/cramping since LMP: _____
Vaginal discharge: _____
Client's belief as to when conception occurred: _____
EDD: _____

Practices breast self-examination (Y/N): _____
Last Pap smear: _____ Results: _____
Recent contraceptive method: _____
Obstetric history: (GPTPAL) Gravida: _____
  Para: _____ Term: _____
  Preterm: _____ Abortions: _____
  Living: _____ Multiple births: _____
Delivery History: Year: _____
  Place of delivery: _____ Length of gestation: _____
  Length of labor: _____ Type of delivery: _____
Born (alive or dead): _____
  Weight: _____ Apgar scores: _____
Complications (maternal/fetal): _____

Objective:

Breast examination: _____ Nipples: _____
Pelvic: Vulva: _____ Perineum: _____
  Vagina: _____ Cervix: _____ Uterus: _____
  Adnexal: _____ Diagonal conjugate: _____
  Transverse diameter: _____
  Outlet (cm): _____
  Shape of sacrum: _____ Arch: _____
  Coccyx: _____ SS notch: _____ Ischial
    spines: _____
  Adequacy of inlet: _____ Mid: _____ Outlet: _____
Prognosis for delivery: _____
Pregnancy test: _____
  Serology test (date): _____

SOCIAL INTERACTIONS:

Subjective:

Relationship status: _____
  Years in relationship: _____ Living with: _____
  Role within family structure: _____
Extended family: _____
  Other support person(s): _____
  Frequency of social contacts: _____
Living in ethnic community (Y/N): _____
  Specify: _____
Concerns/stresses: _____ Coping behaviors: _____
Plans for intra/postpartal period: _____

Objective:

Verbal/nonverbal communication with significant
  other/family: _____
Family interaction (behavioral) pattern: _____

TEACHING/LEARNING:

Subjective:

Dominant language (specify): _____ Secondary: _____
  Literate: _____ Cognitive limitations: _____
Maternal/paternal education levels: _____
  Occupations: _____
Ethnic/cultural background: _____ Where born: _____
  Length of residence in this country if immigrant: _____
  Health/illness beliefs: _____
  Special practices (including religious factors): _____
Familial risk factors (indicate relationship):
  Diabetes: _____ Tuberculosis: _____
  High BP: _____ Epilepsy: _____
  Heart disease: _____ Strokes: _____
  Kidney disease: _____ Cancer: _____
  Blood disorders: _____ Mental illness: _____
  Genetic (congenital) problems: _____
  Cesarean births: _____ Multiple births: _____

Discharge Plan Considerations (when hospitalized)

Date information obtained: _____
Anticipated date of discharge: _____
Home situation: _____
  Resources available: Persons: _____
  Financial: _____ Maternity leave: _____
    Anticipated needs/assistance required: _____

TABLE 3–2. **Prenatal Assessment Tool** (continued)

Prescribed medications: Drug: _____ Dose: _____
  Times: _____ Take regularly: _____
  Purpose: _____
Nonprescription drugs:
  OTC: _____ Street drugs: _____
  Use of alcohol (amount/frequency): _____
  Tobacco/form: _____
Current complaints/symptoms of pregnancy: _____
  Effect on lifestyle: _____ Adaptations made: _____
Relevant illnesses and/or hospitalizations/surgeries: _____
Last physical examination (date and doctor): _____
Expectations of this pregnancy/hospitalization: _____
  Type of delivery: _____ Anesthesia: _____
Infant feeding planned: _____
Education classes attended/resources: _____

SAMPLE MATERNAL CLIENT SITUATION:
Preterm Labor/Prevention of Delivery

Mrs. R.F.M., a 30-year-old gravida 1, para 0, with expected due date (EDD) of 6/26/97 (24 1/7 weeks' gestation), and ultrasound confirmation of 2 fetuses present (office visit 2/5/97), called the physician's office today (3/14/97) at 1400. Beginning at 1340, she had experienced several contractions lasting more than 40 sec each. At 1400 her abdomen remained firm to touch even after she had attempted to diminish the contractions by: (1) drinking two large glasses of water, (2) voiding a moderate amount, and (3) lying on her left side. She was directed to the hospital for evaluation of labor and was admitted with an initial diagnosis of possible preterm labor.

ADMITTING PHYSICIAN'S ORDERS

Have patient drink 480 to 720 ml of fluid now.
Apply continuous external fetal monitor (EFM), document uterine activity and fetal status q1h.
Check cervix for dilatation and effacement.
Nitrazine test, vaginal culture now.
Stat CBC (complete blood count), K^+ (potassium), UA (urinalysis).
Fasting blood glucose per fingerstick in AM.
Terbutaline 0.25 mg SC (subcutaneous) and 5 mg PO now; if contractions do not cease, start
   500 ml $D_5^{1}/_2$ NS and begin magnesium sulfate ($MgSO_4$) drip per protocol.
Betamethasone 12.5 mg (2 ml) IM now and repeat in 12 hr.
VS q4h.
Complete bedrest.
Regular diet.

NURSING HISTORY AND ASSESSMENT

Name: R.F.M.
Age: 30 DOB: 5/6/66. Sex: F. Race: Caucasian.
Admission date: 3/14/97. Time: 1520. From: Home.
Source of information: Client.
Father of Child: R.L.M. Age: 38. Race: Caucasian.
Healthcare provider: Maternal: Dr. C.R.
Infant: Has not chosen yet.

Activity/Rest

Sleep: Hours: 8–10 hr night. Naps: 2/day Aids: None.
Usual activities/hobbies: Needlework and reading.
Limitations imposed by pregnancy: Bedrest, ordered by physician 2/5/97.
Occupation: RN, worked part-time 3–11 shifts in Medical-Surgical until 2/5/97.
Observed response to activity: Cardiovascular: Slight increase in rate (110 beats per minute
   [bpm]). Respiratory: Slight increase in rate (26/min).
Mental status: Outgoing, alert; responds appropriately.
Neuromuscular assessment: Quality of extremities: Moves all four extremities well/equally.
   Posture: Erect. ROM: Full. Tremors: -0-. Strength: Good/equal in all extremities.

Circulation

History of Elevated BP: -0-. Heart trouble: -0-. Rheumatic fever: -0-. Ankle/leg edema: -0-.
   Phlebitis: -0-. Slow healing: -0-.
BP: R: Standing: 122/70. Sitting: 120/66. Lying: 120/62. L: Standing: 124/72. Sitting: 122/68.
   Lying: 120/62.
Peripheral pulses: Radials 3+; pedals 2+.
Heart sounds: No murmurs or rubs. Apical rate: 100 bpm. Rhythm: Regular. Quality: Strong.
Jugular vein distension: -0-.
Extremities: Temperature: Warm to touch. Color: Pink.
Capillary refill: Rapid, under 3 sec.
Homans' sign: -0-. Varicosities: -0-.

Nails: Normal; pink nail beds; nail base firm.
Color/cyanosis: Mucous membranes: Pink; intact. Conjunctiva: Salmon-colored. Sclera: white.

Ego Integrity

Pregnancy planned: Yes.
Client feelings about pregnancy: "We waited several years, so I'm really happy."
Father's feelings about pregnancy: Excited and relieved because conception had been a difficult
  process.
Relationship status: Married.
Financial concerns: Has health insurance coverage and sick leave.
Religion: Maternal/Paternal: Both Protestant. Practicing: Yes.
Cultural factors: Urban white-collar workers, middle-class, western European descent.
Report of stress factors: "It has been frustrating to lie around the house and not be able to do
  things that need to be done. Now I am very concerned about our babies' health."
Ways of handling stress: Previously walking; now relaxation techniques and reading.
Lifestyle: Married, dual-income family. Recent changes: Off work and unable to care for
  husband and self.
Feelings of helplessness: "Sometimes." Hopelessness: No. Powerlessness: "Some right now."
Emotional status: Calm, fearful.
Observed physiological response(s): Remains calm, yet demonstrates appropriate concern; facial
  expression tense; body tense, guarded.

Elimination

Usual bowel pattern: Once per day. Laxative use: 0.
Character of stool: Soft, brown, formed. Last bowel movement: Yesterday.
Bleeding: -0-. Hemorrhoids: -0-.
Usual voiding pattern: Moderate amount every 2–4 hr around the clock; no urgency or
  incontinence.
Frequency: Since third week of pregnancy. Retention: -0-.
Character of urine: Clear, pale yellow.
Pain/burning/difficulty voiding: -0-. History of kidney/bladder disease: -0-.
Abdomen: Slightly tender since 12/96. Soft/firm: Firm. Palpable mass: No abnormalities.
Bowel sounds: Present in all quadrants.
Bladder palpable: -0-. Overflow voiding: -0-.
Urinalysis report: In process.
Albuminuria/glycosuria: Negative per dipstick.

Food/Fluid

Loss of appetite: -0-.
Nausea: -0-. Vomiting: Severe vomiting during first 15 wk of pregnancy.
Heartburn/food intolerance: -0-.
Normal weight: 140 lb.
Use of diuretics: -0-.
Dietary pattern: Eats 3 meals/day.
Last ate/what: Lunch/tomato soup and tuna sandwich, milk, cookie, half an apple.
Current weight: 159 lb. Height: 5 ft 5 in. Body build: Stocky/endomorphic. Skin turgor: Good,
  elastic.
Edema: Dependent/periorbital: -0-. Thyroid enlarged: No.
Condition of teeth/gums: All teeth present and in good condition; gums pink, no bleeding.
Appearance of tongue: Pink; fully mobile within mouth.
Breath sounds: Clear bilateral.
Hb/Hct (anemia): Hb 12.6, Hct 37.8.
Diabetic screening: GTT: N/A. Thyroid studies: N/A.

Hygiene

Activities of daily living: Independent: In all areas until 2/5/97; since then has maintained
  bedrest with bathroom privileges.

Dependent (specify): Husband has done all household tasks and assisted client with self-care activities since client placed on bedrest.

General appearance: Clean and neat, light makeup, hair groomed.

Manner of dress: Maternity dress, low-heeled shoes.

Neurosensory

Fainting spells/dizziness: Dizziness during first trimester.

Headaches: Location: Right temporal area. Frequency: Occasional, "especially when I am under stress." Has right temporomandibular joint (TMJ) disease.

Eyes/vision loss: Nearsighted R/L, corrected with glasses.

Ears/hearing loss: -0-. Nose/epistaxis: "Occasional, especially when humidity is very low."

Sense of smell: Reports no problems/not tested.

Mental status: Alert, oriented to time, person, place.

Pupils: PERLA.

Glasses: Yes. Contacts: -0-. Hearing aid: -0-.

Pain/Discomfort

Location: Suprapubic.

Intensity (0–10): 3–4. Quality: Dull pain; increases when symphysis pubis is touched. Duration: 1 wk.

Precipitating factors: Twin A became engaged; experienced a contraction today, with abdomen remaining tense since.

How relieved: Is not relieved; tried drinking two large glasses of water, voiding, and lying on left side.

Facial grimacing: When area is palpated. Narrowed focus: No.

Guarding affected area: Requests medical staff to use light touch when taking uterine measurements.

Respiration

History: Bronchitis: -0-. Asthma: -0-. Tuberculosis: -0-. Dyspnea: -0-.

Smoker: -0-/nonsmoking household.

Respiratory: Rate: 20/min. Depth: Shallow. Quality: Equal; bilateral.

Breath sounds: Vesicular, clear bilateral.

Safety

Allergies/sensitivity: Penicillin. Reaction: Generalized red rash, occurred when client was a child, has not taken penicillin since.

History of STD (date/type): -0-.

German measles: Immune. Exposure to radiation: Not during pregnancy.

Previous obstetric problems: N/A. ABO/Rh sensitivity: N/A.

Blood transfusion: -0-.

Fractures/dislocations: Nose was fractured at age 4. Arthritis/unstable joints: -0-.

Back problems: -0-.

Impaired: Vision: Wears glasses.

Temperature: 98.8°F (37.1°C), tympanic.

Skin integrity: Intact. Scars: Inner right forearm, old injury from childhood.

Strength (general): Good; equal in all four extremities.

Muscle tone: Firm. Gait: Wide-spaced secondary to pregnancy. ROM: Good.

Fetal: Heart rate: Twin A 150 bpm, Twin B 154 bpm. Location: Twin A left lower quadrant (LLQ) (two-finger breadths above pubic bone), Twin B right upper quadrant (RUQ) (four-finger breadths to R of umbilicus). Method of auscultation: EFM. Fundal height: 22 cm. Estimated gestation: $24^1/_7$ wk. Movement: Frequent; active. Ballottement: Absent; Twin A engaged.

Blood type/Rh: Maternal: A+. Paternal: A+.

Screens: Sickle cell: N/A. Rubella: Immune. Hepatitis: -0-. TB: -0-. AFP: Within normal range at 14 wk.

Serology syphilis: Negative 11/18/96.

Cervical/rectal culture: Pending (done 3/14/97; 1600).

Vaginal warts/lesions: -0-.

Sexuality

Menarche: 10 yr old. Length of cycle: 28 days. Duration: 3–5 days.
Last menstrual period: 9/19/96. Amount: Moderate EDD: 6/26/97.
Vaginal discharge: Odorless, clear, thick.
Bleeding since LMP: Once per month first trimester; spotting.
Practices breast self-examination: Yes. Last Pap smear: 11/18/96.
Recent contraceptive method: Diaphragm.
Obstetric history (GPTPAL): Gravida: 1. Para: -0-. Abortions: -0-.
Pelvic: Vulva: Pink; moist. Perineum: No abnormalities; pink, intact. Vagina: Dark, pink. Cervix:
    Closed; Chadwick's sign present. Uterus: Distended, pear-shaped. Adnexal: Normal.
    Diagonal conjugate: 12.5 cm. Transverse diameter: Outlet: 10.5 cm. Shape of sacrum:
    Normal, average inclination. Coccyx: Movable. Ischial spines: 0.8 cm. Inlet: Adequate. Mid:
    Adequate. Outlet: Adequate.
Prognosis for delivery: Good for vaginal delivery.
Breast examination: Supple, symmetric; no abnormalities.
Nipples: Erect/dark in color; no cracks or fissures; no abnormalities.
Serology test: Negative 10/25/96.

Social Interactions

Relationship status: Married. Yr in relationship: 8. Living with: Husband.
Role within family structure: Housewife; secondary wage earner.
Extended family: Married younger brother/nephew in town; all other relatives live out of town.
Other support person(s): Many close friends in town; mother available to come if client goes
    home on bedrest.
Frequency of social contacts: Family/friends in 2–3 times/wk.
Concerns/stresses: Husband has had to carry all responsibilities for both of them.
Coping behaviors: Maintains open communication, acceptance of situation.
Plans for intra/postpartal period: Mother will be available.
Verbal/nonverbal communication with family/significant others (SOs): Husband sitting beside
    bed, speaks quietly and holds client's hand.

Teaching/Learning

Language dominant: English. Literate: Yes.
Ethnic/cultural background: Anglo-Saxon. Born in the United States. Health/illness beliefs:
    Views pregnancy as normal process requiring minimal intervention. Special practices: -0-.
Education: Client: BSN. Cognitive limitations: -0-.
Husband: MS. Occupation: Certified respiratory therapist.
Familial risk factors (maternal/paternal; indicate relationship): Tuberculosis: Maternal
    grandfather. Diabetes: -0-. High BP: Maternal aunt. Epilepsy: -0-. Heart disease: -0-.
    Stroke: -0-. Kidney disease: -0-. Cancer: Maternal grandmother—colon cancer. Multiple
    births: Maternal: Aunt had twins; father of these babies is a twin. Genetic conditions:-0-.
Prescribed medications: Drugs: Maternal prenatal vitamin/mineral supplement: Takes 1 tablet
    daily at 2200, regularly.
Nonprescription drugs: OTC: -0-. Illicit: -0-.
Use of alcohol (amount/frequency): -0-.
Current complaints/symptoms of pregnancy: Called obstetrician (OB) at 1400, reported having
    contractions that didn't seem to go away and abdomen remained very firm.
Relevant illnesses and/or hospitalization surgery: 12/10/96; short-stay hospitalization for IV
    therapy; experienced 7-lb weight loss in 48 hr because of severe prenatal vomiting.
Last physical examination: Last OB appointment, 3/7/97; uterine measurement, fetal heart tone
    (FHT), and ultrasound done by Dr. C.R.
Ultrasound report: Twin A was shown to be engaged and both babies were growing at the same
    rate. R.M. reported frequent, regular contractions and, the day after the appointment, called
    to report loss of mucous plug.
Expectations of this pregnancy: Full-term, healthy babies.
Type of delivery planned: Vaginal, although twin B is breech, so realizes cesarean birth is
    possible. Type of anesthesia planned: Local, if episiotomy is done; otherwise, none.
Type of infant feeding planned: Breast.

Preparation: Prenatal/intrapartal classes: Prematurity Prevention 2/18/97.
  Infant care/feeding: No formal class yet; was to begin childbirth classes 3/31/97.
  Books: Several medical books dealing with obstetrics and bonding.
  Other (specify): Contacted local chapters of La Leche League International and the Twins
  Club.

Discharge Plan Considerations:

As of 3/14/97:
If delivery delayed: Will require monitoring/periodic visitation; homemaker assistance.
Anticipated discharge: Within 5 days—by 3/19/93.
Resources available: Husband, mother.

SAMPLE MATERNAL CLIENT PLAN OF CARE:
Preterm Labor/Prevention of Delivery

CLIENT DIAGNOSTIC STATEMENT (NURSING DIAGNOSIS):

ANXIETY [MODERATE] related to the possibility of premature delivery, perceived or actual threat of fetuses and self, evidenced by expressions of concern regarding current events, increased tension, apprehension, narrowed focus

DESIRED OUTCOMES/EVALUATION CRITERIA—CLIENT WILL:

Verbalize awareness of feelings of anxiety within 24 hr (3/15 1600).

Appear relaxed and report anxiety is reduced to a manageable level within 24 hr (3/15 1600).

Identify three ways she is effectively dealing with anxieties within 48 hr (3/16 1600).

ACTIONS/INTERVENTIONS	RATIONALE
Introduce self to R.F.M. and family. Maintain "primary caregiver."	Important for couple to feel "connected" to the caregiver to promote a sense of trust.
Explain procedures, nursing interventions, and treatments.	Knowledge of the reasons for these activities can decrease fear of the unknown.
Orient couple to labor suite environment.	Helps client/husband to feel at ease and more comfortable in their surroundings.
Keep communication open; discuss the possible side effects and outcomes, maintaining an optimistic attitude.	Knowing information will be given freely and questions will be answered can help to reduce anxiety, promote hope, and strengthen "working" relationship between client and staff.
Control external stimulation. Review restrictions/rationale (e.g., TV, radio, visitors, phone).	Quiet atmosphere promotes rest and relaxation, which can assist in decreasing muscle tension and may enhance uterine and fetal blood flow. In turn, this may reduce the perceived/actual threat to fetuses.
Encourage use of relaxation techniques (e.g., deep-breathing exercises, visualization, guided imagery).	Enables the client to obtain maximum benefit from rest periods; prevents muscle fatigue and may improve uterine blood flow. Provides opportunity for active participation and enhances sense of control.
Encourage verbalization of fears and concerns.	Helps client to define and become aware of specific problems, providing opportunity for problem solving and thereby reducing anxiety.
Monitor maternal/fetal vital signs.	Vital signs of client and fetuses may be altered by anxiety. Stabilization may reflect reduction of anxiety level.
Assess support systems available to R.F.M./couple.	During this time of stress and uncertainty, availability of the assistance and caring of significant others, including caregivers, is extremely important to decrease anxiety and enhance coping.

CLIENT DIAGNOSTIC STATEMENT (NURSING DIAGNOSIS):	ACTIVITY INTOLERANCE related to muscle/cellular hypersensitivity, evidenced by increased uterine irritability and cervical dilatation; and adverse effect on uteroplacental perfusion evidenced by change in fetal heart rate (FHR).
DESIRED OUTCOMES/EVALUATION CRITERIA—CLIENT WILL:	Report/display cessation of uterine contractions within 12–36 hr (3/15–16 0400).

ACTIONS/INTERVENTIONS	RATIONALE
Expedite the admissions process and institute bedrest using lateral position.	Facilitating reduction of activity and psychological stressors may help decrease tension and relieve uterine contractions. Left or right lateral position improves uterine blood flow and may decrease uterine irritability.
Explain the reasons for requiring bedrest, lying on side, and decreasing activity.	These measures are intended to keep the pressure of the fetus off the cervix and to enhance placental perfusion, decreasing uterine irritability.
Demonstrate/encourage use of relaxation techniques.	Helps reduce muscle tension and client's perception of discomfort.
Provide comfort measures such as changes of position/linen, back rub, and Therapeutic Touch. Decrease stimuli in room (e.g., lighting).	Relieves muscle fatigue and promotes sense of well-being.
Offer diversional activities, such as reading, television, or visits with selected friends or family, as appropriate.	Refocuses attention, reduces boredom, and may enhance coping ability.
Provide uninterrupted periods for rest/sleep.	Promotes rest, prevents fatigue, and may enhance relaxation.
Monitor maternal and fetal vital signs per protocol. Assess uterine contractions per protocol.	Reflects effectiveness of and determines need for further interventions.

CLIENT DIAGNOSTIC STATEMENT (NURSING DIAGNOSIS):	RISK FOR POISONING related to possibility of toxic side effects (cardiovascular) of treatments and medications used to stop labor.
DESIRED OUTCOMES/EVALUATION CRITERIA—CLIENT WILL:	Verbalize understanding of potential dangers, maternal/fetal side effects within 4 hr (3/14 2000). Display no untoward effects/complications (ongoing).

ACTIONS/INTERVENTIONS	RATIONALE
Place in lateral position. Elevate head of bed slightly.	Decreases uterine irritability, increases placental perfusion, and prevents supine hypotension.
Have R.F.M. drink 480–720 ml of fluid now.	Helps rule out preterm labor related to dehydration.
Assist as needed with sterile vaginal examination. Obtain vaginal culture on admission.	Necessary to assess cervical status; however, vaginal examinations are kept to a minimum because they may contribute to uterine irritability. Safety of tocolytic agents when cervix is greater than 4 cm

Apply EFM and assess uterine contractions and FHR electronically on admission and continuously until stable, then bid 0900/2000 (unless MgSO$_4$ infusion in place).

dilated or more than 80% effaced is not documented. Culture is done to rule out infection/STD as cause of uterine irritability.

Tactile and electronic monitoring of uterine contractions and FHR provides ongoing fetal/uterine assessment and basis for altering or maintaining drug administration. Note: External monitors may increase contractions in some clients.

Provide information about the actions and side effects of drug therapy. Obtain release for administration of terbutaline sulfate.

Important for the client/couple to know the purpose of the drug(s) being administered. Terbutaline sulfate is still considered an experimental drug and may cause fetal tachycardia, hyperglycemia, acidosis, and hypoxia.

Administer terbutaline 0.25 mg SC and 5 mg PO now. Document response. Proceed to MgSO$_4$ drip as indicated.

Promotes relaxation of uterine muscle and vessel walls. If unsuccessful, MgSO$_4$ infusion may be required.

Monitor vital signs q4h, noting cardiac rhythm. Auscultate lung sounds. Record intake and output.

Terbutaline sulfate, which stimulates beta$_2$ receptors, may cause complications such as tachycardia/cardiac dysrhythmias and an increase in plasma volume.

Assess deep tendon reflexes (DTRs) q 1 to 2 h, as appropriate.

Adverse effect of MgSO$_4$ infusion is absence of DTRs and respiratory depression, requiring prompt intervention.

Observe for development of side effects (e.g., palpitations, decreased respiratory rate, chest pain, dyspnea, agitation, absence of DTRs). If present, decrease drug rate, give oxygen by mask, start lactated Ringer's infusion (fluid expander), administer calcium gluconate per protocol, and notify Dr. C.R.

Although mild degree of tachycardia and jitteriness may be normal, escalating/persistent symptoms beyond 20 to 40 min on initiation of medication suggest adverse reaction. Prompt action can reverse untoward or toxic effects.

Maintain fluid intake of at least 3500 ml/day.

Amniotic fluid exchange occurs every 3 to 4 hr, so it is advisable for client to drink something every 1 to 2 hr and maintain high daily intake.

Weigh daily, 0730.

Detects fluid shifts/retention, possible alteration in urinary functioning, and adequacy of nutritional intake.

Obtain urine sample for routine urinalysis.

Urinary tract infection may cause/enhance uterine irritability.

Review/monitor laboratory findings: CBC, UA, cultures, serum glucose, and potassium.

Check for anemia, presence of infection (affects treatment options). Terbutaline sulfate causes movement of potassium ions into cells, decreasing plasma K$^+$ levels, increasing blood glucose and plasma insulin levels, and and stimulating release of glycogen from muscle and liver.

CLIENT DIAGNOSTIC STATEMENT (NURSING DIAGNOSIS):

RISK FOR FETAL INJURY related to insufficient development to maintain physiological self outside of uterine environment if delivered prematurely.

DESIRED OUTCOMES/EVALUATION CRITERIA—CLIENT WILL:

Maintain pregnancy until fetal viability is reached (at least 25 wk), or longer if possible.

ACTIONS/INTERVENTIONS	RATIONALE
Perform nitrazine test now.	Verifies spontaneous premature rupture of membranes (SPROM), which presents increased risk of infection and affects choice of interventions and timing of delivery.
Assess for maternal conditions that would contraindicate steroid therapy.	In pregnancy-induced hypertension (PIH) and chorioamnionitis, steroid therapy may aggravate hypertension and mask signs of infection. Steroids may increase blood glucose levels in the client with diabetes.
Assess FHR; note presence of uterine activity or cervical dilation.	Tocolytics can increase FHR. Delivery may be extremely rapid with small infant if persistent uterine contractions are unresponsive to tocolytics, or if cervical changes continue.
Review pros and cons of steroid therapy with R.F.M./couple.	Steroid therapy is most effective between 28 and 34 weeks' gestation to stimulate lung maturity. Long-term effects on the development of the child cannot be known until longitudinal studies have been completed.
Administer betamethasone 12.5 mg (2 ml) IM 1800, repeat × 1 at 0600.	Although steroid therapy has been controversial, research indicates that it prevents or decreases the severity of respiratory distress syndrome (RDS) by stimulating fetal surfactant production.
Stress necessity of follow-up care if discharged without delivering.	If fetuses are not delivered within 7 days of administration of steroids, dose should be repeated weekly.

CLIENT DIAGNOSTIC STATEMENT (NURSING DIAGNOSIS):	KNOWLEDGE DEFICIT [LEARNING NEED] regarding condition, prognosis, treatment, and self-care needs related to lack of information/misinterpretation evidenced by questions and expressions of concerns
DESIRED OUTCOMES/EVALUATION CRITERIA—CLIENT WILL:	Verbalize awareness of implications and possible outcomes of condition and preterm labor within 16 hr (3/15 0800). Ask questions appropriately within 24 hr (3/15 1600). Assume responsibility for own learning and participate in learning process within 48 hr of admission (3/16 1600).

ACTIONS/INTERVENTIONS	RATIONALE
Ascertain knowledge about preterm labor and possible outcomes.	Establishes data base and identifies individual client learning needs.
Determine readiness to learn.	Factors such as anxiety or lack of awareness of need for information (denial) can interfere with readiness to learn.
Include husband in the teaching process.	Support from significant other(s) can help allay anxiety as well as reinforce learning.

Review signs and symptoms of "early" labor.	Helps client to recognize preterm labor so that therapy to suppress this labor can be initiated or reinstituted promptly.
Discuss need for bedrest, limitation of activity, restriction of sexual and nipple activity.	Activity, orgasm, and stimulation of the nipples (which release oxytocin) may stimulate uterine activity.
Determine availability and level of commitment of supportive resources.	Husband may tire of managing total responsibility for client and home, regular role/duties. Enlisting assistance of other resources may reduce risk of burnout and enhance coping ability.
Stress avoidance of use of OTC drugs while tocolytic agents are administered, unless approved by physician.	Concurrent use of OTC drugs may cause deleterious effects, especially if drug has side effects similar to those of tocolytic agent (e.g., antihistamines or inhalers with broncho-dilating effects, such as epinephrine [Primatene Mist]).
Recommend taking oral tocolytic agents with food if drug is continued.	Food improves tolerance to drug and reduces GI side effects.
Provide information about follow-up care, including home monitoring/daily uterine activity record, pump therapy program as appropriate.	Cooperation is enhanced when client understands need for regular monitoring/ongoing treatment.
Arrange for visit to neonatal intensive care unit.	Helps alleviate fears and facilitates adjustment to the potential realities of the situation.
Refer to community health nurse, childbirth education class, and another couple who have experienced a similar episode with a successful outcome.	Additional help may assist client/couple to cope with situation, especially if client returns home to await delivery.
Identify other resources, e.g., Meals on Wheels, telephone visitor (Sidelines), homemaker services.	Community supports may help reduce stress level, enhance coping/problem-solving abilities of client/couple.

EVALUATION

As nursing care is provided, ongoing assessments determine the client's response to therapy and progress toward accomplishing the desired outcomes. This activity serves as the feedback and control part of the nursing process, through which the status of the individual client diagnostic statement is judged to be resolved, continuing, or requiring revision.

This process is visualized in Figure 3–1. Discussion with R.F.M. verifies that she is aware of her feelings of anxiety and is gathering the information she needs to deal more effectively with her concerns. She appears relaxed and states that she feels more in control of her immediate situation. Therefore she is progressing toward resolving and managing her anxiety, and this problem will continue to be addressed, although no revision in the treatment plan is required at this time.

DOCUMENTATION

To date a number of charting formats have been used for documentation. These include block notes, with a single entry covering an entire shift (e.g., 7 AM to 3 PM); narrative timed notes (e.g., 8:30 AM, ate all of breakfast); and the problem-oriented medical record system (POMR or PORS) using the subjective-objective analysis plan (SOAP)/subjective-objective analysis plan, implementation, evaluation, and revision (SOAPIER) format, to name a few. The latter can provide thorough documentation, but it was designed to physicians for episodic care and requires that the entries be tied to a client problem identified from a problem list.

A system format created by nurses for documentation of frequent/repetitive care is FOCUS® Charting. It was designed to encourage looking at the client from a positive rather than a negative (or problem-oriented) perspective by using precise documentation to record the nursing process. Recording assessment, intervention,

CHAPTER 4

PRENATAL CONCEPTS
The Trimesters: Prenatal Assessment

CLIENT ASSESSMENT DATA BASE

Activity/Rest

Lack of/decreased energy/fatigue
Difficulty falling asleep/interrupted sleep (psychological stressors, physical discomforts, nocturia)
Not feeling well rested
Decreased ability to perform/participate in usual activities (as pregnancy progresses)

Circulation

Blood pressure slightly lower than normal (8–12 wk), returning to prepregnancy levels during the last half of pregnancy.
Pulse rate may increase 10–15 beats per minute (bpm).
Short systolic murmur may develop related to increased volume.
Syncopal episodes.
Varicosities.
Slight edema of lower extremities/hands may be present (particularly in last trimester).

Ego Integrity

Expresses changes in perception of self.
Emotional lability.

Elimination

Changes in stool consistency/frequency
Increased frequency of urination
Urinalysis: increased specific gravity
Hemorrhoids

Food/Fluid

Nausea and vomiting, primarily first trimester; heartburn is common.
Weight gain: 2–4 lb first trimester; second and third trimesters, 11–12 lb each (levels below this may suggest eating disorder).
Dry mucous membranes; hypertrophy of gingival tissue may occur and may bleed easily.
Low hemoglobin (Hb) and hematocrit (Hct) may be present (physiological anemia).
Slight dependent edema.
Slight glycosuria may be present.
Diastasis recti (separation of the rectus muscle) may occur late in pregnancy.

The following is an example of documentation of a client need/concern that currently does not require identification as a client problem (nursing diagnosis) or inclusion in the plan of care and therefore is not easily documented in the SOAP format:

DAR Format

Date	Time	Focus	Progress Notes
3/15/97	1920	Gastric distress	D: Reports "indigestion/burning sensation" with hand over epigastric area. Skin warm/dry, color pink, vital signs unchanged. A: Given Mylanta 30 ml PO. Head of bed elevated approximately 15 degrees. R: Reports pain relieved. Appears relaxed, resting quietly. B. Briner, RN

and evaluation information in a *data, action,* and *response* (DAR) format facilitates tracking and following what is happening to the client at any given moment. Charting focuses on client and nursing concerns. The focal point is client status and the associated nursing care. The focus is always stated in a way that reflects the client's concern/need, rather than a nursing task or medical diagnosis.

Thus, the focus can be a client problem/concern or nursing diagnoses; signs/symptoms of potential importance (e.g., fever, blood pressure fluctuations, edema); a significant event or change in status; or specific standards of care/hospital policy. Based on the client situation of R.F.M., the following examples of POMR and FOCUS® documentation are provided:

SOAP/SOAPIER Format

Date	Time	Number/Problem	Progress Notes
3/14/97	1600	No. 1 Anxiety	S: "I feel so helpless. What's going to happen to me and the babies?" O: Crying, hands trembling, voice quivering, pulse 110. A: Moderate anxiety with concern regarding changes in life events and fear of consequences. P: Demonstrate and encourage use of relaxation techniques. Encourage verbalization of fears/concerns. Provide information as indicated re condition/status, expectations. Signed: M. Sickus, RN
3/15/97	0800	No. 5 Knowledge	S: "The signs of early labor include uterine contractions every 10 min or sooner, pelvic pressure, abdominal cramping, low backache, and/or increase in vaginal discharge. Without prompt intervention, labor could progress to the point where my babies will be born prematurely, increasing their risk of complications and threatening their survival. If any of these symptoms occurs, I should empty my bladder, lie down on my side, drink 3 to 4 glasses of water, palpate for uterine contractions, and notify the clinic nurse if symptoms continue." O: Displays relaxed posture, thoughtful expression. A: Has achieved outcome No. 1. P: Continue teaching plan as outlined. Signed: M. Sickus, RN

DAR Format

Date	Time	Focus	Progress Notes
3/15/97	0800	Learning Needs	D: Identified implications/signs of labor, and appropriate responses. Listed available resources/support groups. Verbalized benefits of activity limitations. Appeared relaxed; thoughtful expression as she recounted information. A: Provided positive feedback regarding client's understanding and awareness. R: Demonstrated learning and achievement of outcome No. 1. Signed: M. Sickus, RN
3/15/97	1400	Anxiety	D: Verbalizes awareness of feelings of anxiety. Reports that she is gathering information to deal more effectively with her concerns and feels more in control of situation. Appears slightly tense, no tears. A: Continue open communication and optimistic attitude. Provided information regarding usual home monitoring program. R: Identified additional supports available to self/husband and reported anxiety is manageable. Appeared relaxed and calm. Resting quietly. B. Briner, RN

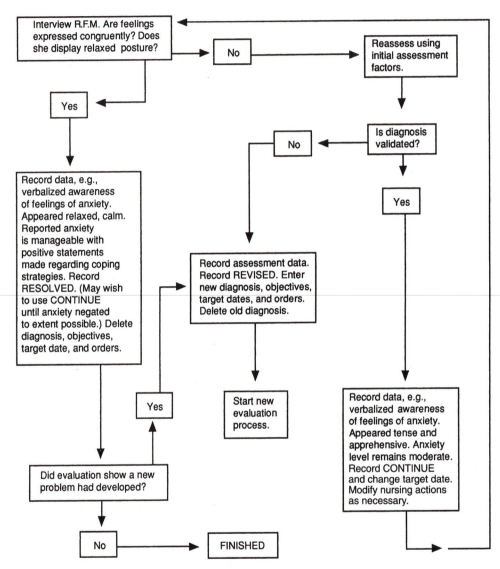

Figure 3–1. Outcome-based evaluation of the client's response to therapy related to nursing diagnosis, Anxiety. (Adapted from Cox, HC, et al: *Clinical Applications of Nursing Diagnosis.* FA Davis, Philadelphia, 1997, p 504.)

Pain/Discomfort

Leg cramps, breast tenderness and swelling; Braxton Hicks contractions noted after 28 wk; back pain, abdominal into groin pain (broad ligament tension)

Respiration

Nasal stuffiness; mucosa redder than normal.
Respiratory rate may increase relative to size/height of uterus; thoracic breathing pattern.

Safety

Temperature 98°F–99.6°F (36.1°C–37.6°C)
Fetal heart tones (FHTs) audible with Doptone (beginning 10–12 wk) or fetoscope (17–20 wk)
Fetal movement noted on examination after 20 wk; quickening (sensation of fetal movement in the abdomen) between 16 and 20 wk
Ballottement present 4th and 5th mo

Sexuality

Cessation of menses.
Change in sexual response/activity.
Leukorrhea may be present.
Progressive increase in uterine size; e.g., fundus slightly above symphysis pubis (at 10–12 wk), at umbilicus (20–22 wk), slightly below ensiform cartilage (36 wk).
Breast changes: Enlargment of adipose tissue, increased vascularity, tenderness on palpation, increase in diameter and pigmentation of areolar tissue, hypertrophy of Montgomery's tubercles; tingling sensation (first and third trimester), possible striae gravidarum; colostrum may appear after 12th wk.
Pigmentation changes: Chloasma, linea nigra, palmar erythema, spider nevi, striae gravidarum.
Positive Goodell's, Hegar's, Chadwick's, Ladin's signs.

Social Interaction

Confusion/questioning of anticipated role changes.
Maturational/development stage varies and may regress with stressor of pregnancy.
Responses of other family members can vary from positive and supportive to dysfunctional.

Teaching/Learning

Individual expectations of pregnancy, labor/delivery dependent on age, level of knowledge, experiences, parity, desire for child, economic stability

DIAGNOSTIC STUDIES

Complete Blood Count (CBC): Identifies anemia, hemoglobinopathies (e.g., sickle cell).
Blood Type: ABO and Rh to identify risk of incompatibility.
Vaginal/Rectal Smear: Tests for *Neisseria gonorrheae*, chlamydia, and beta streptococcus (as indicated by vaginal warts, lesions, abnormal discharge).
Serological Tests: Determine presence of other sexually transmitted diseases (STDs), including syphilis, HIV, hepatitis.
Screening: For tuberculosis.
Rubella Titer: > a:a0 denotes immunity.
Papanicolaou Smear: Identifies neoplasia, herpes simplex type 2.
Urinalysis: Screen for medical conditions (e.g., verification of pregnancy; infection, diabetes, renal disease).
Serum/Urine Testing for Human Chorionic Gonadotrophin (HCG): Positive.
Sonography: Evidence of fetus after 8 weeks' gestation, and verification of estimated date of delivery (EDD)/estimated date of birth (EDB).
Serum Glucose Screen/1-hr Glucose Test: <140 mg/dl (usually done between 24 and 28 wk).
Serum Alpha-Fetoprotein (AFP): Identifies neural tube defects at 16–18 weeks' gestation.

MSAFP$_3$: Maternal serum blood test for AFP, unconjugated estriol, and HCG screen for some birth defects in at risk clients.

Subsequent evaluations and focused assessments are done at each prenatal visit.

Genetic Counseling

Genetic counseling is a communication process that deals with human problems associated with the occurrence or risk of a genetic disorder in a family. Counseling involves genetic screening, whereby a high-risk or general population is analyzed to detect the presence of disease, and case finding for couples at potential risk based on medical/family histories. The process can be prospective (counseling delivered to a client/couple of reproductive age before conception or before the birth of an affected child), or it can be retrospective/postnatal (counseling delivered after the birth of an affected child). In many cases, however, the need for genetic counseling first becomes apparent during the first trimester.

(Refer also to care plan [CP]: The High-Risk Pregnancy, as appropriate.)

CLIENT ASSESSMENT DATA BASE

Circulation

Hypertension
Bleeding

Ego/Integrity

May express feelings of inadequacy

Food/Fluid

Weight gain may be inappropriate for gestational stage (smaller gain may negatively affect fetus).
Maternal insulin-dependent diabetes.
Presence of eating disorders (e.g., anorexia nervosa, bulimia, or obesity).

Safety

Infection (e.g., STDs, pelvic inflammatory disease)
Presence of seizure disorder, degree/method of control
Significant exposure to radiation, toxic chemicals, or infectious teratogens (e.g., rubella, toxoplasmosis, cytomegalovirus [CMV], HIV/AIDS), postnatal infections (e.g., meningitis, encephalitis); postnatal nutritional/stimulatory deprivation
Breech presentation (especially with anencephaly)

Sexuality

History of two or more first-trimester abortions, fetal demise, or previous child with chromosomal abnormality
Birth trauma or identifiable genetically transmitted disorder
Use of ovulation stimulant such as clomiphene (Clomid) or menotropins (Pergonal)

Social Interaction

Interfamily marriage/sexual activity (consanguinity)
Guilt/blame toward self and/or partner who carries defective gene

Teaching/Learning

Positive family history/pedigree of known genetic or inherited disorders (e.g., sickle cell, cystic fibrosis, hemophilia, phenylketonuria, craniospinal defects, renal malformations, thalassemia, Huntington's chorea) familial disorders (cancer, heart disease, diabetes, allergies), congenital abnormalities (Down syndrome, mental retardation, neural tube defects), or inborn metabolic disorder (e.g., maple syrup urine disease, Tay-Sachs disease)
Ethnic background at risk for specific disorder (e.g., black African, Mediterranean, Ashkenazi Jewish)
Maternal age >35 years

Drug usage (alcohol; over-the-counter [OTC], prescribed, or street drugs; anticonvulsant medication)

DIAGNOSTIC STUDIES

Chromosomal Analysis: Using buccal smear/serum.

Prenatal Diagnosis:

Amniocentesis (at 14–16 wk): Determines sex chromatin (rules out sex-linked disorders), karyotype (rules out chromosomal disorders), biochemical studies (rules out inborn errors of metabolism), elevation of AFP levels reflecting neural tube defects (NTDs).

Ultrasonography (using real time) Preceding/During Amniocentesis: Rules out missed abortion, visualizes term pregnancies, and helps to identify genetic/congenital problems. (Current research awaiting validation suggests a scan using a vaginal probe can be done as early as 10 weeks' gestation to screen for Down syndrome by looking for an accumulation of fluid in the neck of the fetus.)

Serum AFP Levels (16–18 wk): Identifies NTDs; if abnormality high/low, test is repeated.

Triple-Screen (MSAFP$_3$): Maternal serum testing at about 16 weeks' gestation measures AFP, unconjugated estriol, and human chorionic gonadatropin (HCG) to detect problems such as open spinal or ventral wall defects, anencephaly, Down syndrome, and trisomy 18.

Amniography/Fetography: Identifies gross problems, such as major soft-tissue abnormalities, esophageal/duodenal atresia, and bone abnormalities, using special x-ray technique (may be potentially teratogenic).

Fetoscopy (considered experimental, of limited availability): Permits direct visual examination of the fetus and sampling of fetal blood/tissue samples to diagnose hereditary blood disorders (e.g., sickle cell anemia, hemophilia).

Chorionic Villi Sampling (CVS) (at 8–10 wk): May replace amniocentesis as a genetic diagnostic tool because it is performed earlier, and results are reported in 7–10 days, which is particularly beneficial if a first-trimester termination is being considered.

NURSING PRIORITIES

1. Assist client/couple/family to recognize and understand specific situation.
2. Facilitate therapeutic use of informational resources.
3. Provide ongoing emotional support.

DISCHARGE GOALS

1. Copes effectively with situation
2. Completes counseling process
3. Understands information specific to individual situation

NURSING DIAGNOSIS:	**Anxiety [specify level]**
May Be Related To:	Presence of specific risk factors (e.g., history of genetic problem, exposure to teratogens), situational crisis, threat to self-concept (perceived/actual), conscious or unconscious conflict about essential values (beliefs) and goals of life
Possibly Evidenced By:	Increased tension, apprehension, uncertainty, feelings of inadequacy, or expressed concern regarding changes in life events, insomnia
DESIRED OUTCOMES/EVALUATION CRITERIA—CLIENT/COUPLE WILL:	Acknowledge awareness of feelings of anxiety. Verbalize realistic concerns related to process of genetic counseling/prenatal diagnosis.

Appear relaxed and report that anxiety is reduced to a manageable level.

Identify and use resources/support systems effectively.

ACTIONS/INTERVENTIONS	RATIONALE

Independent

Assess nature, source, and manifestations of anxiety.	Identifies specific areas of concern and determines direction for and possible options/interventions.
Provide information about specific genetic disorder, risks involved in reproduction, and available prenatal diagnostic measures/options. (Refer to nursing diagnosis [ND]: Knowledge deficit [Learning Need].)	May relieve anxiety associated with the unknown and assist family to cope with stress, make decisions, and adapt positively to choices. Note: A large number of clients at risk of producing a child with a genetic abnormality do not receive prospective counseling/diagnostic services before conception because of ineffective case finding/lack of awareness and often enter counseling, during the first trimester or, retrospectively, after the birth of an affected child. New genetic research at the gene level will have future implications for diagnosis, carrier status, or prenatal detection of genetic disease. Some of the techniques used include restriction endonuclease, DNA probes, polymerase chain reaction (PCR), Southern blot, restriction fragment length polymorphisms (RFLPs).
Promote ongoing sharing of concerns/feelings.	Opportunity for client/couple to begin resolution of situation. Note: Level of anxiety is usually higher in the couple who have already given birth to a child with a chromosomal disorder.
Review procedure and what to expect in terms of discomfort if fetus is affected and couple elects to terminate pregnancy and so on. (Refer to CP: Elective Termination.)	Client/couple may be extremely anxious, guilt-ridden during uncomfortable procedure; information can enhance coping, reduce anxiety.
Visit couple after procedure. Provide anticipatory guidance in terms of physical/psychological changes.	After abortion for genetic indications, follow-up visit by the primary nurse may help to reduce couple's anxiety/depression.
Provide opportunity for discussion of test results on fetus and assist with interpretation of information, especially following abortion.	Helps to confirm the diagnosis; reduces anxiety associated with uncertainty of whether fetus was really affected and whether couple made the "right" choice.
Listen to expressions of concern/feelings about situation.	When concerns and feelings are expressed/listened to, client needs can be identified more readily.

Collaborative

Refer for further counseling (e.g., psychiatric, group).	Anxiety may not be resolved sufficiently, necessitating additional professional assistance.
Assist couple in identifying community agencies to aid in care of their newborn in the event that they elect to continue the pregnancy after fetus is found to be affected, or when diagnosis is made after delivery. (Refer to CP: The Parents of a Child with Special Needs.)	Helps to reduce anxieties regarding how the couple will meet their baby's special needs.

43

NURSING DIAGNOSIS:	Knowledge deficit [Learning Need], regarding purpose/process of genetic counseling
May Be Related To:	Lack of awareness of the purpose/ramifications of genetic counseling, its applicability to their situation, components of the decision-making process necessary for analyzing available options, and available methods of prenatal diagnosis
Possibly Evidenced By:	Verbalization of the problem, statement of misconceptions, request for information
DESIRED OUTCOMES/EVALUATION CRITERIA—CLIENT/COUPLE WILL:	Describe the disorder in question.
	Identify available options.
	Discuss, in own words, purpose and findings of specific prenatal detection methods.
	Estimate risks associated with reproduction.

ACTIONS/INTERVENTIONS

RATIONALE

Independent

ACTIONS/INTERVENTIONS	RATIONALE
Discuss the purpose/goals of genetic counseling.	Serves to educate parents about the risks in their situation and ultimately to help them make educated/informed decisions. Misconceptions may interfere with the decision-making process.
Obtain pertinent family history; create pedigree chart from information. Include both parents in interview.	Provides accurate picture of the proband (afflicted person/index case) in relation to other family members and helps identify other persons similarly affected. Ensures that both parents are provided with the same information.
Identify risk factors in obstetric history, such as maternal age, three or more miscarriages, fetal demise, hypertension, bleeding, infection, significant exposure to radiation, low-level exposure to environmental pollutants (e.g., lead, formaldehyde, anesthetic gases), drug use (OTC, prescribed, street), birth trauma, or identifiable genetically transmitted disorder.	These factors may produce a phenocopy, an imitation of a genetic disorder.
Distinguish between environmental causes of mental retardation and those with a genetic component (e.g., Down syndrome).	Environmental causes include birth trauma, chemical teratogens, infectious teratogens (e.g., rubella, toxoplasmosis, cytomegalovirus), postnatal infections (e.g., meningitis, encephalitis), and postnatal nutritional/stimulatory deprivation.
Define specific genetic disorder in question. Provide prognosis/estimate of risks and probable consequences. Clarify/interpret data; avoid making recommendations or decisions for the client/couple.	Determines the probability of risk and recurrence of risk, allows client/couple to make informed choices incorporating values/goals/personal circumstances, free of biases or recommendations from the nurse.
Carry out ongoing family assessment for available support systems. Note signs of inappropriate coping/maladaptation. Offer information when family is ready to hear it.	Negative coping may interfere with cognitive functioning and hinder educational process. Some families are not ready to listen immediately after a diagnosis is made and many do not listen effectively the first time information is presented.

Arrange for follow-up, telephone calls, visits to home/counseling service.

Provides opportunity to reinforce information when family is "ready" to hear it.

Provide information about readily available/ individually appropriate diagnostic procedures and screenings, such as amniocentesis, serum testing for AFP, and ultrasonography, as well as CVS, fetoscopy, amniography, percutaneous umbilical blood sampling (PUBS) or cordocentesis, computed tomography (CT) scanning, and magnetic resonance imaging (MRI).

Prenatal diagnosis permits preparation for, or offers an alternative to, having children with genetic disorders. Allows couple to make informed choices at their own pace, based on understanding of long-term problems associated with the disorder in question.

Permit couple to arrive at own decision regarding their participation in, or refusal of, prenatal testing procedures.

Although testing may assist in determining whether the fetus at risk for a genetic disorder is actually affected, the client/couple has the right to refuse prenatal evaluation. Their decision needs to be accepted and respected.

Review anticipated follow-up evaluative procedures, especially if client is currently pregnant.

May include regular assessment of fetal heart tones, obtaining 20-min tracing on electronic monitoring, and so forth.

Discuss time element associated with receiving test results.

Prior knowledge of length of time required to obtain results can lessen client's anxiety. Test results may take up to 4 wk to analyze. Although CVS may be limited in its availability, it has advantages over amniocentesis because it can be performed earlier in the pregnancy (first versus second trimester), and results are available quickly (in 1–2 wk versus 2–4 wk). PUBS, or cordocentesis, provides a rapid fetal karyotype.

Encourage participation in community programs, i.e., education/support groups and groups concerned with specific genetic disorders as indicated (Tay-Sachs disease, Down syndrome, and so forth).

Helps client identify with others who have dealt with genetic disorders. Provides role models and information about the identified disorder.

Obtain/coordinate referrals with specialty clinics or adoptive agencies that deal with specific genetic disorders (e.g., cystic fibrosis, hemophilia).

May be needed to provide appropriate care/support that is needed in genetic counseling, especially if genetic component is involved.

Obtain informed consent/surgical permit for procedures/tests. Review risks associated with procedure.

Client needs to be aware of any risks involved to herself or the fetus, especially if the procedure is invasive, such as amniocentesis, CVS, fetoscopy, or PUBS.

Discuss future options, such as preimplantation diagnosis when both partners are identified as carriers of a defective gene.

Several eggs can be fertilized, the embryos evaluated for genetic abnormalities, and then only a healthy embryo is implanted in the uterus.

NURSING DIAGNOSIS:

Family Processes, risk for altered

Risk Factors May Include:

Situational crisis, individual/family vulnerability, difficulty reaching agreement regarding decision

Possibly Evidenced by:

[Not applicable; presence of signs/symptoms establishes an actual diagnosis]

DESIRED OUTCOMES/EVALUATION CRITERIA—CLIENT/COUPLE WILL:

Discuss available options.

Participate in the decision-making process.

Verbalize comfort with final decision.

45

ACTIONS/INTERVENTIONS	RATIONALE

Independent

Determine couple's relationship to one another, strength of intrafamily bonds, and support systems.	Establishes baseline. The threat of a hereditary disorder often results in intrafamily strife, as well as marital disharmony and family disintegration (separation and divorce).
Assess couple's perception of disorder as well as their attitudes/religious beliefs. (Refer to ND: Spiritual Distress.)	The way family members respond depends on the nature of the condition and on their perception of the "burden" (total amount of distress created by the diagnosis/birth of an affected child). Reactions may be more negative in dominant, X-linked disorders in which only one member of the couple is to "blame" or is identified as the carrier.
Provide information about risk estimates for disorder. Assess meaning of "carrier" status to client/couple, especially if couple desires male child and diagnosis is X-linked.	Allows couple to deal with the reality of the situation. For instance, if both parents are carriers of an autosomal recessive disorder for a deleterious gene, the risk is 1 in 4, or 25%, that an offspring will be affected. The nature of the condition influences the family's responses. If the female is a carrier for an X-linked disorder such as hemophilia, male fetuses have a 50% risk of being affected.
Provide opportunity to verbalize concerns. Be truthful and straightforward about genetic transmission.	Helps absolve feelings of guilt by exploring random nature of genetic transmission. Knowledge that everyone has 6–10 defective genes and that it is just chance that spouses have the same recessive deleterious gene may be reassuring/limit "blame."
Review all options available to the client/couple, e.g., adoption, postponing childbearing, artificial insemination by donor sperm, electing to reproduce using prenatal diagnosis, or surrogate parenting. If client is carrying an affected child, options include terminating the pregnancy; refusing aggressive intervention (e.g., not stopping premature labor, no CPR or intensive care); or treating the fetus in utero (if possible), carrying the pregnancy to term and keeping the neonate, or placing the child for adoption/foster care or institutionalization. (Refer to CP: The Parents of a Child with Special Needs.)	Promotes communication between client and partner. Provides opportunity to begin decision-making process based on factual information. Note: Choices may be limited by cultural/religious beliefs (e.g., Catholic, Christian Science, Jehovah's Witnesses and Islamic religions restrict or prohibit abortion).
Assist in problem solving and exploring alternative solutions, weighing impact on family members.	Helps to arrive at a decision, bringing family out of crisis, and facilitates growth of individual members and family as a unit.
Provide emotional support individually and to the couple as a unit.	Sometimes it is helpful to talk to members of the couple independently as well as together to assess individual perceptions of situation. Separate meetings are particularly critical if the couple are not in agreement about possible solutions.

Collaborative

Refer to community support groups, counseling, or social services.	May be necessary to help problem-solve and prevent family disintegration. Situations may arise whereby the couple are unable to agree on a decision when aware of risks/potential outcomes.
Refer to early intervention programs, community groups, or specialists after birth of an affected child.	Assists in management of short- and long-term medical/psychological problems.

NURSING DIAGNOSIS:	Spiritual Distress (distress of the human spirit)
May Be Related To:	Intense inner conflict about the outcome, normal grieving for the loss of a perfect child, anger that is often directed at God, religious beliefs/moral convictions
Possibly Evidenced By:	Verbalization of inner conflict about beliefs, questioning of the moral and ethical implications of therapeutic choices, questioning the meaning of this event, regarding condition as punishment; the development of anger, hostility, and crying
DESIRED OUTCOMES/EVALUATION CRITERIA—CLIENT/COUPLE WILL:	Make informed choices regarding childbearing/childrearing within their religious/moral framework.

Verbalize acceptance/resolution of stress if prenatal diagnosis is positive. |

ACTIONS/INTERVENTIONS

RATIONALE

Independent

Assist in identifying/discussing concerns and analyzing options based on religious beliefs and value system.

Helps couple to recognize their dilemma. The decision regarding the pregnancy outcome and participation in prenatal diagnosis is ultimately the right/responsibility of the prospective parents, with informed decision making dependent on ethical/religious/moral convictions.

Analyze client's/couple's emotional state. Assess for normal or abnormal states of grieving.

Grieving is anticipated, but excessive denial may interfere with progression/resolution of grief work.

Collaborative

Refer to pastor/rabbi/priest or other spiritual counselor as appropriate, especially if client/couple has religious affiliations that might affect decisions regarding conditions such as Tay-Sachs disease or Down syndrome.

May assist in, or be necessary for, resolution of ethical issues. In many religions, such as Catholicism, Orthodox Judaism, and Islam, abortion is viewed as an attack on the sanctity of life, with the mother's endangerment being the only generally permissible reason in some religions, in which case permission from a higher church authority is required.

NURSING DIAGNOSIS:	Self Esteem disturbance
May Be Related To:	Perceived failure at a life event
Possibly Evidenced By:	Denial, self-negating verbalization; feelings of guilt, powerlessness, anger; expressions of the unfairness of the situation, projection of blame/responsibility for problem
DESIRED OUTCOMES/EVALUATION CRITERIA—CLIENT/COUPLE WILL:	Verbalize lessened sense of guilt and restored feelings of self-worth.

Set realistic goals.

Participate actively in conflict resolution process. |

ACTIONS/INTERVENTIONS	RATIONALE

Independent

Determine self-perception of client/couple. Identify and reinforce individual/mutual strengths.

Provides opportunity for nurse to learn about client's/couple's expectations/perceptions of genetic disorder. Helps put feelings/opinions into perspective. When the diagnosis of genetic inheritance is involved, and one or both parents are found to be carriers of the defect, guilt, powerlessness, anger, and feelings of unfairness are normal/universal reactions to be anticipated.

Provide or reinforce information regarding risk estimate, to discuss with client and couple together and separately. Reaffirm inability to control outcome of conception; affirm ability to control decision to reproduce, adopt, or remain childless.

Helps reduce guilt feelings; promotes recognition by couple that some control over outcome is possible. Note: Some cultures believe in external locus of control and client/couple may resign themselves to the belief that they have no control over the events that are occurring.

Arrange for follow-up visit in clinic or office to assess status after abortion.

After discharge from the healthcare setting, feelings of loss/depression/negativism often occur, resulting in alteration of ego functioning.

Assess for recurring unresolved conflicts.

More intensive interventions support may be required to resolve low self-esteem.

Collaborative

Refer for counseling/psychiatric care as needed.

May be necessary to assist in working through the grief process in a healthy manner so that a positive sense of self emerges. Provides opportunity to establish or re-establish family integrity.

NURSING DIAGNOSIS:	Injury, risk for complications of testing procedures
Risk Factors May Include:	Invasive procedure, tissue hypoxia/changes in circulation, teratogenic effects of radiation
Possibly Evidenced By:	[Not applicable; presence of signs/symptoms establishes an *actual* diagnosis]
DESIRED OUTCOMES/EVALUATION CRITERIA—CLIENT/COUPLE WILL:	Identify individual risks and ways of minimizing them.
	Be free of preventable complications.

ACTIONS/INTERVENTIONS	RATIONALE

Independent

Identify the necessity of the specific test(s) and associated risks.

Testing involving radiation, CVS, amniocentesis, and so forth carries with it some degree of risk, i.e., spontaneous abortion/preterm labor, bleeding, infection, rupture of membranes, direct fetal injury/loss. Information helps the client/couple make informed decisions.

Review indications for genetic testing.

Some indications for this procedure are previous birth of a child with a chromosomal disorder or known metabolic defects, identification of client as a carrier of a sex-linked trait; maternal age of 35 or older/paternal age of 45 or older; family history of NTD; both parents carrying an autosomal recessive disease or a chromosomal abnormality; history of environmental teratogenic exposures, e.g., street drugs, dioxin/agent orange.

Review signs/symptoms of complications such as premature labor, infection, and abruptio placentae.

Client needs to recognize these as being important to report to healthcare provider to obtain timely evaluation/intervention.

Collaborative

Assist with obtaining blood or tissue, placental or chromosomal analysis/biopsy.

Determines nature of disorder in the event of a stillbirth/neonatal death/birth of an affected child, which is helpful in counseling couple regarding future pregnancies.

Assist with procedures such as amniocentesis, taking necessary measures (e.g., monitor blood pressure, pulse, respiration, and fetal heart rate). Assess fetal/uterine activity; use external fetal monitor for 20–30 min after procedure.

Testing procedures carry risks to the pregnancy/fetus. Careful monitoring may reduce untoward effects.

Position mother on left or right side.

Increases placental circulation, dilating blood vessels and reducing risk of supine hypotension and uterine irritability.

Administer medications as indicated:
    Rh immune globulin (RhIg) after
    amniocentesis and CVS;

Protects Rh-negative client from sensitization.
    Note: CVS is contraindicated in an Rh-sensitized woman, unless the purpose of the test is to detect an Rh-positive fetus.

    Antibiotics.

Given prophylactically after fetoscopy to prevent amnionitis.

NURSING DIAGNOSIS:	**Health Maintenance, risk for altered**
Risk Factors May Include:	Ineffective coping methods, unresolved grief, disabling distress, lack of material resources.
Possibly Evidenced By:	[Not applicable; presence of signs/symptoms establishes an *actual* diagnosis]
DESIRED OUTCOMES/EVALUATION CRITERIA—CLIENT COUPLE WILL:	Assume responsibility for health care needs.
	Identify factors contributing to condition/situation.
	Verbalize ability to cope adequately with the existing situation.

ACTIONS/INTERVENTIONS

RATIONALE

Independent

Assess level of dependence/independence and ability to make decisions to meet own needs.

May need more help to gain information necessary for problem resolution.

Determine needs (e.g., communication skills, knowledge of resources, motivation).

Initiate/participate in case finding/referral of individuals with real or potential genetic concerns.

Encourage participation in group activities, such as diagnosis-related support groups, March of Dimes, or Easter Seals.

Helps determine extent and type of interventions necessary.

Helps reduce the number of children born with genetic defects.

Can assist client/family in dealing with own situation.

First Trimester

NURSING PRIORITIES

1. Encourage client to adopt health-promoting behaviors.
2. Detect actual or potential risk factors.
3. Prevent/treat complications.
4. Foster client's/couple's positive adaptation to pregnancy.

NURSING DIAGNOSIS:	Nutrition: altered, risk for less than body requirements
Risk Factors May Include:	Changes in appetite, presence of nausea/vomiting, insufficient finances, unfamiliarity with increasing metabolic/nutritional needs
Possibly Evidenced By:	[Not applicable; presence of signs/symptoms establishes an *actual* diagnosis]
DESIRED OUTCOMES/EVALUATION CRITERIA—CLIENT WILL:	Explain the components of a well-balanced prenatal diet, giving food sources of vitamins, minerals, protein, and iron.
	Follow recommended diet.
	Take iron/vitamin supplement as prescribed.
	Demonstrate individually appropriate weight gain (usually a minimum of 3 lb by the end of the first trimester).

ACTIONS/INTERVENTIONS	RATIONALE

Independent

Determine adequacy of past/present nutritional habits using 24-hr recall. Note condition of hair, nails, and skin.	Fetal/maternal well-being depends on maternal nutrition during pregnancy as well as during the 2 yr preceding pregnancy.
Obtain health history; note age (especially less than 17 yr, more than 35 yr).	Adolescents may be prone to malnutrition, eating disorders, anemia; and older clients may be prone to obesity/gestational diabetes. (Refer to CPs: The Pregnant Adolescent; Diabetes Mellitus: Prepregnancy/Gestational.)
Ascertain knowledge level of dietary needs.	Determines specific learning needs. In the prenatal period, the basal metabolic rate (BMR) increases by 20%–25% (especially in late pregnancy), owing to increased thyroid activity associated with the growth of fetal and maternal tissues, creating a potential risk for the client with poor nutrition. An additional 800 mg of iron is necessary during pregnancy for developing maternal/fetal tissue and fetal storage. During the first trimester, the demand for iron is minimal, and a balanced diet meeting increased caloric needs is usually adequate. (Note: Iron preparations are not commonly prescribed in the first trimester because they may potentiate nausea.) Folic acid is crucial to fetal

51

Provide appropriate oral/written information about prenatal diet, food choices, and daily vitamin/iron supplements.

development requiring daily supplement of 0.4 mg of folate to prevent maternal deficiencies.

Reference material can be reviewed at home, increasing the likelihood that the client will select a well-balanced diet.

Review food preparation techniques to preserve nutrients and reduce risk of exposure to contaminants.

Cooking vegetables in large volume of water may cause vitamins to be lost. Microwaving food destroys more folic acid than conventional cooking. Inadequate cooking of meats/eggs increases risk of bacterial/parasitic infection.

Evaluate motivation/attitude by listening to client's comments and asking for feedback about information given.

If client is not motivated to improve diet, further evaluation or other interventions may be indicated.

Elicit beliefs regarding culturally proscribed diet and taboos during pregnancy. Provide alternative choices to meet dietary needs.

May affect motivation to follow recommendations of healthcare provider. For example, some cultures refuse iron, believing that it hardens maternal bones and makes delivery difficult.

Note presence of pica (craving for nonfood substances). Assess choices of substances and degree of motivation for eating them.

The ingestion of nonfood substances in pregnancy may be based on a psychological need, cultural phenomenon, response to hunger, and/or a bodily response to the need for nutrients (e.g., chewing on ice may indicate anemia). Note: Ingestion of laundry starch may potentiate iron deficiency anemia, and ingestion of clay may lead to fecal impaction.

Weigh client; ascertain usual pregravid weight. Provide information about optimal prenatal gain.

Inadequate prenatal weight gain and/or below normal prepregnancy weight increases the risk of intrauterine growth retardation (IUGR)/restriction in the fetus and delivery of low-birth-weight (LBW) infant. Research studies have found a positive correlation between pregravid maternal obesity and increased perinatal morbidity rates (e.g., hypertension and gestational diabetes) associated with preterm births and macrosomia.

Review frequency and severity of nausea/vomiting. Rule out pernicious vomiting (hyperemesis gravidarum). (Refer to CP: The High-Risk Pregnancy; ND: Nutrition: altered, risk for less than body requirements.)

First-trimester nausea/vomiting can have a negative impact on prenatal nutritional status, especially at critical periods in fetal development.

Test urine for acetone, albumin, and glucose.

Establishes baseline, is performed routinely to detect potential high-risk situations such as inadequate carbohydrate ingestion, diabetic ketoacidosis, and pregnancy-induced hypertension (PIH).

Measure uterine growth.

Maternal malnutrition may negatively affect fetal growth and contribute to reduced complement of brain cells in the fetus, which results in developmental lags in infancy and possibly beyond.

Collaborative

Obtain baseline Hb/Hct levels.

Identifies presence of anemia and potential for reduced maternal oxygen-carrying capacity. Clients with Hb levels less than 12 g/dL or Hct levels less than or equal to 37% are considered anemic in the first trimester.

Make necessary referrals as indicated (e.g., dietitian, social services).

May need additional assistance with nutritional choices; may have budget/financial constraints.

Refer to Women, Infants, Children (WIC) food program as appropriate.

Supplemental federally funded food program helps promote optimal maternal/fetal nutrition.

NURSING DIAGNOSIS:	[Discomfort]
May Be Related To:	Physical changes and hormonal influences
Possibly Evidenced By:	Verbalizations, restlessness, alteration in muscle tone
DESIRED OUTCOMES/EVALUATION CRITERIA—CLIENT WILL:	Identify measures that provide relief.
	Assume responsibility for alleviation of discomfort.
	Report absence/successful management of discomfort.

ACTIONS/INTERVENTIONS

RATIONALE

Independent

Note presence/degree of minor discomfort.

Provides information for selection of interventions; is clue to client's response to discomfort and pain.

Evaluate degree of discomfort during internal examination. Use extreme gentleness and pictures or models, especially for the client with infibulation, female circumcision, or adolescents, those with history of sexual abuse.

Discomfort during internal examination may occur, especially in the foreign client who has had a female circumcision or infibulation (whereby, after removal of the clitoris, labia minora, and medial aspect of the labia majora, the raw areas are drawn over the vagina to heal closed). Although many foreign women are intimidated by the American healthcare system and male physicians, it is important to anticipate the discomfort experienced by these clients because they may not ask questions or express discomfort/pain, especially when the husband is present at the procedure. Adolescents may be self-conscious during an examination, which may further increase discomfort. In addition, women with a history of childhood or adult sexual abuse may experience a variety of physical and emotional discomforts with vaginal examination.

Recommend wearing of supportive bra. Review nipple care (e.g., expose to air for 20 min daily; avoid soaps).

Provides proper support for enlarging breast tissues; toughens areolar tissue.

Stress importance of avoiding excessive nipple manipulation.

Stimulation may contribute to preterm labor through the release of oxytocin.

Recommend wearing of hard plastic cup (e.g., Woolrich breast shields) in bra for flat/inverted nipples.

Use of specially designed breast shields helps to break adhesions and cause flat/inverted nipple to evert and to become more erect.

Assess for hemorrhoids: note reports of itching, swelling, bleeding.

Reduced gastrointestinal (GI) motility and displacement of bowel and pressure on vasculature by enlarging uterus can predispose client to the development of hemorrhoids.

Instruct in use of ice packs, heat, or topical anesthetics; teach how to reinsert hemorrhoid with lubricated finger; encourage diet high in fiber, fruits/vegetables, noncaffeinated fluids; suggest

Reduces discomfort and swelling; promotes GI motility.

53

periodically elevating buttocks on pillow. (Refer to ND: Constipation.)

ACTIONS/INTERVENTIONS	RATIONALE
Instruct client to dorsiflex foot with leg extended and to reduce amount of cheese, yogurt, and milk ingested if leg cramps develop.	Increases blood supply to the leg. Excess intake of dairy products results in greater levels of phosphorus than calcium, creating an imbalance that may result in muscle cramping.
Encourage frequent bathing and perineal care, use of cotton underwear, and a dusting of cornstarch to absorb discharge (leukorrhea). Tell client to avoid the use of talcum powder.	Promotes hygiene by removing/absorbing excess vaginal secretions. Application of talcum powder in the genital area is believed to contribute to development of cervical cancers.
Recommend increasing carbohydrate intake on arising (e.g., eating dry toast), eating small and frequent meals, and avoiding strong odors if nausea/vomiting is a recurrent problem. (Refer to ND: Fluid Volume, risk for deficit.)	Reduces likelihood of gastric disturbances that may be caused by the effects of hydrochloric acid on the empty stomach or by increased sensitivity/aversion to odors, spices, or certain foods.
Suggest humidification of air and avoidance of nasal sprays and decongestants to treat nasal congestion.	Increased estrogen levels contribute to nasal congestion. Although humidification of air may be of limited benefit, sprays/decongestants absorbed systemically can be harmful to the fetus.
Review physiological changes resulting in urinary frequency. Recommend avoidance of caffeinated beverages.	Although normal, urinary frequency caused by pressure of the enlarging uterus on the bladder can be a cause of irritation. Caffeine has diuretic properties that can further aggravate the problem of frequency.
Assess fatigue level and nature of family/work commitments. (Refer to NDs: Fatigue and Family Coping: potential for growth.)	Encourages client to set priorities and include time for rest.

Collaborative

Substitute daily calcium supplements if intake of dairy products is reduced.	Assists in restoring calcium/phosphorus balance and reducing muscle cramping.

NURSING DIAGNOSIS:	Fluid Volume risk for deficit
Risk Factors May Include:	Impaired intake and/or excessive losses (vomiting), increased fluid needs
Possibly Evidenced By:	[Not applicable; presence of signs/symptoms establishes an *actual* diagnosis]
DESIRED OUTCOMES/EVALUATION CRITERIA—CLIENT WILL:	Identify and practice measures to reduce frequency and severity of episodes of nausea/vomiting.
	Ingest individually appropriate amounts of fluid daily.
	Identify signs and symptoms of dehydration necessitating treatment.

ACTIONS/INTERVENTIONS	RATIONALE

Independent

Auscultate FHT.	Presence of a fetal heart tones confirms presence of a fetus and rules out gestational trophoblastic disease (hydatidiform mole).

Determine frequency/severity of nausea/vomiting.

Provides data regarding extent of condition. Increased levels of HCG, changes in carbohydrate metabolism, and reduced gastric motility contribute to first-trimester nausea and vomiting.

Review history for other possible medical problems (e.g., peptic ulcer, gastritis, cholecystitis).

Assists in ruling out other causes and in identifying interventions to address specific problems.

Recommend that client maintain diary of intake/output, urine testing, and weight loss. (Refer to CP: The High-Risk Pregnancy; ND: Nutrition: altered, risk for less than body requirements.)

Helpful in determining presence of pernicious vomiting (hyperemisis gravidarum). Initially, vomiting may result in alkalosis, dehydration, and electrolyte imbalance. Untreated or severe vomiting may lead to acidosis, necessitating further intervention.

Assess skin temperature and turgor, mucous membranes, blood pressure (BP), temperature, intake/output, and urine specific gravity. Obtain client weight and compare with pregravid weight.

Indicators assisting in evaluation of hydration level/needs.

Encourage increased intake of noncaffeinated carbonated beverages, six small meals per day, and foods high in carbohydrates (e.g., plain popcorn, dry toast before arising).

Helpful in minimizing nausea/vomiting by reducing gastric acidity.

NURSING DIAGNOSIS:	Knowledge deficit [Learning Need] regarding natural progression of pregnancy, self care needs
May Be Related To:	Lack of understanding of normal physiological/psychological changes and their impact on the client/family
Possibly Evidenced By:	Request for information, statement of misconceptions
DESIRED OUTCOMES/EVALUATION CRITERIA—CLIENT WILL:	Explain normal physiological/psychological changes associated with the first trimester. Display self-care behaviors that promote wellness. Identify danger signs of pregnancy.

ACTIONS/INTERVENTIONS

RATIONALE

Independent

Establish an ongoing and supportive nurse-client relationship.

The role of teacher/counselor can provide anticipatory guidance and promote individual responsibility for wellness.

Evaluate current knowledge and cultural beliefs regarding normal physical/psychological changes of pregnancy, as well as beliefs about activities, self-care, and so forth.

Provides information to assist in identifying needs and creating a plan of care.

Clarify misconceptions.

Fears usually arise out of misinformation and may interfere with further learning.

Determine degree of motivation for learning.

Client may have difficulty learning unless the need for it is clear.

55

Identify who provides support/instruction within the client's culture (e.g., grandmother/other family member, cuerandero/Doula, other healer). Work with support person(s) when possible, using interpreter as needed.

Helps ensure quality/continuity of care because support person(s) may be more successful than the healthcare provider in communicating information.

Maintain open attitude toward beliefs of client/couple.

Acceptance is important to developing and maintaining relationship, supporting independence.

Determine attitude of client toward care given by male provider versus Certified Nurse-Midwife (CNM) or female practitioner.

Some cultures view the medical doctor as someone seen for illness and use midwives/cueranderos for healthy state of childbirth. Modesty or cultural demands may prohibit care by males and/or may require that husband remain in room when care is being given.

Explain office visit routine and rationale for interventions (e.g., urine testing, BP monitoring, weight). Reinforce importance of keeping regular appointments.

Reinforces relationship between health assessment and positive outcome for mother/baby. Different cultures put emphasis on different phases of pregnancy (e.g., prenatal, delivery, or postnatal), and the client's cultural group may not consider prenatal visits as important.

Provide anticipatory guidance, including discussion of nutrition, exercise, comfort measures, rest, employment, breast care, sexual activity, and health habits/lifestyle.

Information encourages acceptance of responsibility and promotes willingness to assume self-care.

Review need for prenatal vitamins, ferrous sulfate, and folic acid.

Helps maintain normal Hb levels. Folic acid deficiency contributes to megablastic anemia, possible abruptio placentae, abortion, and fetal malformation. Research indicates that iron supplements may not be necessary until the second and third trimester, when fetal demand is great. Note: Because of the possibility of overload, iron may be contraindicated in the presence of sickle cell anemia; however, client may require increased folic acid during and after sickle cell crisis.

Using pictures, discuss fetal development.

Visualization enhances reality of child and strengthens learning process.

Elicit/answer questions about infant care and feeding.

Provides information that can be useful for making choices.

Identify danger signals of pregnancy, such as bleeding, cramping, acute abdominal pain, backache, edema, visual disturbance, headaches, and pelvic pressure.

Helps client to distinguish normal from abnormal findings, thus assisting her in seeking timely, appropriate healthcare. (Adverse signs and symptoms may be viewed as "normal" occurrences in pregnancy, and assistance may not be sought.)

Identify agents harmful to the fetus. Assess client's use of drugs (nicotine, alcohol, cocaine, marijuana, and so forth). Stress the need to avoid all medications until the healthcare provider is consulted.

The fetus is most vulnerable in the first 3–8 wk, which is the period of organogenesis.

Refer client/couple to childbirth preparation class. Provide a list of suggested readings.

Knowledge gained helps reduce fear of unknown and increases confidence that couple can manage their preparation for the birth of their child.

NURSING DIAGNOSIS:	**Injury, risk for fetal**
Risk Factors May Include:	Maternal malnutrition, exposure to teratogens/infectious agents, presence of genetic disorders

Possibly Evidenced By:	[Not applicable; presence of signs/symptoms establishes an *actual* diagnosis]
DESIRED OUTCOMES/EVALUATION CRITERIA—CLIENT WILL:	Initiate behaviors that promote health for self and fetus.
	Refrain from self-medication without first contacting the obstetric health practitioner.
	Abstain from smoking and use of alcohol or illicit drugs.

ACTIONS/INTERVENTIONS	RATIONALE

Independent

Discuss importance of maternal well-being.	Fetal well-being is directly related to maternal well-being, especially during the first trimester, when developing organ systems are most vulnerable to injury from environmental/hereditary factors.
Discuss normal activity level and exercise practices. Encourage client to engage in moderate, non–weight-bearing exercise (e.g., swimming, bicycling).	Blood flow to the uterus can decrease by 70% with strenuous exercises, producing transient bradycardia, possible fetal hyperthermia, and IUGR. Yet nonendurance antepartal exercise regimens tend to shorten labor, increase likelihood of a spontaneous vaginal delivery, and decrease need for oxytocin augmentation.
Encourage client to engage in safer sex practices, proper use of condoms. (Refer to CP: Prenatal Infection.)	Failure to use condoms during intercourse may increase risk of transmission of STDs, especially HIV, if client does not know sexual history or contacts of partner.
Review dietary habits and cultural practices. Weigh client. Discuss normal weight gain curve for each trimester.	Malnutrition in the mother is associated with IUGR in fetus and low-birth-weight infants. Pregravid maternal obesity has been linked to preterm births.
Note protein intake. Monitor Hb and Hct. (Refer to ND: Nutrition: altered, risk for less than body requirements.)	Protein intake is essential to development of fetal brain tissue; Hb is essential for oxygen transport.
Review obstetric/medical history for high-risk factors (e.g., lifestyle, abusive relationship, altitude, culture, emotional stressors, use of medications, potential teratogens such as alcohol or nicotine or environmental toxins, or exposure to STDs, including HIV and other viruses).	Identifies physical and psychological risk factors and need for additional evaluation and/or intervention.
Assess for possible high-risk situation associated with genetic disorders (e.g., advanced maternal age for Down syndrome, Jewish background for Tay-Sachs disease). Discuss options, including CVS in first trimester or amniocentesis in second trimester. (Refer to CP: Genetic Counseling.)	Clients at risk for certain genetic disorders may desire testing to determine whether fetus is affected.
Provide information about potential teratogens, such as x-rays, alcohol, nicotine, live attenuated viruses, STORCH group of viruses (syphilis, toxoplasmosis, other, rubella, cytomegalovirus, herpes simplex), and HIV.	Helps client make decisions/choices about behaviors/environment that can promote healthy offspring.
Discuss mode of transmission of certain infections. Stress need to wash hands after animal contact.	In the United States, *Toxoplasma gondii* is most frequently transmitted in cat feces; other cultures

57

Advise against changing cat's litter box or eating improperly cooked meat. Recommend wearing gloves while gardening. Determine history of *Listeria monocytogenes* infection. (Refer to CP: Prenatal Infection.)

may acquire it through ingestion of raw or improperly cooked meat. Therapeutic abortion may be considered if disease is diagnosed before 20 weeks' gestation. *Listeria monocytogenes* is thought to be transmitted via animal contact. Vaginal culture should be obtained from client with fever of nonspecific origin or with history of *Listeria* infection.

Provide information about avoiding contact with persons known to have rubella infection if client is not immune, and about the need to be immunized following delivery. (Refer to CP: Prenatal Infection.)

Approximately 5%–15% of women of childbearing age are still susceptible to rubella, which is spread by droplet infection. Exposure may have negative effects on fetal development, especially in first trimester. Immunization after delivery results in immunity during subsequent pregnancies.

Encourage cessation of tobacco usage.

Smoking negatively affects placental circulation. Low Apgar scores at birth (below 7 at 5 min) are associated with smoking, along with lower-birth-weight and premature delivery. Even smoking fewer than 10 cigarettes per day carries an increased risk of fetal death, damage in utero, abruptio placentae, and placenta previa.

Collaborative

Perform internal examination, and assess uterine growth.

Provides information about gestation of fetus; screens for IUGR; identifies multiple pregnancies.

Obtain vaginal/rectal culture to rule out beta streptococcus, STDs, and *Listeria*; serum should be obtained for HIV testing.

Appropriate treatment may be instituted based on culture report.

Do serological testing.

Positive diagnosis of conditions such as toxoplasmosis can be made.

Treat client appropriately when herpes culture is positive; i.e., for active infection, medication such as acyclovir may be ordered; if inactive, information for self-care is provided.

In cases of herpes simplex virus type II, the client should be free of lesions at the time of labor or rupture of membranes. In the presence of visible lesions, a cesarean birth is indicated.

Evaluate rubella titer for immunity (0.1:10). Note need for postpartum immunization.

Screening for susceptibility allows client to take appropriate precautions, thereby reducing likelihood of prenatal exposure.

Refer to appropriate resources if substance abuse exists. (Refer to CP: Prenatal Substance Dependence/Abuse.)

More help may be needed to deal with resolution of problem and ensure well-being of pregnancy and fetus.

Refer to CVS/other testing as indicated if client is over age 35 or is at risk for a specific genetic disorder. (Refer to CP: Genetic Counseling.)

CVS can detect abnormalities or genetic defects between 9 and 12 weeks' gestation. CVS is an earlier alternative to amniocentesis, which cannot be performed until 14–16 weeks' gestation. Triple screen ($MSAFP_3$), a maternal blood test, can be done at about 16–22 wk to measure AFP, unconjugated estriol, and HCG, to detect problems, such as open spine or ventral wall defects, Down syndrome, and trisomy 18.

Refer to genetic counseling if appropriate.

Additional information may be necessary.

Prepare for/discuss transvaginal sonography.

Can be carried out as early as $4^1/_2$ weeks' gestation as a diagnostic tool for suspected fetal abnormalities or for prompt detection of tubal gestation.

Discuss possible treatment options, such as abortion.

Therapeutic abortion may be considered if disease is diagnosed before 20 weeks' gestation.

NURSING DIAGNOSIS:	Fatigue, risk for
Risk Factors May Include:	Increased carbohydrate metabolism, altered body chemistry, increased energy requirements to perform activities of daily living
Possibly Evidenced By:	[Not applicable; presence of signs/symptoms establishes an *actual* diagnosis]
DESIRED OUTCOMES/EVALUATION CRITERIA—CLIENT WILL:	Identify basis of fatigue and individual areas of control.
	Modify lifestyle to meet changing needs/energy level.
	Report improved sense of energy.

ACTIONS/INTERVENTIONS	RATIONALE

Independent

Determine normal sleep-wake cycle and commitments to work, family, community, and self.	Helps in setting realistic priorities and examining time commitments. Client may need to make adjustments, such as changing work shift to accommodate early-morning nausea (changing to a later morning shift) or provide more rest (changing from night shift to day shift), shifting of household chores/responsibilities, prioritizing and curtailing some outside commitments, and so forth.
Encourage regular exercise in moderation, avoidance of foods/fluids containing caffeine; drinking warm milk/eating a light snack at bedtime, keeping crackers at bedside.	Enhances ability to fall asleep and obtain adequate rest. Fluctuating hormone levels (cortisol, progesterone, estrogen) may limit restful sleep. L-Tryptophan in milk seems to have a sedative effect. A bedtime snack may prevent awakening because of hunger, and crackers may help reduce feelings of nausea on awakening.
Suggest client limit fluid intake 1 or 2 hr before bedtime.	May decrease frequency of nighttime voiding.
Encourage a 1- to 2-hr nap each day, 8 hr of sleep each night in a dark/cool room.	Provides rest to meet metabolic needs associated with growth of maternal/fetal tissues.
Monitor Hb level. Explain role of iron in the body; encourage daily iron supplement to be taken between meals, as indicated.	Low Hb levels result in greater fatigue due to decreased oxygen-carrying capacity. Note: Iron may need to be restricted in the presence of sickle cell anemia.
Recommend use of comfortable bra/jogging top.	Provides support for tender breasts during sleep.

NURSING DIAGNOSIS:	Constipation, risk for
Risk Factors May Include:	Smooth muscle relaxation, increased absorption of water from GI tract, presence of hemorrhoids, ingestion of iron supplements
Possibly Evidenced By:	[Not applicable; presence of signs/symptoms establishes in *actual* diagnosis]
DESIRED OUTCOMES/EVALUATION CRITERIA—CLIENT WILL:	Maintain normal pattern of bowel function.
	Identify individual contributing factors/risk behaviors.
	Report adoption of individually appropriate behaviors to promote elimination.

ACTIONS/INTERVENTIONS	RATIONALE

Independent

Determine pregravid elimination habits, noting alteration with pregnancy.	Usual elimination patterns need to be maintained, when possible. Increasing progesterone level relaxes smooth muscle within the GI tract, resulting in reduced peristalsis and increased reabsorption of water and electrolytes. Iron supplements also contribute to problems of constipation.
Assess for hemorrhoids. (Refer to ND: [Discomfort].)	Varicosities of the rectum frequently develop as a result of prolonged constipation, increased efforts at bearing down, or increased circulating volume and hormonal relaxation of blood vessels. The presence of hemorrhoids can cause pain with defecation, resulting in reluctance of the client to evacuate her bowels.
Provide dietary information about fresh fruits, vegetables, grains, fiber, roughage, and adequate fluid intake (preferably decaffeinated).	Adequate bulk and consistency in diet choices help promote effective bowel pattern.
Encourage regular, nonstrenuous exercise program, such as walking. Tell client to avoid strenuous, prolonged exercise. Note cultural beliefs about exercise.	Promotes peristalsis and assists in prevention of constipation. Strenuous exercise is thought to reduce uteroplacental circulation, possibly resulting in fetal bradycardia, hyperthermia, or growth restriction/retardation. In some cultures, inactivity may be viewed as a protection for mother/child.

Collaborative

Discuss cautious use of stool softener or bulk-producing agent if diet/exercise is not effective.	May be necessary to assist in combatting persistent constipation and establishing a regular routine.

NURSING DIAGNOSIS:	**Infection, risk for urinary tract infection (UTI)**
Risk Factors May Include:	Urinary stasis, poor hygienic practices, insufficient knowledge to avoid exposure to pathogens
Possibly Evidenced By:	[Not applicable; presence of signs/symptoms establishes an *actual* diagnosis]
DESIRED OUTCOMES/EVALUATION CRITERIA—CLIENT WILL:	Identify behaviors to reduce urinary stasis/risk of infection.
	List signs and symptoms requiring evaluation/interventions.
	Be free of *signs* and symptoms of infection.

ACTIONS/INTERVENTIONS	RATIONALE

Independent

Provide information about signs/symptoms of UTI. Stress need to report signs of infection to healthcare provider and to avoid self-medication until after such notification.	Maternal UTIs respond well to treatment and may not be serious; however, they are associated with preterm labor/birth.

Stress need for frequent/thorough hand washing before meals and food handling, and after toileting.

Provide information about other hygiene measures, including wiping vulva from front to back after urinating and voiding after intercourse.

Recommend that client drink 6–8 glasses of noncaffeinated liquid daily. Discuss role of acid residue in diet and addition of cranberry/orange juice.

Encourage practice of Kegel exercise (tightening of the perineum) throughout the day.

Suggest use of cotton underwear and showers instead of tub baths if client has a history of UTI.

Collaborative

Obtain routine urine sample for microscopic examination, pH, presence of white blood cells, and culture and sensitivity, as indicated. Report colony counts of greater than 100,000/ml.

Administer antibiotics (e.g., ampicillin, erythromycin) as appropriate.

Many viruses, such as cytomegalovirus (CMV), can be excreted in the urine for up to 4 yr after exposure and can possibly be transmitted through poor hygienic practices.

Helps prevent rectal *Escherichia coli* contaminants from reaching the vagina. May help to prevent transmission of STDs, especially CMV and nongonococcal urethritis.

Helps prevent stasis in the urinary tract; may acidify urine and help prevent UTI.

Improves support to the pelvic organs, strengthening and increasing elasticity of the pubococcygeus muscle; provides more control over urination.

Urinary stasis and glycosuria can predispose the prenatal client to UTI, especially if history includes urinary/kidney problems. Contributory factors, such as wearing manmade fabrics and sitting in bath water, can add to potential for exposure to infection.

Alkaline urine predisposes client to a possible *Proteus vulgaris* infection. As many as 2%–10% of pregnant women have asymptomatic bacteriuria (colony count greater than 100,000/ml), which increases risk of premature rupture of membranes, preterm labor, and chorioamnionitis.

Treats infection as indicated. Care must be taken in prescribing antibiotics prenatally, owing to potentially negative effects on the fetus.

NURSING DIAGNOSIS:	Cardiac Output [maximally compensated]
May Be Related To:	Increased fluid volume (preload), ventricular hypertrophy, changes in peripheral resistance (afterload)
Possibly Evidenced By:	Variations in blood pressure and pulse, syncopal episodes, presence of pathological edema
DESIRED OUTCOMES/EVALUATION CRITERIA—CLIENT WILL:	Differentiate normal and abnormal changes. Remain normotensive. Be free of pathological edema. Display no more than 1+ albumin in urinalysis.

ACTIONS/INTERVENTIONS

RATIONALE

Independent

Review physiological process and normal or abnormal changes and signs/symptoms.

Prenatally, circulating blood volume in the form of plasma and red blood cells increases 30%–50% to

61

	meet maternal/fetal nutritional and oxygen needs and to act as a safeguard against blood loss during delivery. The body compensates for the increase in fluid volume by increasing cardiac output through ventricular hypertrophy. Hormonal effects of progesterone and relaxin reduce resistance to cardiac output by relaxing smooth muscle within the blood vessel walls. Although this is a normal process, the client is maximally compensated and could be at risk for hypertension and/or circulatory failure as the pregnancy progresses. Prompt recognition and intervention reduce risk of adverse outcome.
Obtain baseline BP and pulse measurement. Report systolic increase of greater than 30 mm Hg or diastolic increase greater than 15 mm Hg. (Refer to CP: Pregnancy-Induced Hypertension, as appropriate.)	An increase in BP may indicate PIH. Pulse increase above 10–15 bpm may indicate cardiac stress.
Auscultate heart sounds; note any murmurs. Review contributory history of cardiac problems or rheumatic fever.	Cardiac ventricles undergo slight hypertrophy to compensate for increase in circulating volume and to maximize output. Systolic murmur may be created by decreased blood viscosity, displacement of the heart, or torsion of great vessels.
Assess for location/degree of edema. Distinguish between physiological and potentially harmful edema. (Refer to CP: Pregnancy-Induced Hypertension, ND: Fluid Volume risk for deficit).	Dependent edema of the lower extremities (physiological edema) often occurs, owing to venous stasis caused by uterine pressure and hormonal effects of progesterone and relaxin, which relax blood vessel walls. Edema of facies and/or upper extremities may indicate PIH.
Assess for varicosities of legs, vulva, rectum.	Increased fluid load and hormonal relaxation of blood vessel walls potentiates risk for vascular engorgement and venous stasis, especially in client whose lifestyle requires prolonged sitting/standing.
Discuss the need to avoid rapid position changes from sitting or lying to standing.	Client may be prone to postural hypotension caused by reduced venous return.

Collaborative

Monitor Hb and Hct levels.	Low Hb may indicate anemia, which can increase heart rate and cardiac workload; elevated Hct may indicate dehydration with PIH fluid shifts.
Test urine for albumin as indicated.	Proteinuria with elevation of albumin above 1+ suggests glomerular edema or spasm (developing PIH), requiring prompt intervention.

NURSING DIAGNOSIS:	**Body Image, risk for disturbance**
Risk Factors May Include:	Perception of biophysical changes; psychosocial, cultural, and spiritual beliefs
Possibly Evidenced By:	[Not applicable; presence of signs/symptoms establishes an *actual* diagnosis]
DESIRED OUTCOMES/EVALUATION CRITERIA—CLIENT WILL:	Verbalize understanding/acceptance of body changes.
	Verbalize acceptance of self in situation.
	Demonstrate a positive self-image by maintaining an overall satisfactory appearance.

ACTIONS/INTERVENTIONS	RATIONALE

Independent

Determine attitude toward pregnancy, changing body image, and job situation, and how these issues are viewed by significant other(s).

Identify basic sense of client's self-esteem in relation to the changes of pregnancy and responsibilities related to this new role.

Assess support systems such as aunt, grandmother, cultural healer, and so on.

Review physiological changes of pregnancy; assure client that mixed feelings are normal. Provide environment in which couple can discuss feelings.

Collaborative

Refer to other resources as indicated (e.g., counseling/therapy).

The client's feelings toward the pregnancy affect her ability to develop positive feelings about her changing body contours, as well as her ability to adapt positively to her parenting roles.

Because of a changing body shape, alterations in body image occur normally in pregnancy and may create a crisis situation that negatively affects both the pregnancy and parenting abilities in clients with poor self-esteem and a weak ego identity.

Adequate support can help client to cope positively with her changing body shape and maintain positive self-esteem.

Helps decrease stress associated with pregnancy. Verbalizing helps sort out feelings, attitudes, and past experiences.

Client may require more intensive intervention to facilitate acceptance of self/pregnancy.

NURSING DIAGNOSIS:	Role Performance, risk for altered
Risk Factors May Include:	Maturational crisis, developmental level (immaturity on the part of the client and/or significant other), history of maladaptive coping, absence of support systems
Possibly Evidenced By:	[Not applicable; presence of signs/symptoms establishes an *actual* diagnosis]
DESIRED OUTCOMES/EVALUATION CRITERIA—CLIENT WILL:	Identify perceived stressors. Verbalize realistic perception and acceptance of self in changing role. Talk with family/significant other about situation and changes that have occurred or may occur. Develop realistic plans for adapting to new role/role changes.

ACTIONS/INTERVENTIONS	RATIONALE

Independent

Evaluate the client's/couple's response to pregnancy, individual and family stressors, and cultural implications of pregnancy/childbirth.

Identifies needs to assist in planning interventions. The client's/couple's ability to adapt positively to this "crisis" depends on support systems, cultural beliefs, resources, and effective coping mechanisms developed in dealing with past stressors. Initially, even if the pregnancy is planned, the expectant mother

ACTIONS/INTERVENTIONS	RATIONALE
	may feel ambivalent toward the pregnancy because of personal/professional goals, financial concerns, and possible role changes that a child will necessitate.
Ascertain from client/couple how stressors have been dealt with in the past.	Provides information regarding client's/couple's ability to deal positively with stress. Learned coping methods, either positive or negative, tend to be used in subsequent crises.
Assess economic situation and financial needs. Make necessary referrals.	Impact of pregnancy on family without adequate resources can create added stress. Members of some cultures may view healthcare as unaffordable and, as a result, may seek abortion or may not seek prenatal care.
Elicit information about preparations or lack of preparations being made for this infant.	May have fears that visible preparations may result in child's death or that planning ahead has the potential of "defying God's will."
Explain emotional lability as characteristic of pregnancy. Discuss normalcy of ambivalence.	Helps client/couple understand mood swings. Partner realizes the need to offer support/affection at these times.
Provide information about, and encourage attendance at, childbirth classes.	Provides an opportunity for formal/informal sharing of problems, feelings, and peer support.
Assess for maladaptive behaviors (e.g., withdrawal, inappropriate anger/reactions, lack of or inappropriate self-care).	Provides information about client's ability to deal with stress and the need for intervention.

Collaborative

Refer for psychological counseling, as necessary.	Further assistance in developing problem-solving skills may be helpful. By the end of the first trimester, the client/couple should have successfully achieved the task of accepting the pregnancy.

NURSING DIAGNOSIS:	Family Coping: potential for growth
May Be Related To:	Client and family needs are sufficiently met; adaptive tasks are effectively addressed to enable goals of self-actualization to surface
Possibly Evidenced By:	Family member/individual makes realistic appraisal of growth impact of pregnancy on own values, priorities, goals, or relationships; moving in direction of health-promoting and enriching lifestyle; chooses experiences that optimize wellness
DESIRED OUTCOMES/EVALUATION CRITERIA—CLIENT/COUPLE WILL:	Explore anticipated role changes.
	Undertake appropriate tasks in preparation for the birth.
	Report feelings of self-confidence and satisfaction with progress being made.

ACTIONS/INTERVENTIONS	RATIONALE

Independent

Identify relationship of family members to one another. Note strengths/stressors (e.g.,	Pregnancy is a crisis situation for client/couple and family members, resulting in a disequilibrium

communication styles, interactions among members).

Determine roles/responsibilities within family unit and use of supportive resources. Identify anticipated adaptations necessitated by pregnancy.

Assess relationship of client/couple to own parents.

Determine availability/involvement of grandparents.

Evaluate sibling responses to pregnancy and upcoming change in family structure.

Provide information about father/sibling or grandparent attendance at childbirth classes and participation in delivery, as client desires.

Encourage father/siblings to attend prenatal office visits and listen to FHT.

Provide list of appropriate reading materials for client, couple, siblings regarding adjusting to newborn.

that necessitates adaptation to new roles and responsibilities.

Family members will need to be flexible in adjusting own roles/responsibilities in order to assist client to meet her needs related to the demands of pregnancy both expected and unplanned, such as prolonged nausea, fatigue, emotional lability.

May provide insight for assisting couple in assuming parenting role. New parents tend to use their own parents as role models and may thus adopt positive or negative parenting behaviors.

May be invaluable in providing support to client/couple although adjustment to role changes may require mutual support.

In the first trimester, young siblings may not be aware of the reality and long-term consequences of pregnancy. Older children may not manifest negative feelings outwardly, yet internally they may begin to fear a change in the security of their relationship with their parent(s). Family members may be concerned about anticipated changes and may express a desire to prepare themselves and siblings for role/life change(s).

Helps family members to realize they are an integral part of the pregnancy and delivery.

Promotes a sense of involvement; helps make baby a reality for family members.

Information helps individual realistically analyze changes in family structure, roles, and behaviors.

Collaborative

Provide information/referral about community resources if client/couple is having concerns about parenting abilities. (Refer to ND: Role Performance, risk for altered.)

Reducing stressors in the home allows the expectant couple to devote emotional energy to the pregnancy.

NURSING DIAGNOSIS:	**Sexuality Patterns, altered**
May Be Related To:	Knowledge/skill deficit about altered body function/structure, changes in comfort level
Possibly Evidenced By:	Reported difficulties, limitations, or changes in sexual response/activities
DESIRED OUTCOMES/EVALUATION CRITERIA—CLIENT/PARTNER WILL:	Share feelings related to changes in sexual desire.
	Take desired steps to remedy situation.
	Report satisfaction with/acceptance of changes or modifications required by pregnancy.

65

ACTIONS/INTERVENTIONS	RATIONALE

Independent

Determine the couple's usual pattern of sexual activity using a sexual assessment tool. Determine the impact of pregnancy on the pattern and the couple's response to the changes.

How the couple copes with changes in sexuality and sexual patterns during pregnancy may affect the relationship. Client/couple may be helped when they know that desire may be diminished because the woman is not feeling well owing to breast tenderness, fatigue, nausea, vomiting, and a changing body image. However, they should know it is all right to continue sexual activity/alternatives as the couple desires.

Review information about the normalcy of these changes; correct misconceptions.

Helps the couple understand the changes from a physiological viewpoint. Reduced libidinal urges in the first trimester are common for the prenatal client. This decreased desire may be difficult for the couple, and especially for the male partner, to understand.

Assess couple's relationship to one another and ability to cope with decrease in frequency of sexual intercourse.

The nature of the relationship before pregnancy affects how well the couple copes during pregnancy.

Note client's/couple's response to changing body shape. Create a teaching plan to discuss sexual changes for prenatal client in the second and third trimester. (Refer to ND: Body Image, risk for disturbance.)

Acceptance of sexuality issues is directly related to a positive self-concept and individual's sense of identity.

Review obstetric history with couple. Assess for vaginal bleeding/spotting.

Intercourse is not usually contraindicated in the first trimester unless the client has experienced complications such as bleeding during this pregnancy or in past pregnancies.

Collaborative

Refer the couple for counseling if sexual concerns are not resolved.

Professional counseling may be necessary to help couples to cope positively with sexuality issues in pregnancy.

Second Trimester

NURSING DIAGNOSIS:	Body Image, risk for disturbance
Risk Factors May Include:	Perception of biophysical changes, responses of others
Possibly Evidenced By:	[Not applicable; presence of signs/symptoms establishes an *actual* diagnosis]
DESIRED OUTCOMES/EVALUATION CRITERIA—CLIENT WILL:	Verbalize gradual acceptance/adaptation to changing self-concept/body image.
	Demonstrate a positive self-image by maintaining an overall satisfactory appearance; dress in appropriately fitting clothes and low-heeled shoes.

ACTIONS/INTERVENTIONS	RATIONALE

Independent

Review/assess attitude toward pregnancy, changing body shape, and so forth. (Refer to CP: First Trimester; ND: Body Image disturbance.)	In the second trimester, the changing body contours are readily visible. Negative responses to such changes may occur in the client/couple whose fragile self-concept is based on physical appearance. Other visible effects caused by prenatal hormones such as chloasma, striae gravidarum, telangiectasia (vascular spiders), palmar erythema, acne, and hirsutism can contribute to the client's emotional changes. These feelings may affect how she deals with the changes that are occurring.
Discuss physiological aspects of, and client's response to, changes. Provide information about normalcy of changes.	Individuals react differently to the changes that occur, and information can help the client understand/accept what is happening.
Suggest styles and available sources of maternity clothing.	Individual circumstances dictate needs for clothing that will enhance the client's appearance for work and leisure activities.
Discuss methods of skin care and makeup (to minimize/hide darkened areas of the skin), the use of support hose, maintenance of posture.	Learning about, and being involved in, ways to look and feel better may be helpful for maintaining positive feelings about the self.

Collaborative

Refer to other resources, such as classes in childbirth education and parenting or counseling.	May be helpful in providing additional support during this period of change; identifies appropriate role models.

NURSING DIAGNOSIS:	Breathing Pattern, ineffective
May Be Related To:	Impingement of the diaphragm by the enlarging uterus
Possibly Evidenced By:	Complaints of shortness of breath, dyspnea, changes in respiratory depth

67

DESIRED OUTCOMES/EVALUATION CRITERIA—CLIENT WILL:	Report decrease in frequency/severity of complaints. Demonstrate behaviors that optimize respiratory function.

ACTIONS/INTERVENTIONS	RATIONALE

Independent

Assess respiratory status (e.g., shortness of breath on exertion, fatigue).	Determines existence/severity of problem, which occurs in approximately 60% of prenatal clients. Even though vital capacity increases, respiratory function is modified as the diaphragm's ability to descend on inspiration is reduced by the enlarging uterus.
Obtain history of and monitor preexisting/developing medical problems (e.g., allergic rhinitis, asthma, sinus problems, tuberculosis). (Refer to CP: The High-Risk Pregnancy; ND: Injury, risk for fetal.)	Other problems may further alter breathing patterns and may compromise maternal/fetal tissue oxygenation.
Note Hb and Hct levels. Stress importance of daily prenatal vitamins/ferrous sulfate intake as appropriate.	Increased plasma levels at 24–32 weeks' gestation further dilute Hb levels, resulting in possible anemia and decreased oxygen-carrying capacity. Note: Iron may be contraindicated for client with sickle cell anemia.
Provide information about rationale for respiratory difficulties and realistic activity/exercise program. Encourage frequent rest periods, providing extra time for certain activities, and participation in mild exercise, such as walking.	Reduces the likelihood of respiratory symptoms caused by overexertion.
Review measures client can take to ease problems; e.g., good posture; avoiding smoking; eating smaller, more frequent meals; using modified semi-Fowler's position for sitting/sleeping if symptoms are severe.	Good posture and small meals help maximize diaphragmatic descent, increasing space available for lung expansion. Smoking reduces oxygen available for maternal-fetal exchange. Semiupright positioning may increase lung expansion as the gravid uterus descends.

NURSING DIAGNOSIS:	**Knowledge deficit [Learning Need], regarding natural progression of pregnancy**
May Be Related To:	Continued need for information as the changes of the second trimester are experienced
Possibly Evidenced By:	Request for information, statement of concerns or misconceptions
DESIRED OUTCOMES/EVALUATION CRITERIA—CLIENT WILL:	Verbalize/demonstrate self-care behaviors that promote wellness. Assume responsibility for her own healthcare. Recognize and act to minimize and prevent risk factors. Identify danger signs/seek medical care appropriately.

ACTIONS/INTERVENTIONS	RATIONALE
Independent	
Review changes to be expected during the second trimester.	Questions continue to arise as new changes occur, regardless of whether changes are expected or unexpected.
Institute/continue a learning program as outlined in CP: First Trimester; ND: Knowledge deficit [Learning Need].	Repetition reinforces learning, and if client has not been seen previously, information is useful at this point. Note: For various reasons (e.g., financial, cultural, denial of condition), many individuals do not seek care until the second or even third trimester.
Provide information about need for ferrous sulfate and folic acid.	Ferrous sulfate and folic acid help maintain normal Hb levels. Folic acid deficiency contributes to megaloblastic anemia, possible abruptio placentae, abortion, and fetal malformation. Note: Clients with sickle cell anemia require increased folic acid during and following crisis episode.
Encourage involvement in a moderate exercise program.	A nonendurance perinatal exercise regimen tends to shorten labor, increase the likelihood of a spontaneous vaginal delivery, and decrease the need for oxytocin augmentation. (Strenuous exercise may result in reduced uterine blood flow/fetal bradycardia.) Note: Exercise may be viewed as inappropriate in some cultures (e.g., Puerto Rican).
Identify possible individual health risks (e.g., spontaneous abortion, hypoxia related to asthma or tuberculosis, heart disease, PIH, kidney disorders, anemia, gestational diabetes mellitus [GDM], STDs). Review danger signs and appropriate actions.	Provides a helpful reminder/information for client about potential high-risk situation requiring closer monitoring and/or intervention. (Refer to CP: High-Risk Pregnancy, as appropriate).
Discuss any medications that may be needed to control or treat medical problem.	Helpful in choosing treatment options because need must be weighed against possible harmful effects on the fetus.
Discuss need for specific laboratory studies, screening, and close monitoring as indicated.	More frequent prenatal visits may be needed to promote maternal well-being. Monitoring Hb and Hct using electrophoresis detects specific anemias and is helpful in determining cause. Screening for GDM at 24–26 weeks' gestation or at 12, 18, and 32 weeks' gestation in high-risk client can detect developing hyperglycemia, which may need treatment with insulin and/or diet. (Refer to CPs: Diabetes Mellitus: Prepregnancy/Gestational; the High-Risk Pregnancy.)

NURSING DIAGNOSIS:	**Injury, risk for fetal**
Risk Factors May Include:	Maternal health problems, exposure to teratogens/infectious agents
Possibly Evidenced By:	[Not applicable; presence of signs/symptoms establishes an *actual* diagnosis]
DESIRED OUTCOMES/EVALUATION CRITERIA—CLIENT WILL:	Verbalize awareness of individual risk factors.
	Avoid factors and/or refrain from behaviors that may contribute to fetal injury.

ACTIONS/INTERVENTIONS	RATIONALE

Independent

Determine understanding of information previously provided. (Refer to CP: First Trimester; ND: Injury, risk for fetal.)

Identifies individual needs/concerns and provides opportunity to clarify misconceptions, especially for clients whose initial prenatal visit occurs at this time.

Review maternal health status; e.g., malnutrition, substance use/abuse. (Refer to CP: First Trimester; ND: Nutrition: altered, less than body requirements.)

These factors can have great impact on developing fetal tissues and organs, and early identification and intervention may prevent untoward results.

Assess for other factors existing in the individual situation that may be harmful to the fetus (e.g., exposure to viruses/other STDs, environmental factors). (Refer to CP: Prenatal Infection.)

Identification enables client and nurse to discuss ways to minimize/prevent injury. STDs or other viruses may be only mildly problematic for the client, but often have a great negative impact on fetal well-being.

Note quickening (maternal perception of fetal movements) and fetal heart tones (FHT). Refer to healthcare provider if problem is detected.

Perceivable fetal movements first occur between 16 and 20 weeks' gestation as fetal size increases; lack of movement may indicate an existing problem. Failure to detect FHT may indicate fetal demise or absence of fetus/presence of hydatidiform mole (gestational trophoblastic disease [GTD]).

Assess uterine growth and fundal height at each visit.

Screens for multiple gestation, normal or abnormal fetal growth; may detect problems related to polyhydramnios or oligohydramnios.

Provide information about diagnostic tests or procedure(s). Review risks and potential side effects.

Having information helps client/couple to deal with situation and make informed decisions. Certain genetic problems such as neural tube defects (NTDs) may be detected at this stage.

Collaborative

Assist with ultrasonographic procedure, and explain its purpose.

Detects presence of fetus as early as 5–6 weeks' gestation and provides information about fetal growth, to confirm gestational age and rule out intrauterine growth retardation/restriction. Also determines placental size and location and may detect some fetal abnormalities such as fetal heart defects when done between 18 and 20 weeks' gestation.

Obtain maternal serum sample for AFP level between 14 and 16 wk.

With an open NTD (most commonly, spina bifida and anencephaly), AFP, a protein produced by the yolk sac and fetal liver, is present in maternal serum at a level 8 times higher than normal at 15 weeks' gestation. Thereafter, it decreases until term.

Assist with amniocentesis when AFP level is abnormal, especially in high-risk population (e.g., clients with possible genetic disorders/previous child having a chromosomal abnormality, older gravidas over age 35 yr), if client has not already had CVS.

Analysis of amniotic fluid detects genetic/chromosomal disorders and NTD.

Follow with genetic counseling as appropriate. (Refer to CP: Genetic Counseling.)

Client/couple will need information to make informed decisions about course of action in this pregnancy as well as future pregnancies.

Screen client for GDM with glucose tolerance test (GTT) at 24–26 weeks' gestation, as indicated. (Refer to CP: Diabetes Mellitus; Prepregnancy/Gestational.)

GDM is associated with macrosomia and problems of dystocia.

NURSING DIAGNOSIS:	Cardiac Output, risk for [decompensation]
Risk Factors May Include:	Increased circulatory demand, changes in preload (decreased venous return) and afterload (increased peripheral vascular resistance), ventricular hypertrophy
Possibly Evidenced By:	[Not applicable; presence of signs/symptoms establishes an *actual* diagnosis]
DESIRED OUTCOMES/EVALUATION CRITERIA—CLIENT WILL:	Remain normotensive during the prenatal course.
	Be free of pathological edema and signs of PIH.
	Identify ways to control and reduce cardiovascular problems.

ACTIONS/INTERVENTIONS	RATIONALE

Independent

Review physiological process and normal and abnormal changes, signs, and symptoms. (Refer to CP: Cardiac Conditions.)	During the second trimester, hypertrophy of the cardiac ventricles ensures increased cardiac output, which peaks at 25–27 weeks' gestation to meet maternal/fetal oxygen and nutrient needs. Normally, the cardiovascular system compensates for increased cardiac output with dilation of blood vessels, which reduces resistance to cardiac output. This lowers the systolic pressure readings approximately 8 mm Hg while the diastolic pressure decrease averages 12 mm Hg. Increases in fluid, stress, and/or preexisting cardiac problems, however, can compromise the system.
Note history of preexisting or potential cardiac/kidney/diabetic problems.	These clients face the greatest risk for cardiac involvement during the second trimester, when cardiac output peaks.
Obtain BP and pulse measurement. Report systolic increase greater than 30 mm Hg and diastolic increase greater than 15 mm Hg above baseline.	An increase in BP may indicate PIH, especially in clients with preexisting cardiac or kidney disease, diabetes, or in the presence of multiple pregnancies or hydatidiform mole.
Auscultate heart sounds; note presence of murmurs.	Systolic murmurs are often benign and may be created by increased volume, decreased blood viscosity, displacement of the heart, or torsion of great vessels. However, a murmur may indicate developing failure.
Assess for presence of ankle edema and varicosities of legs, vulva, and rectum. Distinguish between physiological and potentially harmful edema. (Refer to CP: Pregnancy-Induced Hypertension; ND: Fluid Volume deficit [isotonic].)	Dependent edema of the lower extremities (physiologic edema) often occurs because of venous stasis caused by vasodilation from progesterone activity, heredity, excess fluid retention, and uterine pressure on pelvic blood vessels. This increases the risk of venous thrombus formation. Edema of facies and/or upper extremities may indicate PIH.
Encourage client to avoid crossing legs and sitting/standing for long periods, to put on support hose before arising in the morning, to wear loose, nonconstricting clothing, elevate legs when sitting;	Promotes venous return and reduces the risk of developing edema, varicosities, or venous thrombosis.

71

elevate legs, hips, and vulva vertical to the wall
three times a day for 20 min; and turn feet upward
in dorsiflexion if sitting or standing for long periods.

Dorsiflex foot to test for Homans' sign. If present, refer to healthcare provider.	A positive Homans' sign may indicate thrombophlebitis.
Assess for faintness. Encourage client to avoid changing position rapidly.	Sudden position changes may result in dizziness as blood pools in lower extremities, reducing circulating volume.

NURSING DIAGNOSIS:	**Fluid Volume risk for excess**
Risk Factors May Include:	Changes in regulatory mechanisms, sodium/water retention
Possibly Evidenced By:	[Not applicable; presence of signs/symptoms establishes an *actual* diagnosis]
DESIRED OUTCOMES/EVALUATION CRITERIA—CLIENT WILL:	List ways to minimize problem.
	Identify signs/symptoms requiring medical evaluation/intervention.
	Be free of hypertension, albuminuria, excessive fluid retention, and edema of facies.

ACTIONS/INTERVENTIONS	RATIONALE

Independent

Monitor weight regularly. Have client record weight between visits.	Detects excessive weight gain and invisible fluid retention, which may be potentially pathological. During the second trimester, total body water (plasma and red blood cells) increases by 1000 ml, owing in part to estrogen levels stimulating the adrenal gland to secrete aldosterone, thereby retaining sodium and water. Although up to 5 lb of fluid can be retained with no visible edema, this increase can contribute to cardiac decompensation. Note: Some cultures (e.g., West Indian) believe the more weight gained by the pregnant woman, the healthier the mother and infant will be.
Assess for signs of PIH, noting blood pressure, location/extent of edema, and fluid intake and output. Note reports of visual disturbances, headache, epigastric pain, or presence of hyperreflexia and clonus.	Indicators of pathological edema. Although PIH caused by excessive fluid retention is not usually seen until the last 10 wk of pregnancy, it may develop earlier, especially in the client with predisposing factors, such as diabetes, renal disease, hypertension, multiple gestation, malnutrition (overweight or underweight), or in presence of hydatidiform mole.
Test urine for albumin.	Detects vascular involvement associated with glomerular spasms of the kidney, which reduce resorption of albumin.
Provide information about diet (e.g., increased protein, no added table salt, avoidance of foods and beverages high in sodium).	Adequate nutrition, especially increased protein, reduces likelihood of PIH. Excess sodium may contribute to water retention (too little sodium may result in dehydration.)

Recommend elevating extremities periodically during the day.

Physiological edema of the lower extremities occurring at the end of the day is normal, but it should resolve with simple corrective measures. If it does not resolve, the healthcare provider should be notified.

Review Hct levels. Note effects of variables, such as altitude and race.

In general, Hct levels of 41% (for whites) or 38% (for people of African heritage) indicate intravascular fluid shifts resulting in tissue edema.

Collaborative

Schedule more frequent prenatal visits and institute treatment if PIH exists. (Refer to CP: Pregnancy-Induced Hypertension.)

Treatment helps promote positive maternal/fetal outcomes.

NURSING DIAGNOSIS:	[Discomfort]
May Be Related To:	Changes in body mechanics, effects of hormones, electrolyte imbalances
Possibly Evidenced By:	Reports of back strain, leg cramps, heartburn
DESIRED OUTCOMES/EVALUATION CRITERIA—CLIENT WILL:	Identify and demonstrate appropriate self-care measures.
	Report discomfort is prevented or minimized.

ACTIONS/INTERVENTIONS

RATIONALE

Independent

Note presence of problems related to cardiac output or breathing difficulties and refer to appropriate nursing diagnoses.

Although these conditions are often sources of discomfort, the client usually experiences a sense of physical well-being free of the typical discomforts of the first trimester.

Reassess for changes in bowel elimination and hemorrhoids.

Reduced gastrointestinal motility, the effect of iron supplements, and increasing pressure/displacement from enlarging uterus interfere with normal functioning.

Discuss dietary intake, exercise, and use of stool softener as presented in CP: First Trimester; ND: Constipation, risk for.

Aids in the prevention/management of constipation.

Note presence of heartburn (pyrosis); review dietary history. Explain physiology of problem. Suggest that client avoid fried/fatty foods, chocolate, citrus, spices, or very cold food; refrain from eating immediately before bedtime; eat six small meals per day; assume semi-Fowler's position after meals; and decrease fluid intake with meals.

Fatty foods increase gastric acidity; small, frequent meals neutralize acidity. Semi-Fowler's position, decreased fluid intake, and avoidance of cold food/eating near bedtime help to prevent gastric reflux.

Recommend raising head of mattress or sleeping on a wedge pillow.

Elevating the upper body during sleep helps to reduce incidence of gastric reflux.

Note presence of backache and lower back pressure. Demonstrate exercises (e.g., pelvic tilt, lying flat on back and pressing back to floor).

Relieves strain on lower back caused by increased curvature of the lumbosacral vertebrae and strengthens back muscles.

73

Review proper dress (e.g., low-heeled shoes; loose, comfortable clothing).

Reassess for leg cramps; teach client to extend leg and dorsiflex foot.

Pressure on nerves in the pelvis, as well as low tissue calcium levels, potentiate leg cramps. Extension of the leg and dorsiflexion of the foot increase perfusion/oxygenation of tissue and help relieve pressure on nerves of lower extremities.

Recommend reducing intake of milk products and taking aluminum lactate, or continuing with 1 quart of milk daily and taking aluminum hydroxide, if leg cramps are severe or persist.

Continued intake of calcium-containing foods/products elevates ionized plasma levels. Aluminum hydroxide traps dietary phosphorus in intestinal tract, offsetting calcium-phosphorus imbalances.

Provide information about appropriate choices of OTC antacids. Avoid use of bicarbonate as a neutralizer or calcium products, as appropriate.

May be constipating and/or may contain substances such as sodium, that may be contraindicated in certain situations owing to its water-retaining properties. Frequent use of calcium-containing antacids in addition to intake of high-calcium foods may contribute to calcium-phosphorus imbalance and development of muscle cramps.

Investigate reports of dizziness/lightheadedness or diaphoresis when lying down. Review rest/sleeping position. Recommend use of side-lying position.

Supine position places weight of uterus on major blood vessels interfering with circulation/lowering blood pressure.

Collaborative

Administer low-sodium antacid.

Neutralizes gastric acidity; decreases phosphorus levels.

Give calcium supplements and aluminum gel as appropriate.

Substitutes for milk products in presence of dietary intolerance. Can reduce phosphorus levels.

NURSING DIAGNOSIS:	**Coping, Individual, risk for ineffective**
Risk Factors May Include:	Situational/maturational crisis, personal vulnerability, unrealistic perceptions
Possibly Evidenced By:	[Not applicable; presence of signs/symptoms establishes an *actual* diagnosis]
DESIRED OUTCOMES/EVALUATION CRITERIA—CLIENT WILL:	Express feelings freely.
	Identify individual strengths.
	Display effective problem-solving and coping skills.

ACTIONS/INTERVENTIONS

RATIONALE

Independent

Identify fears/fantasies client/partner may have. Discuss meaning of these thoughts.

Common female/male fears and fantasies may arise at this time. Women may fear the death of their spouses, and the male partners may fantasize about themselves being pregnant (couvade syndrome.)

Reinforce the normalcy of these fears and fantasies.

May result in difficulties for the individual who does not see the normalcy of this experience.

Evaluate degree of dysfunction client/partner is experiencing in relation to changes that are occurring and those that are anticipated.

Clients experiencing difficulty adjusting to the overwhelming tasks associated with pregnancy/parenting may manifest inappropriate follow-through with prenatal healthcare or greater than normal states of emotional lability. The male partner may demonstrate negative coping in preoccupation with work or a new hobby, lack of interest in the pregnancy, or involvement in sexual relations outside the relationship (raising concerns of STDs [including HIV]).

Encourage client/partner to express feelings about pregnancy and parenting.

Acknowledging and expressing feelings can help the individual begin to identify concerns and begin the problem-solving process.

Collaborative

Refer to classes and counseling, as needed. (Refer to CP: First Trimester; ND: Role Performance, risk for altered.)

May need additional help to solve underlying issues.

NURSING DIAGNOSIS:	Sexuality Patterns, altered
May Be Related To:	Conflict regarding changes in sexual desire and expectations, fear of physical injury to woman and/or fetus
Possibly Evidenced By:	Reported difficulties, limitations or changes in sexual behaviors/activities
DESIRED OUTCOMES/EVALUATION CRITERIA—CLIENT/COUPLE WILL:	Discuss sexual concerns.
	Verbalize understanding of possible reasons for changes noted.
	Identify acceptable alternatives to meet individual needs.
	Verbalize mutual satisfaction or seek counseling, if appropriate.

ACTIONS/INTERVENTIONS

RATIONALE

Independent

Discuss impact of pregnancy on normal patterns of sexual intercourse. (Refer to CP: First Trimester; ND: Sexuality Patterns, altered.)

Optimal sexual satisfaction for the prenatal client often occurs in the second trimester as a result of pelvic/perineal vasocongestion increasing orgasmic pleasure. The man may experience mixed feelings in response to his partner's increased arousal and be confused by his own reduced or increased sexual desire in response to his partner's changing body.

Review normalcy of feelings and discuss possible choice of increasing physical contact through hugging and fondling rather than actually engaging in intercourse.

Fear of injuring the fetus during intercourse is another common concern. Reinforcement of the normalcy of these feelings and concerns can help allay anxiety. Other choices are perfectly acceptable if both parties are satisfied.

75

Review possible alterations in position for coitus, which may be useful as the pregnancy progresses, especially in the third trimester.

Assists couple in considering alternatives/making choices, e.g., side-by-side, female superior, vaginal rear entry. Note: Some cultures (e.g., Puerto Rican) support abstinence for the pregnant woman.

Be alert to indications of possible sexual difficulties or inappropriate behaviors by the man.

There appears to be a higher rate of deviations (such as rape, incest, violent crimes, and extramarital affairs), when mate is pregnant.

Collaborative

Refer to clinical nurse specialist/counseling as indicated.

May need additional help to solve underlying problems which may develop as pregnancy progresses, or may be preexisting.

Third Trimester

PRENATAL CONCEPTS: Third Trimester

NURSING DIAGNOSIS:	**[Discomfort]**
May Be Related To:	Physical changes, hormonal influences
Possibly Evidenced By:	Reports of back strain/pain, leg cramps, paresthesia, pruritus, uterine contractions
DESIRED OUTCOMES/EVALUATION CRITERIA—CLIENT WILL:	Use appropriate self-care activities to reduce discomforts.
	Report discomfort minimized/controlled.
	Seek medical attention appropriately.

ACTIONS/INTERVENTIONS	RATIONALE
Independent	
Continue ongoing assessment of client's discomforts and her methods of dealing with problems. (Refer to CP: Second Trimester; ND: Discomfort.)	Updates data base for planning care and evaluates appropriateness of interventions.
Assess client's respiratory status. (Refer to CP: Second Trimester; ND: Breathing Pattern, ineffective.)	Reduced respiratory capacity as the uterus presses on the diaphragm results in dyspnea, especially for the multigravida, who may not experience relief with engagement (lightening) until the onset of labor.
Note reports of back strain and altered gait. Suggest use of low-heeled shoes, pelvic-rock exercise, maternity girdle, heat application, and massage techniques to be used by partner.	Lordosis and muscle strain are caused by the influence of hormones (relaxin, progesterone) on pelvic articulations and a shift in the center of gravity as the uterus enlarges. Multiple interventions are usually more helpful to alleviate discomfort.
Determine presence of leg cramps. Encourage client to extend leg and turn foot upward in dorsiflexion, change position frequently; avoid prolonged standing/sitting; and reduce milk intake appropriately.	Reduces discomfort associated with altered calcium levels/calcium-phosphorus imbalance, or with pressure from enlarging uterus compressing nerves supplying the lower extremities.
Assess for presence/frequency of Braxton Hicks contractions. Provide information regarding physiology of uterine activity.	These contractions may create discomfort for the multigravida in both second and third trimesters. The primigravida usually does not experience this discomfort until the last trimester, when progesterone's protective effect on uterine activity is decreasing and oxytocin levels are increasing.
Note paresthesia of toes and fingers. Suggest client remove constrictive jewelry, maintain adequate intake of prenatal vitamins (take vitamin B_6 supplement with orange juice or banana), use correct posture, exercise limbs regularly throughout the day, and avoid extremes of temperatures.	Reduces effects of extreme lordotic posture (which strains brachial nerves and compresses nerve roots and femoral veins), edema, pressure on carpal tunnel nerves/ligaments, and vitamin B_6 deficiency. Note: Some sources report controversy over the effectiveness of vitamin B_6.
Review reports of urinary frequency and bladder pressure. (Refer to ND: Urinary Elimination, altered.)	Third trimester uterine enlargement reduces bladder capacity, resulting in urinary frequency.

77

Assess for constipation and hemorrhoids.

Increasing displacement of the bowel contributes to problems of elimination.

Discuss dangers of using cathartics during the ninth month, and suggest other means of resolving constipation, such as a high-fiber diet. Note cultural practices that might influence behaviors. (Refer to CP: First Trimester; NDs: [Discomfort]; Constipation, risk for.)

The use of cathartics may stimulate the onset of early labor. Some cultures, such as Hispanic, believe that use of cathartics ensures good delivery of a healthy boy.

Assess for pyrosis (heartburn). Review dietary limitations.

Problem often occurs in second trimester and may continue as gastric emptying time is prolonged, especially when diet is not modified.

Note presence of leukorrhea and pruritus. Encourage client to bathe frequently, use cotton underwear, wear loose clothing, and to avoid long periods of sitting.

As estrogen levels increase, secretions of the cervical glands create an acid medium that encourages proliferation of organisms.

Assess for problems related to diaphoresis; suggest use of lightweight clothing, frequent bathing, and cool environment.

Increased metabolism and body temperature caused by progesterone activity and excess weight gain may create a constant feeling of being overheated and may increase diaphoresis.

Collaborative

Give calcium supplements/calcium-rich antacid as appropriate. Recommend use of aluminum hydroxide gel as needed.

Substitutes for milk products when intolerance is a problem. Gel can reduce phosphorus levels, correcting calcium-phosphorus imbalance.

Refer for Therapeutic Touch or transcutaneous electrical nerve stimulation (TENS), as appropriate.

May be indicated if other comfort measures are insufficient to alleviate severe back pain.

NURSING DIAGNOSIS:	Knowledge deficit [Learning Need], regarding preparation for labor/delivery; infant care
May Be Related To:	Lack of exposure/experience, misinterpretation of information
Possibly Evidenced By:	Request for information, statement of concerns or misconceptions
DESIRED OUTCOMES EVALUATION CRITERIA—CLIENT/COUPLE WILL:	Discuss physical/psychological changes associated with labor/delivery.
	Identify appropriate resources to obtain information about infant care.
	Verbalize preparedness for labor/delivery and infant.

ACTIONS/INTERVENTIONS

RATIONALE

Independent

Continue/institute learning program as outlined in CP: First Trimester.

Builds on previous learning and/or provides new information. Of greatest concern for the couple in this trimester is how to prepare physiologically and psychologically for the event of labor/delivery and issues surrounding infant care. Note: For various reasons (e.g., financial, cultural) clients may delay

Provide information about normal physical/physiological changes associated with third trimester. (Refer to ND: Self Esteem, risk for situational low.)

Review oral/written information about signs of labor onset; distinguish between false and true labor. Discuss when to notify healthcare provider and when to leave for hospital/birth center. Discuss stages of labor/delivery.

Discuss birth plan written by client/partner and provide additional information as needed. Note cultural expectations/references.

Provide oral/written information about infant care, development, and feeding; offer appropriate references. Elicit cultural beliefs.

Determine plan for discharge after delivery and home care support/needs.

Encourage enrollment in childbirth classes (if not already attending) and tour hospital/birth center.

seeking care until pregnancy is well advanced or delivery is imminent, creating a challenge for healthcare providers to provide meaningful education in a timely fashion.

Understanding the normalcy of such changes can reduce anxiety and foster adoption of self-care activities.

Helps client to recognize onset of labor, to ensure timely arrival, and to cope with labor/delivery process.

Helps client to make informed choices that are amenable to the specific care setting and reflect individual needs. Note: Some cultures or personal values may limit male involvement in the delivery process, necessitating the identification of other support person(s).

Helps prepare for new caretaking role, acquiring necessary items of furniture, clothing, and supplies; helps prepare for breastfeeding and/or bottle feeding. Lack of preparation may be culturally linked, indicating belief that preparation may be associated with increased risk of infant's death because they are "defying God's will."

Early planning can facilitate discharge and help ensure that client/infant needs will be met.

Reduces anxiety associated with the unknown; enhances coping mechanisms for labor/delivery.

NURSING DIAGNOSIS:	Sleep Pattern disturbance
May Be Related To:	Changes in level of activity, psychological stress, inability to maintain comfort
Possibly Evidenced By:	Interrupted sleep, awakening earlier/later than desired, difficulty in falling asleep, not feeling well rested, dark circles under eyes
DESIRED OUTCOMES/EVALUATION CRITERIA—CLIENT WILL:	Report improvement in sleep/rest. Report increased sense of well-being and feeling rested.

ACTIONS/INTERVENTIONS

RATIONALE

Independent

Review normal sleep requirement changes associated with pregnancy. Determine current sleep pattern.

Suggest side-lying position with pillow between legs for support, or place bed board under mattress.

Helps identify need for establishing different sleep patterns (e.g., earlier bedtime and naps).

Back discomfort may necessitate change in position, use of multiple pillows/body pillow, or firmer mattress.

Evaluate level of fatigue; encourage client to rest 1–2 hr daily and obtain 8 hr of sleep per night. Give information about normalcy of moderate fatigue. Reassess commitments to work and family. (Refer to CP: First Trimester; ND: Fatigue.)

Increased fluid retention, weight gain, and fetal growth all contribute to feelings of fatigue, especially in the multipara with other children and demands.

Assess for occurrence of insomnia and for client's response to sleep loss. Suggest aids to sleep, such as relaxation techniques/tapes, reading, warm bath, and reduced activity just before retiring.

Excess anxiety, excitement, physical discomforts, nocturia, and fetal activity all may contribute to sleeping difficulties.

Note reports of positional breathing difficulties. Suggest sleeping in a semi-Fowler's position.

In a recumbent position, the enlarging uterus and the abdominal organs compress the diaphragm, thereby restricting lung expansion. Use of semi-Fowler's position allows the diaphragm to descend, fostering optimal lung expansion.

Collaborative

Obtain red blood cell (RBC) count and Hb level.

Rules out organic problems such as anemia. Anemia and reduced Hb/RBC levels result in reduced oxygenation of tissues and contribute to feeling of excessive fatigue.

Refer client for counseling if sleep deprivation/ fatigue is interfering with activities of daily living.

Additional support/guidance may be necessary for client to cope with alterations in sleep-wake cycle, identify appropriate priorities, and modify commitments.

NURSING DIAGNOSIS:	Urinary Elimination, altered
May Be Related To:	Uterine enlargement, increasing abdominal pressure, fluctuation of renal blood flow, and glomerular filtration rate (GFR)
Possibly Evidenced By:	Urinary frequency, urgency; dependent edema
DESIRED OUTCOMES/EVALUATION CRITERIA—CLIENT WILL:	Verbalize understanding of condition.
	Identify ways to prevent urinary stasis and/or tissue edema.

ACTIONS/INTERVENTIONS

RATIONALE

Independent

Provide information about urinary changes associated with third trimester.

Helps client understand the physiological reason for urinary frequency and nocturia. Third-trimester uterine enlargement reduces bladder capacity, resulting in frequency. Positioning affects kidney functioning so that a supine/upright position decreases renal blood flow by 50%.

Encourage client to assume lateral position while sleeping. Note reports of nocturia.

A left or right lateral recumbent position increases GFR and renal blood flow to increase kidney perfusion and mobilize dependent edema. Edema is reduced by morning in cases of physiological edema.

Advise client to avoid long periods in upright or supine position.

These positions potentiate vena caval syndrome and reduce venous return.

Provide information regarding need for fluid intake

Maintains adequate fluid levels and kidney

of 6 to 8 glasses/day (2+ liters), reduction of intake 2–3 hr before retiring, and moderate use of salt- or sodium-containing foods or products.

perfusion, which relies on dietary sodium to maintain an isotonic state.

Provide information regarding danger of taking diuretics and of eliminating sodium from diet.

Sodium losses/restrictions may overstress renin-angiotensin-aldosterone regulators of fluid levels, resulting in severe dehydration and hypovolemia.

Test midstream urine for presence of albumin. Note location and extent of tissue edema and urine output.

May indicate glomerular spasms or decreased kidney perfusion associated with PIH.

Collaborative

Reassess contributory preexisting medical problems (e.g., kidney disease, hypertension, heart disease).

Problems affecting kidney function combined with increased fluid volume and stasis increase the client's risk for circulatory problems affecting the placenta/fetus.

Assess for signs and symptoms of UTI; obtain urine for colony count, and for culture and sensitivity, if count is greater than 100,000/ml.

The prenatal client is susceptible to urinary stasis/UTI due to progesterone's vasodilating effect on ureters and to compression of the ureters by the enlarging uterus. Women with bacteriuria are also at high risk for preterm labor, premature rupture of membranes (PROM), and chorioamnionitis.

NURSING DIAGNOSIS:	***Sexuality Patterns, altered***
May Be Related To:	*Changes in sexual desire, discomfort (shortness of breath, fatigue, abdominal enlargement), misconceptions/fears*
Possibly Evidenced By:	*Reported difficulties, limitations or changes in sexual behavior, concerns about fetal safety*
DESIRED OUTCOMES/EVALUATION CRITERIA—CLIENT/COUPLE WILL:	*Discuss concerns related to sexual issues in the third trimester.*
	Express mutual satisfaction with sexual relationship.

ACTIONS/INTERVENTIONS

RATIONALE

Independent

Continue/initiate sexual assessment, looking for changes in patterns from first and second trimesters.

Diminished interest in sexual activity/intercourse often occurs in the third trimester, owing to physical changes/discomforts.

Assess couple's perception of sexual relationship.

The couple's ability to identify, verbalize and accept changes in sexuality during the third trimester may influence the relationship and their ability to support each other emotionally.

Encourage couple to discuss, separately and with one another, feelings and concerns related to changes in sexual relationship. Provide information as to the normalcy of changes.

Communication between client and partner is critical to constructive resolution of problems. The client may feel less sexually attractive as her body enlarges, and the man's responses to the client's changing shape may vary from increased desire to disinterest or repulsion. In addition, the client often notes changes in orgasmic experience with a single prolonged uterine contraction rather than rhythmic contractions.

81

Provide information about alternative methods of achieving sexual satisfaction to meet needs for intimacy/closeness.

Sexual needs can be met through masturbation, fondling, stroking, and so forth, if mutually desired/acceptable. Client may find that masturbation creates a more intense orgasm than does intercourse. Note: May be contraindicated in women with a history of, or at risk for, preterm labor.

Recommend alternative positions for intercourse other than the traditional male superior position (e.g., side-lying or female superior position).

The client's enlarging abdomen requires change of positioning for comfort and safety.

Discuss importance of not blowing air into the vagina.

Maternal deaths as a result of air embolism have been reported.

Encourage client/couple to verbalize fears that may reduce desire for intercourse.

Misconceptions and fears that intercourse may result in fetal injury, infection, and initiation of labor may also influence sexual desires. Intercourse has not been found to cause fetal injury, premature rupture of membranes (PROM), onset of labor, or infections in most women. Note: Prostaglandins in semen can soften the cervix and orgasm can stimulate uterine contractions in the at-risk client.

Collaborative

Instruct client to discuss with her healthcare provider the safety of intercourse in the last 6–8 wk.

If there is a history of complications or if complications are anticipated, specific instructions may be needed.

Refer for sexual counseling if concerns are not resolved.

May be needed to promote positive adaptation to sexual changes.

NURSING DIAGNOSIS:	Self Esteem, risk for situational low
Risk Factors May Include:	Concern about ability to accomplish tasks of pregnancy/childrearing
Possibly Evidenced By:	[Not applicable; presence of signs/symptoms establishes an *actual* diagnosis]
DESIRED OUTCOMES/EVALUATION CRITERIA—CLIENT WILL:	Discuss reactions to altered body image, dreams.
	Seek positive role models in preparation for parenting.
	Verbalize feelings of confidence in self regarding new role.

ACTIONS/INTERVENTIONS	RATIONALE

Independent

Note client's/couple's verbal and nonverbal cues in discussion of issues related to body change and role expectations. (Refer to CP: First Trimester; ND: Family Coping: potential for growth.)

A crisis situation may result in the last trimester because the client feels anxious, ambivalent, and depressed about her body and the effects of pregnancy on her abilities/activities. She may also fear injury to herself and the fetus and may feel vulnerable to rejection, loss, or insult.

Discuss nature/frequency of dreams.

At this time, dreams and fantasies related to the birth experience, possible abnormalities of the newborn, and role changes intensify.

Evaluate client's/couple's psychological adaptation to pregnancy.	Normal third-trimester tasks focus on preparation for motherhood/fatherhood. If the client and/or her partner have weak egos and do not accomplish the tasks of pregnancy, difficulties coping with the stresses of labor and delivery as well as parenting are possible.
Determine cultural background, including values regarding family.	Society and culture influence the couple's response to pregnancy and to role changes necessitated by the birth of the baby.
Provide information to couple regarding normalcy of introspection, mood swings, and fears.	Turning inward (self-preoccupation) may confuse the man, but allows the client to adjust, adapt, and gain inner strength needed for childbirth, parenting, and role changes. Dreams/fears about labor are common.
Provide/review information about normal physical changes in the third trimester.	Education/communication about how normal body changes can positively affect attitudes and perceptions facilitates understanding and appreciation of the pregnancy by the couple.
Encourage participation in childbirth classes, if not already enrolled.	Allows opportunity for development of peer support group to share emotional reactions to pregnancy and prepare for successful delivery.
Assess availability and nature of support systems, role models, and cultural beliefs.	Availability of sufficient supports can foster positive adjustment to pregnancy and parenting.

NURSING DIAGNOSIS:	**Coping, Individual/Family, risk for ineffective**
Risk Factors May Include:	Situational/maturational crises, personal vulnerability, unrealistic perceptions, inadequate coping methods, absent/insufficient support systems
Possibly Evidenced By:	[Not applicable; presence of signs/symptoms establishes an *actual* diagnosis]
DESIRED OUTCOMES/EVALUATION CRITERIA—CLIENT/COUPLE WILL:	Discuss emotional reaction to third trimester.
	Prepare for birth of baby, in accordance with cultural beliefs, through education/acquisition of furniture and supplies.
	Identify with appropriate role models.
	Ascribe personality characteristics to fetus.

ACTIONS/INTERVENTIONS	RATIONALE
Independent	
Assess preparation for labor, delivery, and arrival of newborn.	Enrollment in childbirth classes and acquisition of nursery equipment and supplies may indicate psychological preparedness. Lack of preparation may be based on cultural beliefs or may indicate financial or psychological problems.
Determine client's/couple's perception of fetus as a separate entity.	Activities such as choosing a name or nicknaming the baby in utero and home preparations indicate completion of psychological tasks of pregnancy.

83

Determine how the man is handling the pregnancy.

As labor and delivery approach, the man who has his own strong dependency needs may have difficulty meeting the client's increasing need for dependence, which may create conflict. In addition, negative coping may be manifested in lack of preparation for labor and/or for the newborn. If he is not accomplishing the tasks of pregnancy, the man may resort to work, hobbies, or an affair.

Note any previous pregnancy loss, genetic factors, or history of stillbirth, and discuss meaning of the incident to the client/couple. (Refer to CPs: Genetic Counseling; Perinatal Loss.)

As a means of protecting themselves from possible loss/injury in the event that the fetus does not survive, the high-risk couple may choose not to undergo appropriate preparation.

Discuss individual concerns, e.g., financial/lack of or inadequate insurance, need to continue employment and/or return to work early, child care, home assistance.

Imminence of delivery makes problem solving a priority that can no longer be postponed. Provides opportunity to identify options.

Evaluate support systems available to client/couple.

Availability of family and friends can help client/couple to manage tasks of upcoming labor/delivery and postpartum period.

Collaborative

Refer to community resources/counseling as indicated.

May require additional support and/or professional counseling to facilitate coping with serious concerns.

NURSING DIAGNOSIS:	Injury, risk for maternal
Risk Factors May Include:	Presence of hypertension, infection, substance use/abuse, altered immune system, abnormal blood profile, tissue hypoxia, PROM
Possibly Evidenced By:	[Not applicable; presence of signs/symptoms establishes an *actual* diagnosis]
DESIRED OUTCOMES/EVALUATION CRITERIA—CLIENT WILL:	Verbalize understanding of potential individual risk factors. Be free of complications.

ACTIONS/INTERVENTIONS

RATIONALE

Independent

Screen for and evaluate preexisting/newly developed high-risk factors (e.g., heart, kidney, or lung conditions; genetic disorders). Monitor BP, pulse, and heart sounds. Screen for signs of PIH, such as edema, albuminuria, and hypertension.

Potential high-risk situations often become problematic and necessitate intervention at this time, when circulatory and metabolic demands are greatest. Varying degrees of cardiovascular involvement (vasoconstriction, vasospasm) occur, with sodium/water retention negatively affecting kidney, uterine circulation, and CNS functioning.

Obtain vaginal culture. Assess for infections and STDs (including *Candida, Trichomonas*, gonorrhea, herpes simplex virus type 2, *Chlamydia*, group B streptococcus, pruritus, and visible warts/lesions). If present, refer for appropriate treatment.

Untreated vaginal infections or STDs create intense discomfort for the client and pose risk for the fetus, either through placental transmission or at the time of delivery.

84

Review need for cesarean birth and schedule the procedure, if within 4 days of delivery and vaginal culture is positive for herpes simplex virus. (Refer to CP: Prenatal Infection.)

Prevents infection of neonate during birth process.

Obtain results of Hb and Hct at 28 weeks' gestation. Determine dietary intake. Verify that client is following prescribed daily iron and prenatal vitamins intake. Screen for genetic problems (e.g., sickle cell anemia, thalassemia) if not previously done. (Refer to CP: The High-Risk Pregnancy.)

Detects anemia with potential problems of hypoxemia/anoxia for client and fetus.

Provide close, ongoing supervision of diabetic client. At 28 weeks' gestation, obtain results of glucose tolerance test. (Refer to CP: Diabetes Mellitus; Prepregnancy/Gestational.)

Diabetic women are most prone to third-trimester problems related to abruptio placentae, UTI, PIH, stillbirths, placental aging, and ketoacidosis.

Provide information about signs of labor onset; review history for PROM or preterm labor.

Positive history increases likelihood of similar problems in subsequent pregnancies.

Determine use of alcohol/other drugs.

Substance use/abuse places client at increased risk for premature labor and the fetus at risk for difficulties following delivery.

Collaborative

Assess for vaginal bleeding, presence of ecchymotic areas, and signs of disseminated intravascular coagulation; refer for appropriate treatment. (Refer to CP: Prenatal Hemorrhage.)

Presents an obstetric emergency, with reduction in fluid volume and decreased oxygen-carrying capacity posing a threat to maternal organs, placental circulation, and fetal systems.

NURSING DIAGNOSIS:	Cardiac Output, risk for [decompensation]
Risk Factors May Include:	Increased fluid volume/altered venous return, changes in capillary permeability
Possibly Evidenced By:	[Not applicable; presence of signs/symptoms establishes an *actual* diagnosis]
DESIRED OUTCOMES/ EVALUATION—CLIENT WILL:	Remain normotensive, free of pathological edema.
	Display albuminuria not greater than 1+.
	Identify abnormal signs requiring further evaluation.

ACTIONS/INTERVENTIONS | RATIONALE

Independent

Review normal physiological changes. Identify signs/symptoms requiring medical evaluation or intervention.

Near term, fluid volume continues to increase by an additional 700 ml, necessitating an accompanying increase in cardiac output (normally 4–7+/min, raises to 5–10+/min during pregnancy). Increased capillary permeability and hydrostatic pressure favors filtration from the vascular bed. Excess fluid retention and initiation of the renin-angiotensone II/aldosterone stress response may cause fluid to leave the cardiovascular system. This may result in "circulatory dehydration," which negatively affects cardiac output.

85

ACTIONS/INTERVENTIONS	RATIONALE
Monitor pulse/heart rate.	Resting heart rate increases normally at this time by as much as 15 bpm to facilitate circulation of the additional fluid volume.
Note signs of PIH; for example, generalized edema/weight gain, albuminuria 2+, and hypertension with systolic increases greater than 30 mm Hg or diastolic increases greater than 15 mm Hg above baseline.	Differentiates between physiologically normal edema and potential for developing problems. (Refer to CPs: Second Trimester, Pregnancy-Induced Hypertension; ND: Cardiac Output, risk for decompensation.)
Determine client's knowledge about the effect positioning has on cardiac functioning.	Supine/recumbent positions and prolonged upright positions severely reduce venous return and cardiac output in the third trimester, negatively affecting flow to the uterus and kidneys. A lateral Sims'/semi-Fowler's position optimizes placental and kidney perfusion.
Recommend frequent position changes.	Promotes venous return, thereby reducing edema.

NURSING DIAGNOSIS: **Gas Exchange, risk for impaired fetal**

Risk Factors May Include: Altered blood flow within decidua, altered oxygen supply/altered oxygen-carrying capacity of blood (anemia, cigarette smoking)

Possibly Evidenced By: [Not applicable; presence of signs/symptoms establishes an *actual* diagnosis]

DESIRED OUTCOMES/EVALUATION CRITERIA—CLIENT WILL: Identify individual risk factors.

Demonstrate techniques to control/alleviate risk factors.

Display normal fetal heart rate (FHR), appropriate daily fetal movements, and progressive fundal growth.

ACTIONS/INTERVENTIONS

RATIONALE

Independent

ACTIONS/INTERVENTIONS	RATIONALE
Evaluate normal growth progression using fundal height measurement and fetal outline size. Investigate measurements greater than or less than expected levels.	Approximate fundal height at 28 weeks' gestation is 28 cm, and it increases approximately 1 cm/wk until lightening occurs from 38 weeks' gestation on. At term, the fetus obtains oxygen from the maternal portion of the placenta at a rate of 20 to 30 L/min. Because the fetus has such critical needs at that time, any maternal condition that affects cardiac functioning within the decidua basalis, such as placental aging, diabetes, hypertension, or a kidney disorder, as well as high altitude, reduces fetal oxygen levels and nutrient transfers.
Help client/couple assess fetal movement. Demonstrate method and review rationale for daily count. Instruct client/couple to notify healthcare provider if less than 10 fetal movements in 3-hr period are felt for 2 consecutive days.	Placental insufficiency can be detected by a reduction in fetal movement, usually before any perceivable alteration in FHR occurs. The fetus with adequate placental perfusion demonstrates peak movement between 29 and 38 weeks' gestation.

Continue ongoing assessment, and encourage cessation of tobacco use (if applicable).

Assess client's prenatal exercise program. Encourage client to engage in moderate, non–weight-bearing exercise (e.g., swimming, bicycling).

Evaluate for other risk factors (e.g., maternal anemia).

Collaborative

Prepare for, and assist with, ultrasonography, if indicated.

Test serum for Rh incompatibility in Rh-negative client. Repeat test every 4 wk until term, or until high titer (greater than 1:8 or 1:16) indicates a need for further intervention, such as amniocentesis or intrauterine transfusion.

Administer Rh-immune globulin (RhIg) at 28 weeks' gestation. (Refer to CP: The High-Risk Pregnancy.)

Tobacco negatively affects placental circulation. Low Apgar scores as well as IUGR are associated with cigarette smoking.

Blood flow to the uterus can decrease by 70% with strenuous exercise, producing transient fetal bradycardia, possible fetal hyperthermia, and intrauterine growth retardation/restriction.

May indicate potential incompatibility problems and decreased placental perfusion.

Comparative biparietal diameter (BPD) measurements, estimated fetal weight, and femur length obtained by ultrasonography can accurately assess growth.

Determines level of anti-D antibodies in serum of Rh-negative client with an Rh-positive partner, permitting early intervention.

In the unsensitized client, may decrease possibility of transplacental bleeding.

NURSING DIAGNOSIS:	Injury, risk for fetal
Risk Factors May Include:	Maternal health problems, exposure to teratogens/infectious agents
Possibly Evidenced By:	[Not applicable; presence of signs/symptoms establishes an *actual* diagnosis]
DESIRED OUTCOMES/EVALUATION CRITERIA—CLIENT WILL:	Identify individual risk factors. Alter lifestyle/behaviors to reduce risks.

ACTIONS/INTERVENTIONS

RATIONALE

Independent

Continue ongoing assessment of maternal nutrition. (Refer to CP: First Trimester; ND: Nutrition: altered, risk for less than body requirements.)

Discourage use of tobacco (if applicable).

Provide information about risks of drug therapy (e.g., sulfonamide, tetracycline, streptomycin) in the event of maternal infection.

Alterations in maternal nutrition can reduce fetal iron stores, limit fat reserves, delay neurological development in the neonate/child, and reduce protein available for brain growth, thereby reducing head circumference in offspring. In addition, elevation of serum glucose levels in gestational diabetes mellitus is associated with macrosomia of the fetus.

May limit maternal weight gain, reduce intrauterine/placental growth, and result in low Apgar scores at birth.

In the third trimester, sulfonamides increase the risk of hyperbilirubinemia by interfering with albumin-bilirubin bond. Tetracycline causes staining

87

of deciduous teeth and inhibits bone growth in premature infants. Streptomycin may cause damage to the auditory nerve, resulting in possible hearing loss. (Note: Review drug literature for all medications prescribed because many agents have adverse effects.)

Collaborative

Monitor fetal biophysical profile.

Helps determine uteroplacental/fetal well-being. (Refer to CP: The High-Risk Pregnancy; ND: Injury, risk for fetal.)

Note condition of membranes; hospitalize client if they are ruptured.

Rupture of membranes places fetus and client at risk for sepsis. Note: In the absence of frank rupture of membranes, client may be considered for monitoring on an outpatient basis.

The High-Risk Pregnancy

This plan of care provides a general framework for assessing and caring for the client and fetus in a high-risk situation during the prenatal period. Specific high-risk problems that occur in 6% or more of the prenatal population are discussed in the individual plans of care that follow. Less common problems can occur, placing both the client and the fetus in a potentially compromised situation. This plan of care focuses on these less common problems, as well as on general psychosocial considerations for all high-risk clients.

(This plan of care is to be used in conjunction with the Trimesters and other plans of care for specific conditions as appropriate.)

CLIENT ASSESSMENT DATA BASE

Activity/Rest

May be pale, listless, fatigued

Circulation

BP, pulse may be elevated.

Ego Integrity

May express concern about own self-esteem regarding problems of pregnancy.
Pregnancy may not be planned/desired.
Stressors may include financial concerns/lack of health insurance.

Elimination

May practice colonic therapy (diminishes normal colon bacteria)

Food/Fluid

May be malnourished/obese or underweight (weight less than 100 lb/greater than 200 lb).
Dietary choices may not include all food groups (may reflect eating disorder).
History of anemia (differentiate iron deficiency, sickle cell trait/disease, hemorrhage).
Edema may be present in the lower extremities, include both upper/lower extremities, or be generalized.

Neurosensory

May have difficulty with muscle function (i.e., multiple sclerosis, myasthenia gravis, paralysis/spinal cord trauma)

Respiration

Breath sounds: crackles, rhonchi, expiratory wheeze

Safety

History of previous obstetric complications, such as PROM, placenta previa, abruptio placentae, miscarriage, two or more episodes of preterm labor/deliveries, Rh incompatibility, previous birth defects, gestational trophoblastic disease (GTD), hyperemesis gravidarum, one or more pregnancy losses due to premature dilation of the cervix, PIH, or postpartal hemorrhage, infection, or phlebitis.
History of STDs, a virus of the TORCH group, or *Listeria*; repeated urinary tract/vaginal infections; bowel problems; diarrhea; or recent influenza.
History of exposure to teratogenic agents, high-risk occupations.

May have history of intrapartal complications (e.g., hemorrhage, dystocia, PIH, meconium staining, fetal distress).

Inadequate/lack of housing (affects safety as well as general well-being), history of prenatal abuse.

May be jaundiced, screening positive for active hepatitis.

Vaginal discharge may have foul odor.

Sexuality

Fundal height may be inappropriate for gestation.

Perineum may have visible lesions.

May be adolescent (age 17 yr or younger); nullipara, age 35 yr or older; multipara age 40 yr or older; conception less than 3 mo after last delivery or have interval of 8 or more yr between pregnancies.

May have history of large-for-gestational-age infant (macrosomia).

May have had a previous cesarean birth, now opting for attempted vaginal birth after cesarean (AVBAC) or planning a repeat cesarean birth if the primary intervention was based on cephalopelvic disproportion.

Pelvic diameter may be smaller than normal.

Vaginal bleeding or spotting may be present.

History of menstrual problems, such as cramping, or irritable uterus.

Social Interaction

May have history of abusive/unstable relationship

Lack of support systems

Teaching/Learning

History of preexisting medical complications (e.g., diabetes, kidney disease, acquired/congenital cardiac problems, asthma, tuberculosis)

History of substance dependency/abuse

DIAGNOSTIC STUDIES

Ultrasonography (Using Real Time): Assesses gestational age of fetus and presence of multiple gestations; detects fetal abnormalities; locates placenta (and amniotic fluid pockets before amniocentesis, if performed).

Biophysical Profile (BPP) Criteria: Assesses fetal well-being through ultrasound evaluation to measure amniotic fluid index (AFI), FHR/nonstress test (NST) reactivity, fetal breathing movement, body movement (large limbs), and muscle tone (flexion/extension).

Amniocentesis: Determines lecithin to sphingomyelin (L/S) ratio, can detect presence of phosphatidyl glycerol (PG), and measures optical density of fluid for detection of hemolysis in Rh incompatibility or infection in fluid.

Glucose Tolerance Test: Screens for GDM.

Platelet Count: Drop may be associated with PIH and *h*emolysis, *e*levated *l*iver enzymes, and *low p*latelet (HELLP) syndrome (hemolysis, elevated liver enzymes, and/or low platelet count).

Serological Studies, VDRL: Screen for hepatitis, human immunodeficiency virus, AIDS, syphilis.

Blood Type, Rh Group, and Screen for Antibodies in Rh-Negative/Du-Negative Client: Identifies incompatibility risks.

Bilirubin, Liver Function Studies (AST, ALT, and LDH levels): Assesses hypertensive liver involvement.

Coagulation Studies (Activated Thromboplastin Time [APPT], Partial Thromboplastin Time [PTT], Prothrombin Time [PT]), Fibrin Split Degradation Products (FSP/FDP): Identifies clotting disorders in presence of hemorrhage.

Urinalysis (or dipstick), Culture/Sensitivity: Determines glucose/protein levels; detects bacteriuria/infecting agent.

Vagina, Cervical, or Rectal Smear: Identifies STDs (e.g., genital herpes, gonorrhea, *Chlamydia*, or *Listeria*).

NURSING PRIORITIES

1. Identify high-risk situations.
2. Minimize risk factors for client and/or fetus.
3. Create ongoing program of education and support.
4. Prevent/minimize deterioration of maternal/fetal status.
5. Counsel client regarding present and/or future pregnancies.

DISCHARGE GOALS

Inpatient care not required, unless complications develop necessitating hospitalization.

NURSING DIAGNOSIS:	Anxiety [specify level]
May Be Related To:	Situational crises, threat of maternal/fetal death (perceived/actual), interpersonal transmission/contagion
Possibly Evidenced By:	Increased tension, apprehension, feelings of inadequacy, somatic complaints, difficulty sleeping
DESIRED OUTCOMES/EVALUATION CRITERIA—CLIENT WILL:	Verbalize fears and concerns related to complication and/or pregnancy.
	Identify healthy ways to deal with anxiety.
	Demonstrate problem-solving skills.
	Use resources/support systems effectively.

ACTIONS/INTERVENTIONS	RATIONAL
Independent	
Note level of anxiety and degree of interference with ability to function/make decisions.	Unresolved stress may interfere with accomplishment of the tasks of pregnancy, with normal acceptance of the pregnancy/fetus, and with decisions regarding future pregnancies versus sterilization.
Provide emotionally warm and supportive atmosphere; accept client/couple as they present themselves.	Facilitates development of trusting relationship. Nonjudgmental acceptance promotes sense of trust.
Assume an unhurried attitude whenever dealing with the client/family.	Fear of the unknown and fear of becoming a burden are incompatible with psychological and emotional rest.
Provide 24-hr access to healthcare team.	Decreases sense of being alone. Anxiety can be reduced when information or help is readily available.
Review possible sources of anxiety (e.g., prior high-risk pregnancy or premature birth, alterations in family life or role performance, financial concerns related to pregnancy, possible delivery of preterm infant, or employment restrictions).	An uncomplicated pregnancy is associated with some anxiety for the client/couple; a medical complication/history of previous poor outcome further intensifies feelings of uncertainty concerning the present pregnancy and may even cause couple to distance themselves emotionally from the fetus. Acknowledgment of the realities of what is happening can provide support.
Assess stress level of client/couple associated with	Poor family relationships and unavailability of

the medical complication, couple's relationship, the relationship of the client/couple to family members, and the availability of a support network.

Encourage client/couple to express feelings of frustration related to therapy regimen and/or lifestyle changes. Explain to client that verbalization is acceptable and important. (Be alert to expressions of concern regarding children at home and "wanting to deliver and get it over with.")

Observe for signs of emotional changes, imbalance, or conflict with family/significant other(s).

Assess physiological response to anxiety (e.g., BP, pulse).

Provide individually appropriate information regarding interventions or treatments (inpatient or outpatient basis) and the potential impact of condition on client and fetus.

Reinforce positive aspects of maternal/fetal condition, if present, such as fetal growth and activity.

Collaborative

Coordinate team conference including client/couple. Create ongoing plan of care.

Refer to community support group, such as the MS Society, American Diabetes or Lung Associations, or to couples who have successfully completed a high-risk pregnancy.

Refer to other resources/counseling, as indicated. (Refer to NDs: Family Processes, risk for altered; Family Coping: potential for growth).

support systems may increase stress level. Client may become dependent on other family members, which may affect her self-esteem and increase her feelings of anxiety, as well as add to the family's level of stress.

Client/couple needs frequent opportunities to vent anger/frustration about changes in family life in order to minimize anxiety levels. Allowing such expression reassures client that these feelings are normal and expressing them is helpful. Anxiety/frustration may interfere with making realistic decisions.

Provides opportunity for early intervention. Anxiety is "contagious" and may be transmitted between client on the one hand, and family and staff members, on the other.

Anxiety/stress may be accompanied by the release of catecholamines, creating physical responses that affect the client's sense of well-being, thus increasing anxiety.

Helps to reduce anxiety associated with the unknown. May enhance cooperation with treatment regimen, promoting optimal pregnancy outcome.

Increases confidence and hope for client and significant other(s).

Promotes continuity of care and team approach to situation. If hospitalization is necessary, stress levels tend to increase further after 2 wk and remain elevated for the remainder of the hospitalization.

Decreases sense of being alone and can help couple develop a positive outlook on pregnancy.

May need help with child care and housekeeping. Counseling or therapy may be necessary to help client/couple verbalize more freely and examine unmanageable anxiety.

NURSING DIAGNOSIS:	Knowledge deficit [Learning Need], regarding high-risk situation/preterm labor
May Be Related To:	Lack of exposure to and/or misinterpretation of information, unfamiliarity with individual risks and own role in risk prevention/management
Possibly Evidenced By:	Request for information, statement of concerns or misconceptions, inaccurate follow-through of instructions

DESIRED OUTCOMES/EVALUATION CRITERIA—CLIENT WILL:	Verbalize awareness of condition(s) placing her at risk.
	Identify signs/symptoms of preterm labor.
	List possible preventive measures.
	Participate in achieving the best possible pregnancy outcome.

ACTIONS/INTERVENTIONS	RATIONALE

Independent

Provide information related to specific high-risk situation, including clear, simple explanations of pathophysiological changes and maternal and fetal implications.	Increases understanding of the impact of pregnancy on the disease process. Client's/ significant other(s)' level of knowledge of, and involvement in, preventive measures appears to have a direct impact on the outcome of an at-risk pregnancy.
Provide appropriate information related to screening and testing methods and procedures.	Understanding of tests can reduce anxiety and may increase client cooperation.
Emphasize the normalcy of pregnancy.	Avoids/limits perception of "sick role" and provides support to client/couple to deal with their specific situation.
Assist client to identify individually appropriate adaptations/self-care techniques: maintaining fluid volume (2–3 L/day), voiding every 2 hr during the day, scheduling rest periods 2–3 times a day using lateral position, avoiding overexertion or heavy lifting, and maintaining contact with family/daily life when bedrest is required.	Preventive problem solving promotes participation in own care and enhances self-confidence, sense of control, and client/couple satisfaction. Note: Bedrest may result in generalized weakness, raising safety concerns when client is out of bed.
Identify danger signals requiring immediate notification of healthcare provider (e.g., PROM, preterm labor, vaginal bleeding).	Recognizing risk situations encourages prompt evaluation/intervention, which may prevent or limit untoward outcomes.
Define labor and review possible symptoms of preterm labor: painless or painful uterine contractions or rhythmic pressure, occurring 10 or fewer min apart; contractions lasting 30 sec or longer for 1 hr (unrelieved by rest, drinking fluids, or emptying bladder); cramps resembling those of menstruation; abdominal cramping with or without diarrhea; and pressure or aching of the low back and/or vulva unrelieved by resting on left side (though may sometimes be relieved by sacral massage).	May help clarify misconceptions regarding "false labor" and aid client in distinguishing between preterm labor and Braxton Hicks contractions. Symptoms of preterm labor may be overlooked by confusing them with normal "aches and pains" of pregnancy.
Describe potential implications of premature birth.	Increases understanding of need for prevention and motivation to follow therapeutic regimen.
Encourage client to assess uterine tone/contractions for 1 hr, once or twice a day.	Although uterine contractions occur occasionally, cervical dilation can occur with contractions every 10 min or less for a period of 1 hr.
Demonstrate technique and specific equipment used when FHR monitoring is done in the home setting.	Provides opportunity for more detailed information regarding fetal well-being in a less stressful environment. Enhances sense of active involvement.

93

Stress importance of reporting increased or altered vaginal discharge.	May reflect cervical changes; indicates need to screen for vaginal infections, which may precipitate preterm labor or may indicate PROM.
Discuss implications of unknown progression of degenerative neurological conditions for client/infant.	Conditions such as multiple sclerosis may occasionally complicate pregnancy or develop afterward; however, exacerbations or remissions seem unrelated to pregnancy. If severely affected, client may elect to interrupt pregnancy or undergo sterilization. Note: Decreased sensation may alter client's ability to sense uterine contractions/presence of labor.
Review significance of symptoms of respiratory difficulty, fatigue, and upper eyelid dropping in client with myasthenia gravis. Discuss implications for care of self and infant after birth.	Peak prevalence of this motor endplate disorder occurs at age 25 yr, and pregnancy may increase severity of symptoms. Myasthenia gravis is not an indication for therapeutic abortion, but adjustments may be required to care for infant and self.
Discuss impact of rheumatoid arthritis on pregnancy/postpartal period, as well as need to avoid nonsteroidal anti-inflammatory drugs such as aspirin.	Severity of symptoms often subside during pregnancy, yet severe exacerbations may occur 1 mo after delivery, making infant care difficult. Aspirin is contraindicated owing to its effect on maternal/fetal platelets, coagulation, and corresponding anemia related to blood loss. Note: Extra rest is important to protect weight-bearing joints.

NURSING DIAGNOSIS:	**Family Coping: potential for growth**
May Be Related To:	Needs sufficiently gratified and adaptive tasks effectively addressed to enable goals of self-actualization to surface
Possibly Evidenced By:	Attempts to describe growth impact of this crisis on own values, priorities, and goals; moving in direction of health-promoting and enriching lifestyle that supports and monitors maturational process; generally chooses experiences that optimize wellness
DESIRED OUTCOMES/EVALUATION CRITERIA—FAMILY WILL:	Verbalize fears/perceived disruptions in family life caused by high-risk pregnancy. Seek assistance/counseling, as needed.

ACTIONS/INTERVENTIONS	RATIONALE
Independent	
Assess perceived impact of complication on client and family members. Encourage verbalization of concerns.	Family stress often occurs in an uncomplicated pregnancy, and it is amplified in a high-risk pregnancy, where concerns focus on the health of both the client and fetus. Family is strengthened if all members have a chance to express fears openly and work cooperatively.
Provide primary caregiver for client and encourage thorough documentation.	Ensures continuity of care, enhances ongoing identification and prevention of additional problems, and ensures appropriate follow-up to assist during postpregnancy readjustment.
Help client/couple plan restructuring of roles/activities necessitated by complication of pregnancy.	Education, support, and assistance in maintenance of family integrity help foster growth of its individual

Include partner/siblings in prenatal office visits or hospital visits if client is hospitalized. Arrange place for family to stay overnight.

members and reduce stress that the client may feel from her dependent role.

Helps family members to view the outcome of the pregnancy as a cooperative effort. Proper management of stress at this time may promote growth within the family and individual members.

Listen for expressions of helplessness and concern about how current situation is affecting the family and home. Problem-solve solutions.

Medical problems necessitating special therapy/restrictions at home or hospitalization significantly disrupt normal routines and cause stress and guilt feelings in the client, partner, and/or siblings. Creative solutions enhance self-esteem, may increase participation/cooperation with medical regimen, and can promote family involvement.

Focus on pregnancy milestones, "countdown to birth."

Promotes sense of hope that modifications/restrictions serve a worthwhile purpose. Helps client/significant others look forward instead of dwelling only on the concerns of the present.

Collaborative

Refer to community service agencies (e.g., visiting nurse, social service); or resources, such as Sidelines.

Community supports may be needed for ongoing assessment of medical problem, family status, coping behaviors, and financial stressors. Sidelines is a national telephone support group for pregnant women on bedrest.

Refer for counseling if family does not sustain positive coping and growth. (Refer to ND: Family Processes, risk for altered.)

May be necessary to promote growth and to prevent family disintegration.

NURSING DIAGNOSIS:	Nutrition: altered, risk for less/more than body requirements
Risk Factors May Include:	Extremes of weight (less than 100 lb/greater than 200 lb), inability to ingest/digest food, excessive/inappropriate intake, limited financial resources
Possibly Evidenced By:	[Not applicable, presence of signs/symptoms establishes an *actual* diagnosis]
DESIRED OUTCOMES/EVALUATION CRITERIA—CLIENT WILL:	Gain 24–28 lb during the pregnancy.
	Follow a well-balanced diet.
	Be free of ketones in urine.

ACTIONS/INTERVENTIONS

RATIONALE

Independent

Ascertain current/past dietary patterns and practices.

Ascertaining the nutritional state before conception is critical to ensuring proper organ development, especially brain tissue, in the early weeks of pregnancy.

Weigh client. Compare current weight with pregravid weight. Have client record weight between visits.

Underweight clients are at risk for anemia, inadequate protein/calorie intake, vitamin/mineral deficiencies, and PIH. Overweight women

95

are at risk for possible changes in the cardiovascular system that create risks for development of PIH, GDM, and hyperinsulinemia of the fetus, resulting in macrosomia. New research indicates increased risk of fetal distress and cesarean delivery. Sudden weight gain of 2+ lb in a week may indicate PIH; a weight loss of 3 lb or more near term suggests postmaturity.

ACTIONS/INTERVENTIONS	RATIONALE
Provide information about risks of weight reduction during pregnancy and about nourishment needs of client and fetus.	Prenatal calorie restriction and resultant weight loss may result in nutrient deficiency or ketonemia, with negative effects on fetal central nervous system (CNS) and possible IUGR.
Test urine for presence of ketones.	Indicates inadequate glucose utilization and breakdown of fats for metabolic processes.
Develop plan with client that provides necessary nutrients, including adequate fluid intake. Recommend at least 2 quarts of noncaffeinated fluid per day.	Prevents malnutrition and dehydration, which appear to compromise optimal uterine and placental functioning and increase uterine irritability, which could potentiate premature labor.
Discuss importance of staying on low-phenylalanine diet for the woman with phenylketonuria (PKU).	This client should have begun the diet before becoming pregnant and continue the diet throughout the pregnancy to prevent elevated phenylpyruvic acid levels and reduce the risk of mental retardation, microcephaly, congenital heart defects, and growth retardation/restriction (IUGR).
Encourage close monitoring of blood glucose levels, as appropriate.	Type I or insulin-dependent diabetes mellitus (IDDM) clients generally need to check blood glucose levels 4–12 times/day because insulin needs may increase 2 to 3 times above pregravid baseline.

(Refer to CPs: First Trimester, Diabetes Mellitus: Prepregnancy/Gestational; ND: Nutrition: altered, risk for less than body requirements.)

NURSING DIAGNOSIS:	Injury, risk for fetal
Risk Factors May Include:	Maternal health problems, substance use/abuse, exposure to teratogens/infectious agents
Possibly Evidenced By:	[Not applicable, presence of signs/symptoms establishes an *actual* diagnosis]
DESIRED OUTCOMES/EVALUATION CRITERIA—CLIENT WILL:	Verbalize understanding of individual risk factors.
	Participate in screening procedures as indicated.
	Display fetal growth within normal limits (WNL).

ACTIONS/INTERVENTIONS

RATIONALE

Independent

Note maternal conditions that affect fetal circulation, such as PIH, diabetes, cardiac or kidney disease, anemia, Rh incompatibility, or hemorrhage, as well as maternal age. (Refer to appropriate plans of care.) Assess for excessive nausea/vomiting.

Any factor that interferes with or reduces maternal circulation/oxygenation has a similar impact on placental/fetal oxygen levels. The fetus who is unable to obtain sufficient oxygen for metabolic needs from maternal circulation resorts to anaerobic metabolism, which produces lactic acid, leading to an acidotic state. Maternal age above 35 is associated with some

Ascertain use of thalidomide before conception.

Determine use/abuse of substances such as tobacco, alcohol, and other drugs. Provide information about negative effects on fetal growth.

Screen for occurrence of abuse during pregnancy.

Note estimated date of birth (EDB).

Assist in screening for and identifying genetic/chromosomal disorders. (Refer to CP: Genetic Counseling.)

Discuss potential negative effects of identified condition (e.g., PKU) on fetus, and review options available to client. (Refer to ND: Nutrition: altered, less/more than body requirements and CP: Genetic Counseling.)

Assess FHR, noting rate and regularity. Have client monitor fetal movement daily as indicated. Note presence of maternal conditions that may also impact FHR (e.g., maternal hyperthyroidism or Graves' disease).

Assess or screen for preterm uterine contractions, which may or may not be accompanied by cervical dilatation. (Refer to CP: Preterm Labor/Prevention of Delivery.)

Monitor FHR during sickle cell crisis.

Collaborative

Monitor maternal laboratory studies:

Serology tests;

increase in risk of abruptio placentae, preterm delivery/stillbirths, fetal chromosomal abnormalities, and IUGR. The most common maternal complications in this age group are PIH and gestational diabetes.

Exposes developing fetus to acidotic state and malnutrition and may contribute to IUGR and poor brain growth. Development of hyperemesis gravidarum may require hospitalization.

Clients with HIV/AIDS may have used this drug to prevent or reverse weight loss; however, it has potential for severe birth defects.

Depending on the extent of use, these substances may result in varying degrees of involvement ranging from an identifiable syndrome such as fetal alcohol syndrome to less specific developmental disorders/delays.

Prenatal abuse is a significant risk factor for low birth weight, preterm delivery, and other poor outcomes.

Placental function is characterized by intense metabolic activity and oxygen consumption, which increases until term and then begins to fall. A post-term placenta becomes calcified and degenerates, thereby reducing surface available for oxygen and nutrient transfer and increasing perinatal mortality.

Disorders such as PKU or sickle cell anemia necessitate special treatment to prevent negative effects on fetal growth.

Intrauterine or postnatal growth retardation/restriction, malformation, or mental retardation may occur in PKU if pregnant woman does not resume diet low in phenylalanine for the duration of the pregnancy.

Tachycardia in a term infant may indicate a compensatory mechanism to reduced oxygen levels and/or presence of sepsis. A reduction in fetal activity occurs before bradycardia. Although fetal thyrotoxicosis is rare, IUGR or tachycardia may result if maternal condition is untreated. Note: Fetal hypothyroidism may result from maternal low-dose antithyroid drug therapy; higher doses may produce a goiter or mental retardation.

Occurs in 6%–7% of all pregnancies and may result in delivery of a preterm infant if tocolytic management is not successful in reducing uterine contractility and irritability.

Maternal acidosis/hypoxia, especially in third trimester, can result in fetal CNS disorders. Repeat crises predispose the client and fetus to increased mortality and morbidity rates.

Assess for presence of TORCH group of viruses and active/carrier state of hepatitis. (Refer to CP: Prenatal Infection.)

97

Blood type/group;

Serum human placental lactogen (HPL), and serum/urinary estriol levels. (Note: Recent studies suggest use of BPP/NST rather than estriol/HPL levels);

MSAFP$_3$ levels at 14–22 weeks' gestation and amniocentesis, if levels are abnormal.

Identifies fetus at risk for isoimmunization. Alterations in placental secretion of HPL/estriol may indicate fetal/placental problems. Low levels occur in toxemia, IUGR, and postmaturity. Elevated levels accompany Rh sensitization, diabetes, maternal sickle cell anemia, and liver diseases.

Triple screen measures alpha-fetoprotein, unconjugated estriol, and human chorionic gonodatropin levels. With a neural tube defect (NTD), most commonly spina bifida and anencephaly, AFP (a protein produced by the yolk sac and fetal liver) is present in maternal serum at a level 8 times higher than normal at 15 weeks' gestation. The AFP level then decreases until term. Also useful in detecting other problems, such as ventral wall defects, Down syndrome, and trisomy 18.

Administer RhIgG to client at 28 weeks' gestation, then again 72 hr postpartum, if indicated.

In Rh-negative clients with Rh-positive partners, RhIgG helps reduce incidence of maternal isoimmunization in nonsensitized mothers and helps prevent erythroblastosis fetalis and fetal red blood cell (RBC) hemolysis.

Prepare client for/review serial testing:

Ultrasonography (Refer to ND: Gas Exchange, risk for impaired maternal and CPs: Diabetes Mellitus: Prepregnancy/Gestational; Pregnancy-Induced Hypertension; Cardiac Conditions);

Monitors clients at risk for reduced/inadequate placental perfusion, such as adolescents, clients older than 35 yr, clients with diabetes, PIH, cardiac/kidney disease, anemia, or respiratory disorders. Inadequate placental perfusion with reduced transfer of oxygen/nutrients may result in fetal IUGR.

NST;

A reactive NST indicates integrity of placental circulation and fetal CNS as evidenced by two or more FHR accelerations of at least 15 bpm lasting 15 sec or longer in a 20-min period during which the baseline rate is WNL and variability is average.

BPP and contraction stress test (CST) (if result of NST nonreactive or unequivocable).

Chronic intrauterine hypoxia caused by vascular changes or postmaturity results in reduced fetal activity, tachycardia, reduced beat-to-beat variability, possibly nonreactive stress test, positive CST, falling estriol levels, and decreased fetal muscle tone and breathing movements. Note: A positive CST with late decelerations indicates a high-risk client/fetus with possible reduced uteroplacental reserves; a negative CST indicates adequate fetal oxygen reserve/placental functioning.

Provide supplemental oxygen as appropriate.

Increases the oxygen available for fetal uptake, especially in presence of severe anemias or sickle cell crisis, or when maternal/fetal circulation is compromised.

Provide information and assist with procedures as indicated, for example:

Aminocentesis;

Aminocentesis may be performed for genetic purposes or to assess fetal lung maturity. Spectrophotometric analysis of the fluid may be done to detect bilirubin after 26 weeks' gestation.

Administer RhIgG after amniocentesis (based on results from Kleihauer-Betke test);

If serum titer is greater than 1:16, sensitization occurs when maternal/fetal cells mix, creating an

Observe external fetal monitor for 20–30 min after amniocentesis, position client on side;

Intrauterine fetal exchange transfusion and repeat transfusion every 2 wk as indicated by titers (Kleihauer-Betke test) followed by administration of RhIgG;

Fetoscopy.

antigen-antibody response with hemolysis of fetal RBCs and release of bilirubin. Kleihauer-Betke test detects presence of fetal blood in maternal system. RhIgG may prevent procedural isoimmunization. Most common complication is preterm labor requiring ongoing monitoring by client following the procedure. Helps detect negative fetal/uterine response to procedure. Lateral position increases uteroplacental perfusion.

If excess fetal RBC hemolysis occurs, transfusion into fetal peritoneal cavity with RhO-negative blood replaces hemolyzed RBCs when fetus is determined at risk of dying before 32 weeks' gestation.

Although it is not widely used, fetoscopy permits fetal blood/skin sampling and direct visualization of the fetus with identification of genetic or developmental problems such as sickle cell anemia, hemophilia, thalessemia major; immunoglogic problems, Rh isoimmunization; and NTD.

Determine fetal maturity when early delivery is anticipated, using results from amniotic fluid analysis for surfactant PG, creatinine, bilirubin, and cytological analysis.

Fetal lung maturity is indicated by an L/S ratio of 2:1 or greater, except in an infant of a diabetic mother. Presence of PG and creatinine levels of 2.0 mg/100 ml reflect kidney maturity. Cornified cells are present at 36 weeks' gestation. Bilirubin levels of 0.025 mg/dl in mothers having no Rh isoimmunization indicate fetal maturity.

Prepare for, and assist with, termination of pregnancy by induction or cesarean delivery as indicated.

Pregnancy may be terminated if desired for such conditions as toxoplasmosis occurring before 20 weeks' gestation, rubella during the first trimester, or elevated AFP levels indicating NTD. In event of post-term placental calcification or deterioration of maternal condition, labor may be induced.

NURSING DIAGNOSIS:	Injury, risk for maternal
Risk Factors May Include:	Preexisting medical conditions, complications of pregnancy
Possibly Evidenced By:	[Not applicable, presence of signs/symptoms establishes an *actual* diagnosis]
DESIRED OUTCOMES/EVALUATION CRITERIA—CLIENT WILL:	Identify signs/symptoms requiring medical evaluation/intervention.
	Verbalize understanding of individual risk factors.
	Be free of maternal injury.

ACTIONS/INTERVENTIONS	RATIONALE

Independent

Review obstetric/medical history. Note maternal age.

Helps identify individual risk factors. Women over age 35 have an increased occurrence of PIH, gestational diabetes, spontaneous abortions, and bleeding problems.

Screen for abuse during pregnancy.	Prenatal abuse is correlated with a low maternal weight gain, infections, anemia, and delay in seeking prenatal care until the third trimester.
Discuss the option of AVBAC in client with incision into the lower uterine segment and potential risks associated with previous classical incision into uterus.	Potential for uterine rupture in subsequent pregnancies exists when incision is a classical (vertical) incision or gestational age is not accurately determined, resulting in overdistension and stimulating onset of labor.
Refer client/couple for AVBAC or cesarean classes, as appropriate.	Provides information/opportunity for asking questions to prepare client for delivery.
Discuss unpredictable effect of pregnancy on epileptic/seizure disorders. Review information regarding medical control with diazepam (Valium), chlordiazepoxide hydrochloride (Librium), and phenytoin (Dilantin).	Pregnancy may cause an increase in seizure activity, especially if complications occur. Note: Dilantin has been associated with cleft lip/palate in the newborn. Other anticonvulsants may impair clotting, requiring prophylactic use of vitamin K during the last month of pregnancy to prevent neonatal hemorrhage.
Assess renal/cardiac involvement in client with systemic lupus erythematosus (SLE). Provide information about the need to continue with corticosteroid intake throughout pregnancy.	Increased rates of spontaneous abortion, cardiac problems, preterm labor, stillbirth, PIH, and even maternal death occur in the client with SLE-related kidney involvement.
Discuss safety concerns related to presence of spinal cord injury/paralysis.	For clients at risk for autonomic dysreflexia, episode may be relieved or prevented by appropriate emptying of the bladder. Other concerns, such as altered mobility/transfer and increased attention to skin care needs, can generally be managed with preventive planning.
Monitor for temperature elevation. Note diaphoresis, tachycardia, fine tremors, weight loss, and altered bowel function.	May indicate onset of hyperthyroidism/thyrotoxicosis, which in addition to deleterious fetal effects (increased mortality and LBW infants), may result in pernicious vomiting and cardiac stress.
Investigate reports of excessive nausea/vomiting in conjunction with elevated BP, pathological edema, and proteinuria.	Hyperemesis gravidarum and PIH before 24 weeks' gestation may develop in association with hydatidiform mole.

Collaborative

Assist with ultrasonography; note absence of fetal heart outline or FHTs. Monitor elevation of HCG titers.	Diagnostic for hydatidiform mole (molar pregnancy), which is most likely to occur in older women or women treated with clomiphene citrate (Clomid). Sequelae of choriocarcinoma may develop if HCG titers remain high after evacuation.
Assist in uterine evacuation by induced abortion, dilation and curettage (D & C), or hysterectomy, as indicated.	Surgery ensures complete removal of all placental fragments. In the presence of excessive bleeding, or in older clients who have increased risk of malignant sequelae, hysterectomy may be the treatment of choice.
Stress need to follow up HCG titers for at least 1 yr.	Pregnancy should be delayed for 1 full year after negative HCG titers are achieved. Chemotherapy is recommended if titers rise/remain high and D & C reveals malignant cells.
Review thyroid profile studies and serum thyroxine values.	Helpful in confirming hypothyroid or hyperthyroid state and identifying treatment needs. Note: Untreated hypothyroidism markedly increases the risk of fetal loss, congenital goiter, and true

cretinism; untreated hyperthyroidism potentiates risk of abortion or fetal demise.

Administer propylthiouracil (PTU) or methimazole as indicated.

Helps reduce effects of Graves' disease and thyrotoxicosis by interfering with synthesis of thyroid hormones. Radioisotope treatment is contraindicated in pregnancy.

NURSING DIAGNOSIS:	**Self Esteem, risk for situational low**
Risk Factors May Include:	Perceived failure at a life event
Possibly Evidenced By:	[Not applicable; presence of signs/symptoms establishes in *actual* diagnosis]
DESIRED OUTCOMES/EVALUATION CRITERIA—CLIENT/COUPLE WILL:	Verbalize thoughts/feelings about situation.
	Express positive self-appraisal.
	Seek appropriate referral as needed.

ACTIONS/INTERVENTIONS

RATIONALE

Independent

Encourage verbalization of feelings. Assess perception of self in nonpregnant state and alteration in perception with pregnancy.

Helps detect problems and determine their severity. Because pregnancy is thought to be a normal physiological process, a high-risk situation can lead to alterations in self-concept, lowered self-esteem, and ego disintegration, especially if one or both members of the couple associate child rearing with success as a woman or man.

Note issues of lack of control.

Client is often frustrated by a loss of control over her body as well as the pregnancy in general, with a sense that all control is in the hands of healthcare providers.

Facilitate positive adaptation to altered self-concept through Active Listening, acceptance, and problem solving.

Helps in successful accomplishment of the psychological tasks of pregnancy, although the high-risk couple may remain ambivalent as a self-protective mechanism against possible loss of the pregnancy/fetal death.

Encourage involvement in decisions about care when possible.

Enhances sense of control and increased self-esteem. Note: Client is often required to undergo many procedures with few—if any—alternatives offered. Pressure may be perceived as implication that the procedure may be the only chance of delivering a viable infant; or if medical option is refused, insurance payor may deny benefits for costs associated with the pregnancy.

Promote attendance at classes/support groups, identify computer-based resources, e.g., E-mail, on-line support groups, as appropriate.

Provides information for client/couple and reassurance that they are not alone.

Collaborative

Refer for individual/group counseling, if indicated.

May be necessary for positive ego integration.

101

NURSING DIAGNOSIS:	Fluid Volume risk for deficit
Risk Factors May Include:	Inability to ingest and retain fluids
Possibly Evidenced By:	[Not applicable, presence of signs/symptoms establishes an *actual* diagnosis]
DESIRED OUTCOMES/EVALUATION CRITERIA—CLIENT WILL:	Maintain adequate circulating volume as evidenced by vital signs WNL, urine output greater than 30 ml/hr, moist mucous membranes, and good skin turgor.

ACTIONS/INTERVENTIONS

RATIONALE

Independent

ACTIONS/INTERVENTIONS	RATIONALE
Determine presence/frequency of excessive or persistent nausea and vomiting/retching.	Pernicious vomiting (hyperemesis gravidarum) results in dehydration, hypovolemia, and metabolic changes, exposing the developing fetus to acidotic state and malnutrition, which may contribute to IUGR and poor brain growth or possibly death.
Note client reports of nervousness or heat intolerance and presence of fine tremors, temperature elevation, excessive diaphoresis, or tachycardia.	Signs suggestive of hyperthyroid state may cause excessive vomiting.
Monitor BP and pulse.	Dehydration/hypovolemia may cause hypotension or tachycardia.
Recommend pacing of activities, adequate sleep, and bedrest, as appropriate.	Conserves energy; allows closer monitoring of physical status.
Record intake/output; measure urine specific gravity.	Provides information regarding hydration and effectiveness of fluid replacement.
Encourage frequent oral care.	Dehydration and acid emesis may cause drying and irritation of mucous membranes.
Note signs of mucosal bleeding or hemorrhage. Recommend use of soft toothbrush, alcohol-free mouthwash, and ingestion of soft foods.	Severe vitamin deficiencies and hypothrombinemia may alter coagulating ability. Preventing trauma to mucous membranes reduces likelihood of bleeding.
Review need for and/or use of antithyroid drugs, such as propylthiouracil (PTU) or methimazole (Tapazole).	Interferes with synthesis of thyroid hormone and helps overcome intractable vomiting (hyperemesis) caused by hyperthyroid state. However, fetal consequences may include hypothyroidism, goiter, or mental retardation.

Collaborative

ACTIONS/INTERVENTIONS	RATIONALE
Monitor laboratory studies as indicated:	
Electrolytes;	Electrolyte/acid-base imbalances are common and may be life-threatening.
Hct;	Elevated in dehydration. May be useful in assessing fluid needs.
BUN;	Hypovolemia reduces renal perfusion and function, elevating BUN.
Thyroid studies and serum thyroxine levels.	Elevated in client with hyperthyroidism/Graves' disease.
Administer prochlorperazine (Compazine) or	Provides sedative action and prevents vomiting,

hydroxyzine (Vistaril) as indicated, or monitor low-dose promethazine (Phenergan) infusion.

Administer parenteral fluids, electrolytes, glucose, or supplemental vitamins, as indicated.

Provide diet as tolerated (may be nothing by mouth [NPO] for 24–48 hr) starting with small/dry feedings followed by clear liquids and progressing to low-fat, soft, then regular foods.

Refer to psychological counseling if no improvement occurs.

Prepare for therapeutic abortion if warranted by patient's condition.

but may have teratogenic effects.

Helps reverse or prevent possible hypokalemia, severe protein/vitamin deficiencies, or acidosis, which may negatively affect maternal/fetal well-being.

Allows the gastrointestinal tract an initial period of rest. Gradually increasing oral feedings may improve food tolerance.

There may be a psychological component to the problem of vomiting.

Early recognition and treatment should prevent such a severe situation from developing, but it may be indicated when mother's life is threatened, as evidenced by jaundice, prolonged fever greater than 101°F (38.3C°), tachycardia, retinal hemorrhage, and delirium.

NURSING DIAGNOSIS: **Gas Exchange, risk for impaired maternal**

Risk Factors May Include: Altered blood flow, alveolar-capillary changes, reduced oxygen-carrying capacity of blood

Possibly Evidenced By: [Not applicable, presence of signs/symptoms establishes an actual diagnosis]

DESIRED OUTCOMES/EVALUATION CRITERIA—CLIENT WILL: Verbalize understanding of individual risk factors.

Identify and use interventions to reduce risks.

Display BP, pulse, respiratory rate, and hemoglobin (Hb) and hematocrit (Hct) within normal limits.

Refer to discussion of circulatory considerations in CPs: Pregnancy-Induced Hypertension; Cardiac Conditions.

ACTIONS/INTERVENTIONS

RATIONALE

Independent

Assess for respiratory disorders that may interfere with lung function, such as asthma or tuberculosis. Note maternal respiratory rate or effort and adventitious lung sounds.

Any condition, either preexisting or developing during the pregnancy, that reduces or interferes with oxygen-carrying capacity impairs normal gas exchange. Such conditions may be a result of problems related to respiration, circulation, or cellular components.

Note conditions potentiating vascular changes/reduced placental circulation (e.g., diabetes, PIH, cardiac problems) or those that alter oxygen-carrying capacity (e.g., anemias, hemorrhage). (Refer to specific plans of care as needed).

Extent of maternal vascular involvement and reduction of oxygen-carrying capacity have a direct influence on uteroplacental circulation and gas exchange. IUGR and birth of an LBW or small-for-gestational-age infant are associated with maternal vascular changes.

Monitor BP and pulse.

Elevated BP may indicate PIH; reduced BP and increased pulse may accompany hemorrhage.

Promote bed/chair rest. Position in upright or semi-Fowler's position when respiratory effort is

Reduces respiratory effort and increases oxygen consumption as diaphragm falls, increasing compromised; otherwise, encourage client to assume lateral position.

vertical chest diameter. Side-lying position increases renal/placental perfusion; either position is effective in preventing supine hypotensive syndrome.

Monitor maternal kidney function, noting overall intake/output, and measure urine-specific gravity, as indicated.

Kidney function may deteriorate during pregnancy, negatively affecting cardiovascular function, elevating BP, and reducing placental circulation.

Encourage increased fluid intake as appropriate/tolerated.

Prevents dehydration, enhances organ perfusion/function, and liquefies respiratory secretions to facilitate expectoration.

Review dietary sources of vitamin C, iron, and protein. Discuss individual need for sufficient calories. Identify substances that foster iron absorption (acid medium, vitamin C) and those that reduce absorption (alkaline medium, milk).

Inadequate nutrition results in iron deficiency anemia and may lead to problems of oxygen transport.

Reduce stressors precipitating allergic/asthmatic response in susceptible client.

Decreases incidence of attacks. Impact of asthma on pregnancy is questionable, although it may be associated with increased incidence of abortion and preterm labor.

Encourage maternal avoidance of potential stressors that may precipitate sickle cell crisis (e.g., hypoxia, dehydration, acidosis, exposure to cold).

Maternal acidosis/hypoxia, especially in third trimester, can result in fetal CNS disorders. Repeat crises predispose the client/fetus to increased rates of mortality/morbidity.

Collaborative

Monitor maternal laboratory studies as indicated:

Hb/Hct using electrophoresis;

Any reduction in Hb levels or circulating blood volume reduces oxygen available for maternal tissues. Treatment depends on the cause of the anemia as diagnosed by electrophoresis.

BUN, creatinine clearance, 24-hr protein, and uric acid levels;
Arterial blood gases (ABGs).

Evaluates adequacy of renal function.

Determines oxygenation and therapy needs.

Administer medications, as indicated:

Theophylline;

Iron dextran (Imferon);

Isoniazid/ethambutol/rifampin.

Assists in bronchial dilation but may be associated with side effects of tachycardia in client/fetus.
Parenteral administration may be necessary in presence of severe iron deficiency anemia to increase maternal oxygen-carrying capacity.
Active tuberculosis requires treatment. Isoniazid crosses the placenta but does not appear to have teratogenic effects. Rifampin also crosses the placenta, but studies of fetal effects are still in progress. Streptomycin is avoided owing to association with vestibular/auditory defects. Note: Isoniazid therapy requires supplementation of pyridoxine (vitamin B_6).

Provide supplemental oxygen.

May be indicated in presence of severe anemias or during sickle cell crisis.

Assist with prophylactic exchange transfusion or crisis/anemia transfusion as indicated.

Helps maintain maternal hemoglobin S (HbS, abnormal sickle cell) level at less than 50%–60% of total Hb, or Hct at 30%, to improve oxygen-carrying capacity.

104

NURSING DIAGNOSIS:	Activity Intolerance, risk for
Risk Factors May Include:	Presence of circulatory/respiratory problems, uterine irritability
Possibly Evidenced By:	[Not applicable; presence of *signs/symptoms* establishes an *actual* diagnosis]
DESIRED OUTCOMES/EVALUATION CRITERIA—CLIENT WILL:	Report an awareness of level of tolerance of activity.
	Plan necessary alterations in lifestyle/daily activities.
	Be free of excessive fatigue or uterine irritability/sustained contractions.

ACTIONS/INTERVENTIONS	RATIONALE

Independent

ACTIONS/INTERVENTIONS	RATIONALE
Encourage client to pace activities and allow sufficient rest.	Conserves energy and avoids overexertion to minimize fatigue/uterine irritability.
Review home/employment situation, noting activity levels and individual responses.	Promotes collaborative problem solving and may enhance participation in modifications of activity.
Discuss activity prescription/limitations.	Therapeutic regimen may dictate specific modifications depending on symptoms and previous history.
Encourage adequate rest and use of lateral position.	Increases uterine blood flow and may decrease uterine irritability/activity.
Instruct client to avoid heavy lifting, strenuous activity/housework, sports, and motor trips longer than 1–2 hr. (Note: Client with cardiac condition may have more severe restrictions.)	Previously tolerated activity may not be indicated for women at risk. Aerobic exercise/abdominal muscle strain may decrease uterine blood flow and increase uterine irritability.
Instruct client to modify or eliminate any type of sexual activity in the presence of symptoms of preterm labor, cervical changes, or bleeding.	Sexual activity, including orgasms and breast stimulation, appears to increase uterine irritability, owing to release of oxytocin.
Recommend avoiding travel and altitude changes in the third trimester.	Motion of travel, prolonged sitting position, and decreased oxygen appear to increase uterine irritability.
Stress importance of quiet diversional activities.	Prevents boredom and enhances cooperation with activity restrictions.

Collaborative

ACTIONS/INTERVENTIONS	RATIONALE
Encourage modified/complete bedrest as indicated.	Activity level may need modification, depending on symptoms of uterine activity, cervical changes, or bleeding. Note: Generalized weakness may develop as a result of prescribed total bedrest with concerns for self-care and independence in the postpartal period.

NURSING DIAGNOSIS:	Coping, Individual/Family, ineffective: risk for compromised
Risk Factors May Include:	Situational crisis, personal vulnerability, inadequate support systems

Possibly Evidenced By:	[Not applicable; presence of signs/symptoms establishes an *actual* diagnosis]
DESIRED OUTCOMES/EVALUATION CRITERIA—CLIENT/FAMILY WILL:	Identify ineffective coping behaviors and consequences.
	Verbalize awareness of own strengths/coping abilities.
	Demonstrate coping by discussing fears and dealing positively with the situation.
	Seek help appropriately.

ACTIONS/INTERVENTIONS	RATIONALE

Independent

Assess past and present coping strategies and emotional response to event/diagnosis.	In coping with a high-risk pregnancy, the client/couple/family often uses denial, then guilt, blame, or feelings of ambivalence, as emotional protection from possible loss of the pregnancy and fetus/newborn.
Evaluate client's/couple's support systems, including ability to comfort one another. Note negative coping, and discuss consequences.	Often, as a protective mechanism, the client and her partner do not form positive emotional attachment ("give of themselves") to the fetus. Lack of adequate support systems and failure to achieve the normal developmental tasks of pregnancy may result in continuation of high-risk situation into the childrearing phase and may create potential problems associated with physical or emotional child abuse and high-risk parenting.
Discuss normalcy of feelings; encourage couple to verbalize (separately and together) their feelings and concerns.	Helps assure client/couple that feelings are appropriate in high-risk situation; promotes open lines of communication. Note: One member of the couple may be reluctant to discuss fears openly in front of partner; may require additional support to facilitate interaction with one another.
Note client reports of increasing fatigue and inability to manage daily household activities.	Lack of family's assistance may indicate a need for help to resolve situation. Client may be reluctant to relinquish responsibilities and/or significant other(s) may be preoccupied with own emotional conflicts/personal suffering and express lack of understanding/knowledge about how to be helpful.
Encourage family restructure daily activities to meet client's needs without negating their own needs.	Family may need assistance in recognition of the importance of time planning to meet such needs as increased rest during pregnancy. However, family needs to work as a group to problem-solve solutions that meet individual needs and prevent negative feelings and "sabotage behaviors."
Obtain/review history of increasing severity of symptoms, especially if hospitalization is necessary.	Problems may require a reduction in activity level and/or hospitalization, necessitating changes in family life.

Collaborative

Identify available community support groups.	Discussion of situation with others who share the same problem can be helpful and can enhance problem solving.

Refer family for homemaker/child care and financial assistance as necessary.	Additional outside assistance with everyday activities, sibling care, and/or financial help may be required for client to cope positively with daily needs/therapy regimen.
Refer for counseling as appropriate.	May be needed in presence of negative coping to assure attachment to pregnancy/fetus/newborn. Helps to resolve concerns and/or develop effective coping skills; may prevent high-risk parenting.

NURSING DIAGNOSIS:	**Family Processes, risk for altered**
Risk Factors May Include:	Situational crisis
Possibly Evidenced By:	[Not applicable; presence of signs/symptoms establishes an *actual* diagnosis]
DESIRED OUTCOMES/EVALUATION CRITERIA—FAMILY WILL:	Express feelings freely and appropriately.
	Direct energies in a purposeful manner to plan for resolution of crisis.
	Seek appropriate help.

ACTIONS/INTERVENTIONS

RATIONALE

Independent

Determine degree of lifestyle change and extent of financial burden/therapeutic restrictions of pregnancy.	Provides information to identify needs and create plan of care. As more high-risk care is managed in the home setting, including therapy for premature delivery, stressors affecting the family may be greatly magnified.
Encourage verbalization and sharing of feelings.	Helps promote integrity of mutual support system.
Assess verbal/nonverbal cues and negative behaviors, such as inappropriate diet, eating improperly; excessive use of alcohol, tobacco, or tranquilizers; and avoidance of discussion of concerns.	The client who does not appropriately verbalize negative feelings or hostility about the complicated pregnancy may express such feelings with nonverbal cues or behaviors.
Provide 1:1 interaction and support of partner. Promote open communication between partners.	Therapeutic restrictions may result in partner assuming multiple roles, caring for client, trying to manage emotional response and personal concerns for client/fetus with limited coping strategies.
Assess partner for behaviors that negatively affect family process.	Expectant fathers may begin working longer hours, spending increased amounts of time away from home, and abusing alcohol, which are signs of negative coping.
Assess siblings for negative, attention-getting behaviors toward parents or authority figures, such as difficulty in school, truancy, or failure to carry out responsibilities.	Such behaviors may signal anger, jealousy, or resentment of changes in lifestyle necessitated by the complicated pregnancy.
Involve in procedures and decisions regarding therapeutic regimen, when possible.	Provides client/family with some degree of control in what is often viewed as an uncontrollable situation.

107

Acknowledge strengths, such as client's effective monitoring for diabetes.

Provides positive reinforcement and helps client/couple to view efforts as worthwhile.

Provide anticipatory guidance.

Knowing what is ahead may decrease stress and allow time for adaptation.

Determine availability of resources, e.g., other caregivers, childcare volunteers, others willing to assist with housekeeping/meal preparation.

Adequate support may help client remain in home setting.

Encourage family to verbalize significance of situation if hospitalization is required.

Monitoring/therapeutic interventions are being done more frequently in the home setting; however, separation necessitated by hospitalization of the client may place stress on family members, who may also experience relief or guilt because the healthcare system has relieved them of the burden of care.

Collaborative

Refer to social worker, hospital chaplain, other families in similar situation, and/or community agencies, support groups.

May assist in providing sources of financial/emotional assistance.

Refer for professional counseling, if necessary.

May be needed to maintain family integrity. Family members who are not positively adjusting to a complicated pregnancy may experience a high level of stress and/or negative coping. Such negative coping may result in family distintegration, separation, or divorce.

NURSING DIAGNOSIS:	Therapeutic Regimen: Individual, risk for ineffective management
Risk Factors May Include:	Patient value system, health beliefs/cultural influences, issues of control, presence of anxiety, complexity of therapeutic regimen, economic difficulties, social support deficits, perceived seriousness/susceptibility
Possibly Evidenced By:	[Not applicable; presence of signs/symptoms establishes an *actual* diagnosis]
DESIRED OUTCOMES/EVALUATION CRITERIA—CLIENT WILL:	Participate in the prescribed regimen during pregnancy. Use appropriate self-care behaviors.

ACTIONS/INTERVENTIONS

RATIONALE

Independent

Identify cause of/contributing factors to perceived lack of cooperation.

The client/couple may find it difficult to follow a prescribed health regimen that significantly alters their lifestyle and requires a great deal of time and energy. In addition, loss of control and anxiety contribute to feelings of helplessness/hopelessness, which increase the possibility of rejection of specific therapeutic interventions. Furthermore, misunderstandings can result in client not following prescribed regimen.

Determine goals that client wants to achieve and the motivating factors.

Review availability and use of resources.

Assist client to reduce/modify causative factors of medical complication. Avoid being judgmental. Encourage an objective problem-solving approach using a cooperative decision-making model.

Discuss and have client demonstrate behaviors/ techniques in question.

Collaborative

Refer to community resources or to a peer who has had a positive outcome with a complicated pregnancy.

Full cooperation and commitment are needed to obtain or maintain control of condition.

Presence or absence of supportive resources can make the difference for the client and family in being able to manage the situation.

Gives a sense of control. Pointing out failure often leads to despair.

During pregnancy, control of condition may require many specific modified or new behaviors. Demonstration allows accurate assessment of learning.

Decreases overwhelming feelings of aloneness; provides role model and opportunity for sharing common experiences. Reinforces idea that efforts can have a positive outcome.

Prenatal Substance Dependence/Abuse

This disorder is a continuum of phases incorporating a cluster of cognitive, behavioral, and physiological symptoms that include loss of control over use of the substance and continued use of the substance, despite adverse maternal/fetal consequences (e.g., poor nutrition/weight gain, anemia, predisposition to infection, PIH, fetal defects/IUGR, fetal alcohol syndrome [FAS]). The drugs most often abused are alcohol, cocaine (crack), heroin, methamphetamine, barbiturates, marijuana, and phencyclidine (PCP). Care depends on the degree of abuse and whether the client is intoxicated or is in the withdrawal phase. The client who is addicted may not seek care during the prenatal period, compounding any existing or developing problems. In addition, negative attitudes on the part of society and often from caregivers affect the pregnant woman and her care.

A return to health consists of gaining a mastery and control over self and environment, and pleasure seeking that does not require the use of drugs.

(This plan of care is to be used in conjunction with the CP: The High-Risk Pregnancy.)

CLIENT ASSESSMENT DATA BASE

Activity/Rest

Lack of energy/fatigue, malaise
Incoordination, unsteady gait
Sleeplessness/insomnia; hyperactivity
Yawning (beyond first trimester)

Circulation

Systemic hypertension; orthostatic hypotension
Tachycardia, palpitations
Ventricular arrhythmias
History of endocarditis, sudden coronary artery spasm, myocardial infarction (rare)

Ego Integrity

Pregnancy usually not planned
May express indecision about pregnancy (i.e., issues of abortion, adoption), concern regarding
    involvement of social/legal agencies
Labile mood, irritability, lack of motivation, denial of problem
Low self-esteem; feelings of guilt regarding substance use, or grandiose behavior
Presence of stressors (financial, changes in lifestyle)
Increased dependency needs
Inadequate coping skills/support systems

Elimination

Diarrhea or constipation
Burning on urination; frequency, hesitancy, lower abdominal or back pain (UTI)

Food/Fluid

Appetite changes, anorexia, nausea, vomiting
Inadequate nutritional/fluid intake
Low weight gain
Pathological edema

Hygiene

Poor oral/body hygiene

Neurosensory

Dizziness
Slurred speech
Hyperactivity; tremors of hands, tongue, eyelids
Pupillary dilation or constriction, nystagmus, diplopia
Decreased attention span, impaired memory
Irritability, depression, confusion, hallucinations, delirium, coma
History of seizure activity

Pain/Discomfort

Low threshold for pain or decreased response to pain
Muscle pain, headache
Early uterine contractions
Pain on urination, vaginal itching

Respiration

Nasal sinus drainage, inflamed mucosa, nosebleeds, septal defect
Tachypnea
Frequent sore throats
Cigarette smoker/exposure to secondhand smoke
History of recurrent pneumonia
Gray mucus expectorated (signs of heavy "crack" cocaine smoking)

Safety

Hyperthermia, diaphoresis
Evidence of needle tracks on extremities
Presence of cellulitis, superficial abscesses, septic phlebitis
History or evidence of traumatic injuries; physical/emotional abuse
Inadequate maintenance of home environment
History of jaundice
Positive screen for hepatitis, STD, or HIV
Previous obstetric problems (e.g., PIH, abruptio placentae, premature rupture of membranes)
Fetal hyperactivity, bradycardia; or decreased fetal movement

Sexuality

Decreased libido
History of multiple sexual partners
Fundal height inappropriate for length of gestation
Vaginal spotting/bleeding; increased vaginal discharge
GPTPAL may reveal spontaneous abortion, premature birth/fetal death, meconium staining, LBW infant, fetal withdrawal/alcohol syndrome, infant death/sudden infant death syndrome (SIDS)

Social Interactions

Lack of support systems; self-imposed/forced isolation
Loss of job; financial problems
Relationship/family discord (manipulative behavior)

Teaching/Learning

Use of alcohol, prescription, OTC, and/or illicit drugs
Difficulty maintaining self drug-free; ineffective recovery attempts; drug hunger
Absence of/limited prenatal care or preparation
Lack of cooperation with therapeutic regimen

DIAGNOSTIC STUDIES

Toxicology Screen: Identifies drug(s) used and current status.
Various Blood Studies (e.g., Complete Blood Count with Differential [CBCD], Serum Glucose, Electrolytes): Determines presence of anemia and nutritional status.
Liver Studies: Detect presence and degree of involvement/damage.
Ultrasonography: Locates placental implantation; assesses fetal size in relation to length of gestation.
Chest X-Ray: Reveals presence of pneumonia, foreign body, emboli, or pulmonary edema.
Screening Tests/Cultures: Determine presence of infectious diseases.
Addiction Severity Index: Produces a "problem severity profile" of the client, including chemical, medical, psychological, legal, family/social, and employment/support aspects, indicating areas of treatment needs.

NURSING PRIORITIES

1. Promote physiological stability and well-being of client and fetus.
2. Support client's acceptance of reality of situation.
3. Facilitate learning of new ways to reduce anxiety; strengthen individual coping skills.
4. Incorporate client into supportive community environment.
5. Promote family involvement in treatment process.
6. Provide information about condition, prognosis, and treatment needs.

DISCHARGE GOALS

1. Free of injury/complications to self and fetus/newborn.
2. Engaged in treatment modalities by identifying and using support systems.
3. Responsibility for own life and behavior assumed.
4. Abstinence from drug(s) maintained on a day-to-day basis.
5. Dependence condition and its impact on pregnancy, prognosis, and therapeutic regimen verbalized.
6. Participation in follow-up care by making and keeping all appointments, managing therapeutic regimen.

NURSING DIAGNOSIS:	Nutrition: altered, less than body requirements
May Be Related To:	Insufficient dietary intake to meet metabolic needs for psychological, physiological, or economic reasons
Possibly Evidenced By:	Low-weight gain, prepregnant weight below norm for height/body build, decreased subcutaneous fat/muscle mass, poor muscle tone, reported altered taste sensation, lack of interest in food; sore, inflamed buccal cavity; laboratory evidence of protein/vitamin deficiencies
DESIRED OUTCOMES/EVALUATION CRITERIA—CLIENT WILL:	Verbalize understanding of effects of substance abuse and reduced dietary intake on nutritional status and pregnancy.
	Demonstrate behaviors and lifestyle changes to regain/maintain appropriate weight for pregnancy.
	Demonstrate progressive weight gain toward goal, with normalization of laboratory values and absence of signs of malnutrition.

ACTIONS/INTERVENTIONS	RATIONALE

Independent

Determine age, height/weight, body build, strength, and activity/rest pattern. Note condition of oral cavity.	Provides information on which to base caloric needs/dietary plan. Type of diet/foods may be affected by condition of mucous membranes and teeth.
Obtain anthropometric measurements, e.g., triceps skinfold.	Calculates subcutaneous fat and muscle mass to aid in determining dietary needs.
Note total daily calorie intake. Encourage client to maintain a diary of intake, times, and patterns of eating.	Information about patient's dietary pattern will identify nutritional strengths, needs, and deficiencies.
Discuss prenatal nutritional needs and develop dietary plan. Assist with developing a grocery budget and provide opportunity to choose foods or snacks to meet dietary plan.	Enhances participation/sense of control and may promote resolution of nutritional deficiencies.
Evaluate energy expenditure (e.g., pregnancy needs, pacing or sedentary activities), and establish an individualized exercise program.	Pregnant state and activity level affect nutritional needs. Exercise enhances muscle tone, may stimulate appetite, and promotes sense of well-being.
Weigh client weekly and record.	Provides information regarding current status/effectiveness of dietary plan.

Collaborative

Consult with dietitian.	Useful in establishing individual dietary needs/plan. Provides additional resource for learning about the importance of nutrition in nonpregnant and pregnant states.
Review laboratory work as indicated; e.g., glucose, serum albumin, and electrolytes.	Identifies anemias, electrolyte imbalances, and other abnormalities that may be present, requiring specific therapy. Note: Toxic vapor abuse of toluene-based solvents (such as spray paint or glue) may cause a distal renal tubular acidosis with resultant hypokalemia, hypophosphatemia, hypomagnesemia, and hypocalcemia as well as rhabdomyolysis.
Refer for dental consultation as necessary.	Teeth are essential to good nutritional intake, and dental hygiene/care is often neglected in this population.

NURSING DIAGNOSIS:	**Denial, ineffective/Coping, individual, ineffective**
May Be Related To:	Personal vulnerability, difficulty handling new situations, previous ineffective/inadequate coping skills with substitution of drug(s), inadequate support systems, anxiety/fear
Possibly Evidenced By:	Denial (one of the strongest and most resistant symptoms of substance abuse), lack of acceptance that drug use is causing the present situation, use of manipulation to avoid responsibility for self, altered social patterns/participation, impaired adaptive behavior and problem-solving skills,

Possibly Evidenced By (cont.):	decreased ability to handle stress of illness/hospitalization, financial affairs in disarray, scholastic or employment difficulties (e.g., losing time on job/not maintaining steady employment, poor work performance, on-the-job injuries)
DESIRED OUTCOMES/EVALUATION CRITERIA—CLIENT WILL:	Verbalize awareness of relationship of substance abuse to current situation.
	Identify ineffective coping behaviors and their consequences.
	Use effective coping skills/problem solving.
	Initiate necessary lifestyle changes.
	Attend support group (e.g., Cocaine/Narcotics/Alcoholics Anonymous) regularly.

ACTIONS/INTERVENTIONS	RATIONALE
Independent	
Determine client's understanding of pregnancy and current situation and previous methods of coping with life's problems.	Provides information about degree of denial; identifies coping skills that may be used in present plan of care.
Remain nonjudgmental. Be alert to changes in behavior; e.g., restlessness, increased tension.	Confrontation can lead to increased agitation, which may compromise safety of client/staff.
Provide positive feedback when client expresses awareness of denial in self and recognizes it in others.	Denial is the major defense mechanism in addictive disease and may block progress of therapy until client accepts reality of the problem. Positive feedback is necessary to enhance self-esteem and to reinforce insight into behavior.
Maintain firm expectation that client will attend recovery support/therapy groups regularly.	Attending is related to admitting need for help, to working with denial and for an optimal outcome of the pregnancy, as well as maintenance of a long-term drug-free existence.
Provide information about addictive use versus experimental, occasional use of drugs; biochemical/genetic disorder theory (genetic predisposition); and use activated by environment, pharmacology of stimulant, or compulsive desire as a lifelong occurrence.	Progression of use continuum in the addict is from experimental/recreational to addictive use. Comprehending this process is important in combatting denial. Education may relieve client of guilt and blame, and may help awareness of recurring addictive characteristics.
Discuss ways to use diversional activities that relate to recovery (e.g., social activities within support group) wherein issues of being chemically free are examined.	Discovery of alternative methods of recreation and methods for coping with drug hunger can remind client that addiction is a lifelong process and that opportunity for changing patterns is available.
Encourage and support client's taking responsibility for own recovery (e.g., development of alternative behaviors to drug use).	When client accepts the reality of own responsibility, denial can be replaced with responsible action.
Set limits and confront efforts to get caregiver to grant special privileges, making excuses for not following through on behaviors agreed on, and attempting to continue drug use.	Client has learned manipulative behavior throughout life and needs to learn a new way of getting needs met. Following through on consequences of failure to maintain limits can help the client to change ineffective behaviors.
Assist client to learn relaxation skills, guided imagery, or visualizations; encourage her to use them.	Helps client to relax and develop new ways to deal with stress and problem-solve.

Be aware of family/staff enabling behaviors and feelings.

Lack of understanding of enabling and codependence can result in nontherapeutic approaches to addicts.

Collaborative

Administer medications as indicated, noting restrictions on use in pregnancy:

Phenobarbital;

Can be used to ease alcohol withdrawal and prevent/reduce frequency and severity of seizures.

Methadone.

This drug is thought to blunt the craving for, and/or diminish the effects of, heroin and is used to assist in withdrawal and long-term maintenance programs. It has fewer side effects than heroin and allows the client to maintain daily activities and ultimately withdraw from drug use.

Encourage involvement with self-help associations; e.g., Alcoholics/Narcotics Anonymous.

Puts client in direct contact with support systems necessary for managing sobriety/drug-free life. Self-help groups are valuable for learning and promoting abstinence in each member with understanding and support as well as peer pressure.

NURSING DIAGNOSIS:	**Powerlessness**
May Be Related To:	Substance addiction with or without periods of abstinence, episodic compulsive indulgence, failed attempts at recovery, lifestyle of helplessness, self-imposed or forced isolation
Possibly Evidenced By:	Ineffective recovery attempts, statements of inability to stop behavior (even with awareness of effects on pregnancy) and/or requests for help, continuous/constant thinking about drug and/or obtaining drug; alterations in personal, occupational, and social life
	Remaining in home, no friends or contact with family
DESIRED OUTCOMES/EVALUATION CRITERIA—CLIENT WILL:	Admit inability to control drug habit, surrender to powerlessness over addiction.
	Involve self in treatment and verbalize awareness that willpower alone cannot maintain abstinence.
	Engage in peer support.
	Demonstrate active participation in program.
	Maintain healthy state during pregnancy with an optimal outcome.

ACTIONS/INTERVENTIONS	RATIONALE

Independent

Use crisis intervention techniques:

Client is more amenable to acceptance of need for treatment in the crisis presented by the pregnancy. Note: Typical binging pattern of cocaine use may promote or inhibit client's responsiveness to intervention.

Assist client to recognize that a problem exists;	While client is hurting and recognizing that substance abuse is harmful to her fetus, it is easier to admit drug use is a problem.
Assess interactions with significant other. Note domination by parents or client's unwillingness to respond in partner's presence;	A woman can experience self-imposed or forced isolation as a result of drug dependence and/or societal rejection of drug use during pregnancy. Potential volatility of situation may require careful consideration of safety issues. Note: Forced isolation is also a form of abuse.
Assist in developing plan to leave abusive environment/situation;	
Identify goals for change;	Helpful in planning direction for care and promoting belief that change can occur.
Discuss alternative solutions;	Brainstorming helps creatively identify possibilities and provides sense of control.
Assist in selecting most appropriate alternative;	As possibilities are discussed, the most useful solution becomes clear.
Support decision and implementation of selected alternative(s).	Helps the client to persevere in process of change.
Discuss need for help in a caring, nonjudgmental way.	A caring, nonconfrontational manner is more therapeutic because the client may respond defensively to a moralistic attitude, blocking recovery.
Discuss ways in which drug use has interfered with life, occupation, and personal/interpersonal relationships.	Awareness of how the drug has controlled the client's life is important in combatting denial/sense of powerlessness.
Assist client to learn ways to enhance health, meet pregnancy needs, and structure healthy diversion from drug use (e.g., a balanced diet, adequate rest, acupuncture, biofeedback, deep meditative techniques, and exercise, such as walking, swimming, or other activity tailored to pregnant state).	Learning to empower self in constructive areas can strengthen ability to continue recovery. These activities help restore natural biochemical balance, aid detoxification, and manage stress, anxiety, and use of free time as well as promote positive pregnancy outcomes. These diversions can increase self-confidence, thereby improving self-esteem. Note: Release of endorphins from sustained exercise can create a feeling of well-being.
Assist in self-examination of spirituality and faith.	Surrendering to a power greater than oneself and faith in that power have been found to be effective in substance recovery; may decrease sense of powerlessness.
Assist client to learn assertive communication.	Effective in assisting in ability to refuse use, to stop relationships with users and dealers, to build healthy relationships, and to regain control of own life.

Collaborative

Refer to/assist with making appointment to treatment program, e.g., partial hospitalization drug treatment programs, Narcotics/Alcoholics Anonymous; shelter for abused women.	Follow-through on appointments may be easier than making the initial contact, and continuing treatment is essential to positive outcome of both substance abuse problem and pregnancy. Note: To date, treatment programs admitting pregnant clients have been very limited in number, reducing treatment options and jeopardizing client/fetal outcomes.
Discuss possibility of private addiction counseling.	Private counseling may be needed, especially when isolation has occurred, until client feels comfortable in group setting.

NURSING DIAGNOSIS:	Self Esteem, chronic situational low
May Be Related To:	Social stigma attached to substance abuse, social expectation that one control own behavior (e.g., abuse of drugs, sexual activity, and use of birth control), biochemical body change (e.g., withdrawal from alcohol/drugs), situational crisis of pregnancy with loss of control over life events
Possibly Evidenced By:	Not taking responsibility for self/self-care, lack of follow-through, self-destructive behavior, change in usual role patterns or responsibility (family, job, legal); confusion about self, purpose, or direction in life; denial that substance use is a problem
DESIRED OUTCOMES/EVALUATION CRITERIA—CLIENT WILL:	Identify feelings and methods for coping with negative perception of self.
	Verbalize acceptance of self "as is" and an increased sense of worth.
	Set goals and participate in realistic planning for lifestyle changes necessary to live without drugs and bring pregnancy to the desired outcome.

ACTIONS/INTERVENTIONS	RATIONALE

Independent

Provide opportunity for, and encourage verbalization/discussion of, individual situation.	Client often has difficulty expressing self and even more difficulty accepting the degree of importance substance has assumed in life and its relationship to present situation/pregnancy. Note: Pregnancy may not have been planned, and client may feel indecisive about plans for the future.
Assess mental status. Note presence of other psychiatric disorders (dual diagnosis).	May affect decisions regarding pregnancy. Many clients use substances (alcohol and other drugs) to seek relief from depression or anxiety. Note: Approximately 60% of substance-dependent individuals also have mental illness problems, and treatment for both is imperative for optimal outcome.
Spend time with client. Discuss client's behavior/substance use in a nonjudgmental way.	Presence of the nurse conveys acceptance of the individual as a worthwhile person. Discussion provides opportunity for insight into the problems that substance abuse has created for the client.
Provide reinforcement for positive actions, and encourage client to accept this input.	Failure and lack of self-esteem have been problems for this client, who needs to learn to accept self as an individual with positive attributes.
Observe family/significant other interactions; note dynamics and presence/effectiveness of support.	Substance abuse is a family disease, and how the members act and react to the client's pregnancy and her behavior affects the course of the disease and how client sees herself. Many unconsciously become "enablers," helping the individual to cover up the consequences of the abuse. (Refer to NDs: Family Coping: ineffective, compromised/disabling; Caregiver Role Strain.)
Encourage expression of feelings of guilt, shame, and anger.	The client often has lost respect for self and believes that the situation is hopeless. Expression of

117

Help the client to acknowledge that substance use is the problem and that problems can be dealt with, without the use of drugs. Confront the use of defenses (e.g., denial, projection, rationalization).

these feelings helps the client begin to accept responsibility for self and take steps to make changes.

When drugs can no longer be blamed for the problems that exist, the client can begin to deal with them and live without substance use. Confrontation helps the client accept the reality of the problems as they exist.

Ask the client to list and review past accomplishments and positive happenings, including previous pregnancy experiences.

There are things in everyone's life that have been successful. Often when self-esteem is low, it is difficult to remember these successes or to view them as successes.

Use techniques of role rehearsal.

Assists client to practice the development of skills to cope with new role as a person who no longer uses or needs drugs to handle life's problems.

Collaborative

Involve client in group therapy.

Group sharing helps encourage verbalization because other members of group are in various stages of abstinence from drugs and can address the client's concerns/denial. The client can gain new skills, hope, and a sense of family or community from group participation.

Refer to other resources, such as Narcotics/Alcoholics Anonymous.

One of the oldest and most popular forms of group treatment uses a basic strategy known as the Twelve Steps. The client admits powerlessness over drug, and, although not necessary, may seek help from a higher power. Members help one another, and meetings are available at many different times and places in most communities. The philosophy of "one day at a time" helps attain the goal of abstinence.

Formulate plan to treat other mental illness problems.

Clients who seek relief for other mental health problems through drugs will continue to do so. Both the substance use and the mental health problems need to be treated together to maximize abstinence potential.

Administer antipsychotic medications as necessary, noting precautions of use in pregnancy.

Prolonged/profound psychosis following LSD or PCP use can be treated with antipsychotic drugs because it is probably the result of an underlying functional psychosis that has now emerged. Note: Avoid the use of phenothiazines because they may decrease seizure threshold and cause hypotension in the presence of LSD/PCP.

NURSING DIAGNOSIS:	Family Coping: ineffective, compromised/disabling/Caregiver Role Strain
May Be Related To:	Personal vulnerability of individual family members, codependency issues, situational crises of drug abuse and pregnancy, compromised social systems, family disorganization/role changes, prolonged disease progression that exhausts supportive capability of family members; significant person(s) with chronically unexpressed feelings of guilt, anger, hostility, or despair

Possibly Evidenced By:

Denial, or belief that all problems are caused by substance use; severely dysfunctional family (family violence, spouse/child abuse, separation/divorce, children displaying acting-out behaviors); financial affairs in disarray; school/employment difficulties; altered social patterns/participation; significant other demonstrating enabling or codependent behaviors (avoiding and shielding, attempting to control, taking over responsibilities, rationalizing and accepting, cooperating and collaborating, rescuing and self-serving)

DESIRED OUTCOMES/EVALUATION CRITERIA—FAMILY WILL:

Verbalize understanding of dynamics of codependence and participate in individual and family programs.

Identify ineffective coping behaviors/consequences.

Demonstrate/plan for necessary lifestyle changes.

Take action to change self-destructive behaviors and/or alter behavior that contributes to client's addiction.

ACTIONS/INTERVENTIONS	RATIONALE

Independent

Assess family history; explore roles of family members and circumstances involving drug use, strengths, and areas for growth. Note attitudes/beliefs regarding pregnancy and parenting.	Determine areas for focus and potential for change.
Explore how the family/significant other has coped with the client's habit (e.g., denial, repression, rationalization, hurt, loneliness, projection).	The codependent person suffers from the same feelings as the client (e.g., anxiety, self-hatred, helplessness, low self-worth, guilt) and needs help in learning new/effective coping skills.
Determine understanding of current situation/pregnancy and previous methods of coping with life's problems.	Identifies misconceptions/areas of need on which to base present plan of care.
Assess current level of functioning of family members.	Affects individual's ability to cope with situation.
Determine extent of enabling behaviors being evidenced by family members; explore with individual and client.	Enabling is doing for the client what she needs to do for herself. People want to be helpful and do not want to feel powerless to help their loved one to stop substance use and change the behavior that is so destructive. However, in many cases the substance abuser relies on others to cover up his or her own inability to cope with daily responsibilities.
Provide information about enabling behavior and addictive disease characteristics for both user and nonuser person who is codependent.	Awareness and knowledge provide opportunity for individuals to begin the process of change.
Provide factual information to client and family about the effects of addictive behaviors on the family and what to expect regarding abstinence from drugs and course of pregnancy.	Many individuals are not aware of the nature of addiction, the involvement of the family, and the effects on pregnancy/fetus. Note: If client is using legally obtained drugs, user and family members may believe this does not constitute abuse.
Encourage family members to be aware of their own feelings and to look at the situation with	When the codependent family members become aware of their own actions that perpetuate the

119

perspective and objectivity. They can ask themselves, "Am I being conned? Am I acting out of fear, shame, guilt, or anger? Do I have a need to control?"

Involve significant other in referral plans.

Be aware of staff's enabling behaviors and feelings about client, pregnancy, and partners who are codependent.

addict's problems, they can decide to change themselves. If they change, the client can then face the consequences of her own actions and may choose to get well.

Drug abuse is a family illness. Because the family has been so involved in dealing with the substance abuse behavior, they need help adjusting to the new behavior of sobriety/abstinence. Incidence of recovery is almost doubled when the family is treated along with the client.

Lack of understanding of enabling and codependence can result in nontherapeutic approaches to addicts and their families. Staff members may feel angry toward client who uses or continues to use drug(s), even though she has been given information regarding possibility of damage to the developing fetus.

Collaborative

Encourage involvement with self-help associations (e.g., Alcoholics/Narcotics Anonymous, Al-Anon, Al-Ateen) and professional family therapy.

Puts client/family in direct contact with support systems necessary for continued sobriety and assistance with learning problem resolution.

NURSING DIAGNOSIS:	Knowledge deficit [Learning Need], regarding condition/pregnancy, prognosis, self-care and treatment needs
May be Related To:	Lack/misinterpretation of information, lack of recall, cognitive limitations/interference with learning (other mental illness problems/organic brain syndrome)
Possibly Evidenced By:	Statements of concern, questions/misconceptions, inaccurate follow-through of instructions, development of preventable complications, continued use in spite of complications/bad trips
DESIRED OUTCOMES/EVALUATION CRITERIA—CLIENT WILL:	Verbalize understanding of own condition, prognosis, and treatment plan.
	Identify/initiate necessary lifestyle changes to remain drug-free with optimal pregnancy outcome.
	Participate in treatment program.
	Recognize health problems as they arise and initiate steps to resolve.

ACTIONS/INTERVENTIONS	RATIONALE

Independent

Provide information about effects of drugs on the reproductive system/fetus (e.g., increased risk of STDs, premature birth, brain damage, and fetal malformation). Review drinking/drug history of client/partner.

Awareness of the negative efforts of alcohol/other drugs on reproduction may motivate client to stop using drug(s). When client is pregnant, identification of potential problems aids in planning for future fetal needs/concerns.

Encourage regular physical examination, including vaginal culture to detect presence of STD.

Vaginal cultures can detect the presence of microorganisms that can be potentially fatal to the fetus or newborn group B streptococcus (GBS), chlamydia, syphilis, gonorrhea.

Review results of sonogram.

Assesses fetal growth and development to identify possibility of IUGR or FAS and future needs.

Be aware of, and deal with, anxiety of client and family members.

Anxiety can interfere with ability to hear and assimilate information.

Provide an active role for the client/partner in the learning process through discussions, group participation, and role playing.

Learning is enhanced when people are actively involved.

Provide various information, as indicated. Include list of articles, books, tapes, and videos related to client/family needs, and encourage reading and discussing what they learn.

Helps individuals to make informed choices about future. Bibliotherapy can be a useful addition to other therapy approaches if materials chosen consider the individual's educational and cognitive abilities.

Assess client's knowledge of own situation, i.e., pregnancy, complications, and needed changes in lifestyle.

Assists in planning for long-range changes necessary for maintaining sobriety/drug-free status. Client may have street knowledge of the drug but be ignorant of medical facts and relationship to pregnancy.

Review condition and prognosis/future expectations.

Provides knowledge base on which client can make informed choices.

Time activities to individual needs.

Facilitates learning because information is more readily assimilated when individual learning pace is considered.

In many cases, client has misperception (denial) of real reason for admission to the medical or psychiatric setting when hospitalized.

Discuss relationship of drug use to current situation/pregnancy.

Discuss variety of helpful organizations and programs that are available for assistance/referral.

Long-term support is necessary to maintain optimal recovery and/or assist with pregnancy needs. Psychosocial needs as well as other issues may require addressing.

The Pregnant Adolescent

Statistics for 1995 reveal that 56.9 babies were born for every 1000 females between the ages of 15 and 19. Although these rates appear to be dropping, pregnant adolescents are at risk physically, emotionally, and socially. The impact of adolescent pregnancy on the individual has far-reaching consequences, which may restrict or limit future opportunities for the adolescent and the child(ren). Educational goals may be altered or eliminated, thus limiting potential for a productive life. The client frequently may be of lower socioeconomic status, with the pregnancy perpetuating financial dependence and lowered self-esteem. Statistically, the obstetric hazards for adolescents and their infants include increased mortality and morbidity rates. Therefore, individualized prenatal nursing care for the adolescent client/family/partner that incorporates developmental needs and health education with prenatal needs has the potential to contribute positively to prenatal, intrapartal, and postpartal outcomes. In addition, neonatal outcomes associated with better Apgar scores, lower incidence of resuscitation, and fewer LBW infants can also be expected.

(Refer to CPs: First Trimester, Second Trimester; Third Trimester, for discussion of usual/expected pregnancy needs.)

CLIENT ASSESSMENT DATA BASE

(In addition to Prenatal Client Assessment Data Base)

Circulation

Elevated blood pressure (risk indicator of PIH)

Ego Integrity

Pregnancy may or may not be wanted by client; may be result of abuse.
Varied cultural/religious responses to pregnancy out of wedlock; or as a stressor on teen marriage (note whether client's mother was a teenage mother).
Expressions of worthlessness, discounting self.
Decision making varies from abdicating all responsibility to extreme independence.
May or may not be involved with father of child by own/partner's choice, family demands, or question of paternity.
May feel helpless, hopeless; fear family/peer response.
Emotional status varies; for example, calm, acceptance, denial, hysteria.
History of limited/no financial resources.

Elimination

Proteinuria (risk indicator of PIH)

Food/Fluid

Weight gain may be less than optimal.
Dietary choices may not include all food groups (adolescent eating patterns; presence of eating disorder).
Edema (risk indicator of PIH).
Hb and/or Hct may reveal anemia and hemoconcentration, suggesting PIH.

Hygiene

Dress may be inappropriate for stage of gestation (e.g., wearing restrictive or bulky clothing to conceal pregnancy).

Respiratory

May be a cigarette smoker

Safety

History/presence of STDs.
Fundal height may be less than normal for gestation (indicating IUGR of fetus).
Ultrasonography may reveal inappropriate fetal growth, low-lying placental implantation.

Sexuality

Lack of/incorrect use of contraception.
Pelvic measurements may be borderline/contracted.

Social Interactions

May report problems with family dynamics, lack of available resources/support
Little or no concept of reality of situation; future expectations, potential responsibilities
History of encounters with judicial systems

Teaching/Learning

Level of maturity varies/may regress; barriers of age and developmental stage.
Experimentation with substance use or abuse.
Lack of achievement in school.
Lack of awareness of own health/pregnancy needs.
Fantasies/fears about childbirth.

NURSING PRIORITIES

1. Promote optimal physical/emotional well-being of client.
2. Monitor fetal well-being.
3. Provide information and review the available options.
4. Facilitate positive adaptation to new and changing roles.
5. Encourage family/partner participation in problem-solving.

DISCHARGE GOALS

Inpatient care is not required unless complications develop necessitating hospitalization (refer to appropriate plans of care.)

NURSING DIAGNOSIS:	Nutrition: altered, less than body requirements
May Be Related To:	Intake insufficient to meet metabolic demands
Possibly Evidenced By:	Lack of information, misconceptions, body weight below (or possibly above) ideal, inappropriate uterine/fetal growth; reported intake that does not meet recommended daily allowance (RDA); anemia, PIH
DESIRED OUTCOMES/EVALUATION CRITERIA—CLIENT WILL:	Ingest nutritionally adequate diet.
	Gain prescribed weight.
	Take daily iron/vitamin supplement as appropriate.
	Maintain normal Hb and Hct levels, free of anemia and without signs of PIH.

ACTIONS/INTERVENTIONS	RATIONALE

Independent

Assess dietary intake using 24-hr recall.	Information about current intake is helpful/necessary to planning changes or additions for adequate diet. Adolescents, especially age 17 or younger, are at risk for malnutrition, because their normally increased bodily requirements for growth

123

Weigh client and determine pregravid weight. Provide information about risk of dieting in pregnancy.	are stressed by the metabolic demands associated with pregnancy.
	Weight gain needed during pregnancy is calculated according to normal growth demands and prepregnancy weight. Food idiosyncrasies, which are related to the adolescent's developmental stage, and delayed prenatal care contribute to poor or inadequate intake, possible fetal IUGR and resultant LBW infant, and maternal complications such as PIH and associated uterine ischemia. Weight loss places client and fetus at risk for acidosis.
Provide individual prescription for weight gain based on growth needs and pregravid weight, recognizing adolescent lifestyle and preferences for "fast foods."	Adequate calories are necessary to spare proteins and ensure iron intake. On average, an underweight client needs an additional 500 cal daily; an overweight client needs 17 cal/lb of pregnancy weight.
Stress importance of daily vitamin/iron intake. (Refer to CP: First Trimester; ND: Nutrition: altered, risk for less than body requirements.)	Pregnant adolescents are prone to problems of malnutrition and anemia, owing to incomplete growth and/or dietary habits, which necessitate increased dietary protein, iron, and calories.
Identify individual protein requirement.	Requirements in pregnancy for the client ages 15–18 yr are equal to 1.5 g/kg of pregnant body weight; for clients younger than age 15 yr, requirements equal 1.7 g/kg of pregnant body weight.
Provide information about role of protein in terms of maternal/fetal development.	Low/inadequate protein intake during pregnancy, especially in the first trimester, places fetus at risk for IUGR and lack of brain cell hyperplasia and hypertrophy, and may contribute to development of maternal PIH. (Refer to CP: Pregnancy-Induced Hypertension)
Assess client's situation, and determine who is responsible for food purchasing and meal preparation. Provide information about ways of improving nutritional intake.	Socioeconomic status/financial concerns, cultural issues or lack of experience with grocery shopping and meal preparation may interfere with proper nutrition.

Collaborative

Refer to WIC program through local public health department.	When client qualifies, programs such as this enable the adolescent to manage a better nutritional program.
Assess Hb/Hct initially and again at 7 months' gestation.	Iron deficiency anemia, which is common in the adolescent, places the fetus at risk for lowered Hb/Hct levels and for continuation of low iron stores/iron deficiency anemia in the infant after delivery.

NURSING DIAGNOSIS:	**Knowledge deficit [Learning Need], regarding pregnancy process, individual needs, future expectations**
May Be Related To:	Lack of information, unfamiliarity with resources, information misinterpretation, lack of interest in learning, developmental stage/cognitive deficit, psychological stressors/absence of support systems

Possibly Evidenced By:	Request for information, statement of misconception, inaccurate follow-through of instructions, development of complications
DESIRED OUTCOMES/EVALUATION CRITERIA—CLIENT WILL:	Participate in learning process.
	Verbalize understanding of condition.
	Discuss and adhere to components of adequate prenatal diet.
	Identify potential teratogens, physiological/psychological aspects of reproduction, pregnancy, labor, and delivery.

ACTIONS/INTERVENTIONS	RATIONALE

Independent

Evaluate client's age and stage of adolescent development.	The age and stage of the adolescent will influence the approach to teaching because the late adolescent (aged 17–20 yr) may be better able to conceptualize, process, and synthesize information than the client in early (aged 11–14 yr) or middle (aged 14–17 yr) adolescence.
Note readiness to learn.	Depending on the stage of development, the adolescent is self-focusing. Because of difficulty recognizing the need or importance of learning, the client may not be motivated.
Encourage client to explore options regarding outcomes of pregnancy, including termination of pregnancy (dependent on stage of gestation), keeping the baby, or giving the baby up for adoption. (Note implications of culture on decisions.)	Although currently many adolescents elect to keep their babies, the client must be given freedom of choice based on available options. In some situations and/or cultures (e.g., Cambodian), the family makes decisions about the pregnancy for the adolescent rather than allowing her to make her own decisions.
Assess client's understanding of female/male anatomy and physiology. Provide appropriate information; correct misconceptions.	For the pregnant client in early adolescence, pregnancy and parenthood are often not recognized as possible outcomes of sexual activity.
Assess factors related to high rate of recidivism. Identify community resources and potential support systems.	If pregnancy is not accompanied by emotional maturation, a high rate of recidivism may be anticipated, especially if the teenager uses sexual activity to demonstrate independence or enhance her self-concept. A comprehensive assessment of the adolescent mother and early intervention are helpful in preventing second and subsequent unplanned pregnancies.
Obtain drug use/abuse history; screen for STDs and for HIV risk behaviors. Provide information about possible negative effects on fetus. (Refer to ND: Injury, risk for fetal [following] and in CP: First Trimester; and CPs: The High-Risk Pregnancy, Prenatal Infection.)	Helps prevent fetal complications. Adolescents, however, frequently do not enter the healthcare system until the second trimester, by which time fetal injury may already have occurred. Reasons for this delay include shame, fear of parental reaction, denial, and failure to recognize pregnancy.
Provide information about nutrition, meal planning, and need to avoid empty calories. (Refer to ND: Nutrition: altered, less than body requirements.)	In desiring to achieve independence, adolescents may repeat poor nutritional habits practiced by parents/peers, thereby risking malnutrition, IUGR, and birth of LBW infant.

125

Refer client to adolescent clinic for peer support and informational services, such as prenatal, parenting, and infant care classes.

Adolescent clinics, which are responsive to the unique needs of the teenager, provide information in concrete terms, which is appropriate for the client unable to cope with abstractions or to solve problems based on inference.

Provide information about importance of establishing individual long-range personal and educational goals for client and her offspring. Refer to appropriate social agencies.

Two out of three pregnant adolescents drop out of school, which often results in their being economically dependent on the welfare system, creating a perpetual cycle for the offspring. Establishing realistic educational goals may interrupt or prevent the development of this cycle.

Discuss signs of labor. Identify factors that place the adolescent at risk for preterm labor/delivery.

Client needs to know when to call the healthcare provider and how to differentiate between true and false labor.

Present/discuss available methods of birth control, giving advantages and disadvantages of each. Be realistic and nonjudgmental. Present information appropriate for the adolescent's particular developmental stage.

Information presented prenatally assists client in selection of contraception following delivery. Rates of recidivism tend to decrease if effective contraception material and methods are provided immediately after the pregnancy.

(Refer to CP: The High-Risk Pregnancy, ND: Knowledge deficit [Learning Need].)

NURSING DIAGNOSIS:	Injury, risk for fetal
May Be Related To:	Maternal malnutrition, preexisting health problems and/or maternal complications/susceptibility, inadequate prenatal care and screening
Possibly Evidenced By:	[Not applicable; presence of signs/symptoms establishes an *actual* diagnosis]
DESIRED OUTCOMES/EVALUATION CRITERIA—CLIENT WILL:	Verbalize understanding of individual risk factors.
	Demonstrate behaviors/lifestyle changes to reduce risk factors and protect self and fetus.
	Display fetal growth within normal limits.
	Carry pregnancy to term, with delivery of full-term infant of size appropriate for gestational age (AGA).

ACTIONS/INTERVENTIONS

RATIONALE

Independent

Assess for potential risks to fetus.

Infants born to adolescent mothers are at risk for prematurity, low birth weight, birth trauma, and resultant sequelae of mental retardation, cerebral palsy, and epilepsy.

Weigh client. Provide individual prescription for weight gain based on body structure, prepregnancy weight, and normal growth (anabolic) needs.

Clients who give birth to LBW infants weigh less before pregnancy and gain less prenatally. Statistics suggest that the birth weight of babies born to adolescent mothers averages 94 g less than that of babies born to older mothers.

Provide oral/written information about dietary

Malnutrition contributes to inadequate

requirements, sources of vitamins/minerals, and food groups. Rule out anorexia nervosa. (Refer to CP: The High-Risk Pregnancy; ND: Nutrition: altered, risk for less/more than body requirements.)

Discuss negative impact of dieting on the fetus.

development of neonatal/fetal brain cells during the prenatal hyperplasia phase and the combined hyperplasia/hypertrophy phase of the first 6 mo of life, resulting in fewer total brain cells and smaller individual cell size.

One in 10 adolescents who become pregnant is obese and, in many cases, is dieting during pregnancy, which results in weight loss, maternal/fetal acidosis, and possible CNS damage to the fetus, especially in the third trimester.

Stress importance of ongoing prenatal care.

Adolescents often feel well and do not follow up with prenatal protocols of care, especially if they do not understand the importance of frequent checkups and health promotion. This could result in inadequate screening and/or early intervention, which might impede normal fetal growth and development.

Discuss role and food sources of iron and need to supplement food intake with daily iron/folic acid.

Low maternal iron stores reduce available oxygen-carrying capacity and fetal oxygen uptake, decrease fetal iron stores during third trimester, and result in iron deficiency anemia of the infant.

Obtain sexual history, including STD exposure or episodes and high-risk behaviors for HIV. Note presence of active herpetic lesions or warts, and review culture reports. (Refer to CPs: The High-Risk Pregnancy, Prenatal Infection; ND: Injury, risk for fetal.)

STDs can contribute to fetal developmental problems as well as neonatal infections. STDs (including HIV) can either be transmitted to the fetus transplacentally or contracted during the delivery. Hepatitis and HIV are transmitted in blood products, so infant could contract either disease through vaginal or cesarean birth.

Provide information related to condom use/safer sexual practices if client is engaging in sexual activity outside of a monogamous relationship or with an at-risk partner. Discuss sexual abstinence.

Use of condoms/safer sexual behaviors tend to reduce risk of STD, including HIV infection. Although abstinence may be preferred, once an individual becomes sexually active, it is often difficult to make the decision to abstain.

Obtain history of use of tobacco, alcohol, or other substances; provide information about potentially harmful effects on fetal development. (Refer to CP: Prenatal Substance Dependence/Abuse.)

Adolescents typically have a higher substance abuse rate than nonadolescents, and in many cases, substance abuse occurs during critical periods of fetal development before client suspects she is pregnant. Substance abuse places the client at higher risk for complications of pregnancy and preterm labor.

Screen for PIH at each prenatal visit. (Refer to CP: Pregnancy-Induced Hypertension.)

Adolescents are at risk for developing PIH, possibly because of malnutrition and inadequate protein intake, which may cause placental inadequacies and placental separation (abruptio placentae).

Collaborative

Obtain pelvic measurements; determine prognosis for eutocia. Discuss possibility of cesarean birth if measurements are small.

Inadequate pelvic measurements because of physiological immaturity place the client/fetus at risk for cephalopelvic disproportion and potential fetal injury intrapartally.

Review results of diagnostic/screening studies:

Hb and Hct;

Reflect level of oxygen-carrying capacity and potential iron stores.

RPR; cultures for herpes virus (HV) and gonorrhea/chlamydia, group B streptococcus;

Identifies treatment needs. If HV cultures are positive just before labor/delivery, a cesarean section may be considered. (Refer to CP: Prenatal Infection.)

127

Serial ultrasonography;	Determines fetal growth. IUGR, possibly caused by malnutrition or vascular changes with PIH, is reflected in biparietal diameter, femur length, estimated fetal weight, and abdominal circumference that are below normal limits for gestational age. Assess placental/fetal well-being. A compromised placenta is reflected in a nonreactive NST, necessitating confirmation by CST.
Biophysical profile (BPP), nonstress test (NST), or contraction stress test (CST) if more than two NSTs are nonreactive. (Refer to CP: The High-Risk Pregnancy; ND: Injury, risk for fetal.)	
Refer to appropriate resources/drug program if client needs assistance with withdrawal from substance use/abuse.	Physiological drug addiction/withdrawal increase risks to both client and fetus and thereby require specialized support and monitoring.

NURSING DIAGNOSIS:	**Body Image disturbance/Role Performance, altered/Personal Identity disturbance/Self Esteem (specify)**
May Be Related To:	Situational and maturational crises, fear of failure at life events, biophysical changes, absence of support systems
Possibly Evidenced By:	Self-negating verbalizations, expressions of shame/guilt, hypersensitivity to criticism, fear of rejection, lack of follow-through and/or nonparticipation in care
DESIRED OUTCOMES/EVALUATION CRITERIA—CLIENT WILL:	Identify feelings and methods for coping with negative perception of self/abilities.
	Verbalize increased sense of self-esteem in relation to current situation.
	Demonstrate adaptation to changes/events as evidenced by setting of realistic goals and active participation in meeting own needs.

ACTIONS/INTERVENTIONS	RATIONALE
Independent	
Establish a therapeutic nurse-client relationship.	Adolescent client needs a caring, nonjudgmental adult with whom to talk. Important to establish trust and cooperation so that the client is free to hear the information available.
Assess use of terms/language used by the client/significant other(s).	Terminology may be specific to the adolescent culture, and words may have different meanings for client and nurse.
Determine developmental level and needs relative to age as early, middle, or late adolescence.	Cognitive development during this period moves from concrete to abstract thinking (formal operations). The younger client may see control of the situation as external and beyond her grasp, and have little ability to understand the consequences of her behavior. With maturity, the abilities to understand possible consequences and to accept individual responsibility develop.
Identify client's self-perception as positive or negative.	Helps client become aware of how she views herself and to begin to increase her self-esteem. Until late adolescence, body image is still formative. The

Elicit the client's feelings about sexual identity/roles.	client is dealing with adolescent developmental tasks, establishing an adult identity. Low self-worth may lead to feelings of hopelessness about the future and inability to visualize a successful outcome.
	May have difficulty seeing herself as a mother. The adolescent must make a role transition from child/daughter to adult/mother, which can create conflicts for the client and significant other(s).
Discuss concerns and fears about body image and transitory changes associated with pregnancy; discuss personal value system.	Establishes a basis for future learning. Conflicts may exist regarding how client has previously seen herself, what her expectations of pregnancy had been, and what the realities of pregnancy are. By midpregnancy, the enlarging abdomen and the increasing size of breasts and buttocks may prompt the teenager to try to control her appearance by dieting, with adverse consequences for fetal health and her own growth needs.
Discuss ways to promote positive self-image (e.g., clothing style, makeup) and recognition of positive aspects of the situation.	Assists in coping with changes in appearance and presenting a positive image.
Discuss appropriate adaptation techniques and the communication skills to implement these techniques.	Role playing and active listening can be used to learn skills of communication and adaptation. Helps client learn information necessary to development of improved self-esteem.

NURSING DIAGNOSIS:	**Social Isolation**
May Be Related To:	Alterations in physical appearance, perceived unacceptable social behavior, inadequate personal resources, difficulty in engaging in satisfying personal relationships (developmental or situational)
Possibly Evidenced By:	Expressed feelings of rejection or aloneness imposed by others, seeking solitude, inability to meet expectations of others, absence of effective support system
DESIRED OUTCOMES/EVALUATION CRITERIA—CLIENT WILL:	Remain involved in school and activities at the level of desire and ability.
	Participate in established social, community, and educational programs.

ACTIONS/INTERVENTIONS	RATIONALE

Independent

Ascertain changes in client's relationships with others that have occurred with the pregnancy.	Initial reactions of parents and boyfriend may include shock, anger, guilt, and shame. The pregnant adolescent often finds herself isolated from her peer group. She may be isolated from school and the normal contacts it affords. Her social sphere may be restricted to other pregnant teenagers, her boyfriend (if he remains involved and if circumstances do not force separation), and perhaps her relatives, who may or

129

ACTIONS/INTERVENTIONS	RATIONALE
Discuss resources available for assistance and ways to use them.	may not include an extended family. Extent of isolation may depend on whether client is in early, middle, or late adolescence and circumstances of pregnancy.
	Acquaints the client with potential avenues for help. Client in late adolescence (aged 17–19 yr) may be more resourceful financially.
Involve client with others who have shared interests.	Establishes peer/support group.
Provide positive reinforcement as appropriate.	Helps adolescent develop sense of self-esteem in a situation in which criticism may be overwhelming.
Encourage enrollment in childbirth and parent-education classes.	Provides a learning environment for client with others who share similar circumstances and physical constraints.

Collaborative

Arrange and assist with placement in foster or group home, if necessary.	May provide more positive environment if family is nonsupportive; may also be beneficial in enhancing self-esteem.

NURSING DIAGNOSIS:	Family Processes, altered
May Be Related To:	Situational and developmental crises, faulty family relationships, impaired patterns of communication
Possibly Evidenced By:	Family fails to adapt to, or deal with, situation; verbalizes difficulty coping with situation; expresses confusion about what to do; displays unhealthy decision-making process and inability to express/accept own feelings or feelings of other family members
DESIRED OUTCOMES/EVALUATION CRITERIA—FAMILY WILL:	Express feelings freely, honestly, and appropriately.
	Participate in efforts directed toward establishing and/or re-establishing healthy communication and interaction.
	Provide adequate support for the pregnant adolescent/partner.
	Seek professional counseling as appropriate.

ACTIONS/INTERVENTIONS	RATIONALE

Independent

| Assess family life stressors and involved members within the client's family of origin. (Refer to ND: Family Coping: ineffective, risk for compromised/disabling.) | The reasons adolescents give for becoming pregnant may be directly related to the family unit. For some clients, there may be faulty relationships within the family. The pregnancy may be an act of rebellion toward parental constraints, or it may represent a search for outside nurturance if parents have not satisfied this need appropriately. At the same time, parents of the adolescent may be experiencing their own midlife crisis. Even more destructive to the family, the pregnancy may be the result of incest/abuse. |
| Assess client's relationship with mother. Note cultural impact of pregnancy out of wedlock. | Mother may feel guilty, see daughter as too young to assume responsibility, and take over |

Identify the mode of communication and interaction within the family. Assess role expectations of family members.

Treat family members in a warm, caring way; encourage establishment of support systems.

Encourage discussion of plans for the future of client, infant, and family.

Encourage supportive association with father of the child, if agreeable to both parties.

Provide information and discuss risks of marriage precipitated by the pregnancy alone.

inappropriately. If client does not assume her new role as mother effectively, the mother may have difficulty assuming her new role as grandmother.

Understanding the dynamics of the family and the roles of individual members can assist with change. Family disruption can best be resolved by assessing reasons for role changes and ways to facilitate them.

Acceptance of the situation can strengthen the family and encourage members to extend their support to each other.

At this time of crisis, members are apt to respond with anger, blaming each other, and may need help in focusing energies on practical solutions. The relationships with the baby's father and with family members in relation to future personal or educational goals may be unclear. Furthermore, the decision as to whether client will relinquish or keep the infant will add to the uncertainties.

Father of the child may or may not be known; reaction of various family members may strain/prohibit involvement. However, with some understanding and assistance, in many cases the teen father would like to be involved in this event and can provide support for the client. (Note: When the pregnancy is the result of incest/abuse, personal and legal constraints are likely to preclude inclusion of the father and will have an impact on the support provided by other family members.)

Although 50%–75% of adolescent marriages end in divorce, some teenage couples have a strong love relationship and may eventually marry or maintain a caring relationship.

Collaborative

Refer client/partner/significant others to parenting classes and counseling.

Additional information and assistance with resolution of conflicts and/or coping with stressors may aid family in developing new and positive relationships.

NURSING DIAGNOSIS: **Parenting, risk for altered**

Risk Factors May Include: Chronological age/developmental stage, lack of knowledge, lack of support between/from significant other(s), ineffective role models, unrealistic expectations for self, lack of role identity, presence of stressors

Possibly Evidenced By: [Not applicable; presence of signs/symptoms establishes an *actual* diagnosis]

DESIRED OUTCOMES/EVALUATION CRITERIA—CLIENT WILL: Participate in activities/classes to promote growth.

Identify appropriate parenting role.

Demonstrate behavior/lifestyle changes to reduce risk of short- and long-term problems.

Use appropriate individual, family, and community resources to support the new family unit.

ACTIONS/INTERVENTIONS	RATIONALE
Independent	
Assess client's ego development, educational level, stressors, and understanding of infant capabilities.	Helps identify needs for establishing educational program if client has decided to keep infant. May identify potentially abusive parent(s). Often, ability to master parenting skills effectively is directly related to educational level, socioeconomic factors, stress level, ego development, and social support.
Assess potential parenting capabilities of both teenage mother and father, if present.	Because of their own developmental needs, adolescent mothers and fathers are less likely to be accepting, cooperative, accessible, and sensitive to their child's needs than are more mature parents.
Use visual data, audiovisual aids, film, lecture, and hands-on instruction to give information on bathing and other aspects of caring for a new baby.	Provides information about skills needed by the new parent(s).
Provide opportunity for the adolescent parent to ask questions and communicate freely.	Offers opportunity to clarify misunderstandings and allows for expressions of frustrations, disappointments, and concerns without judgment; can help both mother and father begin to cope with situation.
Make opportunities for client and involved father to interact with infants/toddlers and appropriate role models. Encourage discussion about full-time responsibility associated with children.	Helps adolescent parents to internalize/adopt appropriate parenting behaviors and gain realistic perceptions of infant capabilities/behaviors. The adolescent mother/father is a high-risk parent known to be less responsive to infant cues, to be more likely to use punishment, and to be unrealistic in expectations of infant behavior.
Assist to develop support systems within the family and/or community.	Making contacts that allow freedom to discuss situation, fears, and confusion can help client make decisions appropriate for her and the infant. Social/extended family supports assist the client in her ability to parent effectively.
Provide information about ongoing prenatal/postnatal classes that focus on learning parenting skills and infant capabilities, caretaking, and stimulation.	Will help to promote positive parenting. Children born to adolescent mothers are at greater risk for behavioral, social, and intellectual retardation and possible physical retardation than children born to older mothers.
Assist client with learning methods of relaxation and ways of conserving energy.	Will help the client learn skills for keeping energy level up after the baby is born in order to care adequately for the infant. She may not be aware of her need for time out and fail to care for her own needs.

NURSING DIAGNOSIS:	**Family Coping: ineffective, risk for compromised/disabling**
Risk Factors May Include:	Temporary disorganization of the client's family of origin, family having difficulty providing support for the client/couple, situational and/or developmental crises the father may be facing, insufficient reciprocity of support between client and father of the baby
Possibly Evidenced By:	[Not applicable; presence of signs/symptoms establishes an *actual* diagnosis]

DESIRED OUTCOMES/EVALUATION CRITERIA—FAMILY WILL:	Participate in discussions/decisions regarding the pregnancy.
	Express feelings honestly.
	Identify resources within selves to deal with situation.
	Identify need for outside support and seek appropriate support.

ACTIONS/INTERVENTIONS	RATIONALE

Independent

Assess family constellation/organization and nature of individual relationships to one another.	Family may consist of the client alone or may encompass an extended family, including the adolescent father and his family. By either withdrawing its support or by overcompensating and interfering, the extended family may have a negative impact on the maturity and development of the young couple.
Assess individual and family response to pregnancy.	Response to pregnancy depends on culture, value systems, socioeconomic status, circumstances of pregnancy, and educational level. In some cultures, teenage parenting is common, and the girl's mother may have been a teenage mother.
Assess client's ability to achieve tasks of pregnancy concurrently with developmental tasks.	In many cases, adolescent is unable to achieve pregnancy tasks as well as normal developmental tasks. This may result in long-term psychological effects associated with impaired adult identity formation.
Determine the client's/couple's perception of individual and collective strengths and weaknesses.	Provides opportunity to use strengths to address areas of concern.
Assess father's developmental, educational, and socioeconomic status.	Developmental tasks are disrupted for the male partner as well as for the client. His level of maturation and education may influence his decision to remain in or leave the situation/relationship.
Provide opportunities for the father to talk about his feelings and perceptions. Listen in a nonjudgmental manner.	Helps him to identify and clarify what is happening. The adolescent father needs an opportunity to verbalize his concerns, have his feelings validated, and assume an active role in all aspects of the pregnancy. Note: To provide nonjudgmental listening and care, nurses need to be aware of their own moral and ethical conflicts.
Help father, and couple as a unit, to identify stressors and ways of dealing positively with them.	Awareness of stressors can facilitate growth; effective coping promotes positive outcomes. Note: Father/couple may already possess some effective coping skills, especially if in late adolescence.
Identify available support systems.	The adolescent father may find himself bearing the brunt of family anger and shame.
Involve father in activities related to pregnancy and childbirth.	Helps him to know that he is an integral part of the process and that his support is important to the client.
Discuss with client/couple, individual expectations/plans for the future and the perception of each regarding the response of both families.	The pregnant adolescent may receive appropriate physical/emotional care while the needs of the father/couple go unidentified and/or unmet. The family may have moral/ethical conflict about

133

providing support to a couple who may not be married or may not intend to get married. Although the relationship may not survive the stress of the pregnancy and accompanying decisions, the couple may see it as important at the moment.

Collaborative

Refer for appropriate assistance: counseling, financial, educational, and/or social services.

The father/couple/family may need help for a prolonged period, depending on how stressors are handled and whether client chooses to keep or relinquish infant.

NURSING DIAGNOSIS:	Family Coping: potential for growth
May Be Related To:	Client and family achieving the developmental tasks of the pregnancy, demonstrating readiness to address goals of self-actualization
Possibly Evidenced By:	Participation in prenatal classes, physical preparation for infant, establishment of realistic goals for the future
DESIRED OUTCOMES/EVALUATION CRITERIA—FAMILY WILL:	Participate in activities related to childbearing and childrearing.
	Seek information designed to enhance personal growth.
	Report feelings of confidence and satisfaction with progress being made.

ACTIONS/INTERVENTIONS	RATIONALE

Independent

Assess stage of family development and potential for growth.	Determines necessary steps to assist in further growth. A supportive family is critical to fostering growth and appropriate parenting behavior.
Ascertain impact of cultural and maturational factors.	These factors may hinder a family from expressing or recognizing their readiness to progress. Sensitivity to these issues can facilitate growth.
Listen to client's/family's expressions of hope and plans for the future. Support continuation of formal education as appropriate.	Can build on awareness of possibilities for the situation. Early termination of education has a severe impact on the client's earning capacity throughout life.
Assist client/family with communication skills, and provide experiences in which they can learn ways of supporting one another.	Learning effective communication skills enhances potential for growth.
Discuss feelings about and plans for the future with client who has decided to give infant up for adoption. Include family in discussion, when possible.	Helping this client deal with issues of loss and grieving will enable her to go on with her life in a positive manner. Family understanding of client's feelings/needs can facilitate this process.

Collaborative

Refer to other resources as appropriate (e.g., support group or psychiatric counseling).	May need additional assistance in learning to express feelings, manage crisis situations, and so forth.

NURSING DIAGNOSIS:	Home Maintenance Management, risk for impaired
Risk Factors May Include:	Chronological age/developmental stage, lack of knowledge, inadequate support systems, insufficient finances
Possibly Evidenced By:	[Not applicable; presence of signs/symptoms establishes an *actual* diagnosis]
DESIRED OUTCOMES/EVALUATION CRITERIA—CLIENT/COUPLE OR FAMILY WILL:	Develop a plan for maintaining a clean, safe, growth-promoting environment. Demonstrate appropriate/effective use of resources.

ACTIONS/INTERVENTIONS	RATIONALE

Independent

Assess developmental level; cognitive, emotional, and physical functioning; and financial situation.	These factors may impair functioning and, therefore, influence creation of the plan of care and available options.
Identify support systems available to the client/couple.	Availability of a good supportive network fosters positive adaptation to caretaking roles. Many teenage clients have few resources and depend on either parents and/or social agencies for assistance.
Assist client/significant other(s) to develop a plan for maintaining a clean, healthful environment.	Helps develop responsibility for having an environment conducive to health and growth of mother and child.

Collaborative

Identify resources available for appropriate assistance.	May need help with budget counseling, financial and living arrangements, social work services, and so forth.

Cardiac Conditions

During pregnancy blood volume increases as much as 50% above the nonpregnant level and is accompanied by increases in maternal heart rate and stroke volume necessitating a drop in systemic and pulmonary vascular resistance. The client with heart disease may not be able to readily accommodate the higher workload of pregnancy as a result of decreased cardiac reserves.

(This plan of care is to be used in conjunction with the Trimesters and The High-Risk Pregnancy.)

CLIENT ASSESSMENT DATA BASE

Activity/Rest

Inability to carry on normal activities
Nocturnal/exertion-related dyspnea; orthopnea

Circulation

Tachycardia, palpitations; severe dysrhythmia.
History of congenital/organic heart disease, rheumatic fever.
Upward displacement of the diaphragm and heart proportionate to uterine size.
May have a continuous diastolic or presystolic murmur; cardiac enlargement; loud systolic murmur, associated with a thrill.
BP may be elevated or may be decreased with decreased vascular resistance.
Clubbing of toes and fingers may be present, with symmetric cyanosis in surgically untreated tetralogy of Fallot.

Elimination

Urine output may be decreased.
Nocturia.

Food/Fluid

Obesity (risk factor)
May have edema of the lower extremities

Pain/Discomfort

May report chest pain with/without activity

Respiration

Cough; may or may not be productive.
Hemoptysis.
Respiratory rate may be increased.
Dyspnea/shortness of breath, orthopnea may be reported.
Rales may be present.

Safety

Repeated streptococcal infections

Teaching/Learning

Possible history of valve replacement/prosthetic device, mitral valve prolapse, Marfan's syndrome, surgically treated/untreated (rare) tetralogy of Fallot

DIAGNOSTIC STUDIES

White Blood Cell (WBC) Count: Leukocytosis indicative of generalized infection, primarily streptococcal.

Hemoglobin (Hg)/Hematocrit (Hct): Reveals actual versus physiological anemia; polycythemia.

Maternal Arterial Blood Gases: Provide secondary assessment of potential fetal compromise due to maternal respiratory involvement.

Sedimentation Rate: Elevated in the presence of cardiac inflammation.

Maternal Electrocardiogram (ECG): Demonstrates patterns associated with specific cardiac disorders, dysrhythmias.

Echocardiography: Diagnoses mitral valve prolapse or Marfan's syndrome.

Radionuclide Cardiac Imaging: Evaluates suspected atrial or ventricular septal defects, patent ductus arteriosus, or intracardiac shunts.

Serial Ultrasonography: Detects gestational age of fetus and possible IUGR.

NURSING PRIORITIES

1. Monitor degree/progression of symptoms.
2. Promote client involvement in control of condition and self-care.
3. Monitor fetal well-being.
4. Support client/couple toward culmination of a safe delivery.

DISCHARGE GOALS

Inpatient care not required unless complications develop.

NURSING DIAGNOSIS:	Cardiac Output, risk for [decompensation]
Risk Factors May Include:	Increased circulating volume, dysrhythmias, altered myocardial contractility, inotropic changes in the heart
Possibly Evidenced By:	[Not applicable; presence of signs/symptoms establishes an *actual* diagnosis]
DESIRED OUTCOMES/EVALUATION CRITERIA—CLIENT WILL:	Identify/adopt behaviors to minimize stressors and maximize cardiac function.
	Tolerate the stress of increasing blood volume as indicated by BP and pulse within individually appropriate limits.
	Demonstrate adequate placental circulation, kidney function with FHR and fetal movement WNL, and individually appropriate urine output.

ACTIONS/INTERVENTIONS	RATIONALE
Independent	
Determine/monitor client's functional classification (as outlined by the New York Heart Association):	Useful for identifying client needs/limitations, effectiveness of therapies, and progression/remission of condition.
Class I: No limitation of physical activity, no discomfort during exertion	
Class II: Ordinary activity may cause symptoms of palpitation, dyspnea, and angina	
Class III: Less than ordinary activity causes cardiac symptoms, such as fatigue, dyspnea, and angina	

137

Class IV: Symptoms of cardiac insufficiency occur in the absence of physical activity, and mortality risk per Clark's classification system of risk status for pregnant women.

Provide information about the necessity of adequate rest (e.g., 8–10 hr at night and $1/2$ hr after each meal).	Minimizes cardiac stress and conserves energy. Class IV clients may require bedrest for the duration of the pregnancy. (Refer to ND: Activity Intolerance, risk for.)
Discuss use of left or right lateral position.	The occurrence of supine hypotension possibly to the point of loss of consciousness can be prevented if the client avoids the supine position and adopts the lateral recumbent resting position.
Monitor vital signs.	The beginning stage of decompensation caused by intolerance of circulatory load, infection, or anxiety may first be noted by an insidious change in the vital sign pattern, associated with increased temperature, pulse (110 bpm or greater), respiration (greater than 20–34/min), and BP.
Auscultate client's breath sounds.	Congestive heart failure (CHF) may develop, especially in clients whose functional classification is class III or IV. Conversely, clients with mitral valve prolapse may be symptom-free during pregnancy, owing to the increase in left ventricular volume, yet are at high risk for involvement related to chest pain, palpitations, and possibly death after delivery.
Evaluate FHR, daily fetal movement count, and NST results as indicated. (Refer to CP: The High-Risk Pregnancy; ND: Injury, risk for fetal.)	Fetal hypoxia caused by beginning stage of maternal cardiac decompensation may be noted in the form of tachycardia, bradycardia, or reduction in fetal activity.
Assess for evidence of venostasis with resulting dependent edema of extremities or generalized edema. Instruct client to elevate legs when sitting down and periodically during the day.	Prolonged positioning of legs and ankles below the level of the heart further impairs venous return in an already stressed circulatory system and places the client at risk for PIH.
Instruct client to monitor fluid intake/output. (Refer to ND: Fluid Volume, risk for excess.)	Although intake and output should be approximately the same, cardiovascular involvement may negatively affect kidney function, resulting in oliguria/anuria.
Investigate reports of chest pain and palpitations. Recommend limiting caffeine as appropriate.	Clients with mitral valve prolapse may develop arrhythmias resulting in chest pain and palpitations. Limiting caffeine may reduce frequency of episodes.
Review medication needs and reason for conversion to heparin by warfarin (Coumadin) users.	Because of its large molecular size, heparin sodium does not cross the placenta, as does warfarin; also, heparin may prevent clot formation in the client with valve prosthesis/atrial fibrillation.
Instruct client in self-administration of medication such as heparin. Observe return demonstration of procedure by client.	Involves client in therapeutic process, and promotes self-care.
Assess for/review signs of ecchymosis, epistaxis, and so forth during anticoagulant therapy.	Signs of bleeding may indicate a need to reduce heparin dosage.

Collaborative

Participate in/coordinate multispecialty care conference as appropriate.	Provides opportunity to review management of both pregnancy *and* cardiac condition, and to plan for

Administer medications such as digitalis glycosides (digoxin or digitoxin) or propranolol (Inderal) as indicated. Monitor for early labor.

special needs during intrapartum and postpartum periods.

Cardiac stress brought on by increased demand for output is greatest between 28 and 32 weeks' gestation, then levels off until delivery. Digitalis glycosides maximize ventricular contractions, but increased plasma volume may lower circulating levels of the drug, necessitating increased or more frequent doses. Digitalis has a direct effect on the myometrium, often causing early labor as well as shortening the length of labor. Propranolol may be used to control dysrhythmias associated with mitral valve prolapse. Note: Although these drugs cross the placenta and have no reported teratogenic effects, studies have not yet clearly established their safety in pregnancy. In addition, ACE inhibitors are contraindicated because of the risk of fetal death or intractable neonatal renal failure.

Administer loading dose of heparin.

Warfarin users should have their anticoagulant converted to heparin. Initial dose may be administered intravenously by healthcare provider.

Treat underlying infections as necessary, e.g., respiratory, and provide prophylaxis as necessary. (Refer to ND: Infection, risk for maternal.)

Cardiac decompensation may develop/is worsened by superimposed upper respiratory infection, which is usually associated with coughing and increased secretions, and which may mask deterioration of cardiac function. Prophylactic antibiotics help prevent bacterial endocarditis in client with diseased heart valves.

Using sequential serum/urine estriol levels and CST/NST, assess placental functioning. (Refer to CP: The High-Risk Pregnancy; ND: Injury, risk for fetal.)

Reduced cardiac function may negatively affect placental functioning.

Obtain/review sequential ECGs.

May demonstrate pathological pattern if decompensation is present; may identify type of dysrhythmia.

Monitor laboratory studies, such as clotting times and electrolyte levels.

Prolonged clotting times may indicate need to adjust heparin dosage. Hyponatremia/hypokalemia may occur, owing to reduced sodium intake or diuretic therapy with imbalances potentiating development/aggravation of dysrhythmias.

Encourage use of antithrombotic stockings.

Promotes venous return; limits venous stasis.

Prepare client for hospitalization as warranted by her condition.

Clients with a functional classification of class II through class IV are usually hospitalized 2 wk before expected delivery, because likelihood of decompensation is greatest during the latter part of the third trimester. Clients with class IV function may be hospitalized earlier in the pregnancy, depending on fetal status/developing complications.

Monitor hemodynamic pressures using arterial and central venous pressure (CVP) lines or Swan-

CVP lines measure venous return/circulating volume; the Swan-Ganz catheter may be required

139

Ganz catheter to monitor pulmonary artery wedge pressure as indicated.

to monitor pulmonary pressures and, indirectly, left-sided heart function in client hospitalized for progressive CHF.

NURSING DIAGNOSIS:	Fluid Volume risk for excess
Risk Factors May Include:	Increasing circulating volume, changes in renal function, dietary indiscretion
Possibly Evidenced By:	[Not applicable; presence of signs/symptoms establishes an *actual* diagnosis]
DESIRED OUTCOMES/EVALUATION CRITERIA—CLIENT WILL:	Demonstrate stable fluid balance with vital signs WNL, appropriate weight gain, absence of edema.
	Verbalize understanding of restrictions/therapy needs.
	List signs that require notification of care provider.

ACTIONS/INTERVENTIONS	RATIONALE

Independent

Obtain baseline weight. Instruct client to monitor her weight at home periodically as indicated.	Weight gain exceeding the normal 2–2½ lb/wk may indicate accumulating fluid and potential CHF. If weight gain is sudden, rule out toxemia.
Review dietary intake, noting factors that may contribute to excessive fluid retention; provide information as needed.	Improper diet, specifically a deficiency of protein and excess of sodium, contributes to fluid retention.
Instruct client to monitor amount and color (concentration) of urine. Measure specific gravity as appropriate during home/office visit.	Decreased output, dark amber urine; increasing specific gravity may reflect impaired renal perfusion associated with developing CHF.
Assess for/review signs of CHF with client (e.g., dyspnea, distended neck veins, crackles, hemoptysis, and so forth).	Indicates developing failure and need for immediate treatment. The normal increase of 1300 ml in circulatory volume that occurs in pregnancy can put stress on the cardiac system. Further increase of fluid can be especially dangerous for the client with existing cardiac problems.
Investigate unexplained cough.	Cough unrelated to respiratory problems may indicate developing CHF.

Collaborative

Restrict fluids and sodium in presence of CHF.	Minimizes risk of fluid retention/overload.
Administer diuretics, e.g., chlorothiazide (Diuril), hydrochlorothiazide (HCTZ), furosemide (Lasix), as appropriate.	Helps rid body of excess fluid resistant to conservative treatment of rest and decreased sodium intake.

NURSING DIAGNOSIS:	Tissue Perfusion, risk for altered: uteroplacental
Risk Factors May Include:	Changes in circulating volume, right-to-left shunt

Possibly Evidenced By:	[Not applicable; presence of signs/symptoms establishes an *actual* diagnosis]
DESIRED OUTCOMES/EVALUATION CRITERIA—CLIENT WILL:	Display BP, pulse, ABGs, and WBC count WNL. Demonstrate adequate placental perfusion as indicated by reactive fetus with heart rate ranging from 120–160 bpm and size appropriate for gestational age.

ACTIONS/INTERVENTIONS	RATIONALE

Independent

Note individual risk factors and pregravid state.	Any preexisting cardiac problems complicated by increased circulatory needs during pregnancy may result in impaired tissue oxygenation. Note: Such problems are greater in the older client with obesity and long-standing cardiac involvement.
Assess BP and pulse. Note behavior changes, cyanosis of mucous membranes and nail beds, activity intolerance, and signs of decompensation (i.e., excessive weight gain, unexplained cough, crackles/wheezes, hemoptysis, and increased pulse and respiratory rate).	Tachycardia (heart rate greater than 110 bpm) at rest, increasing BP, and behavior changes may indicate early cardiac failure or hypoxia. A fall in peripheral vascular resistance may result in a worsening of right-to-left shunting and cyanosis. Presence of cyanosis, a late sign of hypoxia, reflects severe problems and indicates severity of tissue damage and cardiac compromise.
Provide information about use of modified upright position for sleeping and resting.	Eases respiratory rate by reducing pressure of the enlarging uterus on the diaphragm and helps increase vertical diameter for lung expansion. Helps prevent venous stasis in lower extremities.

Collaborative

Monitor laboratory studies as indicated:	
Pulse oximetry/ABGs; Hb/Hct;	Reflects adequacy of ventilation and oxygenation. Anemia further reduces oxygen-carrying capacity of blood and may require treatment.
WBC count, culture of upper/lower respiratory secretions.	Any respiratory involvement reduces intake of oxygen. Infection increases metabolic rates and oxygen needs and may have a negative impact on tissue oxygenation.
Assess uterine/fetal blood flow using NST/CST; check estriol levels and FHR. (Refer to CP: The High-Risk Pregnancy; ND: Injury, risk for fetal.)	Uterine/placental hypoxia reduces fetal activity and FHR, and presents as late decelerations on CST. Hypoxia may result in placental deterioration and falling estriol levels.

NURSING DIAGNOSIS:	Infection, risk for maternal
Risk Factors May Include:	Inadequate primary/secondary defenses, chronic disease/condition, insufficient information to avoid exposure to pathogens
Possibly Evidenced By:	[Not applicable; presence of signs/symptoms establishes an *actual* diagnosis]

ACTIONS/INTERVENTIONS	RATIONALE

Independent

Assess for individual risk factors and history of rheumatic fever.	There is increased risk of bacterial endocarditis in the prenatal client with underlying heart disease, such as valvular damage caused by rheumatic or congenital processes, mitral valve prolapse, ventricular septal defect, tetralogy of Fallot, pulmonic stenosis, coarctation of the aorta, or prosthetic valve.
Provide information about risk of bacterial endocarditis during specific medical-surgical procedures.	The client with a prosthetic valve is at high risk for bacterial endocarditis and emboli, even in an uncomplicated vaginal delivery. Transient bacteremia may occur following invasive procedures, including dental work. (About 60%–90% of clients develop bacteremia after dental extraction).
Review signs/symptoms suggestive of infectious processes requiring notification of healthcare provider, e.g., fever, malaise, cough, cloudy/odiferous urine.	Prompt recognition of problem facilitates timely intervention.

Collaborative

Assess urine periodically, note pH, and presence of bacteria.	Bacturia may be asymptomatic and lead to bacteremia if untreated.
Obtain cultures as indicated.	Useful in identifying infecting agent/appropriate therapy.
Administer penicillin PO or IM, when indicated.	Prophylactic antibiotics may be recommended for prevention of streptococal infection during pregnancy, especially in the client with history of rheumatic fever.

NURSING DIAGNOSIS:	Activity Intolerance, risk for
Risk Factors May Include:	Presence of circulatory problems, previous episodes of intolerance, deconditioned status
Possibly Evidenced By:	[Not applicable; presence of signs/symptoms establishes an *actual* diagnosis]
DESIRED OUTCOMES/EVALUATION CRITERIA—CLIENT WILL:	Demonstrate self-responsibility for monitoring activity tolerance/intolerance. Adopt behaviors to maximize tolerance. Take appropriate actions if cardiac/respiratory symptoms arise.

ACTIONS/INTERVENTIONS	RATIONALE

Independent

Assess for development of subjective/objective symptoms (e.g., lessening of tolerance to ordinary physical activity, fatigue, cyanosis, inability to carry on normal daily activities, increasing dyspnea with or without physical activity, nocturnal dyspnea, change in pulse rate, development of respiratory symptoms).

Indicates a worsening of the cardiac condition, evidenced by a decrease in the client's functional capacity.

Review signs/symptoms with the client and significant other(s).

Promotes self-care and timely medical interventions.

Assist client in setting priorities and restructuring daily routine to include needed rest/sleep periods. Determine expectations of client and partner. Explore conflicts/differences.

Circulatory/respiratory impairment may interfere with ability to perform activities of daily living (ADLs) and may result in fatigue. Activity is limited in relation to the extent of cardiac impairment. Clients with class I or II limitation may only need to include midmorning and midafternoon rest periods, whereas class III or class IV clients may need bedrest for much or all of the day.

Identify energy conserving methods to accomplish necessary ADLs.

May enable client to manage activities more effectively.

Ascertain effectiveness of household assistance and available resources.

May be needed to maximize rest, limit fatigue, and preserve cardiac function.

Collaborative

Refer to home care agency, community resources as indicated.

Can provide additional assistance when necessary.

Refer to occupational therapist (OT), physical therapist (PT), as appropriate.

May be helpful in identifying assistive techniques/devices to conserve energy and accomplish desired ADLs.

NURSING DIAGNOSIS:	Knowledge deficit [Learning Need], regarding condition, prognosis, and treatment needs
May Be Related To:	Lack of exposure to and/or misinterpretation of information
Possibly Evidenced By:	Request for information, statement of misconception, inaccurate follow-through of instructions
DESIRED OUTCOMES/EVALUATION CRITERIA—CLIENT WILL:	Verbalize understanding of individual condition and treatment needs.
	Identify symptoms indicating deterioration of cardiac functioning.
	Intervene and/or notify healthcare provider appropriately.

143

ACTIONS/INTERVENTIONS	RATIONALE

Independent

Assess understanding of pathology/complications regarding cardiac condition and pregnancy. Review history, incidence of complications, and so forth.

Establishes data base for health teaching. Increasingly severe cardiac symptoms may indicate client's need for more information and/or assistance to manage necessary self-care.

Discuss necessity for frequent monitoring; i.e., every 2 wk during first 20 wk, then every week until delivery.

Provides for early detection of problems and prompt intervention.

Provide information about symptoms indicative of cardiac involvement, such as shortness of breath, cough, palpitations, unusual or rapid weight gain (i.e., 2.2–4.4 lb or 1–2 kg in a 2-day period), edema, or anorexia.

Symptoms associated with decompensation should be differentiated from symptoms associated with PIH. (Refer to CP: Pregnancy-Induced Hypertension; ND: Fluid Volume deficit.)

Provide information as appropriate regarding diet, rest/sleep, exercise, and relaxation.

Enhances informed decision making, helps reduce likelihood of complications. The impact of pregnancy superimposed on an existing cardiac problem may necessitate changes in lifestyle. An understanding of techniques designed to lessen cardiac stress may require the acquisition of new knowledge.

Review need/techniques to avoid infection.

Resistance may be lowered because of general condition.

Review side effects of both prescription and OTC drugs.

Determines client's level of knowledge and provides current information.

Discuss special considerations, such as need to avoid foods high in vitamin K (raw, deep-green leafy vegetables) when on anticoagulants.

Such foods counteract/alter anticoagulant drug effect.

Include healthcare team in teaching/planning.

Provides continuity and completeness of care.

Provide appropriate information for protocol of care in home/community/hospital setting.

May foster self-responsibility and reduce anxiety.

Identify support groups, community resources.

May serve as role model for necessary adaptations, enhance coping ability, and provide encouragement for a successful outcome.

Pregnancy-Induced Hypertension

The exact etiology of this disorder is unknown, with several theories being advanced. Data have suggested that PIH may be the result of increased peripheral vascular resistance secondary to generalized vasospasm when the vessels are no longer refractory to the effects of pressor agents. New research proposes that elevated cardiac output and associated hyperdynamic vasodilation during the first trimester result in damage to the endothelium with compensatory vascular vasodilation. Regardless of the mechanisms, PIH is a chronic disease process, with a decrease in placental perfusion occurring before the late sign of hypertension is detected.

(This plan of care is to be used in conjunction with the Trimesters and the High-Risk Pregnancy CPs.)

CLIENT ASSESSMENT DATA BASE

Circulation

Persistent increase in BP over pregravid or first-trimester baseline readings after 20 wk of pregnancy (systolic elevation > 30 mm Hg, diastolic elevation > 15 mm Hg or a BP > 140/90 mm Hg on two consecutive readings assessed at least 6 hr apart).
History of chronic hypertension.
Jugular venous distension.
Gallop rhythm may be present.
Pulse may be decreased.
May have spontaneous bruising, prolonged bleeding, or epistaxis (thrombocytopenia).

Elimination

Oliguria/anuria may be present.
Hematuria may be noted.

Food/Fluid

Nausea/vomiting.
Weight gain of 2+ lb in 1 wk, 4 lb or more per month (depending on length of gestation).
Malnourished (overweight or underweight by 20% or greater); poor protein/caloric intake.
Edema may be present, ranging from mild to severe/generalized; and may involve facies, extremities, and organ systems (i.e., liver, brain).
Glycosuria (diabetes mellitus).

Neurosensory

Dizziness, frontal headaches.
Decreased responsiveness/somnolence.
Diplopia, blurred vision, or even loss of visual fields; scotomata (spots before eyes).
Hyperreflexia; clonus.
Convulsions—tonic, then tonic-clonic phases, followed by a period of loss of consciousness.
Funduscopic examination may reveal edema or vascular spasm.

Pain/Discomfort

Epigastric pain (right upper quadrant [RUQ] region)

Respiration

Respirations may be less than 14/min.
Bibasilar crackles may be present.
Dyspnea.

Safety

Rh incompatibility may be present.

Sexuality

Primigravida, multiple gestation, hydramnios, gestational trophoblastic disease (e.g.,: hydatidiform mole), hydrops fetalis (Rh antigen-antibody)
Fetal movement may be diminished
Signs of abruptio placentae may be present (e.g., uterine tetany, tenderness)

Teaching/Learning

Adolescent (under age 15 yr) and older primigravida (age 35 yr or older) are at greatest risk
Family history of pregnancy-induced hypertension (PIH)

DIAGNOSTIC STUDIES

Supine Pressor Test ("rollover test"): May be used to screen for clients at risk for PIH, 28–32 wk gestation, although accuracy is questionable; an increase of 20–30 mm Hg in systolic pressure or 15–20 mm Hg in diastolic pressure indicates a positive test.
Mean Arterial Pressure (MAP): 90 mm Hg at second trimester indicates PIH.
Hematocrit (Hct): Elevated with fluid shifts, or decreased in HELLP syndrome (*h*emolysis, *e*levated *l*iver enzymes, *l*ow *p*latelet count).
Hemoglobin (Hb): Low when hemolysis occurs (HELLP syndrome).
Peripheral Smear: Distended blood cells or schistocytes in HELLP syndrome or intravascular hemolysis.
Serum Platelet Counts: Less than $100,000/mm^3$ in disseminated intravascular coagulation (DIC) or in HELLP syndrome, because platelets adhere to collagen released from damaged blood vessels.
Serum Creatinine Level: Elevated above 1.0 mg/dL and blood urea nitrogen (BUN): Greater than 10 mg/dL reflects severe renal involvement.
AST, LDH, and Serum Bilirubin Levels (indirect particularly): Elevated in HELLP syndrome with liver involvement.
Uric Acid Level: Greater than 5 mg/100 mL. Helpful in distinguishing preeclampsia from uncomplicated chronic hypertension.
Prothrombin time (PT), Partial Thromboplastin Time (PTT), Clotting Time: Prolonged; fibronogen decreased, FSP and FDP positive when coagulopathy occurs (DIC).
Urine-Specific Gravity: Elevated, reflecting fluid shifts/vascular dehydration.
Proteinuria: By dipstick, may be 1+ to 2+ (moderate), 3+ to 4+ (severe), or greater than 500 mg/dL in 24 h.
Creatinine Clearance: Decreased in preeclampsia (before serum BUN/Creatinine elevated).
Urinary/Plasma Estriol Levels: Decline indicates reduced placental functioning. (Estroils are not as useful a predictor as biophysical profile [BPP] because of the lag time between fetal problem and test results.)
Human Placental Lactogen Levels: Less than 4 mEq/ml suggests abnormal placental functioning (not frequently done n PIH screening).
Ultrasonography: At 20–26 weeks' gestation and repeated 6–10 wk later, establishes gestational age and detects IUGR.
Tests of Amniotic Fluid (lecithin sphingomyelin [L/S] ratio, phosphalidylglycerol (PG), saturated phosphatidylcholine levels): Determine fetal lung maturity.
Biophysical Profile (BPP) (amniotic fluid volume, fetal tone, fetal breathing movements [FMB], fetal movements, and fetal heart rate [FHR] reactivity)/Nonstress Test (NST): Determines fetal risk/well-being.
CST: Assesses the response of the fetus to the stress of uterine contractions.

NURSING PRIORITIES

1. Monitor maternal, fetal, and placental status.
2. Prevent or reduce progressive fluid accumulation and other complications.
3. Promote positive maternal/fetal outcome.
4. Provide information to enhance self-care and therapeutic management.

DISCHARGE GOALS

(Inpatient care generally not required, unless fetal compromise or eclampsia develops, or when labor process begins.)

If hospitalized:
1. Hemodynamically stable, free-of-seizure activity
2. Fetus active and in no distress
3. Condition, prognosis, therapeutic regimen understood
4. Participating in care with plan in place for home monitoring/management

NURSING DIAGNOSIS:	Fluid Volume deficit [isotonic]
May Be Related To:	Plasma protein loss, decreasing plasma colloid osmotic pressure, allowing fluid shifts out of the vascular compartment
Possibly Evidenced By:	Edema formation, sudden weight gain, hemoconcentration, nausea/ vomiting, epigastric pain, headaches, visual changes, decreased urine output
DESIRED OUTCOMES/EVALUATION CRITERIA—CLIENT WILL:	Verbalize understanding of need for close monitoring of weight, BP, urine protein, and edema.
	Participate in therapeutic regimen and monitoring, as indicated.
	Display Hct WNL and physiological edema with no signs of pitting.
	Be free of signs of generalized edema (i.e., epigastric pain, cerebral symptoms, dyspnea, nausea/ vomiting).

ACTIONS/INTERVENTIONS

Independent

Weigh client routinely. Encourage client to monitor weight at home between visits.

Distinguish between physiological and pathological edema of pregnancy. Monitor location and degree of pitting.

Note signs of progressive or excessive edema (i.e., epigastric/RUQ pain, cerebral symptoms, nausea, vomiting). Assess for possible eclampsia. (Refer to ND: Injury, risk for maternal.)

Note changes in Hct/Hb levels.

Reassess dietary intake of proteins and calories. Provide information as needed.

RATIONALE

Sudden, significant weight gain (e.g., more than 3.3 lb (1.5 kg)/month in the second trimester or more than 1 lb (0.5 kg)/wk in the third trimester) reflects fluid retention. Fluid moves from the vascular to interstitial space, resulting in edema.

The presence of pitting edema (mild, 1+ to 2+; severe, 3+ to 4+) of face, hands, legs, sacral area, or abdominal wall, or edema that does not disappear after 12 hr of bedrest is significant. Note: Significant edema may actually be present in nonpre-eclamptic clients and absent in clients with mild or moderated PIH.

Edema and intravascular fibrin deposition (in HELLP syndrome) within the encapsulated liver are manifested by RUQ pain; dyspnea, indicating pulmonary involvement; cerebral edema, possibly leading to seizures; and nausea and vomiting, indicating GI edema.

Identifies degree of hemoconcentration caused by fluid shift. If Hct is less than 3 times Hb level, hemoconcentration exists.

Adequate nutrition reduces incidence of prenatal hypovolemia and hypoperfusion; inadequate

147

| | protein/calories increases the risk of edema formation and PIH. Intake of 80–100 g of protein may be required daily to replace losses. |

Monitor intake and output. Note urine color, and measure specific gravity as indicated.

Urine output is a sensitive indicator of circulatory blood volume. Oliguria and specific gravity of 1.040 indicate severe hypovolemia and kidney involvement. Note: Administration of magnesium sulfate ($MgSO_4$) may cause transient increase in output.

Test clean, voided urine for protein each visit, or daily/hourly as appropriate if hospitalized. Report readings of 2+, or greater.

Aids in determining degree of severity/progression of condition. A 2+ reading suggests glomerular edema or spasm. Proteinuria affects fluid shifts from the vascular tree. Note: Urine contaminated by vaginal secretions may test positive for protein, or dilution may result in a false-negative result. In addition, PIH may be present without significant proteinuria.

Assess lung sounds and respiratory rate/effort.

Dyspnea and crackles may indicate pulmonary edema, which requires immediate treatment.

Monitor BP and pulse. (Refer to ND: Cardiac Output, decreased.)

Elevation in BP may occur in response to catecholamines, vasopressin, prostaglandins, and, as recent findings suggest, decreased levels of prostacyclin.

Answer questions and review rationale for avoiding use of diuretics to treat edema.

Diuretics further increase state of dehydration by decreasing intravascular volume and placental perfusion, and they may cause thrombocytopenia, hyperbilirubinemia, or alteration in carbohydrate metabolism in fetus/newborn. Note: May be useful in treating pulmonary edema.

Collaborative

Schedule prenatal visit every 1–2 wk if PIH is mild; weekly if severe.

Necessary to monitor changes more closely for the well-being of the client and fetus.

Review moderate sodium intake of up to 6 g/day. Instruct client to read food labels and avoid foods high in sodium (e.g., bacon, luncheon meats, hot dogs, canned soups, and potato chips).

Some sodium intake is necessary because levels below 2–4 g/day result in greater dehydration in some clients. However, excess sodium may increase edema formation.

Refer to dietitian as indicated.

Nutritional consult may be beneficial in determining individual needs/dietary plan.

Place client on strict regimen of bedrest; encourage lateral position.

Lateral recumbent position decreases pressure onthe vena cava, increasing venous return and circulatory volume. This enhances placental and renal perfusion, reduces adrenal activity, and may lower BP as well as account for weight loss through diuresis of up to 4 lb in 24-hr period.

Refer to home monitoring/day-care program, as appropriate.

Some mildly hypertensive clients without proteinuria may be managed on an outpatient basis if adequate surveillance and support is provided and the client/family actively participates in the treatment regimen.

Replace fluids either orally or parenterally via infusion pump, as indicated.

Fluid replacement corrects hypovolemia, yet must be administered cautiously to prevent overload, especially if interstitial fluid is drawn back into circulation when activity is reduced. With renal involvement, fluid intake is restricted; i.e., if output is reduced (less than 700 ml/24 hr), total fluid intake is restricted to approximate output plus insensible loss. Use of infusion pump allows more accurate control delivery of IV fluids.

When fluid deficit is severe and client is hospitalized:

Insert indwelling catheter if kidney output is reduced or is less than 50 ml/hr.

Assist with insertion of lines and/or monitoring of invasive hemodynamic parameters, such as CVP and pulmonary artery wedge pressure (PAWP).

Monitor serum uric acid and creatinine levels, and BUN.

Administer platelets as indicated.

Allows more accurate monitoring of output/renal perfusion.

Provides a more accurate measurement of fluid volume. In normal pregnancy, plasma volume increases by 30%–50%, yet this increase does not occur in the client with PIH.

Elevated levels, especially of uric acid, indicate impaired kidney function, worsening of maternal condition, and poor fetal outcome.

Clients with HELLP syndrome awaiting delivery of the fetus may benefit from transfusion of platelets when count is below 20,000.

NURSING DIAGNOSIS:	**Cardiac Output, decreased**
May Be Related To:	Hypovolemia/decreased venous return, increased systemic vascular resistance
Possibly Evidenced By:	Variations in blood pressure/hemodynamic readings, edema, shortness of breath, change in mental status
DESIRED OUTCOMES/EVALUATION CRITERIA—CLIENT WILL:	Remain normotensive throughout remainder of pregnancy.
	Report absence and/or decreased episodes of dyspnea.
	Alter activity level as condition warrants.

ACTIONS/INTERVENTIONS	RATIONALE

Independent

Monitor and graph BP and pulse.	The client with PIH does not manifest the normal cardiovascular response to pregnancy (left ventricular hypertrophy, increase in plasma volume, vascular relaxation with decreased peripheral resistance). Hypertension (the second manifestation of PIH after edema) occurs owing to increased sensitization to angiotensin II, which increases BP, promotes aldosterone release to increase sodium/water reabsorption from the renal tubules, and constricts blood vessels.
Assess MAP at 22 weeks' gestation. A pressure of 90 mm Hg is considered predictive of PIH. Assess for crackles, wheezes, and dyspnea; note respiratory rate/effort.	Pulmonary edema may occur, with changes in peripheral vascular resistance and decline in plasma colloid osmotic pressure.
Institute bedrest with client in lateral position.	Increases venous return, cardiac output, and renal/placental perfusion.

149

Collaborative

ACTIONS/INTERVENTIONS	RATIONALE
Monitor invasive hemodynamic parameters.	Provides accurate picture of vascular changes and fluid volume. Prolonged vascular constriction, increased hemoconcentration, and fluid shifts decrease cardiac output.
Administer antihypertensive drug such as hydralazine (Apresoline) PO/IV, so that diastolic readings are between 90 and 105 mm Hg. Begin maintenance therapy as needed, e.g., methyldopa (Aldomet) or nifedipine (Procardia).	If BP does not respond to conservative measures, short-term medication may be necessary in conjunction with other therapies, e.g., fluid replacement and $MgSO_4$. Antihypertensive drugs act directly on arterioles to promote relaxation of cardiovascular smooth muscle and help increase blood supply to cerebrum, kidneys, uterus, and placenta. Hydralazine is the drug of choice because it does not produce effects on the fetus. Sodium nitroprusside is being used with some success to lower BP (especially in HELLP syndrome).
Monitor BP and side effects of antihypertensive drugs. Administer propranolol (Inderal), as appropriate.	Side effects such as tachycardia, headache, nausea, and vomiting, and palpitations may be treated with propranolol.
Prepare for birth of fetus by cesarean delivery, when severe PIH/eclamptic condition is stabilized, but vaginal delivery is not feasible.	If conservative treatment is ineffective and labor induction is ruled out, then surgical procedure is the only means of halting the hypertensive problems.

NURSING DIAGNOSIS:	Tissue Perfusion, altered: uteroplacental
May Be Related To:	Maternal hypovolemia, interruption of blood flow (progressive vasospasm of spiral arteries)
Possibly Evidenced By:	Intrauterine growth retardation, changes in fetal activity/heart rate, premature delivery, fetal demise
DESIRED OUTCOMES/EVALUATION CRITERIA—FETUS WILL:	Demonstrate normal CNS reactivity on nonstress test (NST); be free of late decelerations; have no decrease in FHR on contraction stress test/oxytocin challenge test (CST/OCT). Be full-term, AGA.

ACTIONS/INTERVENTIONS	RATIONALE

Independent

ACTIONS/INTERVENTIONS	RATIONALE
Provide information to client/couple regarding home assessment/recording of daily fetal movements and when to seek immediate medical attention.	Reduced placental blood flow results in reduced gas exchange and impaired nutritional functioning of the placenta. Potential outcomes of poor placental perfusion include a malnourished, LBW infant, and prematurity associated with early delivery, abruptio placentae, and fetal death. Reduced fetal activity indicates fetal compromise (occurs before detectable alteration in FHR and indicates need for immediate evaluation/intervention.
Identify factors affecting fetal activity.	Cigarette smoking, medication/drug use, serum glucose levels, environmental sounds, time of day, and sleep-wake cycle of the fetus can increase or decrease fetal movement.

Review signs of abruptio placentae (i.e., vaginal bleeding, uterine tenderness, abdominal pain, and decreased fetal activity).

Prompt recognition and intervention increases the likelihood of a positive outcome.

Provide contact number for client to ask questions, report changes in daily fetal movements, and so forth.

Provides opportunity to address concerns/misconceptions and intervene in a timely manner, as indicated.

Evaluate fetal growth; measure progressive fundal growth at each office visit or periodically during home visits, as appropriate.

Decreased placental functioning may accompany PIH, resulting in IUGR. Chronic intrauterine stress and uteroplacental insufficiency decrease amount of fetal contribution to amniotic fluid pool.

Note fetal response to medications such as $MgSO_4$, phenobarbital, and diazepam.

Depressant effects of medication reduce fetal respiratory and cardiac function and fetal activity level, even though placental circulation may be adequate.

Monitor FHR manually or electronically, as indicated.

Helps evaluate fetal well-being. An elevated FHR may indicate a compensatory response to hypoxia, prematurity, or abruptio placentae.

Collaborative

Assess fetal response to BPP criteria or CST, as maternal status indicates. (Refer to ND: Injury, risk for maternal.)

BPP helps evaluate fetus and fetal environment on five specific parameters to assess CNS function and fetal contribution to amniotic fluid volume. CST assesses placental functioning and reserves.

Assist with assessment of fetal maturity and well-being using L/S ratio, presence of PG, estriol levels, FBM, and sequential sonography beginning at 20–26 weeks' gestation. (Refer to CP: The High-Risk Frequency; ND: Injury, risk for fetal.)

In the event of deteriorating maternal/fetal condition, risks of delivering a preterm infant are weighed against the risks of continuing the pregnancy, using results from evaluative studies of lung and kidney maturity, fetal growth, and placental functioning. IUGR is associated with reduced maternal volume and vascular changes.

Assist with assessment of maternal plasma volume at 24–26 weeks' gestation using Evans' blue dye when indicated.

Identifies fetus at risk for IUGR or intrauterine fetal demise associated with reduced plasma volume and reduced placental perfusion.

Using ultrasonography, assist with assessment of placental size.

Decreased placental function and size are associated with PIH.

Administer corticosteroid (dexamethasone, betamethasone) IM for at least 24–48 hr, but not more than 7 days before delivery, when severe PIH necessitates premature delivery between 28 and 34 weeks' gestation.

Corticosteroids are thought to induce fetal pulmonary maturity (surfactant production) and prevent respiratory distress syndrome, at least in a fetus delivered prematurely because of condition or inadequate placental functioning. Best results are obtained when fetus is less than 34 weeks' gestation and delivery occurs within a week of corticosteroid administration.

NURSING DIAGNOSIS:	Injury, risk for maternal
May Be Related To:	Tissue edema/hypoxia, tonic-clonic convulsions, abnormal blood profile and/or clotting factors
Possibly Evidenced By:	[Not applicable: Presence of signs/symptoms establishes an *actual* diagnosis]
DESIRED OUTCOMES/EVALUATION CRITERIA—CLIENT WILL:	Participate in treatment and/or environmental modifications to protect self and enhance safety.

ACTIONS/INTERVENTIONS	RATIONALE
Independent	
Assess for CNS involvement (i.e., headache, irritability, visual disturbances or changes on funduscopic examination).	Cerebral edema and vasoconstriction can be evaluated in terms of symptoms, behaviors, or retinal changes.
Stress importance of client promptly reporting signs/symptoms of CNS involvement.	Delayed treatment or progressive onset of symptoms may result in tonic-clonic convulsions or eclampsia.
Note changes in level of consciousness.	In progressive PIH, vasoconstriction and vasospasms of cerebral blood vessels reduce oxygen consumption by 20% and result in cerebral ischemia.
Assess for signs of impending eclampsia: hyperactivity of deep tendon reflexes (3+ to 4+), ankle clonus, decreased pulse and respirations, epigastric pain, and oliguria (less than 50 ml/hr).	Generalized edema/vasoconstriction, manifested by severe CNS, kidney, liver, cardiovascular, and respiratory involvement, precede convulsive state.
Institute measures to reduce likelihood of seizures; i.e., keep room quiet and dimly lit, limit visitors, plan and coordinate care, and promote rest.	Reduces environmental factors that may stimulate irritable cerebrum and cause a convulsive state.
Implement seizure precautions per protocol.	If seizure does occur, reduces risk of injury.
In the event of a seizure: Turn client on side; insert airway/bite block only if mouth is relaxed; suction nasopharynx, as indicated; administer oxygen; remove restrictive clothing; do not restrict movement. Document motor involvement, duration of seizure, and postseizure behavior.	Maintains airway by reducing risk of aspiration and preventing tongue from occluding airway. Maximizes oxygenation. Note: Be cautious with use of airway/bite block, because attempts to insert when jaws are set may result in injury.
Palpate for uterine tenderness or rigidity; check for vaginal bleeding. Note history of other medical problems.	These signs may indicate abruptio placentae, especially if there is a preexisting medical problem, such as diabetes mellitus, or a renal or cardiac disorder causing vascular involvement.
Monitor for signs and symptoms of labor or uterine contractions.	Convulsions increase uterine irritability; labor may ensue.
Assess fetal well-being, noting FHR.	During seizure activity, fetal bradycardia may occur.
Monitor for signs of DIC easy/spontaneous bruising, prolonged bleeding, epistaxis, GI bleeding. (Refer to CP: Prenatal Hemorrhage.)	Abruptio placentae with release of thromboplastin predisposes client to DIC.
Collaborative	
Hospitalize if CNS involvement is present.	Prompt initiation of therapy helps to ensure safety and limit complications.
Administer MgSO$_4$ IM or IV using infusion pump.	MgSO$_4$ a CNS depressant, decreases acetylcholine release, blocks neuromuscular transmission, and prevents seizures. It has a transient effect of lowering BP and increasing urine output by altering vascular response to pressor substances. Although IV administration of MgSO$_4$ is easier to regulate and reduces the risk of a toxic reaction, some facilities may still use the IM route if continuous surveillance

Monitor BP before, during, and after $MgSO_4$ administration. Note serum magnesium levels in conjunction with respiratory rate, patellar/deep tendon reflex (DTRs), and urine output.

is not possible and/or if appropriate infusion apparatus is not available. Note: Adding 1 ml of 2% lidocaine to the IM injection may reduce associated discomfort. (Current research suggests the use of phenytoin infusion may be effective in the treatment of PIH without the adverse side effects, such as respiratory depression, and tocolytic effect on uterine smooth muscle, which can impede labor during intrapartal therapy.)

A therapeutic level of $MgSO_4$ is achieved with serum levels of 4.0–7.5 mEq/L or 6–8 mg/dL. Adverse/toxic reactions develop above 10–12 mg/dL, with loss of DTRs occurring first, respiratory paralysis between 15–17 mg/dL, or heart block occurring at 30–35 mg/dL.

Have calcium gluconate available. Administer 10 ml (1 g/10 ml) over 3 min as indicated.

Serves as antidote to counteract adverse/toxic effects of $MgSO_4$.

Administer amobarbital (Amytal) or diazepem (Valium), as indicated.

Depresses cerebral activity; has sedative effect when convulsions are not controlled by $MgSO_4$. Not recommended as first-line therapy because sedative effect also extends to the fetus.

Perform funduscopic examination daily.

Helps to evaluate changes or severity of retinal involvement.

Monitor test results of clotting time, PT, PTT, fibrinogen levels, and FPS/FDP.

Such tests can indicate depletion of coagulation factors and fibrinolysis, which suggests DIC.

Monitor sequential platelet count. Avoid amniocentesis if platelet count is less than $50,000/mm^3$. If thrombocytopenia is present during operative procedure, use general anesthesia. Transfuse with platelets, packed red blood cells, fresh frozen plasma, or whole blood, as indicated. Rule out HELLP syndrome.

Thrombocytopenia may occur because of platelet adherence to disrupted endothelium or reduced prostacyclin levels (a potent inhibitor of platelet aggregation). Invasive procedures or anesthesia requiring needle puncture (such as spinal/epidural) could result in excessive bleeding.

Monitor liver enzymes and bilirubin; note hemolysis and presence of Burr cells on peripheral smear.

Elevated liver enzyme (AST, ALT) and bilirubin levels, microangiopathic hemolytic anemia, and thrombocytopenia may indicate presence of HELLP syndrome, signifying a need for immediate cesarean delivery if condition of cervix is unfavorable for induction of labor.

Prepare for cesarean birth if PIH is severe, placental functioning is compromised, and cervix is not ripe or is not responsive to induction.

When fetal oxygenation is severely reduced owing to vasoconstriction within malfunctioning placenta, immediate delivery may be necessary to save the fetus.

NURSING DIAGNOSIS:	Nutrition: altered, risk for less than body requirements
May Be Related To:	Intake insufficient to meet metabolic demands and replace losses
Possibly Evidenced By:	[Not applicable; presence of signs/symptoms establishes an actual diagnosis]
DESIRED OUTCOMES/EVALUATION CRITERIA—CLIENT WILL:	Verbalize understanding of individual dietary needs.

ACTIONS/INTERVENTIONS	RATIONALE

Independent

Assess client's nutritional status, condition of hair and nails, and height and pregravid weight.	Establishes guidelines for determining dietary needs and educating client. Malnutrition may be a contributing factor to the onset of PIH, specifically when client follows a low-protein diet, has insufficient caloric intake, and is overweight or underweight by 20% or more before conception.
Provide information about normal weight gain in pregnancy, modifying it to meet client's needs.	The underweight client may need a diet higher in calories; the obese client should avoid dieting because it places the fetus at risk for ketosis.
Provide oral/written information about action and uses of protein and its role in development of PIH.	Daily intake of 80–100 g/day (1.5 g/kg) is sufficient to replace proteins lost in urine and allow for normal serum oncotic pressure.
Provide information about effect of bedrest and reduced activity on protein requirements.	Reducing metabolic rate through bedrest and limited activity decreases protein needs.

Collaborative

Refer to dietitian, as indicated.	Helpful in creating individual dietary plan incorporating specific needs/restrictions.

NURSING DIAGNOSIS:	**Knowledge deficit [Learning Need] regarding condition, prognosis, self care and treatment needs**
May Be Related To:	Lack of exposure/unfamiliarity with information resources, misinterpretation
Possibly Evidenced By:	Request for information, statement of misconceptions, inaccurate follow-through of instructions, development of preventable complications
DESIRED OUTCOMES/EVALUATION CRITERIA—CLIENT/COUPLE WILL:	Verbalize understanding of disease process and appropriate treatment plan.
	Identify signs/symptoms requiring medical evaluation.
	Perform necessary procedures correctly.
	Initiate lifestyle/behavior changes as indicated.

ACTIONS/INTERVENTIONS	RATIONALE

Independent

Assess client's/couple's knowledge of the disease process. Provide information about	Establishes data base and provides information about areas in which learning is needed. Receiving

pathophysiology of PIH, implications for mother and fetus; and the rationale for interventions, procedures, and tests, as needed.

information can promote understanding and reduce fear, helping to facilitate the treatment plan for the client. Note: Current research in progress may provide additional treatment options, such as using low-dose (60 mg/day) aspirin to reduce thromboxane generation by platelets, limiting the severity/incidence of PIH.

Provide information about signs/symptoms indicating worsening of condition, and instruct client when to notify healthcare provider.

Helps ensure that client seeks timely treatment and may prevent worsening of preeclamptic state or additional complications.

Keep client informed of health status, results of tests, and fetal well-being.

Fears and anxieties can be compounded when client/couple does not have adequate information about the state of the disease process or its impact on client and fetus.

Instruct client in how to monitor her own weight at home, and to notify healthcare provider if gain is in excess of 2 lb/wk, or 0.5 lb/day.

Gain of 3.3 lb or greater per month in second trimester or 1 lb or greater per week in third trimester is suggestive of PIH.

Assist family members in learning the procedure for home monitoring of BP, as indicated.

Encourages participation in treatment regimen, allows prompt intervention as needed, and may provide reassurance that efforts are beneficial.

Review techniques for stress management and diet restriction.

Reinforces importance of client's responsibility in treatment.

Provide information about ensuring adequate protein in diet for client with possible or mild preeclampsia.

Protein is necessary for intravascular and extravascular fluid regulation.

Review self-testing of urine for protein. Reinforce rationale for and implications of testing.

A test result of 2+ or greater is significant and needs to be reported to healthcare provider. Urine specimen contaminated by vaginal discharge or RBCs may produce positive test result for protein.

Diabetes Mellitus: Prepregnancy/Gestational

This disorder of carbohydrate metabolism of variable severity may be preexisting (pregestational insulin-dependent diabetes mellitus [IDDM] or non–insulin-dependent diabetes mellitus [NIDDM]), or may develop during pregnancy (gestational diabetes mellitus [GDM]).

(This plan of care is to be used in conjunction with the Trimesters and the High-Risk Pregnancy.)

CLIENT ASSESSMENT DATA BASE

Circulation

Pedal pulse and capillary refill of extremities may be diminished or slowed (with diabetes of long duration).
Edema, elevated BP (PIH).

Elimination

May have history of pyelonephritis, recurrent UTI, nephropathy
Polyuria

Food/Fluid

Polydipsia, polyphagia.
Nausea and vomiting.
Obesity; excessive or inadequate weight gain (client with GDM is usually obese; client with IDDM is not usually obese before pregnancy).
Abdominal tenderness.
May report episodes of hypoglycemia, glycosuria.

Safety

Skin integrity/sensation of arms, thighs, buttocks, and abdomen may be altered from frequent injections of insulin.
Visual impairment/retinopathy may be present.
History of symptoms of infection and/or positive cultures for infection, especially urinary or vaginal.

Sexuality

Fundal height may be higher or lower than normal for gestational age (hydramnios, inappropriate fetal growth).
History of large for gestational age (LGA) neonate, hydramnios, congenital anomalies, unexplained stillbirth.

Social Interaction

Socioeconomic concerns/factors can increase risk of complications.
Inadequate or lack of committed support system (may adversely affect diabetic control).

Teaching/Learning

Client's own birth weight may have been 9 lb or more.
May report recent problems/change in stability of diabetic control.
Family history of diabetes, GDM, PIH, infertility problem; LGA infant, history of neonatal death(s), stillbirth, congenital anomalies, spontaneous abortion, hydramnios, macrosomia (greater than 4000 g or 9 lb at birth).

DIAGNOSTIC STUDIES

Glucose Tolerance Test (GTT): Elevated above 140 mg/dL at 24–28 weeks' gestation. Clients with specific risk factors are screened at first prenatal visit. (If screening result is positive, 3-hr glucose challenge or oral glucose tolerance test [OGTT] test done to make diagnosis.)

Glycosylated Hemoglobin (HbA$_{1c}$): Reveals glucose control over previous 4–8 wk. Levels greater than 8.5%, especially before pregnancy, puts the fetus at risk for congenital anomalies.

Random Serum Glucose Level: Determines immediate diabetic control.

Urine Ketone Levels: Determines nutritional state.

Glycosylated Albumin: Reflects glucose control over last several days as possible screening test for GDM.

Urine Culture: Identifies asymptomatic UTI.

Vaginal Culture: May be positive for *Candida albicans* (*Monilia* infection).

Protein and Creatinine Clearance (24 hr): Verify level of kidney function, especially in diabetes of long duration.

Thyroid Function Tests: Establish baseline and/or identify coexisting hypothyroidism or hyperthryoidism.

Hemoglobin (Hb)/Hematocrit (Hct): May reveal anemia.

Triglycerides and Cholesterol Levels: May be elevated.

Estriol Level: Indicates level of placental function.

Electrocardiogram (ECG): May reveal altered cardiovascular function in diabetes of long duration.

Nonstress Test (NST): May demonstrate reduced fetal response to maternal activity.

Serial Ultrasonography: Determines presence of macrosomia or IUGR.

Contraction Stress Test (CST), Oxytocin Challenge Test (OCT): Positive results indicate placental insufficiency.

Amniocentesis: Ascertains fetal lung maturity using lecithin to sphingomyelin (L/S) ratio or presence of phosphatidylglycerol (PG).

BPP Criteria: Assesses fetal well-being/maturity.

NURSING PRIORITIES

1. Determine immediate and previous 8-wk diabetic control.
2. Evaluate ongoing client/fetal well-being.
3. Achieve and maintain normoglycemia (euglycemia).
4. Provide client/couple with appropriate information.

NURSING DIAGNOSIS:	Nutrition: altered, risk for less than body requirements
Risk Factors May Include:	Inability to ingest/utilize nutrients appropriately
Possibly Evidenced By:	[Not applicable; presence of signs/symptoms establishes an *actual* diagnosis]
DESIRED OUTCOMES/EVALUATION CRITERIA—CLIENT WILL:	Gain 24–30 lb prenatally, or as appropriate for prepregnancy weight.
	Maintain fasting serum glucose levels between 60–100 mg/dL and 1 hr postprandial no higher than 140 mg/dL.
	Be free of signs/symptoms of ketoacidosis.
	Verbalize understanding of individual treatment regimen and need for frequent self-monitoring.

ACTIONS/INTERVENTIONS	RATIONALE

Independent

Weigh client each prenatal visit. Encourage client to periodically monitor weight at home between visits.	Weight gain is the key index for deciding caloric adjustments.

Assess caloric intake and dietary pattern using 24-hr recall.

Aids in evaluating client's understanding of and/or adherence to dietary regimen.

Review/provide information regarding any required changes in diabetic management; e.g., switch from oral agents to insulin, use of Humulin insulin only, self-monitoring of serum glucose levels at least 4 times/day (e.g., before breakfast and 2 hr after each meal), and reducing/changing time for ingesting carbohydrates.

Metabolism and fetal/maternal needs change greatly during gestation, requiring close monitoring and adaptation. Research suggests antibodies against insulin may cross the placenta, causing inappropriate fetal weight gain. The use of human insulin decreases the development of these antibodies. Reducing carbohydrates to less than 40% of the calories ingested decreases the degree of the postprandial glucose peak of hyperglycemia. Because pregnancy produces severe morning carbohydrate intolerance, the first meal of the day should be small, with minimal carbohydrates.

Review importance of regularity of meals and snacks (e.g., 3 meals/3 or 4 snacks) when taking insulin.

Small, frequent meals avoid postprandial hyperglycemia and fasting/starvation ketosis. Note: Bedtime snack should contain both protein and complex carbohydrates to prevent nighttime hypoglycemia.

Note presence of nausea and vomiting, especially in first trimester.

Nausea and vomiting may result in carbohydrate deficiency, which may lead to metabolism of fats and development of ketosis.

Assess understanding of the effect of stress on diabetes. Provide information about stress management and relaxation. (Refer to CP: The High-Risk Pregnancy.)

Stress can elevate serum glucose levels, creating fluctuations in insulin needs.

Teach client finger-stick method for self-monitoring of glucose. Have client demonstrate procedure.

Insulin needs for the day can be adjusted based on periodic serum glucose readings. Note: Values obtained by reflectance meters may be 10%–15% lower/higher than plasma values.

Recommend monitoring urine for ketones on awakening and when a planned meal or snack is delayed.

Insufficient caloric intake is reflected by ketonuria, indicating need for an increase of carbohydrates or addition of an extra snack in the dietary plan (e.g., recurrent presence of ketonuria on awakening may be eliminated by a 3 AM glass of milk). Presence of ketones during second half of pregnancy may reflect "accelerated starvation" as diminished effectiveness of insulin results in a catabolic state during fasting periods (e.g., skipping meals), causing maternal metabolism of fat. Adjustment of insulin frequency/dosage/type must then be considered.

Review/discuss signs and symptoms and significance of hypoglycemia or hyperglycemia.

Hypoglycemia may be more sudden or severe in first trimester, owing to increased usage of glucose and glycogen by client and developing fetus, as well as low levels of the insulin antagonist human placental lactogen (HPL). Ketoacidosis occurs more frequently in second and third trimesters because of the increased resistance to insulin and elevated HPL levels. Sustained or intermittent pulses of hyperglycemia are mutagenic and teratogenic for the fetus during the first trimester; may also cause fetal hyperinsulinemia, macrosomia, inhibition of lung maturity, cardiac dysrhythmias, neonatal hypoglycemia, and risk of permanent neurological damage. Maternal effects of hyperglycemia can include hydramnios, UTI and/or vaginal infections, hypertension, and spontaneous termination of pregnancy.

Instruct client to treat symptomatic hypoglycemia, if it occurs, with an 8-oz glass of milk and to repeat in 15 min if serum glucose levels remains below 70 mg/dL.

Using large amounts of simple carbohydrates to treat hypoglycemia causes serum glucose values to overshoot. A combination of complex carbohydrates and protein maintains normoglycemia longer and helps maintain stability of serum glucose throughout the day.

Collaborative

Participate in/coordinate multispecialty care conference as appropriate.

Provides opportunity to review management of both pregnancy *and* diabetic condition, and to plan for special needs during intrapartum and postpartum periods.

Discuss dosage, schedule, and type of insulin (e.g., usually 4 times/day: 7:30 AM—NPH; 10 AM—regular; 4 PM—NPH; 6 PM—regular).

Division of insulin dosage considers maternal basal needs and mealtime insulin-to-food ratio, and allows more freedom in meal scheduling. Total daily dosage is based on gestational age, current maternal body weight, and serum glucose levels. A mix of NPH and regular human insulin helps mimic the normal insulin release pattern of the pancreas, minimizing "peak/valley" effect of serum glucose level. Note: Although some providers may choose to manage clients with GDM with oral agents, insulin is still the drug of choice.

Adjust diet or insulin regimen to meet individual needs.

Prenatal metabolic needs change throughout the trimesters, and adjustment is determined by weight gain and laboratory test results. Insulin needs in the first trimester are 0.7 unit/kg of body weight. Between 18 and 24 weeks' gestation, it increases to 0.8 unit/kg; at 34 weeks' gestation, 0.9 unit/kg, and 1.0 unit/kg by 36 weeks' gestation.

Refer to registered dietitian to individualize diet and counsel regarding dietary questions.

Diet specific to the individual is necessary to maintain normoglycemia and to obtain desired weight gain. In-depth teaching promotes understanding of own needs and clarifies misconceptions, especially for client with GDM. Note: New recommendations (Peterson & Peterson, 1992) set dietary needs at 25 kcal/kg dependent on the client's current pregnant weight.

Monitor serum glucose levels (FBS, preprandial, 1 and 2 hr postprandial) on initial visit, then as indicated by client's condition.

Incidence of fetal and newborn abnormalities is decreased when FBS levels range between 60 and 100 mg/dL, preprandial levels between 60 and 105 mg/dL, 1-hr postprandial remains below 140 mg/dL, and 2-hr postprandial is less than 120 mg/dL.

Ascertain results of HbA_{1c} every 2–4 wk.

Provides accurate picture of average serum glucose control during the preceding 60 days. Serum glucose control takes 6 wk to stabilize.

Prepare for hospitalization if diabetes is not controlled.

Infant morbidity is linked to maternal hyperglycemia-induced fetal hyperinsulinemia.

NURSING DIAGNOSIS:	Injury, risk for fetal
Risk Factors May Include:	Elevated maternal serum glucose levels, changes in circulation
Possibly Evidenced By:	[Not applicable; presence of signs/symptoms establishes an *actual* diagnosis]

ACTIONS/INTERVENTIONS	RATIONALE

Independent

Determine White's classification for diabetes; explain classification and significance to client/couple.	Fetus is at less risk if White's classification is A, B, or C. The client with classification D, E, or F who develops kidney or acidotic problems or PIH is at high risk. As a means of determining prognosis for perinatal outcome, White's classification has been used in conjunction with (1) evaluation of diabetic control or lack of control and (2) presence or absence of Pederson's prognostically bad signs of pregnancy (PBSP), which include acidosis, mild/severe toxemia, and pyelonephritis. The National Diabetes Data Group Classification, which includes diabetes mellitus (type I, insulin-dependent; type II, non–insulin-dependent), impaired glucose tolerance, and gestational diabetes mellitus, has not yet had prognostic significance in predicting perinatal outcomes.
Note client's diabetic control before conception.	Strict control (normal HbA_{1c} levels) before conception helps reduce the risk of fetal mortality and congenital anomalies.
Assess fetal movement and FHR each visit as indicated. (Refer to CP: Third Trimester, ND: Injury, risk for fetal.) Encourage client to periodically count/record fetal movements beginning about 18 weeks' gestation, then daily from 34 weeks' gestation on.	Fetal movement and FHR may be negatively affected when placental insufficiency and maternal ketosis occur.
Monitor fundal height each visit.	Useful in identifying abnormal growth pattern (macrosomia or IUGR, small or large for gestational age [SGA/LGA]).
Monitor urine for ketones. Note fruity breath.	Irreparable CNS damage or fetal death can occur as result of maternal ketonemia, especially in the third trimester.
Provide information and reinforce procedure for home blood glucose monitoring and diabetic management. (Refer to NDs: Knowledge Deficit [Learning Need]; Nutrition: altered, risk for less than body requirements.)	Decreased fetal/newborn mortality and morbidity complications and congenital anomalies are associated with optimal FBS levels between 70 and 96 mg/dL, and 2-hr postprandial glucose level of less than 120 mg/dL. Frequent monitoring is necessary to maintain this tight range and to reduce incidence of fetal hypoglycemia or hyperglycemia.
Monitor for signs of PIH (edema, proteinuria, increased blood pressure).	About 12%–13% of diabetic individuals develop hypertensive disorders owing to cardiovascular changes associated with diabetes. These disorders negatively affect placental perfusion and fetal status.
Provide information about possible effect of diabetes on fetal growth and development.	Helps client to make informed decisions about managing regimen and may increase cooperation.
Review procedure and rationale for periodic NSTs (e.g., weekly NST after 30 weeks' gestation, twice-weekly NST after 36 weeks' gestation).	Fetal activity and movement are good predictors of fetal wellness. Activity level decreases before alterations in FHR occur.

Discuss rationale/procedure for carrying out periodic OCT/CST beginning at 30–32 weeks' gestation, depending on diagnosis of IDDM or GDM. (Refer to CP: Third Trimester; ND: Injury, risk for fetal.)

CST assesses placental perfusion of oxygen and nutrients to fetus. Positive results indicate placental insufficiency, in which case fetus may need to be delivered surgically.

Review procedure and rationale for amniocentesis using L/S ratio and presence of PG. (Refer to CP: Second Trimester; ND: Injury, risk for fetal.)

When maternal/placental functioning is impaired before term, fetal lung maturity is criterion used to determine whether survival is possible. Hyper-insulinemia inhibits and interferes with surfactant production; therefore, in the diabetic client, testing for presence of PG is more accurate than using L/S ratio.

Collaborative

Assess HbA_{1c} every 2–4 wk, as indicated.

Incidence of congenitally malformed infants is increased in women with high Hb_{A1c} level (greater than 8.5%) early in pregnancy or before conception. Note: HbA_{1c} is not sensitive enough as a screening tool for GDM.

Assess glycolysated albumin level at 24–28 weeks' gestation, especially for client in high-risk category (history of macrosomic infants, previous GDM, or positive family history of GDM). Follow with OGTT if test results are positive.

Serum test for glycolysated albumin reflects glycemia over several days and may gain acceptance as screening tool for GDM because it does not involve potentially harmful glucose loading as does OGTT.

Verify AFP levels are obtained at 14–16 weeks' gestation.

Although AFP screen is recommended for all clients, it is especially important in this population because the incidence of neural tube defects is greater in diabetic clients than in nondiabetic clients, particularly if poor control existed before pregnancy.

Prepare for ultrasonography at 8, 12, 18, 28, and 36–38 weeks' gestation, as indicated.

Ultrasonography is useful in confirming gestation date and helps to evaluate IUGR.

Perform NST and OCT/CST, as appropriate.

Assesses fetal well-being and adequacy of placental perfusion.

Review periodic creatinine clearance levels.

There is a slight parallel between renal vascular damage and impaired uterine blood flow.

Obtain sequential serum or 24-hr urinary specimen for estriol levels after 30 weeks' gestation.

Although estriol levels are not used as often now, falling levels may indicate decreased placental functioning, leading to possibility of IUGR and stillbirth.

Assist as necessary with BPP assessment.

Provides a score to assess fetal well-being/risk. The criteria include NST results, fetal breathing movements, amniotic fluid volume, fetal tone, and fetal body movements. For each criterion met, a score of 2 is given. A total score of 8–10 is reassuring, a score of 4–7 indicates need for further evaluation and retesting, and a score of 0–3 is ominous.

Assist with preparation for delivery of fetus vaginally or surgically if test results indicate placental aging and insufficiency.

Helps ensure positive outcome for neonate. Incidence of stillbirths increases significantly with gestation more than 36 wk. Macrosomia often causes dystocia with cephalopelvic disproportion (CPD).

NURSING DIAGNOSIS:	Injury, risk for maternal
Risk Factors May Include:	Changes in diabetic control, abnormal blood profile/anemia, tissue hypoxia, altered immune response

Possibly Evidenced By:	[Not applicable; presence of signs/symptoms establishes in *actual* diagnosis]
DESIRED OUTCOMES/EVALUATION CRITERIA—CLIENT WILL:	Remain normotensive.
	Maintain normoglycemia, free of signs/symptoms of ketoacidosis.
	Be free of complications (e.g., infection, placental separation).

ACTIONS/INTERVENTIONS	RATIONALE

Independent

Note White's classification for diabetes. Assess degree of diabetic control (Pederson's criteria). (Refer to ND: Injury, risk for fetal.)	Client classified as D, E, or F is at higher risk for complications, as is client with PBSP.
Assess client for vaginal bleeding and abdominal tenderness.	Vascular changes associated with diabetes place client at risk for abruptio placentae.
Monitor for signs and symptoms of preterm labor.	Overdistension of uterus caused by macrosomia or hydramnios may predispose client to early labor.
Assist client in learning home monitoring of blood glucose, to be done a minimum of 4 times/day. (Refer to NDs: Nutrition: altered, risk for less than body requirements; Knowledge deficit [Learning Need].)	Allows greater accuracy than urine testing because renal threshold for glucose is lowered during pregnancy. Facilitates tighter control of serum glucose levels.
Request that client check urine for ketones daily.	Ketonuria indicates presence of starvation state, which may negatively affect the developing fetus.
Identify for hypoglycemic episodes occurring at home.	Hypoglycemic episodes occur most frequently in the first trimester, owing to continuous fetal drain on serum glucose and amino acids, and to low levels of HPL. In the presence of hypoglycemia, vomiting may lead to ketosis.
Identify for episodes of hyperglycemia.	Diet/insulin regulation is necessary for normoglycemia, especially in second and third trimesters, when insulin requirements often double (may quadruple in third trimester).
Assess for and/or monitor presence of edema. (Refer to CP: Pregnancy-Induced Hypertension; ND: Fluid Volume deficit.)	Because of vascular changes, the diabetic client is prone to excess fluid retention and PIH. The severity of the vascular changes before pregnancy influences the extent and time of onset of PIH.
Determine fundal height; check for edema of extremities and dyspnea.	Hydramnios occurs in 6%–25% of pregnant diabetic clients; may possibly be associated with increased fetal contribution to amniotic fluid, because hyperglycemia increases fetal urine output.
Assess for, and review with client, signs and symptoms if UTI.	Early detection of UTI may prevent pyelonephritis, which is thought to contribute to premature labor.
Determine nature of any vaginal discharge.	If glycosuria is present, client is more likely to develop monilial vulvovaginitis, which is caused by *Candida albicans* and may result in oral thrush in newborn.
Monitor client closely if tocolytic drugs are used to arrest labor.	Tocolytic drugs may elevate serum glucose and insulin levels.

Collaborative

Monitor serum glucose levels each visit.

Detects impending ketoacidosis; helps determine times of day during which client is prone to hypoglycemia.

Obtain HbA_{1c} every 2–4 wk, as indicated.

Allows accurate assessment of glucose control for past 60 days.

Assess Hb/Hct on initial visit, then during second trimester and at term.

Anemia may be present in client with vascular involvement.

Instruct in insulin administration, as required. Ensure that client is adept at self-administration, either subcutaneously (SC) or with pump, depending on client's needs or care setting.

Insulin requirements are decreased in first trimester, then double and may even quadruple as the pregnancy progresses. Highly motivated and capable clients may do well with a continuous subcutaneous insulin infusion pump to more naturally meet insulin needs.

Obtain urinalysis and urine culture; administer antibiotic as indicated.

Helps prevent or treat pyelonephritis. Note: Some antibiotics might be contraindicated because of danger of teratogenic effects.

Obtain culture of vaginal discharge, if present.

Candida vulvovaginitis can cause oral thrush in the newborn.

Collect specimens for total protein excretion, creatinine clearance, BUN, and uric acid levels.

Progressive vascular changes may impair renal function in clients with severe or long-standing diabetes.

Schedule ophthalmologic examination during first trimester for all clients, and in second and third trimesters if client is class D, E, F.

Owing to severe vascular involvement, background retinopathy may progress during pregnancy. Laser coagulation therapy may improve client's condition and reduce optic fibrosis.

Prepare client for ultrasonography at 8, 12, 18, 26, and 36–38 weeks' gestation as indicated.

Determines fetal size using biparietal diameter, femur length, and estimated fetal weight. Client is at increased risk for CPD and dystocia due to macrosomia.

Start IV therapy with 5% dextrose; administer glucagon SC if client is hospitalized with insulin shock and is unconscious. Follow with protein-containing fluids/foods, e.g., 8 oz skim milk when client is able to swallow.

Glucagon is a naturally occurring substance that acts on liver glycogen and converts it to glucose, which corrects hypoglycemic state. (Note: Hypertonic glucose [D_{50}] administered IV may have negative effects on fetal brain tissue because of its hypertonic action.) Protein helps sustain normoglycemia over a longer period of time.

NURSING DIAGNOSIS:	Knowledge deficit [Learning Need], regarding diabetic condition, prognosis, and self care treatment needs
May Be Related To:	Lack of exposure to information, misinformation, lack of recall, unfamiliarity with information resources
Possibly Evidenced By:	Questions, statement of misconception, inaccurate follow-through of instructions, development of preventable complications
DESIRED OUTCOMES/EVALUATION CRITERIA—CLIENT WILL:	Participate in the management of diabetes during pregnancy.

ACTIONS/INTERVENTIONS	RATIONALE

Independent

Assess client's/couple's knowledge of disease process and treatment, including relationships between diet, exercise, illness, stress, and insulin requirements.	Clients with either preexisting diabetes or GDM are at risk for ineffective glucose uptake within the cells, excess utilization of fats/proteins for energy, and cellular dehydration as water is drawn from the cell by a hypertonic concentration of glucose within the serum. Pregnancy alters insulin requirements drastically and necessitates more intense control, requiring the client/couple to take a very active role. Informed decisions can be made only when there is a clear understanding of both the disease process and the rationale for management.
Discuss importance of home serum glucose monitoring using reflectance meter, and the need for frequent readings (at least 4 times/day), as indicated. Demonstrate procedure, then observe return demonstration by the client.	Frequent blood glucose measurements allow client to recognize the impact of her diet and exercise on serum glucose levels and promote tighter control of glucose levels.
Review reasons why oral hypoglycemic medications should be avoided, even though they may have been used by the class A client, to control diabetes before pregnancy.	Although insulin does not cross the placenta, oral hypoglycemic agents do and are potentially harmful to the fetus, necessitating a change in diabetic management. Although some clinical sources report use of oral agents in clients with GDM, this is not recommended during pregnancy.
Provide information about action and adverse effects of insulin. Assist client to learn administration by injection, insulin pump, or nasal spray (experimental technique) as indicated.	Prenatal metabolic changes cause insulin requirements to change. In the first trimester, insulin requirements are lower, but they double and then may quadruple during second and third trimesters.
Explain normal weight gain to client. Encourage home monitoring between visits.	Total gain in the first trimester should be 2.5–4.5 lb, then 0.8–0.9 lb/wk thereafter. Caloric restriction with resulting ketonemia may cause fetal damage and inhibit optimal protein utilization. (Refer to ND: Injury, risk for fetal.)
Provide information about need for regular daily mild exercise program (regularly, 20 min after meals). Warn against exercising if glucose exceeds 300 mg/dL.	Regular exercise may decrease insulin requirements, while radical fluctuations in physical activity can adversely affect glucose control. Client should exercise after meals to help prevent hypoglycemia and to stabilize glucose excursion, unless excessive elevation of glucose is present, in which case exercise promotes ketoacidosis.
Provide information regarding the impact of pregnancy on the diabetic condition and future expectations.	Increased knowledge may decrease fear of the unknown, may increase likelihood of participation, and may help reduce fetal/maternal complications. About 70% of clients diagnosed with GDM will develop NIDDM within 15 yr.

Discuss how client can recognize signs of infection. Caution client not to treat self with OTC vaginal creams.

Recommend client maintain a diary of home assessment of serum glucose levels, insulin dosage, diet, exercise, reactions, general feelings of well-being, and any other pertinent thoughts.

Provide contact numbers for health team members.

Review Hb/Hct levels. Provide dietary information about sources of iron and the need for iron supplements.

Assist client/family to learn glucagon administration. Instruct client to follow with protein source, such as 8 oz of milk, then recheck glucose level in 15 min.

Important to seek medical help early to avoid complications. Choice of self-treatment may be inappropriate/mask infection.

When reviewed by healthcare practitioner(s), client's diary can assist with evaluation and alteration of therapy.

Client needs to be assured that questions will be answered and problems dealt with immediately on a 24-hr–day basis.

Anemias are of greater concern in clients with pre-existing diabetes because elevated glucose levels replace oxygen in the Hb molecule, resulting in reduced oxygen-carrying capacity.

Presence of symptoms of hypoglycemia (diaphoresis, tingling sensation, palpitations) with a serum glucose level under 70 mg/dL requires prompt intervention. Use of glucagon in combination with milk can increase the serum glucose level without the risk of rebound hyperglycemia. Glucagon is also useful during periods of morning sickness/vomiting when food intake is curtailed and serum glucose levels fall.

Prenatal Hemorrhage

Hemorrhage may occur early or late in pregnancy, owing to certain physiological problems, each with its own signs and symptoms, which help in establishing a differential diagnosis and in creating the plan of care. This general guide for care is meant to treat hemorrhage in the antepartal client. Where appropriate, interventions specific to each physiological problem are identified.

CLIENT ASSESSMENT DATA BASE: GENERAL FINDINGS

Circulation

Hypertension or hypotension may be present.
Pallor.
Dizziness.

Ego Integrity

Anxious, fearful, apprehensive

Food/Fluid

Nausea/vomiting

Safety

Pelvic inflammatory disease; repeated episodes of gonorrhea

Sexuality

Multiparity and advanced maternal age (>35).
Previous cesarean sections.
Repeated second- or third-trimester abortions.
Cervical scarring from lacerations, cervical conization, elective abortions, or dilation and
    curettage (D & C).
Specific conditions with appropriate signs and symptoms are listed in the prenatal time
    sequence in which they might appear.

Ectopic Pregnancy

Timing of rupture depends on location of fetus; i.e., isthmus of fallopian tube may rupture after 4–5 wk; an interstitial implantation may not rupture until the beginning of the second trimester. (Note: Enhanced diagnostic techniques are helping to identify the anomaly prior to tubal rupture.)

Circulation

Hypotension
Tachycardia
Delayed capillary refill
Cold, clammy skin
Faintness, syncope

Food/Fluid

Abdomen may be tender.

Pain/Discomfort

Colicky abdominal pain.
Referred shoulder pain may be noted as abdomen fills with blood.
Severe one-sided pain may occur in presence of tubal rupture.

Safety

Normal or subnormal temperature

Sexuality

Abdominal tenderness.
Uterine enlargement may be noted.
Adnexal mass is palpable on pelvic examination.
History of infertility/assisted reproductive techniques; use of progestin as only
contraceptive/intrauterine device; prior tubal surgery.
Abortion: can occur at any time prior to 20 weeks' gestation. (Refer to CP: Spontaneous
Termination.)

Hydatidiform Mole (Gestational Trophoblastic Disease)

May occur as early as the 4th week or as late as the second trimester

Circulation

Hypertensive symptoms and/or edema may have developed before 20 weeks' gestation (PIH).

Food/Fluid

Severe nausea/vomiting (hyperemesis gravidarum).
Urine may be positive for protein.

Sexuality

Uterus may be enlarged out of proportion to gestation or may be smaller than anticipated;
bilateral ovarian enlargement.
No FHTs or fetal outline palpable; no fetal activity noted.
Clear, grapelike vesicles passed vaginally.
Decrease in breast tissue.

Placenta Previa

Generally occurs after 20 weeks' gestation, usually third trimester; commonly the 8th mo
(34 wk).

Circulation

Painless vaginal bleeding (amount dependent on whether previa is marginal, partial, or total);
profuse bleeding may occur during labor.

Sexuality

Fundal height 28 cm or greater.
FHT within normal limits (WNL).
Fetus may be in transverse lie or unengaged.
Uterus soft.
Multiple gestation; increasing parity.
History of prior placenta previa, uterine surgery.

Abruptio Placentae

Premature separation of placenta usually occurs during third trimester, often during labor.

Circulation

Hypertension (predisposing factor).
Bleeding may be dark or bright; may be concealed.

Food/Fluid

Abdomen hard, boardlike; uterus tense with symmetric or asymmetric enlargement

Pain/Discomfort

May have pain with retroplacental hemorrhage; usually sudden onset, constant, marked tenderness to severe general or localized pain; low back pain

Sexuality

Rising uterine fundus, and tender to palpation.
Uterine tone may be increased; progressive decrease of relaxation between contractions.
Hyperactive fetus.
FHT may be WNL or may demonstrate bradycardia or tachycardia.

DIAGNOSTIC STUDIES

Culdocentesis: Positive for free blood.
Complete Blood Count (CBC): May reveal elevated WBC count, lowered Hb and Hct.
Human Chorionic Gonadotropin (HCG) Titers: Lowered with ectopic pregnancy, elevated with hydatidiform mole.
Activated Partial Thromboplastin Time (APTT), Partial Thromboplastin Time (PTT), Prothrombin Time (PT), and Platelet Count: May reveal prolonged coagulation, developing DIC.
Fibrinogen Levels: Decreased.
Fibrin Split Products and Fibrin Degradation Products: Present if DIC develops.
Estrogen and Progesterone Levels: Decline in spontaneous abortion.
Ultrasonography: Verifies the presence of a fetus, localizes the placenta, and reveals degree of separation; determines fetal age (based on measurement of biparietal diameter, length of femur, crown to rump).
Amniocentesis: Determines L/S ratio in cases of placenta previa.
Kleihauer-Betke Test on Maternal Serum, Vaginal Fluids, Amniotic Fluid, Gastric Lavage; or APT Test of Amniotic Fluid: Determines maternal versus fetal blood in amniotic fluid; estimates fetal blood loss.

NURSING PRIORITIES

1. Determine client/fetal status.
2. Maintain circulating fluid volume.
3. Assist with efforts to sustain the pregnancy, if possible.
4. Prevent complications.
5. Provide emotional support to the client/couple.
6. Provide information about possible short- and long-term implications of the hemorrhage.

DISCHARGE GOALS

1. Homeostasis achieved
2. Pregnancy maintained
3. Free of complications
4. Client/couple dealing constructively with situation
5. Condition, prognosis, and treatment needs understood

NURSING DIAGNOSIS:	**Fluid Volume deficit [isotonic]**
May Be Related To:	Excessive vascular loss
Possibly Evidenced By:	Hypotension, increased pulse rate, decreased pulse pressure, decreased/concentrated urine, decreased venous filling, change in mentation

168

DESIRED OUTCOMES/EVALUATION CRITERIA—CLIENT WILL:	Demonstrate stabilization/improvement in fluid balance as evidenced by stable vital signs, prompt capillary refill, appropriate sensorium, and individually adequate urine output and specific gravity.

ACTIONS/INTERVENTIONS

Independent

Evaluate, report, and record amount and nature of blood loss. Initiate pad count; weigh pads/underpad.

Institute bedrest. Instruct client to avoid Valsalva's maneuver and intercourse or any sexual activity that could lead to orgasm.

Position client appropriately, either supine with hips elevated or in semi-Fowler's position for placenta previa. Avoid Trendelenburg position.

Note vital signs, capillary refill of nailbeds, color of mucous membranes/skin, and temperature. Measure CVP, if available.

Monitor uterine activity, fetal status, and any abdominal tenderness.

Ascertain religious practices and preferences.

Avoid rectal or vaginal examination.

Record intake/output. Obtain hourly urine samples; measure specific gravity.

Auscultate breath sounds.

Save expelled tissue or products of conception.

Collaborative

Obtain/review stat blood work: CBC, type and crossmatch, Rh titer, fibrinogen levels, platelet count, APTT, PT, and HCG levels.

Insert indwelling catheter.

RATIONALE

Estimation of blood loss helps in differential diagnosis. Each gram of increased pad weight is equal to approximately 1 ml of blood loss.

Bleeding may stop with a reduction in activity. Increased abdominal pressure or orgasm (which increases uterine activity) may stimulate bleeding.

Ensures adequate blood available to the brain. Elevating hips avoids compression of the vena cava, while semi-Fowler's position allows the fetus to act as a tampon, controlling bleeding in placenta previa. Trendelenburg position may compromise maternal respiratory status.

Helps determine severity of blood loss, although cyanosis and changes in BP and pulse are late signs of circulatory loss and/or developing shock. Also monitors adequacy of fluid replacement.

Helps determine nature of the hemorrhage and possible outcome of hemorrhagic episode. Tenderness is usually present in ruptured ectopic pregnancy or abruptio placentae.

May prohibit use of blood products and establish need for alternative therapy.

May increase hemorrhage, especially if marginal or total placenta previa is present.

Determines extent of fluid losses and reflects adequacy of renal perfusion.

Adventitious breath sounds suggest excessive/inappropriate replacement. (Refer to ND: Fluid Volume risk for excess.)

Physician needs to evaluate for possible tissue/membrane retention; histologic examination may be necessary.

Determines amount of blood loss and may provide information regarding cause. Hct should be maintained above 30% to support oxygen and nutrient transport.

Output of less than 30 ml/hr indicates decreased renal perfusion and possible development of tubular necrosis. Appropriate output is determined by individual degree of deficit and rate of replacement.

169

ACTIONS/INTERVENTIONS	RATIONALE
Administer IV solutions, plasma expanders, whole blood, or packed cells, as indicated.	Increases circulating blood volume and reverses shock symptoms.
Prepare for laparotomy in the case of ruptured ectopic pregnancy.	Removal of the ruptured fallopian tube, and possibly the ovary, stops the hemorrhage. Note: If tube is not ruptured, treatment with medication to lyse the products of conception may preserve the tube.
Prepare for D & C in the presence of hydatidiform mole or incomplete abortion. (Refer to CP: Spontaneous Termination.)	Removes any chorionic vessels or products of conception that may adhere to endometrium.
Prepare for cesarean delivery if any of the following are diagnosed: severe abruptio placentae, DIC; or placenta previa when fetus is mature, vaginal delivery is not feasible, and bleeding is excessive or unresolved by bedrest.	Hemorrhage stops once the placenta is removed and venous sinuses are closed.

NURSING DIAGNOSIS:	Tissue Perfusion, altered uteroplacental
May Be Related To:	Hypovolemia
Possibly Evidenced By:	Changes in FHR and/or activity
DESIRED OUTCOMES/EVALUATION CRITERIA—CLIENT WILL:	Demonstrate adequate perfusion, as evidenced by FHR and activity WNL and reactive NST.

ACTIONS/INTERVENTIONS	RATIONALE
Independent	
Note maternal physiological circulatory status, and blood volume.	An episode of bleeding is potentially damaging to the outcome of the pregnancy, possibly causing uteroplacental hypovolemia or hypoxia.
Auscultate and report FHR; note bradycardia or tachycardia. Note change in fetal activity (hypoactivity or hyperactivity).	Assesses extent of fetal hypoxia. Initially, the fetus responds to decreased oxygen levels with tachycardia and increased movements. If deficit persists, bradycardia and decreased activity occurs.
Record maternal blood loss and any uterine contractions.	Excess maternal blood loss reduces placental perfusion. If uterine contractions are accompanied by cervical dilatation, bedrest and medications may not be effective in maintaining the pregnancy.
Note expected date of birth (EDB) and fundal height.	Provides an estimate for determining fetal viability.
Encourage bedrest in lateral position.	Relieves pressure on the inferior vena cava and promotes placental/fetal circulation and oxygen exchange.
Collaborative	
Administer supplemental oxygen to client.	Increases oxygen available for fetal uptake. The fetus has some inherent capacity to cope with hypoxia in that (1) fetal Hb dissociates (releases oxygen at the cellular level) more rapidly than adult Hb, and (2) the fetal red blood cell count is greater than that of the adult, so fetal oxygen-carrying capacity is increased.

ACTIONS/INTERVENTIONS	RATIONALE
Carry out/repeat NST, as indicated.	Electronically evaluating the FHR response to fetal movements is useful in determining fetal well-being (reactive test) versus hypoxia (nonreactive).
Replace maternal fluid/blood losses.	Maintains adequate circulating volume for oxygen transport. Maternal hemorrhage negatively affects uteroplacental oxygen transfer, leading to possible loss of pregnancy or worsening fetal status. If oxygen deprivation persists, the fetus may exhaust coping mechanisms, and CNS damage/fetal demise can occur.
Assist with ultrasonography and amniocentesis. Explain procedures.	Determines fetal maturity and gestational age. Aids in determining viability and realistically predicting outcome.
Obtain vaginal specimen for APT test, or use Kleihauer-Betke test to evaluate maternal serum, vaginal blood, or products of gastric lavage.	When vaginal bleeding is present, differentiates maternal from fetal blood in amniotic fluid; provides rough quantitative estimate of fetal blood loss and indicates implications for fetal oxygen-carrying capacity, and maternal need for Rh immune globulin G (RhIgG) injections, once delivery occurs. The Kleihauer-Betke test is more sensitive and quantitatively accurate than the APT test, but is time consuming and may be impractical if the specimen is sent to an outside laboratory.
Prepare client for appropriate surgical intervention as indicated.	Surgery is necessary if placental separation is severe; or if bleeding is excessive, fetal oxygen deprivation is involved, and vaginal delivery is impossible, as in cases of total placenta previa (a low-lying placenta), where surgery may be indicated to save the life of the fetus.

NURSING DIAGNOSIS:	**Fear**
May Be Related To:	Threat of death (perceived or actual) to self, fetus
Possibly Evidenced By:	Verbalization of specific concerns, increased tension, sympathetic stimulation
DESIRED OUTCOMES/EVALUATION CRITERIA—CLIENT WILL:	Discuss fears regarding self, fetus, and future pregnancies, recognizing healthy versus unhealthy fears.
	Verbalize accurate knowledge of the situation.
	Demonstrate problem solving and use resources effectively.
	Report/display lessened fear and/or fear behaviors.

ACTIONS/INTERVENTIONS	RATIONALE
Independent	
Discuss situation and understanding of situation with client and partner.	Provides information about individual reaction to what is happening.
Monitor client's/couple's verbal and nonverbal responses.	Indicates the degree of fear the client/couple is experiencing.

171

Listen and Active-Listen to client concerns.	Promotes sense of control over situation and provides opportunity for client to develop own solutions.
Determine religious/cultural practices. (Refer to CP: Spontaneous Termination ND: Spiritual Distress.)	Client may desire, or refuse, baptism and burial of products of conception in event of inevitable abortion.
Provide information in verbal and written form, and make opportunity for client to ask questions. Answer questions honestly.	Knowledge will help client to cope more effectivelywith what is happening. Written information allows for review later because client may not be able to assimilate information due to level of anxiety. Honest answers promote better understanding and can reduce fear.
Involve client in planning and participating in care as much as possible.	Being able to do something to help control the situation can reduce the fear.
Explain procedures and what symptoms mean.	Knowledge can help to reduce fear and promote sense of control over situation.

Collaborative

Contact clergy/spiritual advisor, as appropriate.	May be helpful in addressing some fears.

NURSING DIAGNOSIS:	**Injury, risk for maternal**
Risk Factors May Include:	Tissue/organ hypoxia, abnormal blood profile, impaired immune system
Possibly Evidenced By:	[Not applicable; presence of signs/symptoms establishes an *actual* diagnosis]
DESIRED OUTCOMES/EVALUATION CRITERIA—CLIENT WILL:	Remain afebrile.
	Display normal blood profile with WBC count, Hb, and coagulation studies WNL.
	Maintain urine output appropriate for individual situation.

ACTIONS/INTERVENTIONS

RATIONALE

Independent

Assess amount of blood loss. Monitor for signs/symptoms of shock. (Refer to ND: Fluid Volume deficit [isotonic].)	Persistent, excessive hemorrhage may be life-threatening to the client or may result in postpartal infection, postpartal anemia, DIC, renal failure, or pituitary necrosis attributable to tissue hypoxia and malnutrition.
Note temperature, WBC count, and odor and color of vaginal discharge, obtain culture if appropriate.	Excessive blood loss with decreased Hb increases the client's risk of developing an infection. (Refer to CP: Prenatal Infection.)
Record intake/output. Note urine specific gravity.	Reduced kidney perfusion results in reduced output. When hemorrhage occurs, the anterior pituitary lobe, which enlarges during pregnancy, is at risk for Sheehan's syndrome. (Refer to CP: Postpartal Hemorrhage; ND: Tissue Perfusion, altered.)
Monitor for adverse response to administration of blood products, such as allergic or hemolytic reaction; treat per protocol.	Early recognition and intervention may prevent life-threatening situation.

Inspect client for petechiae or for bleeding from gums/mucous membranes or IV site.

Indicates deficiencies or alterations in coagulation.

Provide information about risks of receiving blood products.

Complications such as hepatitis and HIV/AIDS may not be manifested during hospitalization, but may require treatment at a later date.

Collaborative

Obtain blood type and crossmatch.

Assures correct product will be available if blood replacement required.

Administer fluid replacement.

Maintains circulatory volume to counteract fluid losses/shock.

Monitor coagulation studies (e.g., APTT, platelet count, fibrinogen levels, FSP/FDP).

DIC with an associated drop in fibrinogen levels and a buildup of FSP may occur in response to the release of thromboplastin from placental tissue and/or dead fetus. In order for clot formation to occur, fibrinogen level must be at least 100 mg/dL.

Administer cryoprecipitate and fresh frozen plasma, as indicated. Avoid administration of platelets if consumption is still occurring (i.e., if platelet level is dropping).

In clients with DIC, cryoprecipitate replaces most clotting factors. Administration of platelets during period of continued consumption is controversial, because it may perpetuate the clotting cycle, resulting in further reduction of clotting factors and increasing venous congestion and stasis.

Administer heparin, if indicated.

Heparin may be used in DIC in cases of fetal death, or of death of one fetus in a multiple pregnancy, or to block the clotting cycle by preserving clotting factors and reducing hemorrhage until surgical correction occurs.

Administer antibiotic parenterally.

May be indicated to prevent or minimize infection.

Treat underlying problem (e.g., surgery for abruptio placentae or ectopic pregnancy, bedrest at home for placenta previa).

Stops hemorrhage; reduces likelihood of maternal injury.

NURSING DIAGNOSIS:	Pain [acute]
May Be Related To:	Muscle contractions/cervical dilatation, tissue trauma (fallopian tube rupture)
Possibly Evidenced By:	Reports of pain, distraction behaviors, autonomic responses (changes in pulse/BP)
DESIRED OUTCOMES/EVALUATION CRITERIA—CLIENT WILL:	Report pain/discomfort relieved or controlled.
	Demonstrate use of relaxation skills/diversional activities.

ACTIONS/INTERVENTIONS

RATIONALE

Independent

Determine nature, severity (using 0–10 scale), location, and duration of pain. Assess for uterine contractions, retroplacental hemorrhage, or abdominal tenderness.

Aids in diagnosis and choice of treatment. Discomfort associated with spontaneous abortion and hydatidiform mole is due to uterine contractions, which may be augmented by oxytocin

Assess client's/couple's psychological stress and emotional response to event.

Provide quiet environment and diversional activities. Instruct client in relaxation methods (e.g., deep breathing, visualization, distraction).

Explain procedures, answer questions honestly. Encourage expression of feelings/concerns.

Collaborative

Administer narcotics or sedatives, as appropriate.

Prepare for surgical procedure, administer preoperative medications if indicated.

infusion. In ectopic pregnancy, rupture results in extreme pain, caused by concealed hemorrhage. The hemorrhage occurs when the fallopian tube ruptures into the abdominal cavity. Abruptio placentae is accompanied by severe pain, especially when concealed retroplacental hemorrhage occurs.

Anxiety in response to the emergency situation may intensify the degree of discomfort owing to the fear-tension-pain syndrome.

May lower stimuli, refocus attention, thereby contributing to the reduction of discomfort.

Information, knowing what to expect can assist in lowering level of anxiety which can enhance perception of pain.

Promotes rest/alleviates pain.

Treatment of underlying disorder should alleviate pain.

NURSING DIAGNOSIS:	Fluid Volume risk for excess
Risk Factors May Include:	Excessive/rapid replacement of fluid losses
Possibly Evidenced By:	[Not applicable; presence of signs/symptoms establishes an *actual* diagnosis]
DESIRED OUTCOMES/EVALUATION CRITERIA—CLIENT WILL:	Display BP, pulse, urine specific gravity, and neurological signs WNL, without respiratory difficulties.

ACTIONS/INTERVENTIONS

RATIONALE

Independent

Monitor for increasing BP and pulse; note respiratory signs such as dyspnea, crackles, or rhonchi.

If fluid replacement is excessive, symptoms of circulatory overload and respiratory difficulties may occur. In addition, the client with abruptio placentae who may already have hypertension is at risk for manifesting negative response to fluid replacement, as is the client with compromised cardiac function.

Carefully monitor infusion rate manually or electronically. Record intake/output. Measure urine specific gravity.

Intake and output should be approximately equal because circulating fluid volume is stabilizing. Urine output increases and specific gravity decreases as kidney perfusion and circulatory volume return to normal.

Assess neurological status, noting behavior changes or increasing irritability.

Behavior changes may be an early sign of cerebral edema owing to water retention.

Collaborative

Assess Hct level.

May indicate amount of blood loss and can be used to determine needs and adequacy of replacement.

NURSING DIAGNOSIS:	Knowledge deficit [Learning Need], regarding reason for hemorrhage, prognosis, and treatment needs
May Be Related To:	Lack of exposure to, and unfamiliarity with, information resources
Possibly Evidenced By:	Request for information, statement of misconceptions, inappropriate or exaggerated behaviors
DESIRED OUTCOMES/EVALUATION CRITERIA—CLIENT/COUPLE WILL:	Participate in learning process.
	Verbalize, in simple terms, the pathophysiology and implications of the clinical situation.

ACTIONS/INTERVENTIONS	RATIONALE

Independent

Explain prescribed treatment and rationale for hemorrhagic condition. Reinforce information provided by other healthcare providers.	Provides information, clarifies misconceptions, and may aid in reducing associated stress.
Allow client opportunity to ask questions and verbalize misconceptions.	Provides for clarification of misconceptions, identification of problems, and opportunity to begin to develop coping skills.
Discuss possible short-term maternal/fetal implications of bleeding episode.	Provides information about possible complications, promotes realistic expectations, and enhances follow through with treatment regimen.
Review long-term implications for situations requiring follow-up and additional treatment; e.g., hydatidiform mole, dysfunctional cervix, or ectopic pregnancy. (Refer to CP: Premature Dilation of the Cervix.)	After expulsion of a hydatidiform mole, HCG levels must be monitored for 1 yr. If levels remain high, chemotherapy is indicated, owing to risk of choriocarcinoma. A client with repeated second-trimester spontaneous abortion may have a Shirodkar-Barter procedure performed. A client with an ectopic pregnancy may have difficulty conceiving after removal of the affected tube/ovary.

175

Prenatal Infection

CLIENT ASSESSMENT DATA BASE

Activity/Rest

Malaise, fatigue
Generalized weakness
May report difficulty sleeping
Poor muscle tone/muscle wasting

Circulation

May be jaundiced

Elimination

Dysuria, urinary frequency, decreased urine output, hematuria

Food/Fluid

Nausea, vomiting, anorexia, weight loss.
Tongue may have visible lesion or sore (hairy leukoplakia seen in AIDS).
May report indigestion, altered taste.
Loss of subcutaneous fat.
Poor skin turgor.

Pain/Discomfort

Backache, flank pain, colicky pain noted with acute pyelonephritis.
Chest pain may occur with tuberculosis.
Severe itching, burning pain with lesions.
May complain of pruritus with active (infectious) hepatitis A or B.

Respiration

Dyspnea with exertion.
Cough may be productive of thick/purulent/blood-tinged sputum or may be nonproductive.
Crackles (rales), wheezes, bronchial breath sounds; tubular breath sounds, diminished/absent
    breath sounds over areas of pleural effusion or pneumothorax (tuberculosis).

Safety

Temperature elevation dependent on type of infection, e.g., low-grade in cystitis, high fever in
    pyelonephritis
Chills, night sweats
History of UTI
Positive cultures, elevated titers, positive screening for infectious disease
Exposure to body fluids or blood products through professional practice or through receiving a
    transfusion parenterally as a patient; carrier of group B beta-hemolytic streptococci (GBS) or
    of hepatitis B virus (HbsAg, anti-HBcAg)
Exposure to infectious agents through employment/environmental contact

Sexuality

May have history of early trimester pregnancy loss(es).
May currently have, or have previous exposure to, numerous heterosexual/bisexual partners,
    which increases risk for exposure to HIV and STDs; sexual partner may be hemophiliac,
    necessitating blood transfusions and placing him at risk for acquisition of HIV.
Vaginal discharge may be frothy, gray-green (trichomonal infection); whitish (candidal
    infection); thin, watery, yellow-gray, foul-smelling, "fishy" (*Gardnerella vaginalis* infection).
Strawberry patches on vaginal walls/cervix (trichomonal infection).

May have visible perineal or genital warts, lesions, or chancres.

Fundal height may not be AGA, possibly indicating IUGR associated with rubella or toxoplasmosis, or may correspond with gestational age of less than 37 wk, indicating increased risk for GBS.

Membranes may rupture prematurely (PROM).

Social Interaction

Immigrants from Africa or Haiti may have increased risk of AIDS; immigrants from Southeast Asia, Central America, or the Caribbean islands may have increased risk of infectious or carrier state of hepatitis B virus (HBV); Native Americans, inner city, lower socioeconomic population, and immigrants from underdeveloped countries also have increased risk of tuberculosis.

Teaching/Learning

Risk factors include diabetes, malnutrition, drug/alcohol addiction, anemia.

DIAGNOSTIC STUDIES

Urinalysis/Serum, Culture and Sensitivity: Detects UTI, asymptomatic bacteremia, or GBS.

RPR or VDRL: Tests for syphilis.

Vaginal, Rectal, and Cervical Smears: Determines presence of gonorrhea, chlamydial infection, bacteria, GBS, or genital herpes.

Viral Titers: Identify presence of rubella and CMV.

Mantoux Skin Test with Purified Protein Derivative (PPD): Significant positive reaction suggests tuberculosis but does not distinguish between an active/dormant infection, or an infection caused by a different mycobacteria.

Hepatitis/HIV Screening: Done in presence of high-risk behaviors.

ELISA: Screens for HIV.

Western Blot Test: Confirms HIV infection.

Complete Blood Count (CBC): Reveals anemia and indicators of infection (elevated WBC, differential shifted to the left).

Nucleic Acid Probe Test: Detects *Mycobacterium tuberculosis.*

Chest X-Ray: Visualizes nodular lesions, patchy infiltrates, cavitation, scar tissue, calcium deposits (tuberculosis).

Histology/Tissue Analysis, Needle Biopsy: To verify stage of tuberculosis.

Serial Ultrasonography: Detects IUGR.

Specimen of Vaginal Pool: Determines PROM.

NURSING PRIORITIES

1. Identify/screen for prenatal infection.
2. Provide information about protocol of care.
3. Promote client/fetal well-being.

DISCHARGE GOALS

1. Individual risks/conditions understood
2. Condition, prognosis, treatment needs understood
3. Participates effectively in therapeutic regimen
4. Pregnancy maintained as appropriate/desired

NURSING DIAGNOSIS:	Infection, risk for maternal/fetal
May Be Related To:	Inadequate primary defenses (e.g., broken skin, stasis of body fluids), inadequate secondary defenses (e.g., decreased hemoglobin,

177

May Be Related To (cont.):	immunosuppression), inadequate acquired immunity, environmental exposure, malnutrition, rupture of amniotic membranes
Possibly Evidenced By:	[Not applicable; presence of signs/symptoms establishes an *actual* diagnosis]
DESIRED OUTCOMES/EVALUATION CRITERIA—CLIENT WILL:	Verbalize understanding of individual causative/risk factors.
	Review techniques and lifestyle changes to reduce risk of infection.
	Achieve timely healing, free of complications.

ACTIONS/INTERVENTIONS	RATIONALE
Independent	
Review lifestyle and profession for presence of associated risk factors.	Drug abusers and healthcare professionals are at risk for exposure to HIV/AIDS and HBV through contact with contaminated needles, body fluids, and blood products; tuberculosis through air-borne droplets.
Obtain information about client's past/present sexual partners and exposure to STDs.	Multiple sexual partners or intercourse with bisexual men increases risk of exposure to STDs and HIV/AIDS.
Assess client's cultural background for risk factors.	Recent arrivals from Asia, South America, and the Caribbean islands have increased risk of exposure to HBV. In Africa, male-to-female ratio of HIV is 1:1 owing to cultural sexual practices, poor hygiene, and inadequate healthcare.
Assess for specific signs and symptoms; notify healthcare provider if present:	Identifiable signs of infection assist in determining mode of treatment. Some organisms have a predilection for the fetoplacental unit and the neonate, although the client may be asymptomatic; i.e., *Mycoplasma* and *Ureaplasma* organisms affect a significant number of pregnant women and have been cultured in aborted fetuses, even though the mothers have been free of symptoms.
Visible lesions/warts;	May indicate herpes simplex virus type II (HSV-II)/condyloma, which can be transmitted to newborn at time of delivery if lesion is present at term or if viral shedding is occurring.
Urinary frequency; dysuria; cloudy, foul-smelling urine;	May be associated with *Escherichia coli* or GBS, or client may have asymptomatic bacteriuria.
Change in color, consistency, and amount of vaginal discharge.	Gray-green discharge may indicate trichomoniasis; thick white discharge may indicate *Candida albicans* infection; thin, watery, yellow-gray foul-smelling ("fishy") discharge suggest *Gardnerella*; thin or purulent drainage may reflect *Chlamydia*.
Determine if viral infection is primary or recurrent.	Both herpes viruses (CMV and herpes simplex virus II [HSV-II]) recur in times of stress. Yet only primary CMV is problematic to the fetus, and only 50% of fetuses exposed are affected. Although recurrent HSV-II is associated with reduced viral shedding time, the newborn, if exposed to the virus at delivery, can be affected with either visible lesions or a disseminated type of the disease.

178

Determine status of maternal membranes. If they are ruptured, monitor for signs of blood cell count and FHR; or vaginal discharge having an odor).

Collaborative

Monitor progressive growth of fundal height based on serial ultrasonography.

Obtain appropriate specimens and laboratory/ diagnostic studies as indicated:
    Urine for routine urinalysis, culture, and sensitivity;

Vaginal/rectal culture for gonococci/chlamydiae;

Vaginal/cervical culture for *Listeria monocytogenes* and GBS;

Rubella titer;

Serum for hepatitis B screen for clients in high-risk group (e.g., Asians, Central Americans, natives of Caribbean islands);

Serum for HIV screen if high-risk behaviors are present (injection drug users; healthcare professionals, laboratory technicians, dialysis workers; those having exposure to bisexual partners, recipients of blood or blood product transfusions);
Serum for CD4+, T-lymphocyte count;

Assist as necessary with sputum collection and chest x-rays for client with respiratory symptoms.

Infectious organisms transmitted via the ascending route including *Chlamydia*, mycoplasmas, *Ureaplasma urealyticum*, develop bacteremia and pneumonia or possibly meningitis.

Evaluates fetal growth infections such as rubella and toxoplasmosis, which can result in IUGR.

Asymptomatic bacteriuria (colony count greater than 100,000/mL) occurs in as many as 12% of prenatal clients and has been associated with acute and chronic pyelonephritis, preterm delivery, chorioamnionitis, postpartal maternal sepsis, and congenital defects. From 1%–5% UTIs are linked to GBS, which is the leading cause of neonatal meningitis.

Approximately 40%–60% of patients with culture-positive gonococcus have concomitant chlamydial infection, the most common STD associated with conjunctivitis and pneumonia of the newborn. Other than ophthalmia neonatorum, gonorrheal infection of the newborn is infrequent, but does increase rate of neonatal mortality associated with overwhelming infection.

Fever of nonspecific origin and history of abortions, neonatal meningitis, sepsis, congenital listeriosis, or postpartal maternal sepsis may indicate recurrent listerial infections requiring treatment. From 5%–30% of women have positive cultures for GBS, yet may be asymptomatic. Although antipartum treatment for GBS carriers is not recommended, intrapartal treatment with antibiotics is indicated for all women with positive cultures.

From 5%–15% of women of childbearing age are still susceptible to rubella, which has identifiable teratogenic effects on the fetus. If rubella is contracted in the first trimester, the fetus has no chance of escaping teratogenic effects. If rubella is contracted in the second trimester, the fetus has a 50% chance of being affected.

Hepatitis in the first and second trimesters rarely affects the fetus. Women who contract hepatitis in the third trimester have a 60% chance of transmitting it to offspring coming in contact with blood products at the time of delivery. Carrier status can be passed on to infants if they are not treated at birth. This can possibly result in cirrhosis and hepatocellular carcinoma.

AIDS destroys the immune system, causing a variety of problems, including HSV-II, CMV, toxoplasmosis, candidiasis, Kaposi's sarcoma, and pneumonia.

Determines number of T_4 helper cells to monitor progression of HIV.

Helps in identifying causative organism in bacterial pneumonia and active tuberculosis. Note: Tuberculosis is not exacerbated by pregnancy.

Administer antibiotics/medications as indicated:
Penicillin/penicillin G, erythromycin and Ceftriaxone or spectinomycin;

UTI, listeriosis, gonorrhea, syphilis, bacterial pneumonia, all respond to antimicrobial treatment. Note: Prenatal treatment of client who is carrier of GBS is not effective, because recolonization can occur before birth, with infant still at risk for neonatal sepsis or meningitis.

Acyclovir (Zovirax) capsules;

Generally not recommended in treatment of HSV-II, unless primary infection disseminates.

HPA-23 and zidovudine (Retrovir, formerly AZT);

Although controversial, these drugs are approved by the FDA and have been shown to reduce transmission to the fetus by 68% and to prolong life in HIV-positive clients. Research suggests ZVD administration in the second trimester can reduce maternal transmission of HIV to the neonate by over 60%.

Pyrimethamine (Daraprim) and sulfadiazine;

Controls active disease progression in toxoplasmosis, but have known tetratogenic effects on fetus during the first and probably second trimesters.

Folic acid;

Counteracts side effects of pyrimethamine.

Miconazole (Monistat), tioconazole (Vagistat) or clotrimazole (Mycelex) suppositories/ vaginal tablets;

Indicated for treatment of *Candida albicans*. Note: Diabetic client is prone to monilial infection, which may be extremely resistant to prenatal treatment.

Metronidazole (Flagyl);

Indicated for treatment of trichomonal infections after 20 weeks' gestation. Treatment in the first 20 weeks' is symptomatic; the trichomonal infection may be receptive to Mycelex vaginal suppositories. Note: Both partners must be treated to prevent reinfection.

Isoniazid (INH) in combination with rifampin (Rifadin) and the addition of ethambutol (Myambutol) when INH resistance is suspected;

Treatment of choice for tuberculosis (or seroconversion to positive PPD in last 2 yr), with no known teratogenic effects. Streptomycin is avoided, owing to its association with vestibular and auditory defects, and pyrazinamide is also contraindicated. If time of seroconversion is unknown and chest x-ray is negative, treatment is begun after pregnancy; or if client is over age 35 with unknown or prolonged positive PPD, INH prophylaxis is not recommended in the absence of active disease because of risk of hepatotoxicity. Note: Pyridoxine (vitamin B_6) is recommended for any pregnant woman receiving INH.

Hepatitis A or B immune globulin (HAIB/HBIG).

Recommended for exposure to hepatitis A or B.

Prepare for/assist in transfer to tertiary care center as indicated. (Refer to CP: The High-Risk Pregnancy.)

Availability of staff and equipment ensures optimal care of high-risk client and fetus/ newborn.

Prepare for termination of pregnancy or labor induction, as indicated. (Refer to CP: Labor: Induced/Augmented.)

Pregnancy may be terminated for such conditions as toxoplasmosis occurring prior to 20 wk gestation or rubella in the first trimester. Note: AZT in combination with cesarean birth decreases neonatal HIV infection rate, allowing pregnancy to be carried to term as appropriate, in presence of maternal HIV infection.

NURSING DIAGNOSIS:	Knowledge deficit [Learning Need], regarding treatment/prevention, prognosis of condition
May Be Related To:	Lack of exposure to information and/or unfamiliarity with resources, misinterpretation

Possibly Evidenced By:	Verbalization of problem, inaccurate follow-through of instructions, development of preventable complications/continuation of infectious process
DESIRED OUTCOMES/EVALUATION CRITERIA—CLIENT WILL:	Identify appropriate preventive practices.
	Adopt behaviors/lifestyle changes as indicated.
	Follow-through with individual treatment regimen.
	List signs and symptoms that necessitate evaluation/intervention.
	Verbalize understanding of importance of providing necessary information for data collection.

ACTIONS/INTERVENTIONS	RATIONALE
Independent	
Identify signs/symptoms of infection. Discuss importance of prompt reporting to healthcare provider.	Maternal infection may not be serious, but can have serious implications for the fetus. Timely intervention may prevent complications and enhance likelihood of a positive outcome.
Discuss mode of transmission of specific infections, as appropriate.	Provides information to assist the client in making decisions relative to lifestyle/behavioral changes; reinforces need for partner to be treated.
Provide information concerning identified risks associated with client's employment or profession. Stress use of gloves and need for washing hands when client must handle blood products, saliva, or urine.	Dialysis workers and healthcare professionals who handle body fluids or blood products are at high-risk for exposure to HSV-II, HIV, and HBV, and need to use universal precautions.
Identify risk factors associated with client's lifestyle.	Injection drug users are susceptible to percutaneous transmission of HSV-II, HBV, HIV/AIDS, and other STDs. Involvement with multiple sex partners also increases risk of being infected.
Discuss importance of avoiding contact with persons known to have infections, such as upper respiratory infections, tuberculosis, rubella (if not immune), and hepatitis. Stress the need for immunization for rubella after delivery as indicated.	Preventing exposure helps reduce the risk of acquiring infection. From 5%–15% of women of childbearing age are still susceptible to rubella, which is spread by droplets. Immunization after delivery results in immunity during subsequent pregnancies.
Review hygiene measures, including wiping vulva from front to back after urinating and washing hands frequently (including after animal contact.)	Helps prevent rectal *E. coli* contaminants from reaching the vagina and reduces contamination with other viruses/bacteria that may be transmitted by poor hygiene practices. Listerial infection is thought to be transmitted via animal contact.
Encourage client to drink 6–8 glasses of fluid per day and to void regularly. Discuss results of urine test.	May help prevent UTI associated with stasis. Client with asymptomatic bacteriuria (colony count greater than 100,000/ml) may be at risk for premature delivery, congenital defects in offspring, or anemia.
Suggest client void following intercourse.	May prevent/reduce risk of UTI and transmission of STD, especially CMV, and nongonococcal urethritis.
Recommend wearing gloves while gardening, avoiding contact with cat litter boxes while	Helps prevent toxoplasmosis, most commonly acquired in the United States through contact with

181

pregnant, and cooking meats to appropriate internal temperatures.

Suggest alternative means of sexual gratification for client with active HSV-II, HIV/AIDS, or HBV.

Provide information about possible effects of infection on client/fetus.

cat feces. Some French and Japanese meat dishes are eaten raw or undercooked, thereby increasing the risk of acquiring toxoplasmosis.

Fondling or masturbation for sexual gratification helps prevent spread of infection to sexual partner.

Infection affects approximately 15% of all pregnancies. For some infections, such as rubella, the outcome may be fairly predictable, if the gestational age at which the fetus was exposed is known. For other maternal infections, such as those caused by *Ureaplasma*, *Mycoplasma*, or *Listeria* organisms, it is more difficult to predict the fetal/neonatal outcome, especially because the client may be asymptomatic. Most infections do not pose serious problems to the mother, but can have varying effects on the fetus. Two thirds of these exposed infants are infected in utero, with resultant effects on the liver and brain. Ascending tract infections have a greater chance of resulting in neonatal bacteremia and pneumonia.

Discuss necessary treatments that may have serious fetal implications, such as sulfadiazine and pyrimethamine (used to treat toxoplasmosis), or oral sulfonamides (used to treat UTI during the latter weeks of gestation).

These medications have known teratogenic effects on newborn. When toxoplasmosis is present, the fetus can be damaged by either the disease or the treatment. Neonatal hyperbilirubinemia and kernicterus may occur with the use of oral sulfonamides.

Review available options in cases of known teratogenic effects.

Fetus is more susceptible to effects of rubella early in gestation. HBV poses more risks for the fetus in the third trimester. Teratogenic effects of toxoplasmosis include growth retardation, CNS calcification, microcephaly, hydrocephaly, and chorioretinitis. In cases of rubella infection or toxoplasmosis, client/couple may elect to terminate the pregnancy, depending on stage of gestation in which exposure occurs.

Discuss possible effects of infection on type and timing of delivery.

Operative delivery may be indicated in the case of certain infections, such as HSV-II if client has active herpes with intact membranes or if membranes are ruptured for more than 4–6 hr. If client or fetus has developed an ascending tract infection following PROM, fetus may need to be delivered prior to term to prevent maternal/fetal sepsis.

Discuss implications of PROM for client and fetus/neonate.

Membrane rupture more than 18 hr before delivery increases the risk of ascending tract infection, with resultant chorioamnionitis and maternal/neonatal sepsis. Common causative organisms in ascending tract infections include GBS, *Chlamydiae*, and *Haemophilus influenzae*.

Discuss implications of specific disease process/ treatment as appropriate:

    UTIs;

Client may have asymptomatic bacteriuria with large colony counts (greater than 100,000/ml), and culture may be positive for GBS, *Ureaplasma* organisms, or *Mycoplasma* organisms, placing client at risk for sepsis during and following delivery, and placing the newborn at risk for early- or late-onset infection.

    Listeriosis and treatment with penicillin;

It is uncertain how the fetus/infant contracts listeriosis; however, the infection can result in

	abortion if it is contracted between 17 and 28 weeks' gestation, or cause newborn problems such as meningitis, mental retardation, or hydrocephaly if it is contracted after 28 weeks' gestation.
GBS and antibiotic treatment for the chronic carrier;	Occurring in 5%–30% of pregnant women, GBS is the leading cause of neonatal meningitis and is associated with neonatal sepsis, and with chorioamnionitis if it occurs at < 37 weeks' gestation and is accompanied by PROM. Treating client with antibiotics (penicillin) prior to 38 weeks' gestation is ineffective because the bacteria will probably recolonize before delivery. Antibiotics given after 38 weeks' gestation effectively treat the client, but not the fetus. However, intrapartal treatment for clients with positive GBS culture (between 35 and 37 wk) or prophylaxis for at-risk clients may be useful in preventing GBS disease in the neonate.
Chlamydial infection and prenatal treatment with antibiotics;	Chlamydia transmitted to the fetus through the ascending route can cause conjunctivitis or pneumonia in the first 3–4 mo after birth.
Neisseria gonorrheae;	Transmission by sexual contact requires that both partners be treated, that condoms be used, and that orogenital sex is avoided until post-treatment cultures are negative at two consecutive follow-up visits.
Hepatitis A or B, including designation of hepatitis B carrier state (involving HBV, HBsAg, anti-HbcAg);	Exposure to hepatitis A or B may result in fetal anomalies, preterm birth, intrauterine fetal death, or fetal/neonatal hepatitis. Chronic HBV carrier states can result in cirrhosis and hepatocellular cancer.
HSV-II;	Spread occurs through sexual contact during viral shedding, which lasts 21 days in active primary infections and 12 days in recurrent infections. A stressor such as pregnancy may cause viral shedding.
Positive HIV status;	Incubation periods for HIV range from 6 mo to 5 or more yr. Because of its immunosuppressive properties, HIV/AIDS results in opportunistic infections, which include pneumonia, meningitis, and encephalitis, caused by CMV, herpes viruses, *Toxoplasma, Histoplama, Candida,* or *Pneumocystis carinii.*
Primary, secondary, and tertiary stages of syphilis and treatment with penicillin;	Administration of penicillin effectively treats the fetus/newborn. The spirochete does not cross the placenta until 16–18 weeks' gestation. Primary and secondary stages of untreated syphilis may lead to stillbirth; tertiary stage results in congenital syphilis of the newborn.
Primary CMV infection during pregnancy;	Although CMV can recur in times of stress, only primary CMV can potentially cause cytomegalic inclusion disease in 50% of the offspring of affected mothers.
Supplemental pyridoxine (vitamin B$_6$).	Helps prevent peripheral neuropathy when INH is used to treat active tubercolsis.
Discuss newborn care and the need for follow-up in infants born to mothers in active or carrier state of HBV.	Bathing the newborn immediately after delivery and administering HBIG and hepatitis B vaccine will prevent the newborn from contracting the virus. Follow-up immunizations of the newborn with hepatitis B vaccine at 1 and 6 mo are then necessary.
Provide information, specific to infection, regarding possible long-term effects and incubation period	For example, longitudinal studies of children at age 3.5–7 yr show that effects of CMV are ongoing,

Identify self-help groups and sources of community supports.

May help client in gathering information and resolving issues.

resulting in learning disabilities, motor deficits, deafness, and lower than normal IQs.

NURSING DIAGNOSIS:	[Discomfort]
May Be Related To:	Body response to infective agent, properties of infection (e.g., skin/tissue irritation, development of lesions)
Possibly Evidenced By:	Verbal reports, restlessness, withdrawal from social contact
DESIRED OUTCOMES/EVALUATION CRITERIA—CLIENT WILL:	Identify/use individually appropriate comfort measures.
	Report discomfort is relieved/controlled.
	Demonstrate use of relaxation skills and diversional activities.

ACTIONS/INTERVENTIONS	RATIONALE

Independent

Identify source, location, and extent of discomfort; note signs and symptoms of infectious process.	Determines course of treatment and individual interventions.
Suggest increasing fluid intake and voiding in warm sitz bath for client with UTI.	Helps prevent stasis; warmth relaxes perineum and urinary meatus to facilitate voiding.
Provide information about hygienic measures such as frequent bathing, use of cotton underwear, and application of cornstarch for client with vaginal discharge associated with STDs (chlamydial infection or gonorrhea).	Helps promote dryness and prevent skin breakdown.
Provide information regarding use of warm sitz baths, use of hair dryer on genital area, urinating through an empty toilet paper tube, and wearing loose-fitting jeans/pants and cotton underwear for client with HSV-II.	Helps keep genital area dry/clean; prevents discomfort associated with urine coming in contact with lesions.
Encourage rest for client who has tuberculosis or flulike symptoms associated with listeriosis, rubella, or toxoplasmosis.	Reduces metabolic rate; facilitates response of individual immune system to infection.
Suggest use of humidified air, increased fluid intake, and use of semi-Fowler's position during sleep for clients with respiratory infections, such as tuberculosis.	Helps liquefy secretions and facilitates respiratory functioning. Upright position allows diaphragm to descend, thereby facilitating lung expansion.

Collaborative

Administer medications as indicated: Analgesics (e.g., acetaminophen, codeine);	Relieves discomfort associated with backache, neuralgia, cervical lymphadenopathy, and perineal lesions. Note: In toxic levels, acetaminophen can

	cause liver damage. Use of acetylsalicylic acid (ASA) can result in alteration of fetal clotting.
Antipyretics;	Reducers fever and chills. Note: In client with PROM, administration of analgesic that may have antipyretic properties (e.g., acetaminophen) should be avoided because it may mask temperature rise that would signal infection.
Antibiotics specific to organisms cultured;	Eradicates organisms associated with UTI, bacterial pneumonia, STDs (gonorrhea, syphilis, chylamydial infection), and listeriosis. Relieves flulike symptoms associated with listeriosis.
HPA-23;	An experimental anti-AIDS drug that may help reduce discomforts associated with HSV-II, candidiasis, pneumonia, and Kaposi's sarcoma.
Lidocaine hydrochloride (Xylocaine) ointment.	Helps provide local anesthesia to herpetic lesions.

Premature Dilation of the Cervix (Incompetent/Dysfunctional Cervix)

Premature dilation of the cervix often occurs in the 4th or 5th mo and is associated with repeated second-trimester spontaneous abortions accounting for 15%–20% of second-trimester pregnancy losses.

CLIENT ASSESSMENT DATA BASE

Ego Integrity

Feelings of failure at a life event; expressions of shame/guilt
Expressions/manifestations of anxiety and/or fear

Elimination

Urinary frequency/urgency

Pain/Discomfort

Absence of pain, although lower abdominal pressure may be noted

Safety

May present with premature rupture of membranes (PROM) during second trimester

Sexuality

History of repeated, relatively painless, bloodless, second-trimester fetal loss (habitual spontaneous aborter).
Premature shortening, effacement, and dilation of cervix during current pregnancy.
Cervical trauma associated with previous deliveries with D & C, conization, cauterization, abortions (therapeutic, elective), or cervical lacerations.
Sterile vaginal examination reveals dilation, cervical effacement.
Membranes may be felt or seen protruding though cervical os.

Social Interaction

Concern about response of others; report of conflicted relationship with mother (e.g., especially if she used diethylstilbestrol [DES]).

Teaching/Learning

Reported previous occurrence of spontaneous abortion
Family history of DES use by mother

DIAGNOSTIC STUDIES

Diagnosis is usually made on basis of history of repeated second-trimester abortions.
Serial Ultrasonography: Beginning at 6–8 weeks' gestation can detect cervical shortening and premature dilation and aid in diagnosis, especially in women without clear-cut history of cervical dysfunction.
Nitrazine and/or Fern Test: Detects presence of amniotic fluid, indicating ruptured membranes.

NURSING PRIORITIES

1. Evaluate client/fetal status.
2. Assist with efforts to maintain the pregnancy, if possible.
3. Provide emotional support.
4. Provide appropriate instruction/information.

DISCHARGE GOALS

1. Client/fetal condition stable following procedure
2. Uterine contractions absent
3. Therapeutic needs and concerns understood

NURSING DIAGNOSIS:	Anxiety [specify level]
May Be Related To:	Situational crisis, threat of death/fetal loss
Possibly Evidenced By:	Increased tension, apprehension, feelings of inadequacy, sympathetic stimulation, and repetitive questioning
DESIRED OUTCOMES/EVALUATION CRITERIA—CLIENT/COUPLE WILL:	Verbalize fears and concerns.
	Report anxiety is reduced to a manageable level.
	Use individually appropriate coping mechanisms to deal with the short- and long-term outcomes of the situation.

ACTIONS/INTERVENTIONS	RATIONALE
Independent	
Provide primary nurse, if possible.	Facilitates continuity of care and increases client's/couple's confidence in care providers.
Review obstetric history.	The degree of anxiety depends on the nature of the situation, the history of fetal loss, the client's understanding of the events and proposed interventions, and the client's coping behaviors, both past and present.
Identify client's perception of the threat represented by this occurrence.	The ambiguity of the outcome can aggravate anxiety.
Determine availability of support systems and psychological response to event.	Establishes data base and plan of care. Degree of negative response and lack of/inadequate support contributes to heightened levels of anxiety, possibly to the point of affecting overall outcome.
Assess physiological indicators of anxiety: BP, pulse, respiratory rate, and diaphoresis.	Physiological changes in vital signs may have psychological origin.
Remain with couple. Explain what is happening and what can be expected. Provide factual information about causes, implications, and proposed treatment.	May reduce anxiety by increasing awareness of the circumstance.
Provide information on an ongoing basis.	Can allay anxiety.
Collaborative	
Refer to other sources for support or counseling if anxiety is excessive or support systems are inadequate.	May aid in long-term adjustment to situation.

NURSING DIAGNOSIS:	Injury, risk for maternal
Risk Factors May Include:	Surgical intervention, use of tocolytic drugs
Possibly Evidenced By:	[Not applicable; presence of signs/symptoms establishes an *actual* diagnosis]
DESIRED OUTCOMES/EVALUATION CRITERIA—CLIENT WILL:	Carry pregnancy to stage of fetal viability.
	Be free of complications.

ACTIONS/INTERVENTIONS	RATIONALE

Independent

Assess for presence of contraindications for cerclage procedure.	The procedure is not done if vaginal bleeding or cramping is present, if membranes are ruptured, if cervical dilation greater than 3 cm occurs, or if the diagnosis of cervical dysfunction is in question because situation has progressed and spontaneous abortion is inevitable.
Review implication of cerclage procedure on outcome of delivery at term.	A cesarean birth may be planned if the suture is left intact, or the suture may be removed, allowing a vaginal delivery. Note: Scar tissue may interfere with normal intrapartal cervical dilation and effacement.
Note presence of vaginal bleeding, leaking amniotic fluid, or uterine contractions after surgery.	Vaginal bleeding other than slight spotting may be sign of cervical dilatation. Leaking membranes may herald impending delivery and place client at greater risk for infection. Client may experience mild cramping after surgery, but strong uterine contractions may be indication of labor.
Monitor vital signs closely.	Changes in vital signs (e.g., elevated temperature or pulse, decreasing BP) may indicate infection or shock.
Notify physician of abnormal findings or signs of labor.	Prompt intervention lessens likelihood of complications.
Monitor for side effects of drugs used to prevent labor. Provide information to client.	A common side effect is maternal/fetal tachycardia; rare side effects include flushing, pulmonary edema, and congestive heart failure.

Collaborative

Prepare for cerclage procedure (Shirodkar-Barter or McDonald's modification), if indicated. Review information.	Between 14 and 18 weeks' gestation, insertion of a purse-string suture into the cervix may prolong the pregnancy.
Ensure continued bedrest in supine or Trendelenburg position for 24–48 hr after surgery.	Reduces pressure of presenting part on cervix.
Administer tocolytics as indicated. (Refer to CP: Preterm Labor/Prevention of Delivery.)	Reduces uterine irritability by relaxing smooth muscle.
Avoid contraction stress tests (CST or OCT) for duration of the pregnancy.	CST is contraindicated because it may result in trauma to the uterus and cervical sutures.

NURSING DIAGNOSIS:	Injury, risk for fetal
Risk Factors May Include:	Premature delivery, surgical procedure

Possibly Evidenced By:	[Not applicable; presence of signs/symptoms establishes an *actual* diagnosis]
DESIRED OUTCOMES/EVALUATION CRITERIA—CLIENT WILL:	Maintain pregnancy until fetal viability is assured.

ACTIONS/INTERVENTIONS

RATIONALE

Independent

Auscultate and report FHTs, noting strength, regularity, and rate. Note any changes in fetal movement. Note EDB and fundal height.

Indicates fetal well-being. EDB provides rough estimate of fetal age to help determine chance of viability.

Assess maternal condition and presence of uterine contractions or other signs of impending delivery. (Refer to CP: Spontaneous Termination.)

If advanced cervical dilation (4 cm or more) or regular uterine contractions occur, likelihood of preserving pregnancy is small.

Collaborative

Prepare mother for surgical procedure, as indicated. (Refer to ND: Injury, risk for maternal.)

Placement of cervical suture may preserve pregnancy until fetus reaches stage of viability.

Assist with ultrasonography, if indicated.

Provides more accurate picture of fetal maturity and gestational age.

NURSING DIAGNOSIS:	**Grieving, anticipatory**
May Be Related To:	Perceived potential fetal loss
Possibly Evidenced By:	Expression of distress, guilt, anger, and choked feelings
DESIRED OUTCOMES/EVALUATION CRITERIA—CLIENT/COUPLE WILL:	Identify and express feelings.
	Demonstrate effective coping behaviors to adjust to situation.
	Maintain positive self-esteem.

ACTIONS/INTERVENTIONS

RATIONALE

Independent

Assess client's/couple's emotional response to situation.

The client who has been diagnosed as having premature dilation of cervix may have previously experienced fetal loss. Should delivery occur at this time, fetal survival is extremely doubtful. Previous loss may have left the couple grief-stricken, with feelings of guilt.

Note presence of support systems.

Support from family, friends, and others can assist with adjustment to situation.

Encourage client/couple to verbalize feelings surrounding previous/current event.

Opens lines of communication and facilitates progress toward successful resolution of feelings.

Discuss normalcy of individual feelings/ grief reaction.

Client may suffer loss of self-esteem related to her difficulty in carrying a pregnancy to term. Feelings of

Review information about event, and discuss possibility for future pregnancies.

Provide information about community support groups.

inadequacy and role failure are frequently present and can have a negative impact on client's future and couple's relationship.

May lessen feelings of guilt and promote future adaptation to situation.

Participation in group activities with others who have been through similar experiences may help client/couple successfully work through grief process.

NURSING DIAGNOSIS:	Knowledge deficit [Learning Need], regarding nature of condition, self care needs
May Be Related To:	Lack of exposure/recall or misinterpretation of information
Possibly Evidenced By:	Request for information, statement of misconception, inappropriate or exaggerated behaviors
DESIRED OUTCOMES/EVALUATION CRITERIA—CLIENT WILL:	Verbalize understanding of her own circumstances and treatment.
	Demonstrate self-care behavior to maintain the pregnancy.

Independent

Determine level of client's knowledge.

Provides opportunity to clarify what has been learned previously, to identify cultural myths, and to correct misconceptions.

Assess degree of anxiety.

Anxiety can interfere with learning process.

Involve significant other(s) in discussions.

Helps to reinforce understanding of all individuals involved.

Provide information about future expectations.

Client may experience concern about whether difficulties may be encountered.

Identify signs/symptoms to be reported to the healthcare provider. (Refer to CP: The High-Risk Pregnancy.)

Prompt evaluation/intervention may prevent or limit complications.

Refer to other resources, such as counseling, group therapy, and childbirth education.

May need additional help to deal with individual concerns.

Spontaneous Termination

This plan of care applies to the client whose pregnancy is being, or has been involuntarily, terminated.

(To be used in conjunction with CP: Perinatal Loss.)

CLIENT ASSESSMENT DATA BASE

(Refer to "Client Assessment Data Base" section in CP: Prenatal Hemorrhage.)

Circulation

History of essential hypertension, vascular disease, ABO incompatibility

Ego Integrity

Pregnancy may/may not have been planned.
May be very anxious/fearful.

Elimination

Chronic nephritis

Food/Fluid

Poor maternal nutritional status

Pain/Discomfort

Pelvic cramping, backache

Safety

Exposure to toxic/teratogenic agents
History of pelvic inflammatory disease, STDs, or exposure to contagious diseases such as rubella, CMV, or active herpes

Sexuality

Vaginal bleeding, ranging from dark spotting to frank bleeding.
Examination may reveal premature dilation of cervix, bicornate or septate uterus, uterine fibroid tumors (leiomyoma), or other abnormalities of the maternal reproductive organs.
Note EDB (80% of spontaneous abortions occur in first trimester).

Teaching/Learning

Family history of genetic conditions

DIAGNOSTIC STUDIES

(Refer to CP: Prenatal Hemorrhage.)

NURSING PRIORITIES

1. Evaluate client status.
2. Prevent complications.
3. Support the grief process.
4. Provide appropriate instruction/information.

DISCHARGE GOALS

1. Free of complications following procedure
2. Support resources identified/contacted
3. Specific therapeutic needs and concerns understood

NURSING DIAGNOSIS:	Injury, risk for maternal
Risk Factors May Include:	Abnormal blood profile (decreased hemoglobin, altered clotting factors)
Possibly Evidenced By:	[Not applicable; presence of signs/symptoms establishes an *actual* diagnosis]
DESIRED OUTCOMES/EVALUATION CRITERIA—CLIENT WILL:	Report any bleeding.
	Be free of negative side effects from termination.

ACTIONS/INTERVENTIONS	RATIONALE

Independent

Assess vital signs and urine output. Note skin color/temperature. Estimate blood loss; conduct pad count/weight.	Early recognition of developing problems is important for prompt treatment.
Assess for and review signs/symptoms of DIC: abnormal clotting factors, elevated fibrin degradation products levels.	Fetal autolysis of the products of conception, which release thromboplastin, can cause DIC.

Collaborative

Prepare client for hospitalization.	For client with missed abortion, hospitalization is necessary if products of conception are not expelled spontaneously within 1–6 wk after fetal death.
Provide IV/oral fluids as appropriate. Administer volume expanders/blood products as indicated.	Prevents complications associated with blood loss. Note: Religious beliefs may limit therapeutic options.
Assist with necessary therapeutic procedures, (e.g, D & C, labor induction with oxytocin or prostaglandin).	The client with incomplete or missed abortion may need D & C to stop bleeding and to remove products of conception. If labor does not spontaneously follow fetal death, induction may be required in the second trimester.

NURSING DIAGNOSIS:	Spiritual Distress (distress of the human spirit), risk for
Risk Factors May Include:	Need to adhere to personal religious beliefs/practices; blame for loss directed at self or God
Possibly Evidenced By:	[Not applicable; presence of signs/symptoms establishes an *actual* diagnosis]
DESIRED OUTCOMES/EVALUATION CRITERIA—CLIENT/COUPLE WILL:	Discuss values/beliefs.
	Express feelings of self-worth/belief in self.
	Acknowledge responsibility without self-blame.

ACTIONS/INTERVENTIONS	RATIONALE

Independent

Determine client's/couple's religious preferences.	Establishes base for creating plan of care.
Ascertain client's specific needs; i.e., baptizing products of conception and/or formal burial.	If the individual preferences for/or refusal of religious rites is not honored or if desired support

is not offered, the client/couple may suffer additional distress. Note: Some religions (e.g., Catholic) require baptism. In the Islamic religion, a fetus aborted before 130 days' gestation is discarded like any other tissue. In addition, individual state laws may affect disposition of the fetus.

ACTIONS/INTERVENTIONS	RATIONALE
Provide information in nonjudgmental manner.	Because of emotional state or lack of knowledge, client may not realize that baptism may be performed.
Be aware of own biases and beliefs about events that are occurring.	Nurses must be aware of their own beliefs and prejudices about religious practices and not impose them on the client.
Provide opportunity for expressions of anger or concern.	Allows detection of self-blame or of alienation from God and/or previously held religious beliefs and values.
Note expression of hopelessness and/or helplessness.	These feelings may be normal initially. However, they may indicate a need for further evaluation and possible intervention to prevent or treat depression.
Encourage client's participation in development of treatment plan.	Can provide client with sense of control over difficult situation.

Collaborative

Offer clerical support and notify clergy/spiritual advisor, as desired.	Client may not recognize/verbalize own need for spiritual support.

NURSING DIAGNOSIS:	Knowledge deficit [Learning Need], regarding cause of abortion, self-care, contraception/future pregnancy
May Be Related To:	Lack of exposure to, or misinterpretation of, information
Possibly Evidenced By:	Request for information, statement of misconception, development of preventable complication
DESIRED OUTCOMES/EVALUATION CRITERIA—CLIENT WILL:	Verbalize the implications of the loss for future pregnancies.
	Explain proper use of desired contraceptive methods.
	Demonstrate appropriate follow-through with treatment and aftercare.
	Receive $Rh_o(D)$ immune globulin within 72 hr of termination, when appropriate.

ACTIONS/INTERVENTIONS	RATIONALE

Independent

Provide/review information about the cause of the spontaneous abortion when known, e.g., genetic anomalies, infection, Rh incompatibility.	May enhance understanding and promote positive self-care. Helps client prepare for future pregnancies.

193

Discuss alternative methods of contraception. Provide written information.

Client needs information to be able to choose a method that will meet her needs. Ovulation may occur before menses resume, so contraception needs to be considered at this time. Because of the anxiety and stress associated with the termination, verbal information may not be retained.

Identify signs/symptoms to be reported to healthcare providers.

Prompt evaluation/intervention may prevent or limit complications.

Review need for RhIgG dependent on client's Rh status.

For the Rh_o(D)-negative client, RhIgG prevents formation of anti–Rh-positive antibody so that adverse effects on future pregnancies are avoided.

Identify local support group or couple who have experienced a similar occurrence.

Provides opportunity to share experience with peers; may promote acceptance of loss/hope for the future.

Discuss option of genetic counseling, as appropriate.

May be necessary if the possibility of genetic involvement exists.

NURSING DIAGNOSIS:	Sexuality Patterns, risk for altered
Risk Factors May Include:	Increasing fear of pregnancy and/or repeat loss, impaired relationship with significant others, self-doubt regarding own femininity
Possibly Evidenced By:	[Not applicable; presence of signs/symptoms establishes an *actual* diagnosis]
DESIRED OUTCOMES/EVALUATION CRITERIA—CLIENT/COUPLE WILL:	Discuss sexual issues/concerns openly.
	Resume sexual activity at a pace agreeable to couple.
	Use contraception appropriately, if needed/desired.

ACTIONS/INTERVENTIONS

RATIONALE

Independent

Provide open discussion about sexual activities and future pregnancies.

Client may be reluctant to initiate discussion.

Discuss concerns/expectations about future plans, including pregnancies and feelings about self in this situation.

Because of the client's inability to maintain the pregnancy, one or both partners may have doubts regarding the client's femininity and may fear trying to maintain a pregnancy again.

Let client/couple know it is all right to feel what they are feeling and be where they are.

Physiological healing and grieving need to take place at some point in time.

Discuss resuming sexual activity, including alternative means of gratification, as indicated.

Safety of resuming sexual activity may depend on the medical regimen. Although the client/couple may find it difficult to talk about this topic, they usually appreciate this information.

Determine past methods of contraception.

Previously used methods of contraception may need to be replaced; client may need new information about contraception in the current situation.

Provide information about contraceptive alternatives, if needed.

Provide specific information about contraceptive method chosen.

Collaborative

Refer for further counseling, as indicated.

May need additional information to make informed decision. Some physicians advise avoiding pregnancy for 2–3 mo following an abortion.

Client needs to know how to use the method and what the possible side effects are.

May need additional help to resolve deep-seated conflicts.

Elective Termination

Therapeutic abortion may be done to safeguard the woman's health, or a voluntary abortion may be a woman's reproductive decision.

CLIENT ASSESSMENT DATA BASE

Circulation

Preexisting maternal health problems placing client at risk

Ego Integrity

Pregnancy often unplanned; may be result of incest/rape.
May express concern about decision and future expectations.
Possible feelings of abandonment, i.e., loss of contact with male partner.
Stress factors may include inadequate finances, cultural/religious conflicts, and individual plans for the future.
May have strong feelings/beliefs regarding abortion that may be in conflict with present situation (e.g., conception is result of incest or rape); lack of support, or family/other pressures to have abortion.

Food/Fluid

Severe nausea and vomiting

Safety

History of pelvic inflammatory disease, STDs, or exposure to contagious diseases, such as rubella
Exposure to toxic/teratogenic agents

Sexuality

Lack of, or inadequate use of, birth control measures.
Menstrual history may include problems such as endometriosis, heavy flow, or irregular periods.
Uterus may be in extreme flexion or version.
Absence of adnexal masses (rules out ectopic pregnancy).
Vaginal bleeding may be present.

Social Interaction

Possible lack of support systems or conflict within the family/couple.

Teaching/Learning

Family history of genetic conditions.
Client's perception of reasons for pregnancy termination, influencing factors, and anticipated effects may/may not be clear; alternatives may not have been considered/discussed or explored.

DIAGNOSTIC STUDIES

Complete Blood Count (CBC), Blood Type, and Rh Determination: Identifies individual needs.
Urine or Radioimmunoassay of Serum for Human Chorionic Gonadotropin (HCG): Verifies pregnancy.
Papanicolaou Smear: Rules out dysplasias.
Gonorrheal Culture, Rapid Plasma Reagin (RPR): Determine presence of STD.
Ultrasonography: May be done to confirm the pregnancy, to date the pregnancy, or to localize the placenta, if there is some discrepancy between uterine size and estimated date of birth.

Genetic Testing/Screening: Identifies affected fetus, which may be reason for decision to terminate pregnancy.

NURSING PRIORITIES

1. Evaluate biopsychosocial status.
2. Promote/augment coping strategies.
3. Provide emotional support.
4. Prevent postprocedural complications.
5. Provide appropriate instruction/information.

DISCHARGE GOALS

1. Free of complications following procedure
2. Coping effectively with situation
3. Specific therapeutic needs and concerns understood

NURSING DIAGNOSIS:	**Decisional Conflict, risk for**
Risk Factors May Include:	Unclear personal values/beliefs, lack of experience or interference with decision making, lack of relevant sources of information or information from multiple or divergent sources, support system deficit
Possibly Evidenced By:	[Not applicable; presence of signs/symptoms establishes an *actual* diagnosis]
DESIRED OUTCOMES/EVALUATION CRITERIA—CLIENT WILL:	Acknowledge feelings of anxiety/distress related to making difficult decision.
	Verbalize confidence in the decision to terminate the pregnancy.
	Meet psychological needs as evidenced by appropriate expression of feelings, identification of options, and use of resources.
	Display relaxed manner and/or calm demeanor, free of physical signs of distress.

ACTIONS/INTERVENTIONS	RATIONALE
Independent	
Ascertain circumstances of conception and response of family/significant other. Encourage client to talk about the issues and process used to problem-solve and make decision regarding termination.	Allows the nurse to determine whether the client/couple has explored alternatives. The decision to terminate a pregnancy may have been based on an inability to problem-solve or a lack of support and resources.
Note expressions of indecision and dependence on others.	May indicate ambivalence about decision and need for further information and discussion.
Assist client to look at alternatives and use problem-solving process to validate decision. Involve significant others as appropriate.	Helps client to reinforce reasons for decision and to be comfortable that this is the course she wants to pursue.
Provide explanations about the procedure desired by the client, pre-procedural and post-procedural tests, examinations, and follow-up.	Lack of knowledge about the procedures, reproduction, or self-care may contribute to the client's/family's inability to cope positively with this

197

Evaluate the influence of family and significant other(s) on the client.

Remain with the client during examinations and the procedure. Provide both physical and emotional support.

Act as a liaison and lend support to significant other(s).

Collaborative

Review safe options available based on gestation.

Obtain/review informed consent.

Refer for additional counseling or resources, if needed.

event, which may be behaviorally manifested by the client canceling appointments or verbalizing ambivalence. By eliminating fear of the unknown and by reinforcing reasons for and appropriateness of decision, ongoing verbalization can foster positive decision making.

Conflict can arise within the client herself as well as within the family. Allows the nurse to encourage positive forces or provide support where it is lacking.

Physical presence of nurse can help client feel accepted and reduce stress.

Helps reduce stress and encourages significant other(s) to be supportive of the client.

Assists client in making informed decision.

Depends on agency guidelines. No procedure should be performed unless the client freely consents to it.

Some clients may be more affected by the decision and may require additional support and/or education or genetic counseling.

NURSING DIAGNOSIS:	Knowledge deficit [Learning Need], regarding reproduction, contraception, self-care, Rh factor
May Be Related To:	Lack of exposure/recall or misinterpretation of information
Possibly Evidenced By:	Request for information, statement of misconception, inaccurate follow-through of instructions, development of preventable events/complications
DESIRED OUTCOMES/EVALUATION CRITERIA—CLIENT WILL:	Verbalize accurate information about the reproductive system.
	Explain proper use of desired contraceptive methods.
	Demonstrate appropriate follow-through with treatment and aftercare.
	Receive $Rh_o(D)$ immune globulin within 72 hr of termination, if appropriate.
	Verbalize the implications of the Rh factor for planning future pregnancies or for receiving blood transfusions.

ACTIONS/INTERVENTIONS	RATIONALE

Independent

Assess level of client knowledge, and provide information about reproduction. Use charts and diagrams.

Knowledge is essential to prevention of future unplanned pregnancies. Written and visual materials are more concrete and easily understood.

Discuss alternative methods of contraception.

Client needs information to be able to choose a method that is right for her. Ovulation may occur before menses resume, so contraception needs to be considered at this time.

Give specific instructions, preferably written, about the contraceptive chosen.

Client may have a method of contraception prescribed prior to discharge. Because of the anxiety and stress associated with the termination, verbal information may not be retained.

Reinforce postabortion instructions concerning the use of tampons and resumption of sexual activity, exercise, and prescribed antibiotics, if applicable. Provide written instructions.

The stress/anxiety caused by the procedure can diminish the client's ability to retain information. Written instructions can be reviewed when necessary. Note: Specific time frames vary according to practitioner.

Provide information about the implications of Rh_o (D)-negative blood and the need for RhIgG administration.

The client may not be aware of her blood type or the implications for future pregnancies if she is Rh_o(D)-negative. Understanding may promote positive self-care, enhance cooperation, and help prepare client for future pregnancies.

Identify signs/symptoms to be reported to healthcare provider.

Prompt evaluation/intervention may prevent or limit complications.

Collaborative

Verify Rh-negative status and administer RhIgG. Give 50 mg for early abortion; otherwise, dosage is the same as for delivery or fetal hemorrhage in the nonsensitized client.

For the Rh_o(D)-negative client, RhIgG prevents anti-Rh-positive antibody formation, so that negative effects on future pregnancies are avoided. Microdoses are given for early abortions, and this dose is sufficient up to 12 weeks' gestation. Fetal RBCs may be noted as early as 38 days after conception.

NURSING DIAGNOSIS:	Spiritual Distress (distress of the human spirit), risk for
Risk Factors May Include:	Perception of moral/ethical implications of therapy
Possibly Evidenced By:	[Not applicable; the presence of signs/symptoms establishes an *actual* diagnosis]
DESIRED OUTCOMES/EVALUATION CRITERIA—CLIENT WILL:	Discuss beliefs/values about spiritual issues.
	Verbalize acceptance of self/decision.

ACTIONS/INTERVENTIONS

RATIONALE

Independent

Note comments indicating feelings of guilt, negative self-concept/self-esteem, and ethical or religious value conflicts.

There may be conflict with family/significant other(s) regarding the morality of the client's decision, which can create confusion for the client.

Discuss alternatives to abortion with the client and significant other(s), if present. Maintain nonjudgmental attitude.

A decision based on a rational choice is less likely to result in conflict.

Assist with problem solving within the client's ethical and religious framework.

The ability to project the consequences of a decision or to explore alternatives may be hampered by anxiety and emotion.

199

Support the client's decision.	Client may have few, if any, support systems available at this time and may need a nonjudgmental resource.
Explain the grief response that may occur.	Client may not expect to feel loss.
Stress the importance of follow-up visits.	There may be delayed psychological reactions, which can be assessed at the follow-up visit along with the physical status.

Collaborative

Refer to clergy/spiritual advisor, or professional counseling. (Refer to CP: The High-Risk Pregnancy; ND: Coping, Individual/Family, ineffective.)	Some clients may need additional counseling before and after abortion to help them resolve feelings of conflict or guilt.

NURSING DIAGNOSIS:	**Anxiety [specify level]**
May Be Related To:	Situational/maturational crises, unmet needs, unconscious conflict about essential values/beliefs
Possibly Evidenced By:	Increased tension, apprehension, fear of unspecific consequences, sympathetic stimulation, focus on self
DESIRED OUTCOMES/EVALUATION CRITERIA—CLIENT WILL:	Recognize the presence of anxiety.
	Identify the cause of anxiety.
	Begin to use positive coping strategies to adjust to the situation.
	Report anxiety reduced to a manageable level.

ACTIONS/INTERVENTIONS

RATIONALE

Independent

Acknowledge the client's anxiety. Encourage ventilation of feelings.	Client may need assistance in recognizing reactions.
Be empathic and nonjudgmental.	Conveys a caring attitude.
Provide instruction in breathing and relaxation techniques.	Holding the breath and tightening the muscles may influence physiological responses (BP, pulse, and respiration). Tense muscles may interfere with the procedure.
Explain procedures before they are performed, and stay with the client to provide concurrent feedback.	A physical presence is reassuring and can increase cooperation and promote a sense of security.
Have a support person remain with the client, particularly if she is undergoing a second-trimester procedure requiring induction of labor.	The presence of a familiar person can help reduce anxiety and promote relaxation and coping.

NURSING DIAGNOSIS:	Pain/[Discomfort]
May Be Related To:	Aftereffects of procedure/drug effect
Possibly Evidenced By:	Report of discomfort, distraction behaviors, changes in muscle tone, autonomic responses/change in vital signs
DESIRED OUTCOMES/EVALUATION CRITERIA—CLIENT WILL:	Identify/use methods that provide relief. Report discomfort is minimized and/or controlled.

ACTIONS/INTERVENTIONS	RATIONALE

Independent

Explain to client the nature of discomfort expected.	Knowledge helps the client to cope with reality. Cramping pain during, and for 1 wk after, a first-trimester termination is expected. Clients treated with prostaglandins may experience nausea, vomiting, and diarrhea.
Determine the extent/severity and location of discomfort.	Although some discomfort is expected, severe cramping and abdominal tenderness may indicate complications.
Provide instruction in relaxation and breathing techniques.	May help break the cycle of fear, tension, and pain; provide distraction; and enhance coping.

Collaborative

Administer narcotic/nonnarcotic analgesics, sedatives, and antiemetics, as indicated.	These drugs promote relaxation, decrease pain awareness, and control side effects of treatment (drug therapy).
Provide information about the use of prescription or nonprescription analgesics.	Specific instructions about the use of any drugs increases awareness of safe use and side effects.

NURSING DIAGNOSIS:	Injury, risk for maternal
Risk Factors May Include:	Surgical procedure/anesthesia
Possibly Evidenced By:	[Not applicable; presence of signs/symptoms establishes an actual diagnosis]
DESIRED OUTCOMES/EVALUATION CRITERIA—CLIENT WILL:	Recognize and report signs/symptoms of complications. Institute appropriate corrective measures.

ACTIONS/INTERVENTIONS	RATIONALE

Independent

Monitor and assess blood loss. Count and weigh or estimate peripads.	Bleeding is normally like a heavy menstrual period. Excessive loss (more than 1 large pad per

Monitor vital signs, noting increased pulse rate, severe headache, or flushed face.

Note dyspnea, wheezing, or agitation.

Evaluate level of discomfort.

Instruct client to report symptoms indicating complications (e.g., temperature 100.4° F (40.0°C) or greater, chills, malaise, abdominal pain or tenderness, severe bleeding, heavy flow with clots, foul-smelling and/or greenish vaginal discharge).

Provide information about person to contact in case of emergency.

Stress importance of returning for a follow-up examination.

hour for 4 hr) may indicate retained tissue or uterine perforation.

Changes in vital signs are often a late sign of hypovolemic shock from blood loss. If hypertonic saline solution is used in second-trimester procedure and is inadvertently injected into the circulatory system, convulsions and death can occur.

Prostaglandins may cause vasoconstriction or bronchial constriction.

Abdominal pain, tenderness, and severe cramping may indicate retained tissue or uterine perforation.

Clients are in the healthcare facility for a short time. Complications, including bleeding and infection, may be manifested days or weeks after the procedure.

A specific phone number encourages contact; can save time and anxiety.

Follow-up is necessary to assess healing. A repeat pregnancy test is sometimes done after early first-trimester procedures to assure procedure was complete.

Collaborative

Assist with/review results of ultrasonography before procedure as indicated.

Determine cervical status before procedure. Assist as needed with insertion of *Laminaria* tent or prostaglandin (lamicel) gel.

Assist with any additional treatment or procedures necessary to control complications.

(Refer to CP: Labor: Induced/Augmented.)

Helps in confirming gestational age and the size of products of conception.

Aids in softening cervix; may be inserted 24–48 hr before procedure.

IV therapy may need to be instituted, with or without oxytoxics. Additional surgery (D & C or hysterectomy) may be needed to control bleeding.

Preterm Labor/Prevention of Delivery

Preterm labor refers to labor that occurs after the fetus has reached the period of viability (at least 20 weeks' gestation but before the completion of the 37th wk). Carrying the pregnancy to term may be contraindicated if associated client or fetal risks outweigh the risks of delivering a preterm infant.

(To be used in conjunction with CP: The High-Risk Pregnancy.)

CLIENT ASSESSMENT DATA BASE

Note: Etiology is unknown in 70%–80% of cases; PROM occurs in the remaining 20%–30%.

Activity

Works outside home, job heavy/stressful
Unusual fatigue

Circulation

Hypertension, pathological edema (signs of PIH)
Preexisting cardiovascular disease

Ego Integrity

Moderate anxiety apparent

Elimination

Dark amber urine, decreased frequency/amount

Food/Fluid

Inadequate or excessive weight gain
Inadequate fluid intake
Dry mucous membranes

Pain/Discomfort

Intermittent to regular contractions (may not be painful) less than 10 min apart and lasting at
least 30 sec for 30–60 min

Respiratory

May be heavy smoker (7–10 cigarettes/day), although any smoking during pregnancy is a risk
factor

Safety

Infection may be present (i.e., UTI and/or vaginal infection).

Sexuality

Cervical os softening/dilated/effacing.
Bloody show may be noted.
Membranes may be ruptured (PROM).
Third-trimester bleeding.
Previous abortions, preterm labor/delivery, history of cone biopsy, less than 1 yr since last birth.
Uterus may be overdistended, owing to polyhydramnios, macrosomia, or multiple gestation.

Social Interaction

May be low socioeconomic status

Teaching/Learning

Inadequate or no prenatal care
May be under age 18 or over age 40
Alcohol/other drug use, diethylstilbesterol (DES) exposure

DIAGNOSTIC STUDIES

Ultrasonography: Assesses gestation (with fetal weight of 500–2499 g).
Nitrazine Test or "Ferning" Slide: Determines PROM.
White Blood Cell (WBC) Count: Elevation indicates presence of infection.
Plasma/Cervicovaginal Oncofetal Fibronectin (onfFN): Elevated risk level associated with risk of preterm delivery, as well as pre-eclampsia and other abnormalities. (Currently under investigation as a clinical indicator or predictor of true/preterm labor.)
Urinalysis and Culture: Rule out UTI.
Vaginal Culture, RPR: Identify infection.
Amniocentesis: L/S ratio detects phosphatidyl glycerol (PG) for fetal lung maturity; or amniotic infection.
Electronic Monitoring: Validates uterine activity/fetal status.

NURSING PRIORITIES

1. Ascertain maternal condition/presence of labor and fetal well-being.
2. Assist with efforts to maintain pregnancy, if possible.
3. Prevent complications.
4. Provide emotional support.
5. Provide necessary information.

DISCHARGE GOALS

1. Cessation of uterine contractions
2. Free of complications and/or untoward effects
3. Dealing with situation in a positive manner
4. Signs of preterm labor/complications and therapy needs understood

NURSING DIAGNOSIS:	Anxiety [specify level]/Fear
May Be Related To:	Situational crisis, perceived or actual threats to self and fetus
Possibly Evidenced By:	Increased tension, apprehension, sympathetic stimulation, and extraneous movements
DESIRED OUTCOMES/EVALUATION CRITERIA—CLIENT WILL:	Verbalize understanding of individual situation and possible outcomes.
	Report anxiety is reduced/manageable.
	Appear relaxed; with maternal vital signs within normal limits.

ACTIONS/INTERVENTIONS	RATIONALE

Independent

Explain procedures, nursing interventions, and treatments. Keep communication open;	Knowledge of the reasons for these activities can decrease fear of the unknown.

discuss with client the possible side effects and outcomes, maintaining an optimistic attitude.

Orient client and partner to labor suite environment.

Helps client and significant other(s) feel at ease and more comfortable in their surroundings.

Answer questions honestly, including information regarding contraction pattern and fetal status.

Providing clear information can help the client/couple understand what is happening and may reduce anxiety.

Encourage use of relaxation techniques.

Enables the client to obtain maximum benefit from rest periods; prevents muscle fatigue and improves uterine blood flow.

Encourage verbalization of fears or concerns.

Can help reduce anxiety and stimulate identification of coping behaviors.

Monitor maternal/fetal vital signs.

Vital signs of client and fetus may be altered by anxiety. Stabilization may reflect reduction of anxiety level.

Assess support systems available to the client/couple, whether client remains hospitalized or is to return home to await delivery.

The assistance and caring of significant others, including caregivers, are extremely important during this time of stress and uncertainty. If client is to return home, additional support will be required to meet self-care needs and homemaker activities as well as child care, as appropriate.

Collaborative

Administer sedative if other measures are not successful.

Provides soothing and tranquilizing effect.

NURSING DIAGNOSIS:	Activity intolerance [specify level]
May Be Related To:	Muscle/cellular hypersensitivity (contracted plasma volume/dehydration, prolonged physical activity and stress)
Possibly Evidenced By:	Continued uterine contractions/irritability
DESIRED OUTCOMES/EVALUATION CRITERIA—CLIENT WILL:	Reduce activity level.
	Identify/engage in activities appropriate to situation.
	Demonstrate reduction/cessation of uterine contractions.

ACTIONS/INTERVENTIONS

RATIONALE

Independent

Explain the reasons for requiring bedrest, use of lateral recumbent/side-lying position, and decreasing activity.

These measures are intended to keep the fetus off the cervix and to enhance uterine perfusion; bedrest may decrease uterine irritability.

Provide comfort measures such as back rubs, changes of position, or decreased stimuli in room (e.g., low lighting).

Decreases muscle tension and fatigue and helps promote sense of well-being.

Group activities together as much as possible, such as medication administration, vital signs, and assessments.	Promotes longer opportunities for client to rest between interruptions.
Provide uninterrupted periods for rest/sleep.	Promotes rest, prevents fatigue, and may enhance relaxation.
Offer diversional activities, such as reading, radio, and television, or visits with selected friends or family.	Assists client in coping with decreased activity.
Assess uterine contractions per protocol.	Reflects effectiveness of and determines need for further interventions.

NURSING DIAGNOSIS:	**Poisoning, risk for**
Risk Factors May Include:	Dose-related toxic/side effects of tocolytics
Possibly Evidenced By:	[Not applicable; presence of signs/symptoms establishes an *actual* diagnosis]
DESIRED OUTCOMES/EVALUATION CRITERIA—CLIENT WILL:	Display no evidence of untoward effects of tocolytic therapy.
	Prevent or minimize maternal injury.
	Demonstrate cessation of uterine contractions, dependent on fetal well-being.

ACTIONS/INTERVENTIONS

RATIONALE

Independent

Place client in lateral recumbent position. Elevate head during infusion of IV drug.	Decreases uterine irritability, increases placental perfusion, and reduces supine hypotension.
Monitor vital signs. Auscultate lung sounds; note cardiac irregularities and investigate reports of dyspnea/chest tightness.	Complications, such as pulmonary edema, cardiac dysrhythmias/tachycardia, agitation, dyspnea, chest pain, and increase in plasma volume may occur with administration of beta-receptor agonists, e.g., terbutaline sulfate (Brethine) or ritodrine (Yutopar), which stimulate beta$_2$ receptors (especially with concomitant use of steroids to stimulate fetal lung maturity).
Measure intake and output. Encourage fluid intake between 2000 and 3000 ml/day, unless restricted (e.g., during administration of magnesium sulfate [MgSO$_4$]).	Promotes adequate hydration and prevents fluid excess, especially when MgSO$_4$ is administered. MgSO$_4$ is excreted through the kidneys, therefore, urine output must be maintained. Initial therapy may cause transient increase in output, and intake may be restricted in presence of generalized edema.
Weigh client daily.	Detects potential alteration in urinary functioning/retention of fluid.
Monitor for drowsiness, hot flashes, visual disturbances, respiratory depression, and depressed deep tendon reflexes, as appropriate.	Signs of neuromoscular depression, indicating increasing serum levels of MgSO$_4$.

206

Have antidote available (calcium gluconate for MgSO$_4$; propranolol for terbutaline sulfate).

Administration of antidote may be necessary to reverse or counteract effects of tocolytic agent.

Collaborative

Assist as needed with sterile vaginal examination.

To assess cervical status. Vaginal examinations are kept to a minimum, because they may contribute to uterine irritability and infection. Safety of tocolytics when cervix is more than 4 cm dilated or 80% effaced is not documented and is generally contraindicated.

Administer IV solution or fluid bolus as indicated.

Hydration may decrease uterine activity. Before beginning drug therapy, hydration promotes renal clearance and minimizes hypotension.

Administer IV solutions containing tocolytic agents (e.g., MgSO$_4$; terbutaline sulfate) by infusion pump or microdrip equipment, or by subcutaneous route. (Note: Experimental studies are evaluating the efficacy of prostaglandin synthesis inhibitors, such as indomethacin [Indocin], and other beta sympathomimetics, such as hexaprenaline.)

MgSO$_4$ acts directly on myometrial tissue to promote relaxation; therefore, there are fewer side effects than other drug choices. For example, unlike IV ritodrine, it produces no change in blood pressure, maternal heart rate or cardiac output. Terbutaline sulfate relaxes uterine muscle as well as bronchioles and blood vessel walls. Only ritodrine is currently approved by the FDA as a tocolytic agent; however, terbutaline sulfate is preferred because of its efficacy and lower cost.

Obtain serum potassium level prior to initiation of IV terbutaline and periodically per protocol. Monitor serum glucose and potassium levels.

Terbutaline sulfate (and ritodrine) cause movement of potassium ions into cells, decreasing plasma levels; elevated blood glucose and plasma insulin levels, and release of glycogen from muscle and liver may result in hyperglycemia.

Administer nifedipine (Procardia) to be chewed and swallowed with food or drink. Nifedipine may occasionally be alternated with terbutaline sulfate.

Nifedipine, a calcium channel blocker, has been used experimentally when other drugs fail to suppress uterine activity.

Monitor nifedipine levels as appropriate. Note development of tachycardia, hypotension, peripheral edema, or proteinuria.

The therapeutic dosage of nifedipine for preterm labor has not been established. Periodic monitoring may prevent development of adverse/toxic effects, such as congestive heart failure.

Apply antiembolic hose as indicated, and provide passive range of motion exercises to legs every 1–2 hr.

Prevents pooling of blood in lower extremities, which can occur because of smooth muscle relaxation.

Monitor serum magnesium levels per protocol during administration of MgSO$_4$. (Refer to CP: Pregnancy-Induced Hypertension.)

Therapeutic level is 4–7 mEq/L, or 6–8 mg/dL. Toxic signs and symptoms develop above 10 mg/dL.

Insert indwelling catheter, as indicated.

Urine output must be monitored and maintained when administering MgSO$_4$. Output should be at least 30 ml/hr, or 100 ml in a 4-hr period.

Assess uterine contractions and FHR electronically while IV tocolytic agents are administered, or at least twice a day when oral route is used.

Tactile and electronic monitoring of uterine contractions and FHR provides a continuous fetal/uterine assessment and basis for altering or maintaining rate of drug administration. Note: External monitors may increase contractions with some patients.

Decrease IV dose of tocolytics and gradually wean client to subcutaneous or oral dose, as indicated.

IV therapy should continue for at least 12 hr after contractions cease. Oral/subcutaneous therapy should begin 30 min before stopping IV infusion. Note: Intermittent subcutaneous administration of terbutaline may be preferred over oral route because

207

Arrange for transfer of client to high-risk facility or tertiary care center, if uterine activity persists following administration of tocolytics.

of significantly lower dosages, continued effectiveness, and uninterrupted sleep.

Helps ensure availability of appropriate intensive care, which may be needed by newborn following preterm delivery. (Refer to other CPs as appropriate; e.g., Cesarean Birth; Preterm Infant.)

NURSING DIAGNOSIS:	Injury, risk for fetal
Risk Factors May Include:	Delivery of preterm/immature infant
Possibly Evidenced By:	[Not applicable; presence of signs/symptoms establishes an *actual* diagnosis]
DESIRED OUTCOMES/EVALUATION CRITERIA—CLIENT WILL:	Maintain the pregnancy at least to the point of fetal maturity.

ACTIONS/INTERVENTIONS	RATIONALE

Independent

Assess for maternal conditions that would contraindicate steroid therapy to facilitate fetal lung maturity.	In PIH and chorioamnionitis, steroid therapy may aggravate hypertension and mask signs of infection. Steroids may increase serum glucose levels in the patient with diabetes. Drug will not be effective if unable to delay birth for at least 48 hr.
Assess FHR; note presence of uterine activity or cervical changes. Prepare for possible preterm delivery.	Tocolytics can increase FHR. Delivery may be extremely rapid with small infant if persistent uterine contractions are unresponsive to tocolytics, or if cervical changes continue.
Provide information about the actions and side effects of the drug therapy.	Important for the client/couple to know the purpose of the drug(s) being administered. Beta-agonist therapy may cause fetal tachycardia, hyperglycemia, acidosis, and hypoxia. Steroid therapy is most effective for increasing lung surfactant when the fetus is between 30 and 32 weeks' gestation (but may be used between 26 and 34 weeks' gestation).
Review potential side effects of steroid therapy with client/couple.	Short-term effects may include hypoglycemia, increased risk of sepsis, and possible suppression of aldosterone for up to 2 wk following delivery. Long-term effects on the development of the child will not be known until longitudinal studies have been completed.
Stress necessity of follow-up care.	If fetus is not delivered within 7 days of administration of steroids, dose should be repeated weekly.

Collaborative

Assist as needed with analysis of amniotic fluid from amniocentesis or vaginal pool specimen; test for ferning.	L/S ratio, presence of PG, and shake test results indicate fetal lung status. Ferning indicates rupture of membranes with increased risk of infection.
Administer betamethasone (Celestone) deep IM.	This synthetic cortisol can accelerate fetal lung maturity by stimulating surfactant production and

thereby preventing or decreasing the severity of respiratory distress syndrome. Note: Administration into the deltoid muscle may result in local atrophy.

Administer antibiotics, as indicated.

In the event of PROM and fetal lung immaturity, antibiotics may be used to prevent/reduce risk of infection, while allowing an additional 24–28 hr to elapse after administration of Celestone.

Initiate tocolytic therapy, as ordered.

Helps reduce myometrial activity to prevent/delay early delivery.

NURSING DIAGNOSIS:	Pain [acute]/[Discomfort]
May Be Related To:	Muscle contractions, effects of medications
Possibly Evidenced By:	Reports of pain/discomfort, muscle tension, narrowed focus
DESIRED OUTCOMES/EVALUATION CRITERIA—CLIENT WILL:	Report of discomfort is minimized, controlled.
	Use relaxation techniques, effectively.
	Appear relaxed, resting appropriately.

ACTIONS/INTERVENTIONS

RATIONALE

Independent

Expedite the admissions process and institute bedrest for client, using lateral recumbent position.

Side-lying position improves uterine blood flow and may decrease uterine irritability.

Review relaxation techniques, e.g., deep breathing exercises, visualization, guided imagery, soft music.

Helps client refocus attention, decreases muscle tension, reduces perception of discomfort and promotes sense of control. (Refer to ND: Anxiety [specify level]/Fear.)

Use nursing comfort measures such as changes of linen and position, back rug, and Therapeutic Touch.

Relieves muscle tension and fatigue.

Encourage routine inspection of mucous membranes for ulceration or reaction to chewing of nifedipine, if used.

Nifedipine may be irritating to oral cavity, in which case it should be swallowed whole.

Monitor maternal and fetal vital signs.

Reflects effectiveness of interventions.

Collaborative

Administer analgesics, as indicated.

Mild analgesics decrease muscle tension and discomfort.

NURSING DIAGNOSIS:	Knowledge deficit [Learning Need], regarding preterm labor, treatment needs, and prognosis
May Be Related To:	Misinterpretation or lack of information
Possibly Evidenced By:	Verbalization of questions/concerns, statements of misconceptions
DESIRED OUTCOMES/EVALUATION CRITERIA—CLIENT WILL:	Verbalize awareness of implications and possible outcomes of preterm labor.

ACTIONS/INTERVENTIONS	RATIONALE

Independent

ACTIONS/INTERVENTIONS	RATIONALE
Ascertain client's knowledge about preterm labor and possible outcomes.	Establishes data base and identifies needs.
Assess client readiness to learn.	Factors such as anxiety or lack of awareness of need for information can interfere with readiness to learn. Retention of information is enhanced when client is motivated and ready to learn.
Include significant other(s) in teaching-learning process.	Support from significant others can help allay anxiety as well as reinforce principles of teaching and learning.
Provide information about follow-up care when client is discharged.	Client may need to return on a regular basis for monitoring and/or treatments.
Identify signs/symptoms that should be reported immediately to healthcare provider, i.e., sustained uterine contractions, clear drainage from vagina.	Prompt evaluation and interventions may improve the outcome of the pregnancy.
Review signs/symptoms of "early" labor. (Refer to CP: The High-Risk Pregnancy; ND: Knowledge deficit [Learning Need]).	Assists client to recognize preterm labor so that therapy to suppress this labor can be instituted or reinstituted promptly.
Demonstrate how client is to evaluate contraction activity after discharge, e.g., lying down, tilted to one side with a pillow to the back; placing fingertips on the fundus for approximately 1 hr to note hardening/tightening of the uterus; or via use of electronic recorder.	Although uterine contractions commonly occur periodically, contractions occurring 10 min or less apart for an hour can result in cervical dilation and labor without prompt intervention. Self-monitoring is usually adequate and has no cost; however, some healthcare providers may require electronic monitoring, which necessitates data be transmitted via telephone lines and interpreted by a nurse upon receipt.
Stress importance of maintaining daily record of uterine activity and other pertinent information as individually appropriate.	Periodic review of data will be used to adjust therapy.
Arrange for client to visit neonatal intensive care unit.	Helps alleviate fears and facilitates adjustment to situation.
Discuss need to restrict lifestyle by stopping smoking and probably by restricting sexual activity and nipple stimulation.	Nicotine has adverse effect on fetoplacental growth and on uterine circulation. Orgasm or release of oxytocin may stimulate uterine activity.
Encourage regular rest periods 2–3 times daily in side-lying position. If bedrest is to be continued after discharge, suggest client spend part of day on couch/recliner.	Enhances relaxation and reduces fatigue. If client is up and about, resting in the bedroom may maximize rest; however, the client on full bedrest may feel isolated and bored without a "change of scenery."
Review daily routine, employment, and activity schedule to identify alternatives and ways to compensate for limitations.	Pacing activities, avoidance of heavy chores/lifting, and modification in work duties or cessation of employment may help prevent recurrence of preterm labor.

Determine availability and level of commitment of supportive resources.	Division of homecare responsibilities helps reduce risk of caregiver burn-out when one individual attempts to take on responsibilities of the client in addition to own role.
Recommend client empty bladder every 2 hr while awake.	Prevents pressure of a full bladder on the irritable uterus.
Review daily fluid need, i.e., 2–3 quarts of liquid and avoidance of caffeine.	Dehydration and caffeine both lead to increased uterine muscle irritability.
Obtain permit, if necessary, for administration of terbutaline.	Currently only ritodrine is FDA-approved as a tocolytic agent but is not generally used; terbutaline sulfate, which is usually the drug of choice, is still considered an experimental drug.
Stress avoidance of OTC drugs while tocolytic agents are administered unless approved by physician.	Concurrent use of OTC drugs may cause deleterious effects, especially if OTC drug has similar side effects to tocolytic agent (e.g., antihistamines or inhalers with bronchodilating effects such as epinephrine [Primatene Mist]).
Recommend adhering to a predetermined schedule for oral drug therapy.	Maintains blood level of drug for optimum effect. Note: Recent studies are evaluating the effectiveness and safety of low-dose continuous subcutaneous infusion and intermittent high-dose bolus administration of terbutaline in place of oral therapy.
Provide information about taking oral tocolytics with food.	Food improves tolerance to drug and reduces side effects.
Instruct in proper use of infusion pump when used and need to count/record pulse before bolus doses are administered.	Promotes safe use of drug, enhances participation in therapeutic regimen and supports self-care/independence.
Identify drug side effects requiring medical evaluation.	Pulse rate greater than 120 bpm; presence of tremors, palpitations, chest pain, or dyspnea; or feelings of nervousness and agitation may require alteration/discontinuation of drug.
Establish routine schedule for homecare nurse visitation. Provide regular telephone contact.	Weekly or biweekly visits provide opportunity for regular physical assessment, review of uterine activity record, additional education, and timely problem solving. Between visits, daily contact may be maintained via telephone, with a 24-hr "hot line" number also available for emergencies.
Identify other resources, as indicated (e.g., community or home health nurse, childbirth preparation classes, groups such as Parents of Twins, or other couple who have had a successful outcome, Internet support groups).	May need additional help in coping with situation, especially if client returns home to await delivery.

CHAPTER 5

INTRAPARTAL CONCEPTS

Intrapartal Assessment Tool

At the time of admission, the client should undergo a basic assessment because not all clients will arrive with a prenatal history/physical or will have been seen prenatally. Furthermore, with the increase in early release, discharge planning must be implemented at the time of admission, as feasible.

Date:_____ Time:_____ Admitted from:_____

Name:_____ Date of birth (DOB):_____ Age:_____ Race:_____

Reason for admission:_____

Healthcare provider: Maternal:_____ Infant:_____

Father of child:_____ Age:_____ Race:_____

Source of information:_____ Reliability:_____ (1–4 with "4" very reliable)

ACTIVITY/REST

Subjective

Sleep/rest last 24 hr:_____
Occupation: _____
Usual activities/hobbies:_____

Objective

Neuromuscular assessment: Quality of
   extremities:_____
   Posture:_____ Tremors:_____
   Range of motion (ROM):_____ Strength_____
   Deformity:_____ Other:_____

CIRCULATION

Subjective

History of: Elevated blood pressure (BP):_____
   Heart trouble:_____
   Rheumatic fever:_____
   Ankle/leg edema:_____
   Phlebitis:_____ Slow healing:_____
Extremities: Numbness:_____
   Tingling:_____
Cough/character of sputum:_____

Objective

BP: R: Sitting:_____ Lying:_____
   L: Sitting:_____ Lying:_____
Pulse (palpation): Carotid:_____
   Temporal:_____ Jugular:_____
   Peripheral:_____
Heart sounds:_____ Rate:_____
   Rhythm:_____ Quality:_____
Extremities: Temperature:_____ Color:_____
   Capillary refill:_____
   Homans' sign:_____ Varicosities:_____
Color/cyanosis: Mucous membranes:_____
   Nail beds:_____
   Conjunctiva:_____ Sclera:_____

EGO INTEGRITY

Subjective

Pregnancy planned (Y/N):_____
Previous childbirth experience:_____

Objective

Response to labor (check those that apply):
   Calm:_____ Anxious:_____ Excited:_____

Attitude toward this pregnancy:
    Client:_____
    Father:_____
Client's perceptions of her mother's
    childbirth experience:_____
Support person(s) (identify):_____
Expectations during labor/delivery of:
    Self:_____
    Support person(s):_____
    Primary nurse:_____
    Physician/Certified Nurse–Midwife (CNM):_____
Relationship with father of the
    baby:_____
Financial concerns:_____
Religions: Maternal:_____
    Paternal:_____
Cultural factors:_____
Presence of risk factors:_____
Preparation for childbirth:_____

Depressed:_____   Fearful:_____   Irritable:_____
Restive:_____   Intense:_____   Tired:_____
Observed interaction with support person(s):_____
    Physical contact:_____   Verbal:_____
Management of labor:_____
    Frequency of coaching required:_____
    Use of support person(s):_____
    Breathing/relaxation techniques:_____
    Copes with contraction effectively:_____

ELIMINATION

Subjective

Usual bowel pattern:_____
    Last bowel movement (BM):_____
    Laxative use:_____
    Character of stool:_____
    Bleeding:_____
    Hemorrhoids:_____
Character of urine:_____
Pain/burning/difficulty voiding:_____
History of kidney/bladder disease:_____

Objective

Bowel sounds:_____
Hemorrhoids (per pelvic examination): Internal:_____
    External:_____
Bladder palpable:_____   Overflow voiding:_____
Urinalysis report:_____   Albuminuria:_____

FOOD/FLUID

Subjective

Oral intake last 4 hr:_____
Nausea/vomiting:_____
Dentures:_____
Headache:_____
    Visual disturbance:_____
Epigastric pain:_____
Use of diuretics:_____
Diabetes/onset:_____
Thyroid disorder:_____

Objective

Current weight:_____   Total prenatal gain:_____
    Height:_____
Skin turgor:_____
Edema (degree): Legs:_____   Sacrum:_____
    Hands:_____   Face:_____
Deep tendon reflexes: L:_____   R:_____
    Clonus:_____
Jugular distension:_____
Appearance of tongue:_____
    Mucous membranes:_____
    Teeth/gums:_____
Breath sounds:_____
Hb/Hct (anemia):_____
Diabetic screening: GTT:_____
Urine sugar/acetone:_____
Thyroid studies:_____

HYGIENE

Subjective

Activities of daily living (ADLs):
    Independent:_____
    Dependent (specify):_____

Objective

General appearance:_____
Body odor:_____   Condition of scalp:_____
Presence of vermin:_____

NEUROSENSORY

Subjective

Fainting spells/dizziness:_____

Objective

Mental status (e.g., alert/oriented):_____

Tingling/numbness (location):_____
Seizures:_____   How controlled:_____
Eyes: Vision loss: R:_____   L:_____
Ears: Hearing loss: R:_____   L:_____

Pupils: R:_____   L:_____   Glasses:_____
    Contacts:_____
Hearing aid:_____
Unusual speech pattern/impairment:_____

PAIN/DISCOMFORT

Subjective

Uterine contractions began:_____
    Became regular:_____
Location of contractile pain:
    Front:_____   Sacral area:_____
Degree of discomfort: Mild:_____
    Moderate:_____   Severe:_____
How relieved:
    Breathing/relaxation techniques:_____
    Positioning:_____   Sacral rubs:_____
    Effleurage:_____

Objective

Facial expression:_____   Narrowed focus:_____
Physical response:_____

RESPIRATORY

Subjective

Dyspnea/cough:_____
History:
    Bronchitis:_____   Asthma:_____
    Tuberculosis:_____   Other:_____
Smoker:_____   Packs/day:_____   No. of yr:_____

Objective

Respiratory status: Rate:_____   Depth:_____
    Quality:_____
Breath sounds:_____
Sputum characteristics:_____
Chest x-ray results:_____

SAFETY

Subjective

Allergies/sensitivity:_____
    Reaction (specify):_____
History of STD (date/type):_____
Month of first prenatal visit:_____
Previous/current obstetric problems and
        treatment:
    PIH:_____   Kidney:_____
    Hemorrhage:_____   Cardiac:_____
    Diabetes:_____
    Infection (specify)/UTI:_____
    ABOs/Rh sensitivity:_____
    Uterine surgery:_____
    Anemia:_____
Length of time since last pregnancy:_____
Type of previous delivery:_____
Health status of living children:_____
Blood transfusion:_____   When:_____
    Reaction (describe):_____
Maternal stature/build:_____
Fractures/dislocations:_____
Pelvis:_____
Arthritis/unstable joints:_____
Spinal problems/deformity:
    Kyphosis:_____   Scoliosis:_____
    Trauma:_____   Surgery:_____
Prosthesis:_____
Ambulatory devices:_____

Objective

Temperature:_____
Skin integrity:_____   Rashes:_____   Sores:_____
    Bruises:_____   Scars:_____
Paresthesia/paralysis:_____
Fetal status: Heart rate:_____   Location:_____
    Method of auscultation:_____
    Fundal height:_____   Estimated gestation:_____
    Activity/movement:_____
    Fetal assessment testing (Y/N):_____
        Date:_____
        Test:_____   Results:_____
Labor status: Cervical dilation:_____
    Effacement:_____
    Fetal descent:_____   Engagement:_____
    Presentation:_____   Lie:_____
    Position:_____
Membranes: Intact:_____   Ruptured (time):_____
    Nitrazine test:_____   Amount of drainage:_____
    Character:_____
Blood type/Rh: Maternal:_____   Paternal:_____
Screens: Sickle cell:_____   Rubella:_____
    Hepatitis:_____   HIV:_____   Tuberculosis (TB):_____
Serology: Syphilis: Positive_____   Negative_____
Cervical/rectal culture: Positive_____   Negative_____
Vaginal warts/lesions:_____
Perineal varicosities:_____

SEXUALITY

Subjective

Last menstrual period:_____
    Estimated date of birth (EDB):_____

Objective

Breast examination:_____   Nipples:_____
Pelvis: Adequate:_____   Borderline:_____

Practices breast self-examination (Y/N):_____
Obstetric history: GTPAL:
 Gravida:_____ Para:_____
 Abortions:_____
 Living children:_____
 Full term:_____ Premature:_____
 Multiple births:_____
Delivery history:
 Year:_____ Place:_____
 Length gestation:_____
 Length labor:_____
 Type delivery:_____
 Born A/D:_____ Weight:_____
 Complications Maternal/Fetal:_____

Contracted:_____
Inlet:_____ Mid:_____ Outlet:_____
Pelvimetry:_____
Prognosis for delivery:_____

SOCIAL INTERACTION

Subjective

Marital status:_____ No. of yr in
 relationship:_____
 Members of family:_____
Living with:_____ Extended family:_____
 Other support person(s):_____
Report of problems:_____

Objective

Verbal/nonverbal communication with
 family/SOs:_____
Family interaction (behavior) pattern:_____

TEACHING/LEARNING

Subjective

Education level:
 Maternal:_____ Paternal:_____
 Occupations:_____
Dominant language (specify):_____
Literate:_____ Cognitive limitations:_____
Familial risk factors (maternal/paternal;
 indicate relationship):
 TB:_____ Diabetes:_____
 High BP:_____ Epilepsy:_____
 Heart disease:_____ Stroke:_____
 Kidney disease:_____ Cancer:_____
 Multiple births:_____
 Genetic problems (specify):_____
 Other (specify):_____
Prescribed medications (note last dose):
 Drug:_____ Dose:_____
 Schedule:_____
 Take regularly (Y/N):_____
Nonprescription drugs: Over the counter
 (OTC):_____
 Street drugs:_____
 Use of alcohol (amount/frequency):_____
Relevant illnesses and/or hospitalizations/
 surgeries:_____
Plans/expectations for: Labor site (choice):_____
 Support person(s) for labor:_____
 For delivery:_____
 Medications: During labor:_____
 During delivery:_____
 Position: During labor:_____
 During delivery:_____
 Procedures: Intravenous (IV) fluids:_____
 Saline lock:_____
 Fetal monitor:_____
 Enema:_____ Episiotomy:_____

Discharge Plan Considerations

Date information obtained:_____
Anticipated date of discharge:_____
Home situation:_____
Resources available: Persons:_____
 Financial:_____Maternity leave:_____
Anticipated needs/assistance required:_____

215

Type of delivery:_____
Type of infant feeding:_____
Preparation for:
Prenatal/intrapartal period and infant
care/feeding:
Classes:_____ Books:_____
Other (specify):_____
Support person(s) preparation:_____

LABOR: Stage I—Latent Phase

The latent phase, or the first phase of stage I labor, begins with the onset of true labor and ends with the cervix dilated 4 cm. The phase averages approximately 8–10 hr, up to 20 hr for nulliparas and 3–6 hr, up to 14 hr for multiparas. It usually occurs with client at home, unless specific concerns necessitate inpatient care, e.g., spontaneous rupture of membranes (SROM), history of rapid labor, unsafe weather conditions/distance from facility.

CLIENT ASSESSMENT DATA BASE

Ego Integrity

May be excited or anxious

Pain/Discomfort

Regular contractions, increasing in frequency, duration, and severity.
Contractions are mild to moderate, 10–20 min apart, progressing to 5–7 min apart, lasting 15–20 sec, progressing to 30–40 sec.

Safety

Fetal heart tones best heard below level of umbilicus (dependent on fetal position)

Sexuality

Membranes may or may not have ruptured.
Cervix dilates from 0 to 4 cm.
Fetus may be at station −1 to 0 (primigravida) or from 0 to +2 cm (multigravida).
Scant vaginal discharge, may be pink or brownish mucus ("show"), or may consist of mucous plug.

NURSING PRIORITIES

1. Enhance client's/couple's/other involved family members' emotional and physical preparedness for labor.
2. Promote and facilitate normal labor progress.
3. Support client's/couple's/involved family members' coping abilities.
4. Prevent maternal/fetal complications.

DISCHARGE GOALS

(Inpatient care is not required in early labor, unless complications develop necessitating hospitalization.)

1. Displays only early, or no, signs of active progression of labor.
2. Demonstrates appropriate coping behaviors.
3. Understands self-care needs and signs of labor progression requiring re-evaluation.

NURSING DIAGNOSIS:	Anxiety, risk for
Risk Factors May Include:	Situational crisis, interpersonal transmission, unmet needs
Possibly Evidenced By:	[Not applicable; presence of signs/symptoms establishes an *actual* diagnosis]

217

DESIRED OUTCOMES/EVALUATION CRITERIA—CLIENT WILL	Report anxiety is at a manageable level.
	Use breathing and relaxation techniques proficiently.
	Appear relaxed appropriate to the labor situation.
	Remain normotensive.

ACTIONS/INTERVENTIONS	RATIONALE

Independent

Provide primary nurse or continuous in trapartum professional support as indicated.	Continuity of care and assessment may decrease stress. Research studies suggest that these clients require less pain medication, which may result in shorter labor.
Orient client to environment, staff, and procedures. Provide information about psychological and physiological changes in labor, as needed.	Education may reduce stress and anxiety and promote labor progress.
Assess level and causes of anxiety, preparedness for childbirth, cultural background, and role of significant other/partner.	Provides baseline information. Anxiety magnifies pain perception, interferes with use of coping techniques, and stimulates the release of aldosterone, which may increase sodium and water resorption.
Monitor BP and pulse as indicated. (If BP is elevated on admission, repeat procedure in 30 min to obtain true reading once client is relaxed.)	Stress activates the hypothalamic-pituitary-adrenocortical system, which increases retention and resorption of sodium and water and increases excretion of potassium. Sodium and water resorption may contribute to development of intrapartal toxemia/hypertension. Loss of potassium may contribute to reduction of myometrial activity.
Monitor uterine contractile pattern; report dysfunctional labor. (Refer to CP: Dysfunctional Labor/Dystocia.)	A hypertonic or hypotonic contractile pattern may develop if stress persists and causes prolonged catecholamine release.
Encourage client to verbalize feelings, concerns, and fears.	Stress, fear, and anxiety have a profound effect on the labor process, often prolonging the first phase because of utilization of glucose reserves; causing excess epinephrine release from adrenal stimulation, which inhibits myometrial activity; and increasing norepinephrine levels, which tends to increase uterine activity. Such an imbalance of epinephrine and norepinephrine can create a dysfunctional labor pattern.
Demonstrate breathing and relaxation methods. Provide comfort measures. (Refer to CP: Labor: Stage I—Active Phase; ND: Pain [acute].)	Reduces stressors that might contribute to anxiety; provides coping strategies.
Promote privacy and respect for modesty; reduce unnecessary exposure. Use draping during vaginal examination.	Modesty is a concern in most cultures. Support person may or may not desire to be present while client is examined or care provided.
Be aware of client's need or preference for female caregivers/support persons.	Cultural practices may prohibit presence of men (even father of the child) during labor and/or delivery.
Provide opportunity for conversation to include choice of infant names, expectations of labor, and perceptions/fears during pregnancy.	Presents opportunity for client to verbalize excitement about herself, the pregnancy, and her baby. Serves as a diversion to help pass time during what is commonly the longest phase of labor.

218

Determine diversional needs; encourage variety of activities (e.g., television, books, cards, walking, rocking, showering, massage, music, aroma therapy).	Helps divert attention away from labor, making time pass more quickly. If condition permits, walking usually promotes cervical dilatation, shortens labor, and lowers the incidence of fetal heart rate (FHR) abnormalities.
Prepare for, and/or assist with, discharge from hospital setting, as indicated.	During very early latent phase with no apparent progress of labor, the comfort and familiarity of the home environment may decrease anxiety and allow opportunity for a variety of acceptable diversional activities, thereby hastening the labor process.

NURSING DIAGNOSIS:	**Knowledge deficit [Learning Need], regarding progression of labor, available options**
May Be Related To:	Lack of exposure/recall, information misinterpretation
Possibly Evidenced By:	Questions, statements of misconception, inaccurate follow-through of instruction
DESIRED OUTCOMES/EVALUATION CRITERIA—CLIENT WILL:	Verbalize understanding of psychological and physiological changes.
	Participate in decision-making process.
	Demonstrate appropriate breathing and relaxation techniques.

ACTIONS/INTERVENTIONS	RATIONALE
Independent	
Assess client's preparation, knowledge level, and expectations/birth plan.	Helps establish information/learning needs and set priorities.
Provide information about procedures (especially fetal monitor and telemetry) and normal progression of labor.	Antepartal education can facilitate the labor and delivery process, assist the client in maintaining control during labor, help promote a positive attitude and/or sense of control, and may decrease reliance on medication.
Discuss options for care during the labor/ delivery process. Provide information about birthing alternatives, if available and appropriate.	Necessary for the client/couple to participate actively in the decision-making process.
Review roles of staff members.	Identifies resources for specific needs/situations.
Demonstrate breathing/relaxation techniques appropriate to each phase of labor; teach and review pushing positions for stage II.	Unprepared couples need to learn coping mechanisms on admission to help reduce stress and anxiety. Couples with prior preparation can benefit from review and reinforcement.
Review appropriate activity levels and safety precautions, whether client remains in hospital/ clinic or returns home.	Provides guidelines for client to make appropriate self-care choices; allows client to engage in safe diversional activities to refocus attention/pass time.
Obtain informed consent for procedures, e.g., invasive monitoring, episiotomy. Explain usual procedures and the possible risks associated with labor and delivery.	When procedures involve client's body, it is necessary for client to have appropriate information to make informed choices.

(Refer to ND: Coping, Individual, risk for ineffective, for further discussion of coping techniques.)

219

NURSING DIAGNOSIS:	Fluid Volume risk for deficit
Risk Factors May Include:	Decreased intake, increased losses (e.g., nausea/vomiting, mouth breathing, hormonal shifts)
Possibly Evidenced By:	[Not applicable; presence of signs/symptoms establishes an *actual* diagnosis]
DESIRED OUTCOMES/EVALUATION CRITERIA—CLIENT WILL:	Maintain fluid intake as able.
	Demonstrate adequate hydration (e.g., moist mucous membranes, yellow/amber urine of appropriate amount, absence of thirst, afebrile, stable vital signs/FHR).

ACTIONS/INTERVENTIONS	RATIONALE

Independent

Monitor intake/output. Note urine specific gravity. Encourage client to empty bladder at least once every 1½–2 hr.	Intake and output should be approximately equal, dependent on degree of hydration. Concentration of urine increases as urine output decreases and may warn of dehydration. Fetal descent may be impaired if bladder is distended.
Monitor temperature every 4 hr, more frequently if elevated. Monitor vital signs/FHR as indicated.	Increases in temperature, BP, pulse, respirations, and FHR may reflect presence of dehydration.
Assess production of mucus, amount of tearing within eyes, and skin turgor.	Additional signs of adequacy of hydration or development of dehydration.
Provide clear fluids (e.g., juice, broth, popsicles, jello) and ice chips, as permitted.	Helps promote hydration and may provide some calories for energy production.
Determine cultural practices regarding intake.	Some cultures (e.g., some African immigrants, residents of the southern region of the United States) drink special teas, believing they stimulate continued progression of labor, or avoid certain foods believed to inhibit labor.
Provide mouth care and hard candy, as appropriate.	Reduces discomfort of a dry mouth.

Collaborative

Administer bolus of parenteral fluids, as indicated.	May be needed if oral intake is inadequate or restricted. Acts as a safeguard in the event of dehydration or hemorrhage; counteracts some negative effects of anesthesia/analgesia.
Monitor Hct level.	Hct increases as the plasma component decreases in the presence of severe dehydration.

NURSING DIAGNOSIS:	Coping, Individual, risk for ineffective
Risk Factors May Include:	Situational crisis, personal vulnerability, inadequate support systems and/or coping methods
Possibly Evidenced By:	[Not applicable; presence of signs/symptoms establishes an *actual* diagnosis]
DESIRED OUTCOMES/EVALUATION CRITERIA—CLIENT WILL:	Verbalize awareness of own coping abilities.
	Identify individually appropriate behaviors to maintain control.
	Use medication appropriately.

ACTIONS/INTERVENTIONS	RATIONALE

Independent

Determine client's cultural background, coping abilities, and verbal and nonverbal responses to pain. Determine past experiences and antepartal preparation.

Each client responds in a unique manner to the stresses of labor and associated discomfort based on these factors. The appearance of appropriate or inappropriate coping may actually be a manifestation of one's culture; e.g., Asian or Native American women may be stoic because of fear of shaming self or family, whereas Hispanic and Middle Eastern cultures typically encourage verbal expression of suffering. For this reason, it is important to compare both verbal and nonverbal responses when assessing coping ability.

Note age of client and presence of partner/ support person(s).

Negative coping may result in increased anxiety, in which case the client may request medication too early in the labor process. Younger clients and those unattended may exhibit more vulnerability to stress/discomfort and have difficulty maintaining composure/control.

Stay with/provide companion (e.g., doula [woman's servant]) for client who is alone.

At a time of increased dependence, unmet needs and fear of being abandoned may interfere with ability to focus on the task at hand. Note: Doula describes an individual who provides emotional, physical, and informational support to the pregnant woman but does not perform clinical tasks. These childbirth companions may be volunteers or may be paid for their services. Research suggests that using doulas during labor and delivery results in shorter labors, decreased use of forceps and epidural anesthesia, reduced oxytocin use, fewer cesarean births, better infant outcomes, and enhanced client/partner satisfaction.

Reinforcing breathing and relaxation techniques during contractions.

Provides support for client/couple. Reduces anxiety and provides distraction, which may block perception of pain impulses within the cerebral cortex.

Establish rapport and accept behavior without judgment. Make verbal contract about expected behaviors of client and nurse.

Facilitates cooperation; provides an opportunity for the client to leave the experience with positive feelings and enhanced self-esteem. Nurse may need to assist the client in maintaining/regaining control of breathing and relaxation, or set limits if inappropriate (unsafe) behavior occurs.

Assess uterine contraction/relaxation pattern, fetal status, vaginal bleeding, and cervical dilatation.

Rule out possible complications that could be causing or contributing to the discomfort/reduced coping ability.

Collaborative

Discuss types of systemic/regional analgesics or anesthetics when available in birth setting.

Helps client make informed choice about methods to relieve pain/promote comfort and maintain control.

Discuss administration of sedatives such as secobarbital (Seconal), pentobarbital (Nembutal), or hydroxyzine (Vistaril).

Occasionally, a barbiturate or ataractic may be administered during early labor to promote rest/sleep, so that the client enters the active phase more relaxed and rested and better able to cope. Note: Because barbiturates can have a prolonged depressant effect on the newborn, Vistaril may be the drug of choice.

221

ACTIONS/INTERVENTIONS	RATIONALE
Independent	
Emphasize importance of/demonstrate good hand washing.	Reduces risk of acquiring/spreading infective agents.
Use aseptic technique during vaginal examination.	Helps prevent growth of bacteria; limits contaminants from reaching the vagina.
Perform initial vaginal examination; repeat only when contractile pattern or client's behavior indicates significant progress of labor.	Repeated vaginal examinations contribute to the incidence of ascending tract infections.
Provide/encourage perineal care after elimination and prn as indicated; change underpad/linen when wet.	Reduces risk of ascending tract infection.
Assess vaginal secretions using phenaphthazine (nitrazine paper). Perform microscopic examination for positive ferning.	Spontaneous rupture of membranes 1 hr or more before onset of labor increases risk of chorioamnionitis during the intrapartal period. Color changes of nitrazine paper from yellow to dark blue indicate presence of alkaline amniotic fluid; ferning indicates rupture of membranes. Note: Excess bloody show, which is more alkaline than vaginal secretions, may cause similar changes on nitrazine paper.
Monitor and describe character of amniotic fluid.	With infection, amniotic fluid becomes thicker and yellow-tinged and has a strong, detectable odor.
Monitor temperature, pulse, respirations, and white blood cell (WBC) count, as indicated.	Within 4 hr after rupture of membranes, the incidence of chorioamnionitis increases progressively with the passage of time, reflected by elevations of vital signs and WBC count.
Collaborative	
Provide oral and parenteral fluids, as indicated.	Maintains hydration and general sense of well-being.
Carry out perineal preparation, as appropriate.	Some providers believe it may facilitate perineal repair at delivery and cleaning of perineum in the postpartal period, thereby reducing risk of infection.
Administer cleansing enema, if indicated.	Although not often done, bowel evacuation may promote progression of labor and prevent or reduce risk of infection caused by contamination of the sterile field during delivery.
Administer prophylactic antibiotic IV, if indicated.	Although antibiotic administration in the intrapartal period is controversial because of antibiotic load for

Administer oxytocin infusion, as ordered. (Refer to CP: Labor: Induced/Augmented.)

Obtain blood cultures if symptoms of sepsis are present.

the fetus, it may help protect against development of chorioamnionitis in the client at risk.

If labor does not ensue within 24 hr after rupture of membranes, infection may occur. If client is at 36 weeks' gestation, onset of labor reduces risk of negative effects on client/fetus.

Detects and identifies causative organism(s).

NURSING DIAGNOSIS:	Injury, risk for fetal
Risk Factors May Include:	Tissue hypoxia/hypercapnia or infection
Possibly Evidenced By:	[Not applicable; presence of signs/symptoms establishes an *actual* diagnosis]
DESIRED OUTCOMES/EVALUATION CRITERIA—CLIENT WILL:	Display FHR and beat-to-beat variability within normal limits, with no ominous periodic changes in response to uterine contractions.

ACTIONS/INTERVENTIONS

RATIONALE

Independent

Perform Leopold's maneuvers to determine fetal position, lie, and presentation.

A transverse lie or breech presentation may necessitate cesarean birth. Other abnormalities, such as face, chin, and posterior presentations, may also require special interventions to prevent prolongation of labor/fetal harm.

Obtain baseline FHR manually and/or electronically. Evaluate frequently per protocol. Note FHR variability and periodic changes in response to uterine contractions.

FHR should range from 120–160 bpm with average variability, accelerating in response to maternal activity, fetal movement, and uterine contractions.

Note progress of labor.

Prolonged/dysfunctional labor with an extended latent phase can contribute to problems of maternal exhaustion, severe stress, infection, and hemorrhage caused by uterine atony/rupture, placing the fetus at greater risk for hypoxia and injury.

Inspect maternal perineum for vaginal warts, herpetic lesions, or chlamydial discharges.

STDs can be acquired by the fetus during the delivery process; therefore, cesarean birth may be **to** indicated, especially for clients with active herpes simplex virus type II. (Refer to CP: Prenatal Infection.)

Administer perineal care to mother according to protocol; change underpad when wet.

Helps prevent growth of bacteria; eliminates contaminants that might contribute to maternal chorioamnionitis or fetal sepsis.

Note FHR when membranes rupture, reassess per protocol, obtain 30-min EFM strip for record. Evaluate periodic changes in FHR.

Changes in amniotic fluid pressure with rupture, and/or variable decelerations of FHR after rupture, may reflect compression of the umbilical cord, which reduces oxygen transfer to the fetus.

Assess for visible cord prolapse at vaginal introitus. If present:
    Calm client/partner, explain the prolapse and
        its implications;

Helps couple understand the significance of prolapse, and promotes cooperation with emergency measures.

223

Elevate client's hips (elevated Sims' position), or help client to assume knee-chest position, push presenting part off of cord and hold off while summoning help;

Check cord for pulsations; wrap cord in sterile gauze soaked in saline solution.

Relieves pressure of presenting part on cord. This is an emergency situation requiring surgical intervention.

Keeps cord moist and helps decrease chance of uterine infection.

Monitor FHR and periodic changes if a problem is detected with fetoscopy or external monitor. Note presence of bradycardia/tachycardia or sinusoidal pattern.

Any decrease in baseline FHR variability—severe and untreatable variable decelerations, recurrent late decelerations, or persistent bradycardia—indicates fetal decompensation, hypoxia, or acidosis resulting from anaerobic metabolism. Sinusoidal pattern is often associated with fetal anemia or severe fetal hypoxia just prior to fetal demise.

Position client in lateral recumbent position.

Increases placental perfusion; prevents supine hypotensive syndrome.

Collaborative

Prepare for transfer to a level 2 or 3 hospital setting as indicated, if client is at home, or in free-standing birth setting.

Compromised fetal status or identification of maternal conditions such as STD requires closer observation and may indicate need for therapeutic interventions such as cesarean birth.

Rule out maternal problems or medications that could effect an increase in FHR;

Factors such as fever, anxiety, anemia, or use of beta-sympathomimetic drugs can increase maternal and fetal heart rate.

Turn off oxytocin if infusing, and increase plain IV solution;

Promotes greater periods of uterine relaxation and increases uteroplacental blood flow; increases circulating blood volume available for oxygen transfer within maternal circulation of the placenta.

Administer oxygen via face mask;

Increases maternal oxygen available for fetal uptake.

Assist as needed with obtaining fetal scalp blood sample when indicated.

Direct measurement of fetal pH is occasionally indicated to determine fetal metabolic reserve and to differentiate fetal respiratory acidosis from metabolic or mixed acidosis. Fetal pH between 7.20 and 7.25 may reflect intermittent umbilical cord compression, necessitating constant monitoring and/or possibly immediate surgical intervention.

Prepare for surgical intervention, as indicated. (Refer to CP: Cesarean Birth.)

CNS damage occurs if fetal hypoxia/acidosis persists for more than 30 min. To avoid fetal compromise/demise, cesarean birth is treatment of choice for prolapsed cord prior to full cervical dilatation.

LABOR: Stage I—Active Phase

As contractions increase to moderate intensity in the active phase, and as the cervix dilates from 4 to 8 cm, the client becomes more involved and focused on the labor process. The active phase lasts approximately 1–2 hr in the multipara and 3–4 hr in the nullipara. The fetus descends in the birth canal at approximately 2 cm/hr in the multipara and 1 cm/hr in the nullipara.

CLIENT ASSESSMENT DATA BASE

Activity/Rest

May show evidence of fatigue

Ego Integrity

May appear more serious and absorbed with labor process
Apprehensive about ability to control breathing and/or perform relaxation techniques

Pain/Discomfort

Contractions are moderate, occurring every 2.5–5 min and lasting 45–60 sec.

Safety

Fetal heart tones (FHTs) detected slightly below umbilicus in vertex position
FHR variability and periodic changes commonly noted in response to contractions, abdominal palpation, and fetal movement

Sexuality

Cervix dilates from approximately 4–8 cm (1.5 cm/hr multipara, 1.2 cm/hr nullipara).
Moderate amount of bloody show present.
Fetus descends to 11–12 cm below ischial spines.

NURSING PRIORITIES

1. Promote and facilitate normal progression of labor.
2. Support client's/couple's coping abilities.
3. Promote maternal and fetal well-being.

NURSING DIAGNOSIS:	Pain [acute]
May Be Related To:	Tissue dilation/muscle hypoxia, pressure on adjacent structures, stimulation of both parasympathetic and sympathetic nerve endings
Possibly Evidenced By:	Verbalizations, distraction behaviors (restlessness), muscle tension
DESIRED OUTCOMES/EVALUATION CRITERIA—CLIENT WILL:	Identify/use techniques to control pain/discomfort.
	Report discomfort is minimized.
	Appear relaxed/resting between contractions.
	Be free of untoward side effects if analgesia/anesthetic agents are administered.

ACTIONS/INTERVENTIONS	RATIONALE

Independent

Assess degree of discomfort through verbal and nonverbal cues; note cultural influences on pain response.

Attitudes and reactions to pain are individual and based on past experiences, understanding of physiological changes, and cultural expectations.

Assist in use of appropriate breathing/relaxation techniques and in abdominal effleurage.

May block pain impulses within the cerebral cortex through conditioned responses and cutaneous stimulation. Facilitates progression of normal labor.

Assist with comfort measures (e.g., back/leg rubs, sacral pressure, back rest, mouth care, repositioning, shower/hot tub use, perineal care, and linen changes).

Promotes relaxation and hygiene; enhances feeling of well-being. Note: Lateral recumbent position reduces uterine pressure on the vena cava, but periodic repositioning prevents tissue ischemia and/or muscle stiffness, and promotes comfort.

Encourage client to void every 1–2 hr. Palpate above symphysis pubis to determine distension, especially after nerve block.

Keeps bladder free of distension, which can increase discomfort, result in possible trauma, interfere with fetal descent, and prolong labor. Epidural or pudendal analgesia may interfere with sensations of fullness.

Provide information about available analgesics, usual responses/side effects (client and fetal), and duration of analgesic effect in light of current situation.

Allows client to make informed choice about means of pain control. Note: If conservative measures are not effective and increasing muscle tension impedes progress of labor, minimal use of medication may enhance relaxation, shorten labor, limit fatigue, and prevent complications.

Support client's decision about the use or nonuse of medication in a nonjudgmental manner. Continue encouragement for efforts and use of relaxation techniques.

Helps reduce feelings of failure in the client/couple who may have anticipated an unmedicated birth and did not follow through with that plan. Enhances sense of control and may prevent/decrease need for medication.

Time and record the frequency, intensity, and duration of uterine contractile pattern per protocol.

Monitors labor progress and provides information for client. Note: Anesthetic agents may alter uterine contractile pattern. (Refer to CP: Dysfunctional Labor/Dystocia.)

Assess nature and amount of vaginal show, cervical dilation, effacement, fetal station, and fetal descent.

Cervical dilation should be approximately 1.2 cm/hr in the nullipara and 1.5 cm/hr in the multipara; vaginal show increases with fetal descent. Choice and timing of medication is affected by degree of dilation and contractile pattern.

Provide safety measures; e.g., encourage client to move slowly, keep siderails up after drug administration, and support legs with position changes.

Regional block anesthesia produces vasomotor paralysis, so that sudden movement may precipitate hypotension. Analgesics alter perception, and client may fall trying to get out of bed.

Assess BP and pulse every 1–2 min after regional injection for first 15 min, then every 10–15 min for remainder of labor. Elevate head approximately 30 degrees, alternate position by turning side to side and use of hip roll.

Maternal hypotension, the most common side effect of regional block anesthesia, may interfere with fetal oxygenation. Elevating head prevents block from migrating up and causing respiratory depression. Lateral positioning increases venous return and enhances placental circulation.

Monitor FHR variability.

Agents such as bupivacaine (Marcaine) and fentanyl (Sublimaze) reportedly have little effect on FHR variability (but in practice may decrease variability); alterations should be investigated thoroughly. Note:

Using alcohol pad or cotton swab on both sides of abdomen, assess and record level of sensation q 30 min.

Engage client in conversation to assess sensorium; monitor breathing patterns and pulse.

Assess for warmth, redness of large toe or ball of foot, and equal distribution of spinal medication if used.

Monitor FHR electronically, and note decreased variability or bradycardia.

Collaborative

Assist with complimentary therapies as indicated, e.g., acupressure/acupuncture.

Administer analgesic such as butorphanol tartrate (Stadol) or meperidine hydrochloride (Demerol) by IV or deep intramuscular (IM) during contractions, if indicated.

Administer oxygen, and increase plain fluid intake if systolic pressure falls below 100 mm Hg or falls more than 30% below baseline pressure.

Obtain fetal scalp sample if bradycardia persists for 30 min or more per electronic monitor.

Administer IV bolus of 500–1000 ml of lactated Ringer's solution just before administration of lumbar epidural block.

Assist with epidural or caudal block anesthesia using an indwelling catheter.

Risks associated with caudal anesthesia include perforation of fetal scalp, as well as maternal rectum, and is rarely used.

Increasing loss of sensation following when epidural block indicates migration of anesthesia. Level above T-9 may alter respiratory function while loss of sensation at level of breastbone (approximately 7–6) increases risk of profound hypotension.

Systemic toxic responses with altered sensorium occur if medication is absorbed into the vascular system. Altered sensorium may also be an early indicator of developing hypoxia. Interference with respiratory functioning occurs if analgesia is too high, paralyzing the diaphragm.

Ensures proper placement of catheter for continuous block and adequate levels of anesthetic agent.

Decreased FHR variability is a common side effect of many anesthetics/analgesics. These side effects can begin 2–10 min after administration of anesthetic, and may last for 5–10 min, on occasion.

Some clients and healthcare providers may prefer a trial of alternative therapies to mediate pain before pursuing invasive techniques.

IV route is preferred because it ensures more rapid and equal absorption of analgesic. Medication administered by IM route may require up to 45 min to reach adequate plasma levels, and maternal uptake may be variable, especially if drug is injected into subcutaneous fat instead of muscle. Administering IV drug during uterine contraction decreases amount of medication that immediately reaches the fetus. Note: Stadol is used with caution when drug dependence is suspected, and is contraindicated for clients with opiate dependency because drug interaction may precipitate withdrawal in drug-dependent clients.

Increases circulating fluid volume, placental perfusion, and oxygen available for fetal uptake.

Prolonged fetal bradycardia may indicate need to determine pH for evaluation of hypoxia.

Increased circulating fluid level helps prevent side effects of hypotension associated with block.

Provides relief once active labor is established; reinforcement through catheter provides sustained comfort during delivery. Such analgesia does not interfere with uterine activity and/or Ferguson reflex. While it relaxes the cervix and facilitates the labor process, it may alter internal fetal rotation and diminish client's ability to bear down when needed.

ACTIONS/INTERVENTIONS	RATIONALE
	Note: A new technique of ultra–low-dose epidural is being used to achieve pain control without negative effect on client's ability to sense contractions and push effectively. With this approach, the client is not restricted to bedrest but may even be up walking as able.
Administer emergency medications as indicated, e.g., nalaxone (Narcan) or ephedrine (Ephedra).	Narcan is used to reverse opiate-induced respiratory depression. Adrenalin may be required for hypotensive episodes not responsive to IV fluid bolus.
Succinylcholine chloride, and assist with intubation, as appropriate.	Systemic toxic reaction to epidural anesthetic may alter sensorium or cause convulsions if medication is absorbed into the vascular system.

NURSING DIAGNOSIS:	**Urinary Elimination, altered**
May Be Related To:	Altered intake, fluid shifts, hormonal changes, mechanical compression of bladder, effects of regional anesthesia
Possibly Evidenced By:	Changes in amount/frequency of voiding, urinary urgency, urine retention, slowed progression of labor
DESIRED OUTCOMES/EVALUATION CRITERIA—CLIENT WILL:	Empty bladder appropriately.
	Be free of bladder injury.

ACTIONS/INTERVENTIONS

RATIONALE

Independent

ACTIONS/INTERVENTIONS	RATIONALE
Palpate above symphysis pubis.	Detects presence of urine in bladder and degree of fullness. Incomplete emptying of the bladder may occur because of decreased sensation and tone.
Record and compare intake and output. Note amount, color, concentration, and specific gravity of urine.	Output should approximate intake. Increased output may reflect excessive fluid retention prior to the onset of labor and/or effects of bedrest; i.e., increased glomerular filtration rate and decreased adrenal stimulation. Specific gravity reflects kidney's ability to concentrate urine and the client's hydration status. Decreased output may occur with dehydration, hemorrhage, and pregnancy-induced hypertension (PIH). (Refer to CP: Intrapartal Hypertension.)
Encourage periodic attempts to void, at least every 1–2 hr.	Pressure of the presenting part on the bladder often reduces sensation and interferes with complete emptying. Regional anesthesia (especially in conjunction with IV fluid infusion and use of Stadol) also may contribute to voiding difficulties/bladder distension.
Position client upright, run water from the faucet, pour warm water over the perineum, or have client blow bubbles through a straw.	Facilitates voiding/enhances emptying of bladder.

Take temperature and pulse, noting increases. Assess dryness of skin and mucous membranes.	Helps monitor degree of hydration.

Collaborative

Catheterize as indicated.	An overdistended bladder can cause atony, impede fetal descent, or become traumatized by presenting part of the fetus.

NURSING DIAGNOSIS:	**Anxiety, risk for**
Risk Factors May Include:	Situational crisis, interpersonal transmission from other(s), unmet needs
Possibly Evidenced By:	[Not applicable; presence of signs/symptoms establishes an *actual* diagnosis]
DESIRED OUTCOMES/EVALUATION CRITERIA—CLIENT WILL:	Report anxiety minimized/manageable.
	Appear relaxed and/or in control.
	Self-initiate breathing/relaxation techniques.
	Follow instructions of partner/nurse.

ACTIONS/INTERVENTIONS	RATIONALE

Independent

Assess client's anxiety level through verbal and nonverbal cues.	Identifies level of intervention necessary. Excess anxiety increases pain perception and can have negative impact on the outcome of labor.
Provide continuous intrapartal professional support/doula. Inform client that she will not be left alone.	Fear of abandonment can intensify as labor progresses. The client may experience increased anxiety and/or loss of control when left unattended. Doulas can provide client with emotional, physical, and informational support as an adjunct to primary nurse.
Encourage use of breathing and relaxation techniques. Breathe with client/couple as necessary.	Assists in reduction of anxiety and of perception of pain within the cerebral cortex, enhancing sense of control.
Monitor FHR and its variability; monitor maternal BP.	Prolonged anxiety can result in endocrine imbalances, with excess release of epinephrine and norepinephrine, elevating BP and pulse. Note: Medications relaxing smooth muscle may reduce FHR variability and maternal BP.
Evaluate contractile pattern/progression of labor.	Increasing force/intensity of uterine contractions can heighten client's concerns about personal capabilities and outcome of labor. In addition, increased levels of epinephrine may also inhibit myometrial activity. Excess anxiety and stress levels can deplete glucose reserves, thereby decreasing the amount available for adenosine triphosphate (ATP) synthesis, which is necessary for uterine contractions.
Refer to CP: Labor: Stage I—Latent Phase; ND: Anxiety, risk for.	If client is admitted during the active phase, interventions usually accomplished during the latent phase need to be addressed at this time.

229

Collaborative

| Administer combination of narcotic and sedative (e.g., meperidine hydrochloride [Demerol] and promethazine [Phenergan] IM. | Addition of mild sedative potentiates the action of the narcotic, reducing anxiety, and assisting client in focusing on breathing/relaxation techniques. |

NURSING DIAGNOSIS:	Coping, Individual/Couple, risk for ineffective
Risk Factors May Include:	Situational crises, personal vulnerability, inadequate support systems
Possibly Evidenced By:	[Not applicable; presence of signs/symptoms establishes an *actual* diagnosis]
DESIRED OUTCOMES/EVALUATION CRITERIA—CLIENT/COUPLE WILL:	Identify effective coping behaviors.
	Engage in activities to maintain/enhance control.

ACTIONS/INTERVENTIONS	RATIONALE

Independent

Ascertain client's understanding and expectations of the labor process.	The client's/couple's coping skills are most challenged during the active and transition phases as contractions become increasingly intense. Lack of knowledge, misconceptions, or unrealistic expectations can have a negative impact on coping abilities.
Encourage verbalization of feelings.	Helps nurse gain insight into individual needs, and assists client/couple to deal with concerns.
Reinforce use of positive coping mechanisms and relaxation techniques.	Assists client in maintaining or gaining control. Enhances feelings of competence, and fosters self-esteem. The stressors that accompany labor can be threatening to a woman's self-esteem, especially if she has not coped positively with past experiences and/or successfully accomplished the tasks of pregnancy.
Note withdrawn behavior.	Adolescents, in particular, may become withdrawn and not express needs to be nurtured. This may also be true for some cultures (such as Native American or Vietnamese) where the woman is encouraged to be stoic/suffer in silence.
Assess effectiveness of labor partner. Provide role modeling as indicated.	The client is influenced by those around her and may respond positively when others remain calm and in control.
Demonstrate behaviors and techniques partner can use to assist with pain control and relaxation. Provide information regarding water, music, imagery, aromatherapy, and correct misconceptions.	Encourages choice of multiple options, enhances coping and self-esteem of partner/couple.
Limit verbalization/instruction during contractions to a single "coach."	Allows client to focus attention and may enhance ability to follow directions. Multiple coaches may actually result in decreased concentration, confusion, and loss of control.
Provide positive reinforcement for efforts. Use touch and soothing words of encouragement.	Encourages repetition of appropriate behaviors. Enhances individual's confidence in own ability to cope with or handle labor, while also meeting her needs for dependency.

NURSING DIAGNOSIS:	Injury, risk for maternal
Risk Factors May Include:	Effects of medication, delayed gastric motility, physiological urges
Possibly Evidenced By:	[Not applicable; presence of signs/symptoms establishes an *actual* diagnosis]
DESIRED OUTCOMES/EVALUATION CRITERIA—CLIENT WILL:	Verbalize understanding of individual risks and reasons for specific interventions.
	Follow directions to protect self/fetus from injury.
	Be free of preventable injury/complications.

ACTIONS/INTERVENTIONS	RATIONALE

Independent

Monitor uterine activity manually and/or electronically, noting frequency, duration, and intensity of contraction. (Refer to CP: Dysfunctional Labor/Dystocia.)	The uterus is susceptible to possible rupture if a hypertonic contractile pattern develops spontaneously or in response to oxytocin administration. Placental separation and hemorrhage can also occur if contraction persists.
Institute bedrest and use of siderails (as labor intensifies) or following administration of medication. Avoid leaving client unattended.	Promotes safety should dizziness or precipitous delivery occur following administration of medication.
Place client in lateral recumbent or semi-upright position.	Increases placental perfusion and reduces supine hypotensive syndrome. Note: Some women may prefer an upright position during the phase of maximum slope of labor (i.e., 4–9 cm dilation). Studies suggest this position may shorten this phase of labor without increasing discomfort or producing adverse effects on fetal well-being.
Administer perineal care after defecating or urinating.	Reduces risk of ascending infection, which can occur, especially with prolonged rupture of membranes.
Monitor temperature and pulse.	Elevations are indicators of developing infection.
Offer client clear liquids or ice chips, as appropriate; avoid solid foods.	Delayed gastric motility inhibits digestion during labor, placing the client at risk for aspiration. However, client can benefit from intake of calories in PO fluids to help generate energy for work of labor.
Monitor urine for ketones.	Urinary ketones indicate metabolic acidosis resulting from a deficiency in glucose metabolism, which may reduce uterine activity and cause myometrial fatigue that prolongs labor.
Note time of rupture of membranes and characteristics of amniotic fluid.	The incidence of ascending infection increases with the passage of time.
Have client pant or blow out if she feels the premature urge to bear down.	Panting during the active phase or the transition phase prevents bearing down too early and can thereby reduce risk of lacerations or edema of the cervix/birth canal.

Collaborative

Discontinue or decrease flow rate of oxytocin when used if contraction lasts longer than 90 sec, or if the	Helps to prevent hypertonic contractile pattern with resultant decreased placental blood flow and

231

uterus fails to relax completely between contractions.

Administer IV antibiotics, if indicated.

risk of uterine rupture. (Refer to CP: Dysfunctional Labor/Dystocia.)

Administration of antibiotics during labor is controversial, but on occasion may protect against infection in cases of prolonged rupture of membranes.

NURSING DIAGNOSIS:	**Gas Exchange, risk for impaired fetal**
Risk Factors May Include:	Altered oxygen supply/blood flow
Possibly Evidenced By:	[Not applicable; presence of signs/symptoms establishes an *actual* diagnosis]
DESIRED OUTCOMES/EVALUATION CRITERIA—FETUS WILL:	Display FHR and beat-to-beat variability within normal limits (WNL).
	Be free of adverse effects of hypoxia during labor.

ACTIONS/INTERVENTIONS

RATIONALE

Independent

Assess for presence of maternal factors or conditions that compromise uteroplacental circulation (e.g., diabetes, PIH, kidney or cardiac disorders). Note prenatal testing of placental functioning by nonstress test (NST) or contraction stress test (CST).

High-risk situations that negatively affect circulation are likely to be manifested in late decelerations and fetal hypoxia.

Monitor FHR every 15–30 min if WNL. Monitor FHR electronically if it is less than 120 bpm, or greater than 160 bpm. Periodically compare client's apical heart rate with FHR.

Fetal tachycardia or bradycardia is indicative of possible compromise, which may necessitate intervention. Note: External monitoring device may inadvertently record maternal rather than fetal heart activity.

Check FHR immediately if membranes rupture, and then again 5 min later. Observe maternal perineum for visible cord prolapse.

Detects fetal distress due to visible or occult cord prolapse.

Instruct client to remain on bedrest if presenting part does not fill the pelvis (station 14).

Reduces risk of cord prolapse.

Note and record color, amount, and odor of amniotic fluid and time of membrane rupture.

In a vertex presentation, prolonged hypoxia results in meconium-stained amniotic fluid owing to vagal stimulation, which relaxes the fetal anal sphincter. Hydramnios may be associated with fetal anomalies and poorly controlled maternal diabetes.

Monitor fetal descent in birth canal through vaginal examination. In cases of breech presentation, assess FHR more frequently.

Prolonged head compression stimulates vagal responses and may result in fetal bradycardia if the rate of descent is not at least 1 cm/hr for primiparas or 1.5 cm/hr for multiparas. Fundal pressure in breech presentation may cause vagal stimulation and head compression.

Assess FHR changes during a contraction, noting decelerations and accelerations.

Detects severity of hypoxia and possible cause. The fetus is vulnerable to potential injury during labor, owing to situations that reduce oxygen levels, such as cord prolapse, prolonged head compression, or uteroplacental insufficiency.

Monitor uterine activity manually or electronically.

Talk to client/couple as care is being given, and provide information about situation, as appropriate.

Collaborative

If late or persistent variable decelerations occur:
  Transfer to level 2 or 3 hospital setting as indicated:
  Discontinue oxytocin if it is being administered;

  Place client in lateral recumbent position;

  Turn client from side to side as indicated;

  Increase plain IV infusion rate;

  Administer oxygen to client via mask;
  Prepare for and assist with fetal scalp sampling, repeating as indicated;

  Prepare for delivery by the most expeditious means or by surgical intervention, if no improvement occurs.

Development of hypertonicity can compromise uteroplacental circulation and fetal oxygenation.

Provides psychological support and assurance to reduce anxiety related to increased monitoring.

May require specialized monitoring/interventions.

Strong contractions caused by oxytocin may inhibit or reduce uterine relaxation and lower fetal oxygen levels.
Increases placental perfusion, which may correct problem if caused by uteroplacental insufficiency.
Helps take pressure from the presenting part off the umbilical cord, if cord is being compressed.
Increases circulating fluid volume and placental perfusion.
Increases available oxygen for placental transfer.
Prolonged, decreased variability may indicate acidosis. On occasion, determining fetal pH value may be helpful in identifying fetal respiratory acidosis and metabolic reserves.
Repetitive late decelerations over a 30-min period accompanied by decreased variability may warrant a cesarean birth to prevent fetal injury and/or death from hypoxia.

(Refer to CP: Labor Stage I—Latent Phase; NDs: Knowledge deficit [Learning Need]; Infection, risk for maternal; Injury, risk for fetal; and Fluid Volume risk for deficit.)

LABOR: Stage I—Transition Phase (Deceleration)

The transition phase is typically the most intense of the three phases of stage I labor. It is also the shortest phase, lasting an average of 2–3 hr in nulliparas and 1 hr in multiparas. The cervix dilates 8–10 cm as the fetus descends approximately 1 cm/hr in nulliparas and 2 cm/hr in multiparas.

CLIENT ASSESSMENT DATA BASE

Circulation

BP elevated 5–10 mm Hg above client's normal level
Pulse elevated

Ego Integrity

Irritable behavior, difficulty communicating/answering queries
May have difficulty maintaining control, requiring reminders about breathing/comfort techniques
May state, "I can't stand it anymore," or may desire to "leave the hospital and come back later"
May be amnesic

Elimination

Urge to void or defecate throughout phase (may indicate fetus in posterior position)

Food/Fluid

Nausea or vomiting may occur
Belching/hiccuping

Pain/Discomfort

Strong uterine contractions occurring every 2–3 min and lasting 60+ sec (unmedicated state).
Intense level of discomfort in abdominal/sacral area.
May become very restless, thrash with pain, or be fearful.
May report being "too hot"; tingling sensation of fingertips, toes, and face.
Leg tremors may occur.

Safety

Diaphoretic
FHTs heard just above symphysis pubis.
FHR may display variable decelerations (cord compression), late decelerations (uteroplacental insufficiency), or early decelerations (head compression).

Sexuality

Cervix dilates 8–10 cm.
Fetus descends 12–14 cm.
Copious amounts of bloody show.

NURSING PRIORITIES

1. Promote fetal and maternal well-being.
2. Provide physical and emotional support.

NURSING DIAGNOSIS:	Pain [acute]
May Be Related To:	Mechanical pressure of presenting part; tissue dilation/stretching and hypoxia; stimulation of parasympathetic and sympathetic nerves; emotional and muscular tension
Possibly Evidenced By:	Verbalizations, distraction behavior (e.g., restlessness), facial mask of pain, narrowed focus, autonomic responses
DESIRED OUTCOMES/EVALUATION CRITERIA—CLIENT WILL:	Verbalize perceived or actual reduction of pain.
	Use appropriate techniques to enhance comfort and maintain control of labor process.
	Rest between contractions.

ACTIONS/INTERVENTIONS	RATIONALE
Independent	
Assess degree of discomfort through verbal and nonverbal cues. Assess personal and cultural implications of pain.	Attitudes toward pain and reactions to pain are individual and based on past experiences, cultural background, and self-concept.
Assess client's need for physical touch during contractions.	Touch may serve as a distraction, provide supportive reassurance, and encouragement, and may aid in maintaining control/reducing pain. Note: Desire for touch may change from one contraction to the next.
Monitor frequency, duration, and intensity of uterine contractions.	Detects progress and screens for abnormal uterine response.
Inform client of onset of contractions, as appropriate.	Client may "sleep" and/or encounter partial amnesia between contractions. This can be a problem for some clients, impairing her ability to recognize contractions as they begin and thus have a negative impact on her sense of control. For others, the brief rest may "energize" them for the next contraction.
Assist client and partner with changing to more rapid breathing; (i.e., pant-blow).	Redirects and focuses attention; helps reduce perception of pain within the cerebral cortex.
Provide for a quiet environment that is adequately ventilated, dimly lit, and free of unnecessary personnel. Carry out nursing procedures between contractions whenever possible.	Nondistracting environment provides optimal opportunity for rest and relaxation between contractions.
Assist client with comfort measures, including sacral/back rubs, positioning, mouth care, perineal care, change of pads/linens, hot/cold compresses, sponge baths to face and neck, or bath/whirlpool.	Such measures promote hygiene, relaxation, and physical comfort. Note: Individual needs/preference can change quickly during transition; i.e., client may request sacral rub, then the next moment demand everyone move away from her.
Monitor cervical dilation. Note perineal bulging or vaginal show.	Discomfort levels increase as cervix dilates, fetus descends, and small blood vessels rupture.
Encourage client to void.	May enhance labor progress and reduce risk of trauma to bladder.
Offer encouragement, provide information about labor progress, and provide positive reinforcement for client's/couple's efforts.	Provides emotional support, which can reduce fear, lower anxiety levels, and help minimize pain.

235

Provide break for partner as appropriate.

Support person may be reluctant to leave, but does need a break for renewal of energy and relaxation, which can enhance ability to help partner.

Evaluate client for tingling of lips, face, hands, or feet. If present, have client breathe into cupped hands or paper bag.

Discomfort caused by respiratory alkalosis can be relieved by increasing carbon dioxide levels through the rebreathing process.

Monitor maternal vital signs and FHR variability after drug administration. Note drug's effectiveness and the physiological response.

Narcotics can have a depressant effect on the fetus, particularly when administered 2–3 hr before delivery. Therefore, use may be limited/restricted, or naloxone hydrochloride (Narcan) may be administered to reverse adverse drug effects.

Collaborative

Administer analgesic as ordered. Assist anesthesiologist if epidural or caudal anesthetic is to be used.

Judicious use of a pharmacologic agent assists the client in coping with contractions and may facilitate labor.

NURSING DIAGNOSIS:	Cardiac Output, risk for decreased
Risk Factors May Include:	Decreased venous return, hypovolemia, changes in systemic vascular resistance
Possibly Evidenced By:	[Not applicable; presence of signs/symptoms establishes an *actual* diagnosis]
DESIRED OUTCOMES/EVALUATION CRITERIA—CLIENT WILL:	Maintain vital signs appropriate for stage of labor, free of pathological edema and excessive albuminuria.
	Display FHR within normal limits.

ACTIONS/INTERVENTIONS

RATIONALE

Independent

Assess BP and pulse between contractions, as indicated. Note abnormal readings.

During contractions, blood pressure usually increases 5–10 mm Hg, except during transition phase, when the blood pressure remains elevated. Increased resistance to cardiac output can occur if intrapartal hypertension develops, further elevating blood pressure. Finally, cardiac output/blood pressure may be negatively affected by uterine pressure on the inferior vena cava, reducing venous return, or by a decrease in circulating blood volume caused by dehydration or occasionally hemorrhage.

Note presence and extent of edema. Monitor FHR during and between contractions.

Excess fluid retention places the client at risk for circulatory changes, with possible uteroplacental insufficiency manifested as late decelerations.

Accurately record parenteral/oral intake, and output. Measure specific gravity if kidney function is decreased.

Bedrest promotes increases in cardiac and urine output with a corresponding decrease in urine specific gravity. An elevation of specific gravity and/or reduction in urine output suggests dehydration or possibly developing hypertension.

Test urine for albumin. Report levels above 12.

Indicates glomerular spasms, which reduce the reabsorption of albumin. Levels greater than 12

Monitor BP and pulse per protocol or continually if hypotension is severe after administration of analgesia.

Note any hypertensive responses to oxytocin administration. (Refer to CPs: Labor: Induced/Augmented; Intrapartal Hypertension.)

indicate kidney involvement; levels 11 or lower may be due to muscle catabolism occurring with activity (contraction) or to increased metabolism in the intrapartal period.

Analgesics relax smooth muscles within the blood vessels, reducing resistance to cardiac output and lowering BP and pulse.

Oxytocin increases cardiac circulating volume (sodium/water absorption) and cardiac output, and may also increase BP and pulse.

NURSING DIAGNOSIS:	Fluid Volume, risk for deficit/excess
Risk Factors May Include:	Excess fluid loss/hemorrhage, reduced intake, excess fluid retention, rapid parenteral fluid administration
Possibly Evidenced By:	[Not applicable; presence of signs/symptoms establishes an *actual* diagnosis]
DESIRED OUTCOMES/EVALUATION CRITERIA—CLIENT WILL:	Maintain vital signs and urine output/concentration WNL.
	Be free of thirst.

ACTIONS/INTERVENTIONS

Independent

Monitor BP and pulse every 15 min and more frequently during oxytocin infusion.

Assess client's anxiety level.

Take temperature every 4 hr, as indicated (every 2 hr after membranes rupture). Assess skin and mouth for dryness.

Record intake and output. Note concentration of urine. Measure urine specific gravity, as indicated.

Measure amount and character of emesis.

Remove excess clothing, keep environment cool, and wipe client's face/body with cool washcloth.

Assess amount and location of edema, Hct level, changes in behavior, and reflex irritability. (Refer to CP: Intrapartal Hypertension.)

RATIONALE

Increased BP and pulse may indicate fluid retention; decreased BP and increased pulse may be late signs of fluid volume loss or dehydration.

Anxiety may alter BP and pulse, affecting assessment findings.

Dehydration can result in elevated body temperature, dry skin, and reduced production of saliva.

Bedrest results in decreased adrenal cortex activity, increased glomerular filtration rate, and increased urine output. When fluid volume is decreased, aldosterone acts to reabsorb water and sodium from the kidney tubules, reducing urine output.

Nausea and vomiting contribute to fluid losses. With reduced gastric motility, food may remain in the stomach for up to 12 hr after ingestion and pose a risk for aspiration.

Limits diaphoreses; provides comfort.

Intrapartal hypertension can develop, causing fluid shifts from the intravascular spaces and increasing Hct levels. Cerebral edema/vasospasms/hypoxia can cause increased reflex irritability and/or behavior changes.

237

Assess amount of vaginal bloody show; observe for excess blood loss.	Bloody show increases as the presenting part moves down in the birth canal; excess bleeding may indicate placental separation.
Position client on side, as appropriate.	Increases venous return by taking pressure of the gravid uterus off the inferior vena cava and descending aorta.

Collaborative

Administer and monitor IV fluid infusion, as indicated.	Maintains hydration by replacing fluid losses. Rate may be adjusted to meet individual needs, but too rapid administration can lead to fluid overload, especially in a compromised client.

NURSING DIAGNOSIS:	**Fatigue**
May Be Related To:	Discomfort/pain, overwhelming psychological emotional demands, increased energy requirements, changes in energy production, decreased caloric intake (restricted/nothing by mouth [NPO] status)
Possibly Evidenced By:	Verbalizations, impaired ability to concentrate, emotional lability or irritability, lethargy, altered coping ability
DESIRED OUTCOMES/EVALUATION CRITERIA—CLIENT/COUPLE WILL:	Use techniques to conserve energy between contractions.
	Report sense of control.
	Appear moderately relaxed.

ACTIONS/INTERVENTIONS	RATIONALE

Independent

Assess degree of fatigue.	Fatigue may interfere with the client's physical and psychological abilities to maximally participate in labor process and to master and carry out self-care and infant care after delivery.
Provide dimly lit, nondistracting environment.	Reducing stressors helps promote rest.
Keep client informed of progress of labor. Provide encouragement for efforts client makes.	Provides reinforcement for desired behaviors. Realizing that labor is progressing toward goal may help client maintain maximal effort.
Provide comfort measures. (Refer to ND: Pain [acute].)	Promotes relaxation, enhances sense of control, and may strengthen coping.
Plan care to limit interruptions.	Maximizes opportunities for rest.
Encourage client to close eyes, extend legs, and relax between contractions.	A comfortable position facilitates muscle relaxation.
Monitor urine for ketones.	Urinary ketones indicate metabolic acidosis resulting from a deficiency in glucose metabolism, which may reduce uterine activity and cause myometrial fatigue, which can prolong labor.
Monitor energy level of partner. Assume supportive responsibilities as needed.	Allows partner to have a brief break and refresh self, enhancing ability to maintain focus and support client.

Collaborative

Administer an analgesic as ordered.	May help the client cope with contractions and facilitate relaxation between contractions. Use with caution, because analgesics may cause fetal depression.
Provide calorie-rich fluids, e.g., fruit juices, broths.	Calories are necessary to maintain energy level to help with work of labor.

NURSING DIAGNOSIS:	**Coping, Individual/Couple, risk for ineffective**
Risk Factors May Include:	Sense of "work overload," personal vulnerability, inadequate/exhausted support system
Possibly Evidenced By:	[Not applicable; presence of signs/symptoms establishes an *actual* diagnosis]
DESIRED OUTCOMES/EVALUATION CRITERIA—CLIENT/COUPLE WILL:	Identify effective coping behaviors.
	Engage in activities to maintain/enhance control.

ACTIONS/INTERVENTIONS	RATIONALE

Independent

Reinforce information that labor is progressing; encourage client to cope with one contraction at a time.	Provides reassurance that baby will soon be born. A natural response in the transition phase is for the client to feel that she has had enough and wants to "quit and go home."
Inform client/partner of initiation of each contraction.	Allows client to rest/relax and still maintain control of breathing pattern as contraction begins.
Ensure that client, under direction of partner, initiates breathing patterns. Breathe with client if necessary.	A more complex breathing pattern initiated at the beginning of a contraction is necessary as a distraction and helps reduce pain perception within the cerebral cortex. Client may have difficulty understanding directions because of inward focus.
Acknowledge reality of both client's and partner's irritable feelings.	The increase in intensity and frequency of contractions and the premature urge to push may add to sense of loss of control. The client's hostility may be manifested as anger at the nurse or support person(s). In addition, general fatigue of both client and partner further impair their ability to cope.
Encourage client and partner to verbalize doubts about ability to continue and fear of being left alone (even if this fear is unfounded).	When these thoughts are expressed, they can be acknowledged and the client/partner can realize that they are coping to the best of their ability in the situation and can move forward with support.
Provide support to partner.	May feel helpless and require more support as the partner becomes less able to relieve client's pain.

(Refer to CP: Labor Stage I—Active Phase; NDs: Coping, Individual/Couple, risk for ineffective; Infection, risk for maternal; Gas Exchange, risk for impaired fetal.)

LABOR: Stage II (Expulsion)

Stage II of labor, the stage of expulsion, begins with full cervical dilation (10 cm) and ends with the birth of the newborn. Maternal efforts to bear down occur involuntarily during contractions that are 1.5–2 min apart, lasting 60–90 sec. The average rate of fetal descent is 1 cm/hr for nulliparas, 2 cm or more per hr for multiparas.

CLIENT ASSESSMENT DATA BASE

Activity/Rest

Reports of fatigue
May report inability to self-initiate pushing/relaxation techniques
Lethargic
Dark circles under eyes

Circulation

BP may rise 5–10 mm Hg in between contractions.

Ego Integrity

Emotional responses may range from feelings of fear/irritation to relief/joy.
May feel a loss of control or the reverse as she is now actively involved in bearing down.

Elimination

Involuntary urge to defecate/push with contractions, combining intraabdominal pressure with uterine pressure.
May have fecal discharge while bearing down.
Bladder distension may be present, with urine expressed during pushing efforts.

Pain/Discomfort

May moan/groan during contractions.
Amnesia between contractions may be noted.
Reports of burning/stretching sensation of the perineum.
Legs may tremble during pushing efforts.
Uterine contractions strong, occurring 1.5–2 min apart and lasting 60–90 sec.
May fight contractions, especially if she did not participate in childbirth preparation classes.

Respiratory

Respiratory rate increases.

Safety

Diaphoresis often present
Fetal bradycardia appearing as early decelerations on electric monitor during contractions (head compression) or variables (cord compression)

Sexuality

Cervix fully dilated (10 cm) and 100% effaced.
Increased vaginal bloody show.
Rectal/perineal bulging with fetal descent.
Membranes may rupture at this point if still intact.
Increased expulsion of amniotic fluid during contractions.
Crowning occurs; caput is visible just before birth in vertex presentation.

NURSING PRIORITIES

1. Facilitate normal progression of labor and fetal descent.
2. Promote maternal and fetal well-being.
3. Support client's/couple's wishes regarding delivery experience, maintaining safety as a priority.

NURSING DIAGNOSIS:	Pain [acute]
May Be Related To:	Mechanical pressure of presenting part, tissue dilation/stretching, nerve compression, muscle hypoxia, intensified contractile pattern
Possibly Evidenced By:	Verbalizations, distraction behavior (e.g., restlessness), facial mask of pain, narrowed focus, autonomic responses
DESIRED OUTCOMES/EVALUATION CRITERIA—CLIENT WILL:	Verbalize reduction of pain.
	Use appropriate techniques to maintain control.
	Rest between contractions.

ACTIONS/INTERVENTIONS	RATIONALE

Independent

Identify degree of discomfort and its sources.	Clarifies needs; allows for appropriate intervention.
Provide comfort measures, such as mouth care; perineal care/massage; clean, dry linen and underpads; cool environment (68°F–72°F [20°C–22.1°C]), cool, moist cloths to face and neck; or hot compresses to perineum, abdomen, or back, as desired.	Promotes psychological and physical comfort, allowing client to focus on labor, and may reduce the need for analgesia or anesthesia.
Review information with client/couple about type of regional analgesia/anesthesia available at this stage specific to the delivery setting (e.g., local, pudendal block, lumbar epidural reinforcement) or use of transcutaneous electrical nerve stimulation (TENS), acupressure/acupuncture. Review advantages/disadvantages, as appropriate.	Although client is under the stress of labor and discomfort levels may interfere with normal decision-making skills, she still needs to be in control and make her own informed decisions regarding anesthesia. Note: The option of a nerve root block should be restricted to a hospital setting where emergency equipment is available.
Monitor and record uterine activity with each contraction.	Provides information/legal documentation about continued progress; helps identify abnormal contractile pattern, allowing prompt assessment and intervention. (Refer to CP: Dysfunctional Labor/Dystocia.)
Provide information and support related to progress of labor.	Keeps couple informed of proximity of delivery; reinforces that efforts are worthwhile and the "end is in sight."
Encourage client/couple to manage efforts to bear down with spontaneous, rather than sustained, pushing during contractions. Stress importance of using abdominal muscles and relaxing pelvic floor.	Anesthetics may interfere with client's ability to feel sensations associated with contractions, resulting in ineffective bearing down. Spontaneous, rather than sustained, efforts to bear down avoid negative effects of Valsalva's maneuver associated with reduced maternal and fetal oxygen levels. Relaxation of the pelvic floor reduces resistance to pushing efforts, maximizing effort to expel the fetus.
Observe for perineal and rectal bulging, opening of vaginal introitus, and changes in fetal station.	Anal eversion and perineal bulging occur as the fetal vertex descends, indicating need to prepare for delivery.
Assist client in assuming optimal position for bearing down; (e.g., squatting or lateral recumbent, semi-Fowler's position (elevated 30–60 degrees). Assess effectiveness of efforts to bear down. (Refer to ND: Skin/Tissue Integrity, risk for impaired.)	Proper positioning with relaxation of perineal tissue optimizes bearing-down efforts, facilitates labor progress, reduces discomfort, and reduces need for forceps application.

241

Encourage client to relax all muscles and rest between contractions.

Complete relaxation between contractions promotes rest and helps limit muscle strain/fatigue.

Monitor maternal BP and pulse, and FHR. Observe unusual adverse reactions to medication, such as antigen-antibody reactions, respiratory paralysis, or spinal blockage. Note adverse reactions such as nausea/vomiting, urine retention, delayed respiratory depression, and pruritus of face, eyes, or mouth. (Refer to ND: Gas Exchange, risk for impaired fetal.)

Maternal hypotension caused by decreased peripheral resistance as vascular tree dilates is the main adverse reaction to subarachnoid or peridural block. Fetal hypoxia or bradycardia is possible, owing to decreased circulation within the maternal portion of the placenta. Other adverse reactions may occur after administration of spinal or peridural anesthetic especially when morphine is used.

Collaborative

Assess bladder fullness. Catheterize between contractions if distension is noted and client is unable to void.

Promotes comfort, facilitates fetal descent, and reduces risk of bladder trauma caused by presenting part of fetus.

Assist with reinforcement of medication via indwelling lumbar epidural catheter when caput is visible. Monitor vital signs and adverse responses. (Refer to CP: Labor: Stage I—Active Phase; ND: Pain [acute].)

Reduces discomfort associated with episiotomy, forceps application, and fetal expulsion. Adverse reactions include maternal hypotension, muscle twitching/convulsions, loss of consciousness, reduced FHR, and beat-to-beat variability.

Position client in dorsal lithotomy position and assist as necessary with administration of pudendal anesthetic.

Anesthetizes lower two-thirds of vagina and perineum during delivery and for episiotomy repair. May interfere with efforts to bear down but has no effect on maternal BP, FHR, or FHR variability.

Assist as needed with administration of local anesthetic just before episiotomy, if done.

Anesthetizes perineum tissue for incision/repair purposes.

Lumbar, Epidural, or Low Spinal Anesthesia

Administer IV fluid bolus of 500–1000 ml lactated Ringer's as indicated, before administration of agent.

Increases maternal circulating fluid as a means of preventing adverse reactions of anesthetic such as maternal hypotension, fetal hypoxia, and fetal bradycardia.

Position client in sitting or lateral recumbent position for insertion of drug/placement of catheter for continuous infusion. Have client flex head sharply on chest/arch back during intrathecal administration.

Proper alignment of vertebrae maximizes space for needle/catheter placement.

Assist with administration of opiates (e.g., fentanyl [Sublimaze], morphine) into epidural space via indwelling catheter. Have ephedrine, 10 mg, or naloxone (Narcan), 0.4 mg, available as an antidote, depending on agent used.

Intraspinal narcotic, acting on opiate receptors within the spinal column, blocks pain for as long as 11 hr. Literature reveals mixed results regarding use of morphine via indwelling catheter in stage II labor (may be more effective in the active phase of stage I labor). Note: Because of the potential for life-threatening complications, initial and subsequent bolus dosing should be done by anesthesia service or providers specifically trained and certified.

Turn client side to side periodically during continuous infusions.

Promotes even distribution of drug to prevent "one-sided" or unilateral block.

Monitor level of block per protocol.

Migration of decreased sensation from belly button (dermatome T-10) to tip of breastbone (approximately T-6) increases risk of profound hypotension. Necessitates evaluation of drug concentration/infusion rate by anesthesia personnel.

Administer oxygen and increase plain IV fluid. If hypotension occurs, displace uterus to the left and elevate legs.

Enhances venous return and circulating blood volume, increasing placental perfusion and oxygenation.

Administer diphenhydramine (Benadryl), promethazine hydrochloride (Phenergan), or metoclopramide hydrochloride (Reglan) when indicated.

May relieve pruritus, a side effect of morphine administration.

Assist with administration of intrathecal subarachnoid anesthetic. Identify beginning and ending of contractions. Administer anesthetic between contractions when fetal head is on the perineum.

Anesthetizes nerves at lumbar spaces L3–L4 and L4–L5. Administration of medication during a contraction may cause the level of the anesthetic to rise too high, anesthetizing the diaphragm.

Transcutaneous Electrical Nerve Stimulation

Apply two pairs of electrodes on either side of thoracic and sacral vertebrae.

Electrical stimulation of pain receptors (by TENS units) within the skin may block pain sensations by causing release of endorphins. Has no adverse effect on client or fetus and may reduce need for analgesia/anesthesia.

Encourage and assist client/couple with operation of control knobs on battery-operated device.

Ability to turn on mild electrical currents during a contraction promotes a feeling of control for the client.

Complimentary Therapy

Assist with acupressure/acupuncture, moxibustion.

May be used to stimulate/regulate contractions to restore balance to labor and reduce perception of pain.

General Anesthesia

Assist with general anesthesia (inhalation or IV administration), as indicated.

Because of maternal and fetal side effects, general anesthesia should only be used in obstetric emergencies, such as hemorrhage, internal version with a second twin, or delivery of the aftercoming head in a breech presentation.

Assist with monitoring BP, pulse, respirations, FHR, and variability. Watch for vomiting reaction.

General anesthesia has a depressant effect on the client and fetus, and poses a risk of maternal aspiration.

NURSING DIAGNOSIS:	Cardiac Output, altered [fluctuation]
May Be Related To:	Fluctuation in venous return, changes in systemic vascular resistance
Possibly Evidenced By:	Variations in blood pressure, changes in pulse rate, decreased urine output, fetal bradycardia
DESIRED OUTCOMES/EVALUATION CRITERIA—CLIENT WILL:	Maintain vital signs appropriate for stage of labor.
	Use appropriate techniques to sustain/enhance vascular return.
	Display FHR and variability WNL.

ACTIONS/INTERVENTIONS	RATIONALE
Independent	
Monitor BP and pulse frequently (every 5–15 min). Note amount and concentration of urine output; test for albuminuria.	Increases in cardiac output of 30%–50% occur in the expulsion stage, peaking at the acme of uterine contractions and slowly returning to a precontractile state as the contraction diminishes or ceases. Intrapartal toxemia due to stress, excess sodium and fluid retention, or oxytocin administration may be manifested by increased BP, decreased urine output, and increased concentration of urine.
Encourage client to inhale/exhale during bearing-down efforts, using an open glottis technique and holding breath no longer than 5 sec at a time. Instruct client to push only when she feels the urge to do so. Avoid forced pushing.	Repeated, prolonged Valsalva's maneuvers (occurring when the client holds her breath while pushing against a closed glottis) eventually interrupt venous return and reduce cardiac output, BP, and pulse pressure. Avoiding Valsalva's maneuver minimizes fall of maternal PO_2 and rise in PCO_2 levels, which would have a negative impact on fetus.
Monitor FHR after every contraction or bearing-down effort.	Detects fetal bradycardia and hypoxia associated with reduction in maternal circulation and reduced placental perfusion caused by anesthesia, Valsalva's maneuver, or incorrect positioning. (Refer to ND: Gas Exchange, risk for impaired fetal.)
Encourage client/couple to select laboring position that optimizes circulation, such as the lateral recumbent position, Fowler's position, or squatting.	Upright and lateral recumbent positions prevent occlusion of the inferior vena cava and obstruction of the aorta, sustaining venous return and preventing hypotension.
Monitor BP and pulse immediately after administration of anesthesia, and repeat until client is stable. (Refer to ND: Pain [acute] for information about anesthesia and side effects.)	Hypotension is the most common adverse reaction to lumbar epidural or subarachnoid (low spinal) block as vascular dilation slows venous return and reduces cardiac output.
Collaborative	
Regulate IV infusion as indicated; monitor oxytocin administration, and decrease rate if necessary.	IV line (or saline lock access) should be available in case the need to correct hypotension or administer emergency drugs arises. Excess fluid retention (a possible adverse reaction of oxytocin) may contribute to development of intrapartal toxemia.

NURSING DIAGNOSIS:	**Gas Exchange, risk for impaired fetal**
Risk Factors May Include:	Mechanical compression of head/cord, reduced placental perfusion, prolonged labor, maternal hyperventilation
Possibly Evidenced By:	[Not applicable; presence of signs/symptoms establishes an *actual* diagnosis]
DESIRED OUTCOMES/EVALUATION CRITERIA—FETUS WILL:	Be free of variable or late decelerations with FHR WNL.
CLIENT WILL:	Maintain control of respiratory pattern.
	Use positions promoting venous return/placental circulation.

ACTIONS/INTERVENTIONS	RATIONALE
Independent	
Position client in lateral recumbent or upright position, or turn side to side as indicated.	Increases placental perfusion, prevents supine hypotensive syndrome, and takes pressure from presenting part off cord, enhancing fetal oxygenation and improving FHR patterns.
Avoid placing client in dorsal recumbent position.	Contributes to fetal hypoxia and acidosis; reduces baseline variability and placental circulation.
Determine fetal station, presentation, and position. If fetus is in occiput posterior position, place client on her side.	During stage II labor, the fetus is most vulnerable to bradycardia and hypoxia, which are associated with vagal stimulation during head compression. Malpresentations such as face, mentum (chin), or brow may prolong labor and increase risk of hypoxia and the likelihood of the need for a cesarean birth, whereas posterior position increases duration of stage II labor. Placing client in lateral recumbent position facilitates fetal rotation from occiput posterior (OP) position to occiput anterior (OA) position.
Assess client's breathing pattern. Note reports of tingling sensation of face or hands, dizziness, or carpopedal spasms.	Identifies ineffective (inappropriate) respiratory pattern. Initially, hyperventilation results in respiratory alkalosis and an increase in serum pH; toward the end of labor, the pH falls and acidosis develops owing to lactic acid buildup from myometrial activity.
Have client breathe into cupped hands or small paper bag, as indicated.	Increases carbon dioxide levels and corrects respiratory alkalosis caused by hyperventilation.
Assist partner in helping with verbal coaching of respirations. Remind client to focus on an object/mental picture.	Provides opportunity for couple to work together to maintain/regain control of situation and maintain state of relaxation during contractions.
Monitor client for fruity breath odor.	Suggests acidosis associated with hyperventilation. As shifts in acid-base levels occur, fetal status can be compromised with resultant acidosis and hypoxia.
Encourage client/couple to inhale and exhale every 10–20 sec during bearing-down efforts. Monitor response to pushing efforts.	Helps maintain adequate oxygen levels. Exhaling while pushing minimizes physiological effects of Valsalva's maneuver, which can decrease maternal heart rate and PO_2, and increases PCO_2, potentially resulting in placental and fetal hypoxia and acidosis.
Assess FHR, with fetoscope or fetal monitor, during and after each contraction or pushing effort.	Early decelerations due to vagal stimulation from head compression should return to baseline patterns between contractions.
Monitor periodic changes in FHR for severe, moderate, or prolonged decelerations. Note presence of variable or late decelerations.	Variable decelerations indicate hypoxia due to possible cord entrapment or to nuchal or short cord. Late decelerations indicate uteroplacental insufficiency, which should not be allowed to persist for more than 30 min. Late decelerations are more likely to occur in clients with pregnancy-induced hypertension, diabetes, and kidney problems; placental aging; or following maternal anesthesia.
Note short- and long-term FHR variability.	Average beat-to-beat changes should range from 6 to 10 bpm, indicating integrity of fetal CNS.
Collaborative	
Perform sterile vaginal examination, feeling for prolapse. If prolapse is present, lift vertex off cord.	Elevation of vertex helps free umbilical cord, which may be compressed between presenting part and birth canal.

245

ACTIONS/INTERVENTIONS	RATIONALE
Transfer to acute care setting, as indicated, if client is in a free-standing birth center/home setting.	In cases of bradycardia or reduced FHR variability, more invasive monitoring, acute care equipment, or a cesarean birth may be needed.
Monitor FHR electronically with internal lead.	Electronic monitoring allows continued, accurate assessment. Direct scalp electrodes accurately detect abnormal fetal responses and reduction in beat-to-beat variability.
If severe bradycardia, late decelerations, or prolonged variable decelerations appear:	
Position client in lateral recumbent position; increase plain IV fluid; Administer oxygen to client;	Increases maternal circulating blood volume and placental perfusion. Increases circulating oxygen available for fetal uptake. During this stage of labor, enhanced metabolic processes increase oxygen consumption by twice the normal level.
Assist as needed with intermittent fetal scalp sampling, if done;	Determines trends in fetal acid-base status, and presence of fetal acidosis. The pH of fetal blood falls rapidly during stage II labor, and prolonged hypoxia may result in anaerobic metabolism with buildup of lactic acid.
Prepare for surgical intervention if spontaneous vaginal or low forceps delivery is not immediately possible after approximately 30 min, and fetal pH is 7.20 or less.	The fastest means of delivery must be implemented when the fetus has severe or irreversible hypoxia or acidosis.

NURSING DIAGNOSIS:	*Skin/Tissue Integrity, risk for impaired*
Risk Factors May Include:	Precipitous labor, hypertonic contractile pattern, adolescence, large fetus, forceps application
Possibly Evidenced By:	[Not applicable; presence of signs/symptoms establishes an *actual* diagnosis]
DESIRED OUTCOMES/EVALUATION CRITERIA—CLIENT WILL:	Relax perineal musculature during bearing-down efforts. Be free of preventable lacerations.

ACTIONS/INTERVENTIONS

RATIONALE

Independent

ACTIONS/INTERVENTIONS	RATIONALE
Assist client/couple with proper positioning, breathing, and efforts to relax. Ensure that client relaxes the perineal floor while using abdominal muscles in pushing.	Helps promote gradual stretching of perineal and vaginal tissue. If maternal tissue within the birth canal or perineum resists gradual stretching as the presenting part of the fetus descends, trauma or lacerations of the cervix, vagina, perineum, uretha, and clitoris are possible.
Offer use of birthing bed in upright position. Encourage squatting, Fowler's position, or standing while pushing, if these positions are not contraindicated.	Upright positions reduce duration of labor, enhance forces of gravity, reduce need for episiotomy, and maximize uterine contractility.
Place client in left lateral Sims' position for delivery, if desired/comfortable.	Reduces perineal tension, promotes gradual stretching, and reduces need for episiotomy.

Help client as needed in assuming position of choice/transfer to delivery table between contractions. Monitor safety, and support legs, especially if epidural (or caudal) catheter is in place.

Reduces risk of injury, especially if client is unable to assist with transfer.

Lift legs simultaneously, if leg supports/stirrups are used, and place feet and legs properly in low position, supporting feet.

Reduces muscle strain; prevents pressure on calf and popliteal space that could contribute to development of postpartal thrombophlebitis.

Collaborative

Assess for bladder fullness; catheterize prior to delivery, as appropriate. (Refer to CP: Labor: Stage I—Active Phase; ND: Urinary Elimination, risk for altered.)

Reduces bladder trauma from presenting part.

Assist as needed with hand maneuvers; apply pressure to fetal chin through maternal perineum while exerting pressure on the occiput with the other hand (modified Ritgen maneuver).

Allows slow delivery once the fetal head has distended the perineum 5 cm; reduces trauma to maternal tissues.

Assist with midline, or mediolateral episiotomy, if necessary.

Although controversial, episiotomy may prevent tearing of perineum in cases of a large infant, rapid labor, and insufficient perineal relaxation. It may shorten stage I of labor, especially when forceps are used. Note: Research suggests use of midline episiotomy is associated with a fourfold increase of major perineal trauma, including extensive tearing, whereas mediolateral episiotomy reduces likelihood of severe perineal lacerations, the surgical repair is more difficult, and problems with healing may occur.

Maintain accurate delivery records of location of episiotomy and/or lacerations. Record type and timing of forceps if used.

Ensures proper documentation of events occurring during delivery process; identifies specific problems affecting postpartal recovery; e.g., maternal tissue trauma is increased with forceps application, which may result in possible lacerations or extension of episiotomy, increased level of postpartal discomfort.

NURSING DIAGNOSIS:	Fluid Volume risk for deficit
Risk Factors May Include:	Active loss, reduced intake, fluid shifts
Possibly Evidenced By:	[Not applicable; presence of signs/symptoms establishes an *actual* diagnosis]
DESIRED OUTCOMES/EVALUATION CRITERIA—CLIENT WILL:	Maintain vital signs WNL, adequate urine output, moist mucous membranes.
	Be free of thirst.

ACTIONS/INTERVENTIONS	RATIONALE

Independent

Measure intake/output and urine-specific gravity. Assess skin turgor and production of mucus. Note albuminuria.

In presence of dehydration, urine output decreases, specific gravity increases, and skin turgor and mucus production decrease. Proteinuria may be caused by dehydration or exhaustion, or may indicate preeclampsia.

Monitor temperature, as indicated.

Elevated temperature and pulse may indicate dehydration or, on occasion, infection.

Assess FHR and baseline; note periodic changes and variability (if internal scalp electrode is used).

Initially, FHR may become tachycardic with maternal dehydration and fluid losses. Prolonged maternal acidosis may result in fetal acidosis and hypoxia. (Refer to ND: Gas Exchange, risk for impaired fetal.)

Reduce excess clothing, cool body with wet cloths, and maintain cool environment. Protect from chilling.

Cools the body through evaporation; may reduce diaphoretic losses. Muscle tremors associated with chilling increase body temperature and general discomfort. Note: Diaphoresis, blood loss at delivery, hyperventilation, reduced oral intake, and vomiting all contribute to possible alterations in maternal fluid-electrolyte balances.

Place client in upright or lateral recumbent position.

Optimizes placental perfusion.

Collaborative

Administer fluids orally (sips of juices/broth or ice chips), as allowed, or parenterally.

Replaces fluid losses. Solutions such as lactated Ringer's administered intravenously help correct or prevent electrolyte imbalances.

NURSING DIAGNOSIS:	Infection, risk for maternal
Risk Factors May Include:	Repeated invasive procedures, traumatized tissues, exposure to pathogens, prolonged labor, or rupture of membranes
Possibly Evidenced By:	[Not applicable; presence of signs/symptoms establishes an *actual* diagnosis]
DESIRED OUTCOMES/EVALUATION CRITERIA—CLIENT WILL:	Be free of infection.

ACTIONS/INTERVENTIONS

RATIONALE

Independent

Perform perineal care per protocol, using medical asepsis. Remove fecal contaminants expelled during pushing; change linens/underpad as needed.

Helps promote cleanliness; prevents development of an ascending uterine infection and possible sepsis.

Note date and time of rupture of membranes. (Refer to CP: Prenatal Infection.)

Within 4 hr after rupture of membranes, the client and fetus are at increased risk for ascending tract infections and possible sepsis.

Perform vaginal examination only when absolutely necessary, using aseptic technique.

Repeated vaginal examination increases the risk of endometrial infections.

Monitor temperature, pulse, and WBC count, as indicated.

Increased temperature or pulse greater than 100 bpm may indicate infection. Normal protective leukocytosis with WBC count as high as $25,000/mm^3$ must be differentiated from elevated WBC count caused by infection.

Use surgical asepsis in preparing equipment. Clean perineum with sterile water and soap or surgical disinfectant just prior to delivery.

Reduces risk of contamination.

Assist partner with dressing in scrub apparel (if indicated), washing hands, and so forth, as required by setting. Reduce number of persons present at delivery, depending on client's/care provider's wishes.	Reduces risk of infection resulting from cross-contamination.

Collaborative

Administer antibiotics, as indicated.	Used only occasionally; prophylactic antibiotics are controversial and must be used with caution because they may stimulate overgrowth of resistant organisms.
Provide aseptic conditions for delivery.	Helps prevent postpartal infection and endometritis.

NURSING DIAGNOSIS:	**Injury, risk for fetal**
Risk Factors May Include:	Malpresentations/positions, precipitous delivery, or cephalopelvic disproportion (CPD)
Possibly Evidenced By:	[Not applicable; presence of *signs/symptoms* establishes an *actual* diagnosis]
DESIRED OUTCOMES/EVALUATION CRITERIA—FETUS WILL:	Be free of preventable trauma or other complications.

ACTIONS/INTERVENTIONS

RATIONALE

Independent

Assess fetal position, station, and presentation.	Malpresentations such as face, mentum (chin), or brow may prolong labor and increase the likelihood that cesarean delivery will be necessary, because lack of neck flexion increases the diameter of the fetal head as it passes through the pelvic outlet. Breech presentation usually necessitates surgical intervention, owing to the high risk of spinal cord injuries resulting from hyperextension of the fetal head during vaginal delivery.
Monitor labor progress and rate of fetal descent.	Precipitous labor increases the risk of fetal head trauma because skull bones do not have adequate time to adjust to dimensions of the birth canal.
Assess amount of amniotic fluid expelled at the time membranes rupture and then during contractions.	Hydramnios is associated with fetal disorders such as anencephaly, disorders of the gastrointestinal tract, kidney dysfunction, and maternal diabetes. Oligohydramnios is associated with postmaturity and intrauterine growth retardation secondary to placental insufficiency.
Note color of amniotic fluid.	Meconium-stained amniotic fluid, greenish in color, may indicate fetal distress caused by hypoxia in a vertex presentation or to compression of fetal intestinal tract in breech presentation.
Transfer to delivery room, as appropriate, when vertex is visible at introitus in nullipara, or when multipara is 8 cm dilated.	If delivery is to occur in area separate from the labor setting, transfer at this time ensures that infant is born where emergency medications and equipment are available, if needed.

249

Remain with client and monitor pushing efforts as head emerges. Instruct client to pant during process.

Ensures that trained personnel are present and reduces possibility of trauma to fetal vertex; allows gradual accommodation of skull bones to birth canal and overriding of sutures.

Obtain emergency delivery kit if delivery not usually done in labor room. (Refer to CP: Precipitous Labor/Delivery or Unplanned Out-of-Hospital Delivery.) Verify proper functioning of equipment and availability of appropriate supplies.

Assures the availability of needed equipment and supplies in the event that labor progresses too rapidly for a planned delivery. When precipitous delivery is imminent, transfer to the delivery room is postponed until the neonate is delivered and the cord is clamped and cut.

Maintain record of events.

Accurate documentation provides information about neonate/client status and postpartal needs.

Collaborative

Assist with vaginal delivery when fetus is in posterior position.

Posterior position increases possibility of fetal trauma caused by neck injuries.

Assist with vertex rotation from OP to OA (Scanzoni maneuver).

Manual or vacuum rotation from OP to OA is possible (if no CPD exists). Double application of forceps to vertex may increase risk of fetal injury, yet OA position is preferred position for delivery.

Prepare for surgical intervention, if indicated. (Refer to CP: Cesarean Birth.)

May be necessary in cases of CPD, persistent OP position, or deep transverse arrest of the head with prolonged stage II labor or fetal distress, or with breech or shoulder presentation. Fetus with anencephaly may not dilate maternal tissues effectively and may therefore require surgical intervention.

NURSING DIAGNOSIS:	Fatigue, risk for
Risk Factors May Include:	Decreased metabolic energy production, increased energy requirements, overwhelming psychological/emotional demands, presence of pain
Possibly Evidenced By:	[Not applicable; presence of signs/symptoms establishes an *actual* diagnosis]
DESIRED OUTCOMES/EVALUATION CRITERIA—CLIENT WILL:	Effectively participate in bearing-down activities.
	Relax/rest between efforts.

ACTIONS/INTERVENTIONS

RATIONALE

Independent

Assess fatigue level, and note activities/rest immediately before onset of labor.

The amount of fatigue is cumulative, so that the client who has experienced a longer-than-average stage I labor, and/or one who was not rested at the onset of labor, may experience greater feelings of exhaustion.

Encourage rest/relaxation between contractions. Provide environment conducive to rest. (Refer to ND: Pain [acute].)

Conserves energy needed for pushing efforts and delivery. Stage II can be extremely exhausting because of the muscular effort involved in bearing down, the intensity of the emotional response to the birth experience, inadequate rest, and/or length of labor.

Keep client/couple informed of progress.

Helps provide needed psychological energy. Spontaneous efforts to bear down tend to lengthen stage II labor, but do not negatively affect the fetus.

Encourage use of relaxation techniques. Review them with client/partner, as necessary.

Tense muscles increase feelings of exhaustion and resistance to fetal descent and may prolong labor.

Monitor fetal descent, presentation, and position. (Refer to ND: Injury, risk for fetal.)

Malposition and malpresentation may prolong labor and cause/increase fatigue.

Collaborative

Supply fluids with glucose orally as appropriate or parenterally, if ordered. Test urine for ketones, as indicated.

Replenishes reserves that may have been depleted in labor and possibly resulted in hypoglycemia or ketonuria.

Assist with anesthesia or use of forceps if client's efforts do not rotate fetal vertex and promote fetal descent.

Low forceps delivery may be necessary in the event of extreme maternal feelings and/or when maternal efforts to deliver are unsuccessful. Midforceps delivery with rotation (Scanzoni maneuver) helps rotate fetus from OP to OA position. (Refer to ND: Injury, risk for fetal.)

Prepare for cesarean birth if vaginal delivery is not possible.

Maternal fatigue and lack of progress may result from CPD or fetal malposition.

NURSING DIAGNOSIS:	Coping, Individual, risk for ineffective
Risk Factors May Include:	Situational crisis, personal vulnerability, inadequate support system, unrealistic perceptions/expectations
Possibly Evidenced By:	[Not applicable; presence of signs/symptoms establishes an *actual* diagnosis]
DESIRED OUTCOMES/EVALUATION CRITERIA—CLIENT WILL:	Verbalize feelings congruent with behavior.
	Demonstrate effective coping skills by the use of self-directed techniques for bearing-down efforts.

ACTIONS/INTERVENTIONS

RATIONALE

Independent

Determine client's/couple's perception of behavioral response to labor. Encourage verbalization of feelings. Note cultural influences.

Helps nurse gain insight into couple's feelings and identify needs. Depending on ethnic background and childbirth preparation, involvement in the birth process can be ego-enhancing for the father or support person who desires active participation. Conversely, negative feelings or disappointment about performance arise if active involvement is not allowed or supported.

Discuss normal emotional and physical changes as well as variation in emotional responses.

Understanding helps client cope with situation and cooperate with pushing efforts. Emotional responses in this stage of labor vary from excitement at being able to participate more actively/control the forces of labor through pushing efforts, to embarrassment, irritability, or fear resulting from loss of control. This may be manifested by a lack of cooperation or ineffective pushing during contractions.

251

Monitor response to contraction. Provide gentle but firm instructions for efforts to bear down when the urge to push arises.

Active involvement provides positive means of coping and assists in descent of the fetus. Negative coping can result in prolonged labor and increases the likelihood that anesthesia and/or forceps or vacuum may be needed for the delivery.

Discuss options for pain control/reduction. (Refer to ND: Pain [acute].)

Client may require anesthesia or analgesia to promote relaxation and facilitate coping.

Support client/couple in their decision to use analgesia or anesthesia.

The client's perception of her performance may be influenced by her own goals for coping with pain. If she has planned an unmedicated birth, she may feel a sense of failure if she resorts to anesthesia as fatigue and pain become intense. The client may be concerned about the support person's sense of failure as a coach if she resorts to medication. The nurse can reduce these feelings of "failure" by accepting the decision in a nonjudgmental manner.

Point out tense or furrowed brow, clenched fists, and so forth, and suggest that partner touch tense areas.

Helps client focus on tension reduction, and allows couple to work together to regain control of situation.

Provide comfort measures (e.g., applying cool cloths to face, neck, and extremities; eliminating excess clothing; positioning properly; providing perineal care; and providing a quiet, nonstimulating environment).

Reduction of discomforts and distractions allows couple to focus on labor efforts.

Encourage client to rest between contractions with eyes closed.

Conserves strength needed for pushing, thereby facilitating the coping process.

Facilitate partner's participation in meeting client's needs regarding comfort, pushing, and emotional support.

Active participation fosters positive sense of self and may actually strengthen and enhance couple's future relationship and their relationship to the child.

Provide positive reinforcement; inform couple of labor progress, appearance of fetal vertex, and that their efforts are helpful. Provide mirror for visualization of emerging infant or have client reach down and touch baby's head as she pushes.

Helps couple to feel positive about their participation and rewarded for their cooperation. Encourages continuation of efforts.

LABOR: Stage III (Placental Expulsion)

Stage III of labor begins with the birth of the baby and is completed with placental separation and expulsion. Lasting anywhere from 1–30 min, with an average length of 3–4 min in the nullipara, and 4–5 min in the multipara, this stage is the shortest. Careful management and monitoring are necessary, however, to prevent short- and long-term negative outcomes.

CLIENT ASSESSMENT DATA BASE

Activity/Rest

Behaviors may range from excitement to fatigue.

Circulation

BP increases as cardiac output increases; then returns to normal levels shortly thereafter.
Hypotension may occur in response to analgesics and anesthetics.
Pulse rate slows in response to change in cardiac output.

Food/Fluid

Normal blood loss is <500 ml.

Pain/Discomfort

May complain of leg/body tremors/chills, leg cramps

Safety

Manual inspection of uterus and birth canal determines presence of tears or lacerations.
Extension of the episiotomy or birth canal lacerations may be present.

Sexuality

Dark vaginal bleeding beginning as a trickle occurs as the placenta separates from the endometrium, usually within 1–5 min after delivery of the infant.
Umbilical cord lengthens at vaginal introitus.
Uterus changes from discoid to globular shape and rises in abdomen.

NURSING PRIORITIES

1. Promote uterine contractility.
2. Maintain circulating fluid volume.
3. Promote maternal and newborn safety.
4. Support parental-infant interaction.

NURSING DIAGNOSIS:	**Fluid Volume risk for deficit**
Risk Factors May Include:	Lack/restriction of oral intake, vomiting, diaphoresis, increased insensible water loss, uterine atony, lacerations of the birth canal, retained placental fragments
Possibly Evidenced By:	[Not applicable; presence of *signs/symptoms* establishes an *actual* diagnosis]
DESIRED OUTCOMES/EVALUATION CRITERIA—CLIENT WILL:	Display BP and heart rate WNL, palpable pulses.
	Demonstrate adequate contraction of the uterus with blood loss WNL.

253

ACTIONS/INTERVENTIONS	RATIONALE

Independent

Instruct the client to push with contractions; help direct her attention toward bearing down.	Client attention is naturally on the newborn; in addition, fatigue may affect individual efforts, and she may need help in directing her efforts toward assisting with placental separation. Bearing down helps promote separation and expulsion, reduces blood loss, and enhances uterine contraction.
Assess vital signs before and after administering oxytocin.	Hypertension is a frequent side effect of oxytocin.
Palpate uterus; note "ballooning."	Suggests uterine relaxation with bleeding into uterine cavity.
Monitor for signs and symptoms of excess fluid loss or shock (i.e., check BP, pulse, sensorium, skin color, and temperature). (Refer to CP: Postpartal Hemorrhage.)	Hemorrhage associated with fluid loss greater than 500 ml may be manifested by increased pulse, decreased BP, cyanosis, disorientation, irritability, and loss of consciousness.
Place infant at client's breast if she plans to breast-feed.	Suckling stimulates release of oxytocin from the posterior pituitary, promoting myometrial contraction and reducing blood loss.
Massage uterus gently after placental explusion.	Myometrium contracts in response to gentle tactile stimulation, thereby reducing lochial flow and expressing blood clots.
Record time and mechanism of placental separation; i.e., Duncan's mechanism (placenta separates from the inside to outer margins) versus Schulze's mechanism (placenta separates from outer margins inward).	Separation should occur within 5 min after birth. The Duncan's mechanism of separation carries increased risk of retained fragments, necessitating close inspection of the placenta. Failure to separate may require manual removal. The more time it takes for the placenta to separate, and the more time in which the myometrium remains relaxed, the greater the blood loss.
Inspect maternal and fetal surfaces of placenta. Note size, cord insertion, intactness, vascular changes associated with aging, and calcification (which possibly contributes to abruption).	Helps detect abnormalities that may have an impact on maternal or newborn status.
Obtain and record information related to inspection of uterus and placenta for retained placental fragments.	Retained placental tissue can contribute to postpartal infection and to immediate or delayed hemorrhage. If detected, the fragments should be removed manually or with appropriate instruments.

Collaborative

Avoid excessive traction on umbilical cord.	Force may contribute to breakage of the cord and retention of placental fragments, increasing blood loss.
Administer fluids through parenteral route.	If fluid loss is excessive, parenteral replacement helps restore circulating volume and oxygenation of vital organs.
Administer oxytocin (Pitocin) through IM route, or dilute IV drip in electrolyte solution, as indicated. IM methylergonovine maleate (Methergine) or prostaglandins may be given at the same time.	Promotes vasoconstrictive effect within the uterus to control postpartal bleeding after placental explusion. IV bolus may result in maternal hypertension. Water intoxication may occur if electrolyte-free solution is used. Note: Methergine is contraindicated in presence of hypertension/hypotension.

Obtain and record information related to inspection of birth canal for lacerations. Assist with repair of cervix, vagina, and episiotomy extension.

Lacerations contribute to blood loss; can cause hemorrhage.

Assist as needed with manual removal of placenta under general anesthesia and sterile conditions.

Manual intervention may be necessary to facilitate expulsion of placenta and stop hemorrhage.

Elevate fundus by dipping fingers down behind and moving uterine body up away from symphysis pubis.

May be requested by practitioner to facilitate internal examination.

NURSING DIAGNOSIS:	Injury, risk for maternal
Risk Factors May Include:	Positioning during delivery/transfers, difficulty with placental separation, abnormal blood profile
Possibly Evidenced By:	[Not applicable; presence of signs/symptoms establishes an *actual* diagnosis]
DESIRED OUTCOMES/EVALUATION CRITERIA—CLIENT WILL:	Observe safety measures.
	Be free of injury.

ACTIONS/INTERVENTIONS

RATIONALE

Independent

Palpate fundus to note "ballooning" of uterus, and massage gently.

Helps identify relaxation of uterus and subsequent bleeding into the uterus and facilitates placental separation.

Gently massage fundus after placental expulsion. (Refer to ND: Fluid Volume, risk for deficit.)

Enhances uterine contraction while avoiding overstimulation/trauma to fundus.

Assess respiratory rhythm and excursion.

With placental separation, danger exists that an amniotic fluid embolus may enter maternal circulation, causing pulmonary emboli, or that fluid changes may result in emboli mobilization.

Clean vulva and perineum with sterile water and antiseptic solution; apply sterile perineal pad.

Removes possible contaminants that might result in an ascending tract infection during postpartal period.

Remove client's legs simultaneously from leg supports, if used.

Helps avoid muscle strain.

Assist in transfer from delivery bed to recovery cart, as appropriate.

Although many clients remain in labor/delivery bed for recovery period, if transfer is required, client may be unable to move lower limbs due to continued effects from anesthesia/leg "heaviness" or cramping.

Assess client's behavior, noting central nervous system (CNS) changes.

Increased intracranial pressure during pushing and a rapid increase in cardiac output place the client with preexisting cerebral aneurysm at risk for rupture.

Obtain sample of cord blood; send to laboratory for blood typing of newborn and banking as desired. Record information regarding the sample being sent.

If infant is Rh-positive and client is Rh-negative, the client will require immunization with Rh immune globulin (Rh Ig) in the postpartal period. (Refer to CP: The Client at 4 Hours to 2 Days Post Partum.) Note: Banking of cord blood is suggested in presence of strong family history of leukemia/other

255

cancers, or for minorities who are significantly underrepresented in bone marrow donor programs. Cord blood may also be donated for the use of others.

Collaborative

Assist with episiotomy repair, as necessary.

Approximation of edges facilitates healing.

Use ventilatory assistance if needed.

Respiratory failure may occur following amniotic or pulmonary emboli.

If uterine inversion occurs:

Administer volume replacement, insert indwelling urinary catheter; obtain blood type and cross-match; monitor vital signs, and maintain careful intake/output records.

Administer oxytocin IV, replace uterus under anesthesia, and give ergonovine maleate (Ergotrate) IM after replacement. Assist with packing of uterus, as indicated.

Rapid maternal hemorrhage and shock follows inversion, and immediate lifesaving interventions may be necessary. Kidney function is a useful indicator of fluid volume levels/tissue perfusion. Promotes contractility of uterine myometrium.

Administer prophylactic antibiotics.

Limits potential for endometrial infection.

NURSING DIAGNOSIS:	Family Processes, risk for altered
Risk Factors May Include:	Developmental transition (gain of a family member), situational crisis (change in roles/responsibilities)
Possibly Evidenced By:	[Not applicable; presence of signs/symptoms establishes an *actual* diagnosis]
DESIRED OUTCOMES/EVALUATION CRITERIA—CLIENT WILL:	Demonstrate behaviors indicative of readiness to actively participate in the acquaintance process when both mother and infant are physically stable.

ACTIONS/INTERVENTIONS

RATIONALE

Independent

Facilitate interaction between the client/couple and the newborn as soon as possible after delivery.

Fosters the beginning of lifelong emotional ties between family members. Both mother and infant have a critically sensitive period during which interactional capabilities are enhanced.

Provide client and father with the opportunity to hold baby immediately after birth if infant's condition is stable.

Early physical contact helps foster attachment. Fathers are also more likely to participate in infant caretaking activities and feel stronger emotional ties if they are actively involved with the infant soon after birth.

Delay installation of eye prophylaxis ointments (containing erythromycin or tetracycline) until client/couple and infant have interacted, and dim room lights.

(Refer to CP: The First Hour of Life.)

Allows infant to open eyes fully to establish eye contact with parent(s) and actively participate in the interaction, free from the blurred vision caused by medication.

NURSING DIAGNOSIS:	Knowledge deficit [Learning Need], regarding labor process
May Be Related To:	Lack of information and/or misinterpretation of information

Possibly Evidenced By:	Verbalizations of questions/concerns, lack of cooperation
DESIRED OUTCOMES/EVALUATION CRITERIA—CLIENT WILL:	Verbalize understanding of physiological responses.
	Actively engage in efforts to push to promote placental expulsion.

ACTIONS/INTERVENTIONS

RATIONALE

Independent

Discuss/review normal processes of stage III labor.	Provides opportunity to answer questions/clarify misconceptions, enhancing cooperation with regimen.
Explain reason for such behavioral responses as chills and leg tremors.	Understanding helps client accept such changes without anxiety or undue concern.
Discuss routine for recovery period during the first 4 hr following delivery. Orient client to new staff and unit if transfer occurs at the end of this stage.	Provides continuity of care and reassurance; enhances cooperation.

NURSING DIAGNOSIS:	Pain [acute]
May Be Related To:	Tissue trauma, physiological response following delivery
Possibly Evidenced By:	Verbalizations, changes in muscle tone, restlessness
DESIRED OUTCOMES/EVALUATION CRITERIA—CLIENT WILL:	Verbalize management/reduction of pain.

ACTIONS/INTERVENTIONS

RATIONALE

Independent

Assist with use of breathing techniques during surgical repair, as appropriate.	Breathing helps direct attention away from the discomfort, promotes relaxation.
Apply ice bags to perineum after delivery.	Constricts blood vessels, reduces edema, and provides local comfort and anesthesia.
Change wet clothing and bedding.	Promotes warmth, comfort, and cleanliness.
Provide a heated blanket.	Postdelivery tremors/chills may be caused by sudden release of pressure on pelvic nerves or may possibly be related to a fetus-to-mother transfusion occurring with placental separation. Warmth promotes muscle relaxation and enhances tissue perfusion, reducing fatigue and enhancing sense of well-being.

257

Dysfunctional Labor/Dystocia

Dystocia refers to difficult labor which is usually due to uterine dysfunction, fetal malpresentation/abnormality, or pelvic abnormality.

(Refer to CPs: Labor: Stage I—Latent Phase; Labor: Stage I—Active Phase.)

CLIENT ASSESSMENT DATA BASE
Activity/Rest

Report of fatigue, lack of energy
Lethargy, decreased performance

Circulatory

BP may be elevated.
May have received magnesium sulfate ($MgSO_4$) for pregnancy-induced hypertension.

Elimination

Bowel or bladder distension may be evident.

Ego Integrity

May be extremely anxious, fearful

Pain/Discomfort

May have received narcotic or peridural anesthesia early in labor process.
May have noted false labor at home.
Infrequent or irregular contractions, mild to moderate in intensity (fewer than three contractions in a 10-min period).
May occur prior to the onset of labor (primary latent-phase dysfunction) or after labor is well established (secondary active-phase dysfunction).
Latent Phase of Labor May Be Prolonged: 20 hr or longer in nullipara (average is 8½ hr), or 14 hr in multipara (average is 5½ hr).
Myometrial resting tone may be 8 mm Hg or less, and contractions may measure less than 30 mm Hg or may occur more than 5 min apart; or resting tone may be greater than 15 mm Hg, with contractions rising to 50–85 mm Hg with increased frequency and decreasing intensity.

Safety

May have had external version after 34 weeks' gestation in attempt to convert breech to cephalic presentation.
Fetal descent may be less than 1 cm/hr in nullipara or less than 2 cm/hr in multipara (protracted descent), or no progress over 1 or more hr for nullipara or for 30 min in multipara after complete cervical dilation (arrest of descent).
Vaginal examination may reveal fetus to be in malposition (i.e., breech; chin, face, or brow position).
Cervix may be rigid/"not ripe."
Dilation may be less than 1.2 cm/hr in primipara or less than 1.5 cm/hr for multipara, in active phase (protracted active phase), or absence of cervical changes over a 2-hr period (secondary arrest of labor).
Failure to deliver within 2 hr, or 3 hr with regional anesthesia for primipara, or 1 hr/2hr with regional anesthesia for multipara (prolonged stage II).

Sexuality

May be primigravida or grand multipara.
Uterus may be overdistended owing to hydramnios, multiple gestation, a large fetus, or grand multiparity.
May have identifiable uterine tumors.

DIAGNOSTIC STUDIES

Prenatal Testing: May have confirmed polyhydramnios, large fetus, or multiple gestation.
Nonstress Test/Contraction Stress Test (NST/CST): Assesses fetal well-being.
X-ray Pelvimetry or Ultrasound: Evaluates pelvic architecture, fetal presentation, position, and formation.
Fetal Scalp Sampling: Occasionally done to detect or rule out acidosis.

NURSING PRIORITIES

1. Identify and treat abnormal uterine pattern.
2. Monitor maternal/fetal physical response to contractile pattern and length of labor.
3. Provide emotional support for the client/couple.
4. Prevent complications.

NURSING DIAGNOSIS:	**Injury, risk for maternal**
Risk Factors May Include:	Alteration of muscle tone/contractile pattern, mechanical obstruction to fetal descent, maternal fatigue
Possibly Evidenced By:	[Not applicable; presence of signs/symptoms establishes an *actual* diagnosis]
DESIRED OUTCOMES/EVALUATION CRITERIA—CLIENT WILL:	Accomplish cervix dilation at least 1.2 cm/hr for primipara, 1.5 cm/hr for multipara in active phase, with fetal descent at least 1 cm/hr for primipara, 2 cm/hr for multipara.

ACTIONS/INTERVENTIONS	RATIONALE
Independent	
Review history of labor, onset, and duration.	Helpful in identifying possible causes, needed diagnostic studies, and appropriate interventions. Uterine dysfunction may be caused by an atonic or a hypertonic state. Uterine atony is classified as primary when it occurs before the onset of labor (latent phase) or secondary when it occurs after well-established labor (active phase).
Note timing/type of medication(s). Avoid administration of narcotics or of epidural block anesthetics until cervix is 4 cm dilated.	A hypertonic contractile pattern may occur in response to oxytocin stimulation; sedation/analgesia given too early (or in excess of needs) can inhibit or arrest labor.
Evaluate current level of fatigue, as well as activity and rest prior to onset of labor.	Excess maternal exhaustion contributes to secondary dysfunction, or may be the result of prolonged labor/false labor.
Assess uterine contractile pattern manually (palpation) or electronically via external, or internal monitor with internal uterine pressure catheter (IUPC).	Dysfunctional contractions prolong labor, increasing the risk of maternal/fetal complications. A hypotonic pattern is reflected by frequent, mild contractions measuring less than 30 mm Hg via IUPC or "soft as chin" per palpation. A hypertonic pattern is reflected by increased frequency, an elevated resting tone per palpation or greater than 15 mm Hg via IUPC, and possibly decreased intensity of contractions. Note: Intensity of contractions cannot be measured by external monitor.

259

Note condition of cervix. Monitor for signs of amnionitis. Note elevated temperature or WBC; odor and color of vaginal discharge.

A rigid or unripe cervix will not dilate, impeding fetal descent/labor progress. Development of amnionitis is directly related to length of labor, so that delivery should occur within 24 hr after rupture of membranes.

Note effacement, fetal station, and fetal presentation.

These indicators of labor progress may identify a contributing cause of prolonged labor. For example, breech presentation is not as effective a wedge for cervical dilation as is vertex presentation.

Graph cervical dilation and fetal descent against time (i.e., Friedman curve).

May be used on occasion to document progress/prolongation of labor.

Place client in lateral recumbent position and encourage bedrest or sitting position/ambulation, as tolerated.

Relaxation and increased uterine perfusion may correct a hypertonic pattern. Ambulation may assist gravitational forces in stimulating normal labor pattern and cervical dilation.

Encourage client to void every 1–2 hr. Assess for bladder fullness over symphysis pubis.

A full bladder may inhibit uterine activity and interfere with fetal descent.

Assess degree of hydration. Note amount and type of intake. (Refer to ND: Fluid Volume risk for deficit.)

Prolonged labor can result in a fluid-electrolyte imbalance as well as depletion of glucose reserves, resulting in exhaustion and prolonged labor with increased risk of uterine infection, postpartal hemorrhage, or precipitous delivery in the presence of hypertonic labor.

Review bowel habits and regularity of evacuation.

Bowel fullness may inhibit uterine activity and interfere with fetal descent.

Remain with client if possible, arrange for presence of doula as appropriate; provide quiet environment as indicated.

Reduction of outside stimuli may be necessary to allow sleep after administration of medication to client in the hypertonic state. Also helpful in reducing level of anxiety, which can contribute to both primary and secondary uterine dysfunction.

Have emergency delivery kit available.

May be needed in the event of a precipitous labor and delivery, which are associated with uterine hypertonicity.

Palpate abdomen of thin client for presence of pathological retraction ring between uterine segments. (These rings are not palpable through the vagina, or through the abdomen, in the obese client).

In obstructed labor, a depressed pathological ring (Bandl's ring) may develop at the juncture of lower and upper uterine segments, indicating impending uterine rupture.

Investigate reports of severe abdominal pain. Note signs of fetal distress, cessation of contractions, presence of vaginal bleeding.

May indicate developing uterine tear/acute rupture necessitating emergency surgery. Note: Hemorrhage is usually occult since it is intraperitoneal with hematomas of the broad ligament.

Collaborative

Prepare client for amniotomy, and assist with the procedure, when cervix is 3–4 cm dilated.

Rupture of membranes relieves uterine overdistension (a cause of both primary and secondary dysfunction) and allows presenting part to engage and labor to progress in the absence of CPD. Note: Active management of labor (AML) protocols may support anmniotomy once presenting part is engaged to accelerate labor/help prevent dystocia.

Use nipple stimulation to produce endogenous oxytocin, or initiate infusion of exogenous oxytocin (Pitocin) or prostaglandins. (Refer to CP: Labor:

Oxytocin may be necessary to augment or institute myometrial activity for hypotonic uterine pattern. It is usually contraindicated in hypertonic labor

Induced/Augmented.)

Administer narcotic or sedative, such as morphine, pentobarbital (Nembutal), or secobarbital (Seconal), for sleep as indicated.

Prepare for forceps delivery, as necessary.

Assist with preparation for cesarean delivery, as indicated, e.g., malposition, CPD, or Bandl's ring. (Refer to CP: Cesarean Birth.)

pattern because it can accentuate the hypertonicity, but may be tried with amniotomy if latent phase is prolonged and if CPD and malpositions are ruled out.

May help distinguish between true and false labor. With false labor, contractions cease; with true labor, more effective pattern may ensue following rest. Morphine helps promote heavy sedation and eliminate hypertonic contractile pattern. A period of rest conserves energy and reduces utilization of glucose to relieve fatigue.

Excessive maternal fatigue, resulting in ineffective bearing-down efforts in stage II labor, necessitates use of forceps.

Immediate cesarean birth is indicated for Bandl's ring or fetal distress due to CPD. Note: Once labor is diagnosed, if delivery has not occurred within 12 hr, and amniotomy and oxytocin have been used appropriately, then a cesarean delivery is recommended by some protocols.

NURSING DIAGNOSIS:	Injury, risk for fetal
Risk Factors May Include:	Prolonged labor, fetal malpresentations, tissue hypoxia/acidosis, abnormalities of the maternal pelvis, CPD
Possibly Evidenced By:	[Not applicable; presence of signs/symptoms establishes an actual diagnosis]
DESIRED OUTCOMES/EVALUATION CRITERIA—FETUS WILL:	Display FHR within normal limits, with good variability, no late decelerations noted.
CLIENT WILL:	Participate in interventions to improve labor pattern and/or reduce identified risk factors.

ACTIONS/INTERVENTIONS	RATIONALE

Independent

Assess FHR manually or electronically. Note variability, periodic changes, and baseline rate. If in free-standing birth center, check FHTs between contractions using Doptone. Count for 10 min, break for 5 min, and count again for 10 min. Continue this pattern throughout the contraction to midway between it and the following contraction.

Detects abnormal responses, such as exaggerated variability, bradycardia, and tachycardia, which may be caused by stress, hypoxia, acidosis, or sepsis.

Note uterine pressures during resting and contractile phases via intrauterine pressure catheter, if available.

Resting pressure greater than 30 mm Hg or contractile pressure greater than 50 mm Hg reduces or compromises oxygenation within intervillous spaces.

Identify maternal factors such as dehydration, acidosis, anxiety, or vena caval syndrome.

Sometimes, simple procedures (such as turning client to lateral recumbent position) can increase circulating blood and oxygen to uterus and placenta and may prevent or correct fetal hypoxia.

261

Note frequency of uterine contractions. Notify physician if frequency is 2 min or less.	Contractions occurring every 2 min or less do not allow for adequate oxygenation of intervillous spaces.
Assess for malpositioning using Leopold's maneuvers and findings on internal examination (location of fontanelles and cranial sutures). Review results of ultrasonography.	Determining fetal lie, position, and presentation may identify factor(s) contributing to dysfunctional labor.
Monitor fetal descent in birth canal in relation to ischial spines.	Descent that is less than 1 cm/hr for a primipara, or less than 2 cm/hr for a multipara, may indicate CPD or malposition.
Arrange transfer to acute care setting if malposition is detected in client in free-standing birth center without adequate surgical/high-risk neonatal capabilities.	Risk of fetal/neonatal injury or demise increases with vaginal delivery if presentation is other than vertex.
Prepare client for the most expedient method of delivery if fetus is in brow, face, or chin presentation.	Such presentations increase the risk of CPD, owing to a larger diameter of the fetal skull entering the pelvis (11 cm in brow or face presentation, 13 cm in chin presentation, versus 9.5 cm for vertex presentation), often necessitating assisted delivery via forceps or vacuum, or cesarean delivery because of failure to progress and ineffective labor pattern.
Assess for deep transverse arrest of the fetal head.	Failure of the vertex to rotate fully from an OP to an occiput OA position may result in a transverse position, arrested labor, and the need for cesarean delivery.
Have client assume hands-and-knees position, or lateral Sims' position on side opposite that to which fetal occiput is directed, if fetus is in OP position.	These positions encourage anterior rotation by allowing fetal spine to fall toward the client's anterior abdominal wall (70% of fetuses in OP position rotate spontaneously).
Note color and amount of amniotic fluid when membranes rupture.	Excess amniotic fluid causing uterine overdistention is associated with fetal anomalies. Meconium-stained amniotic fluid in a vertex presentation results from hypoxia, which causes vagal stimulation and relaxation of the anal sphincter. Noting characteristics of amniotic fluid alerts staff to potential needs of newborn, e.g., airway/ventilatory support.
Observe for visible cord prolapse when membranes rupture, and occult cord prolapse as indicated by variable decelerations on monitor strip, especially if fetus is in breech presentation.	Cord prolapse is more likely to occur in breech presentation, because the presenting part is not firmly engaged, nor is it totally blocking the os, as in vertex presentation.
Note odor and change in color of amniotic fluid with prolonged rupture of membranes.	Ascending infection and sepsis with accompanying fetal tachycardia may occur with prolonged rupture of membranes.

Collaborative

Administer antibiotic to client, as indicated.	Prevents/treats ascending infection and will protect fetus as well.
If fetus fails to rotate from OP to OA position (face to pubis), prepare for delivery in posterior position. Alternatively, apply vacuum extractor as indicated.	Delivering the fetus in a posterior position results in a higher incidence of maternal lacerations. Vacuum extractor may be used to rotate and expedite delivery of fetus.

Prepare for cesarean delivery of breech presentation if fetus fails to descend, labor progress ceases, or CPD is identified.

Vaginal delivery of an infant in breech position is associated with injury to the fetal spinal column, brachial plexus, clavicle, and brain structures, increasing neonatal mortality and morbidity. Risk of hypoxia caused by prolonged vagal stimulation with head compression, and trauma such as intracranial hemorrhage, can be alleviated or prevented if CPD is identified and surgical intervention follows immediately.

NURSING DIAGNOSIS:	**Fluid Volume risk for deficit**
Risk Factors May Include:	Hypermetabolic state, vomiting, profuse diaphoresis, restricted oral intake, mild diuresis associated with oxytocin administration
Possibly Evidenced By:	[Not applicable; presence of signs/symptoms establishes an *actual* diagnosis]
DESIRED OUTCOMES/EVALUATION CRITERIA—CLIENT WILL:	Maintain fluid balance, as evidenced by moist mucous membranes, appropriate urine output, and palpable pulses.
	Be free of complications.

ACTIONS/INTERVENTIONS	RATIONALE
Independent	
Keep accurate intake/output, test urine for ketones, and assess breath for fruity odor.	Decreased urine output and increased urine specific gravity reflect dehydration. Inadequate glucose intake results in a breakdown of fats and presence of ketones.
Monitor vital signs. Note reports of dizziness with change of position.	Increased pulse rate and temperature, and orthostatic BP changes may indicate decrease in circulating volume.
Assess lips and oral mucous membranes and degree of salivation.	Dry oral mucous membranes/lips and decreased salivation are further indicators of dehydration.
Note abnormal FHR response. (Refer to ND: Injury, risk for fetal.)	May reflect effects of maternal dehydration and decreased perfusion.
Encourage oral fluids as appropriate.	Clear liquids such as fruit juices and broths provide not only fluids but also calories for energy production. Note: PO fluids are not recommended if surgical intervention is contemplated.
Collaborative	
Review laboratory data, e.g.: Hb/Hct, serum electrolytes, and serum glucose.	Increased Hct suggests dehydration. Serum electrolyte levels detect developing imbalances; serum glucose levels detect hypoglycemia.
Administer fluids intravenously.	Parenteral solutions containing electrolytes and glucose can correct or prevent maternal and fetal imbalances and may reduce maternal exhaustion.

263

NURSING DIAGNOSIS:	Coping, Individual, ineffective
May Be Related To:	Situational crisis, personal vulnerability, unrealistic expectations/perceptions, inadequate/exhausted support systems
Possibly Evidenced By:	Verbalizations and behavior indicative of inability to cope (loss of control, inability to problem-solve and/or meet role expectations), irritability, reports of tension/fatigue
DESIRED OUTCOMES/EVALUATION CRITERIA—CLIENT WILL:	Verbalize understanding of what is happening.
	Identify/use effective coping techniques.

ACTIONS/INTERVENTIONS	RATIONALE
Independent	
Determine progress of labor. Assess degree of pain in relation to dilation/effacement.	Prolonged labor with resultant fatigue can reduce the client's ability to cope/manage contractions. Increasing pain when the cervix is not dilating/effacing can indicate developing dysfunction. Extreme pain may indicate developing anoxia of the uterine cells.
Acknowledge reality of client's reports of pain/discomfort.	Discomfort and pain may be misunderstood in the presence of lack of progression that is not recognized as a dysfunctional problem. Feeling listened to and supported can help client relax, reducing discomfort and enhancing ability to cope with situation.
Determine anxiety level of client and partner. Note evidence of frustration.	Excess anxiety increases adrenal activity/release of catecholamines, causing endocrine imbalance. Excess epinephrine inhibits myometrial activity. Stress also depletes glycogen stores, reducing glucose available for adenosine triphosphate (ATP) synthesis, which is needed for uterine contraction.
Discuss possibility of discharge of client to home until active labor is established.	Too early admission fosters a sense of longer/prolonged labor for client. Client may be able to relax better in familiar surroundings. Provides opportunity to divert/refocus attention and to attend to tasks that may be contributing to level of anxiety/frustration.
Provide comfort measures and reposition client/encourage ambulation as appropriate. Demonstrate/encourage use of relaxation techniques, including patterned breathing.	Reduces anxiety, promotes relaxation and sense of control, assisting client to cope positively with the situation.
Provide encouragement for client/couple efforts to date.	May be useful in correcting misconception that client is overreacting to labor or is somehow to blame for alteration of anticipated birth plan.
Give factual information about what is happening.	Reduces the "unknowns" to assist with reduction of anxiety and provides data necessary to make informed decisions.

LABOR: Induced/Augmented

This plan of care concerns the induction of labor for maternal health problems, fetal compromise, or postmaturity (medically indicated inductions), and the augmentation of labor in uterine dysfunction. For optimal use of this plan of care, combine it with the previous plans of care in this chapter, concerning the normal stages of labor and dysfunctional labor, as appropriate.

CLIENT ASSESSMENT DATA BASE

Circulation

BP elevation (possibly anxiety or pregnancy-induced hypertension [PIH]); decrease (suggests supine hypotension or dehydration)

Food/Fluid

Maternal weight loss of 2.5–3 lb (may be associated with postmaturity or fetal weight loss)

Neurosensory

Deep tendon reflexes may be brisk 3+ with PIH; presence of clonus indicates severe excitability.

Pain/Discomfort

Uterine palpation may reveal dysfunctional contractile pattern.

Safety

May experience SROM without contractions.
Elevated temperature (infection in presence of prolonged rupture of membranes).
FHR may be greater than 160 bpm if preterm, hypoxic, or septic.
Fetal size may indicate weight loss; fetal demise.
Greenish amniotic fluid (fetal distress in vertex presentation).
Presenting part below the pelvic inlet.
Fundus may be lower than anticipated for term, with intrauterine growth retardation/restriction (IUGR) associated with maternal vascular involvement.
History/presence of Rh isoimmunization, chorioamnionitis, diabetes, PIH not controlled by medical therapy, chronic hypertension, postmaturity, cyanotic maternal cardiac disease, or renal disease; or previous cesarean delivery with low transverse incision (vertical incision is contraindication).

Sexuality

Precipitous (or rapid) labor with previous pregnancy; client lives a distance from the hospital.
Cervix may be ripe (approximately 50% effacement and 2–3 cm dilated).
Uterine inertia may occur.
Bloody show may be present with dilation.
Increased vaginal bleeding (placenta previa or abruptio placentae are contraindications).
May be 42 weeks' gestational age or more.

DIAGNOSTIC STUDIES

Complete Blood Count with Differential (CBCD): Determines presence of anemia and infection, as well as level of hydration.
Blood type and Rh factor, if not previously done.
Urinalysis: Reveals urinary tract infection, protein, or glucose.
Lecithin to Sphingomyelin Ratio: Determines fetal maturity.
Nitrazine Paper and/or Fern Test: Confirms rupture of membranes.
Scalp pH: Indicates degree of fetal hypoxia/fetal metabolic reserves.
Ultrasonography: Determines gestational age, fetal size, presence of fetal heart motion, and location of the placenta.

Pelvimetry: Identifies deformities of the pelvis, CPD, or fetal malposition (all of which are contraindications for induction/augmentation).
Nonstress Test (NST) or Contraction Stress Test (CST): Evaluates fetal/placental functioning.

NURSING PRIORITIES

1. Promote maternal and fetal well-being.
2. Provide client/couple with information about induction and augmentation of labor.
3. Provide emotional support.
4. Promote comfort.

NURSING DIAGNOSIS:	Knowledge deficit [Learning Need], regarding procedure, possible outcomes
May Be Related To:	Lack of exposure/unfamiliarity with information resources, misinterpretation of information
Possibly Evidenced By:	Verbalization of questions/concerns, exaggerated behaviors
DESIRED OUTCOMES/EVALUATION CRITERIA—CLIENT WILL:	Verbalize understanding of procedures/situation. Participate in decision-making process.

ACTIONS/INTERVENTIONS	RATIONALE

Independent

ACTIONS/INTERVENTIONS	RATIONALE
Review the need for induction or augmentation of labor. Discuss Bishop score.	Informed consent and cooperation depend on the client's understanding of the situation and choices. Bishop score is a numerical score assigned to cervical characteristics (position, consistency, ripeness, effacement, dilation) and fetal station that predicts whether induction will be successful.
Explain the expected procedures to client/couple: Use of prostaglandin gel; continuous monitoring of contractions and FHR; BP checked frequently; administration of oxytocin may result in increased discomfort because contractions will become more intense and onset of labor will be more rapid; analgesics may need to be administered after 5 cm dilation, or when good labor pattern is established.	Anxiety is allayed when client/couple know what is happening and what to expect. Cooperation and involvement are also enhanced.
Review amniotomy procedure (artificial rupture of membranes [AROM]); explain that it is no more uncomfortable than sterile vaginal examination.	Amnihook is guided into the vagina by the examiner's fingers during the sterile vaginal examination. Membranes, which do not contain nerves, are hooked or nicked to rupture, stimulating labor. When used alone or in conjunction with oxytocin, amniotomy can be a successful means of inducing labor. However, amniotomy generally commits the client to delivering within 24 hr.
Demonstrate and explain use of equipment (i.e., external or internal fetal monitor and IV infusion pump). Point out safety features and alarms.	Knowledge can alleviate anxiety, enhance coping with false alarms, and give a sense of control over the situation.
Instruct client/partner in basic interpretation of fetal monitor, differentiating changes in pattern that occur on movement.	Encourages involvement, gives a sense of control, and lessens anxiety regarding normal variations of tracing.

Explain oxytocin infusion.	Oxytocin may be used prior to amniotomy or may be implemented after a trial of amniotomy that fails to induce labor.
Discuss possibility of failed induction and/or operative intervention if fetal distress occurs.	Depending on the degree of cervical ripening and the client's response to procedures, induction may not be successful. If membranes are ruptured, and induction fails, a cesarean birth is indicated. If severe fetal distress is apparent, or if uterine hyperstimulation places client at risk for uterine rupture, induction may be discontinued and cesarean delivery performed. Providing this information to the client/couple in advance can prepare them psychologically and may diminish disappointment.

NURSING DIAGNOSIS:	Fear/Anxiety [specify level]
May Be Related To:	Situational "crisis," perceived threat to client/fetus, unanticipated deviation from expectations
Possibly Evidenced By:	Identification of specific concerns, increased tension, apprehension, feelings of inadequacy, decreased self-awareness, sympathetic stimulation
DESIRED OUTCOMES/EVALUATION CRITERIA—CLIENT WILL:	Use support systems effectively.
	Report anxiety diminished and/or managed.
	Appear relaxed.
	Accomplish successful labor.

ACTIONS/INTERVENTIONS	RATIONALE

Independent

Assess psychological and emotional status.	Any interruption of the normal progression of labor can contribute to feelings of anxiety and failure. These feelings can interfere with client cooperation and hamper the induction process.
Encourage verbalization of feelings.	Client may be frightened or may not clearly understand the need for inducing labor. A sense of failure at being unable to "labor naturally" may occur. Note: In cases of fetal demise, going through labor is especially disturbing and requires extensive support. (Refer to CP: Perinatal Loss.)
Use positive terminology; avoid use of terms that indicate abnormality of procedures or processes.	Helps client/couple accept the situation without self-recrimination.
Listen to client's comments that may indicate loss of self-esteem.	Client may believe that any intervention to aid the labor process is a negative reflection on her own abilities.
Provide opportunities for client input into decision-making process.	Enhances client's sense of control even though much of what is happening may be beyond her control.
Encourage use/continuation of breathing techniques and relaxation exercises.	Helps to reduce anxiety and enables client to participate actively.

267

ACTIONS/INTERVENTIONS	RATIONALE
Independent	
Review prenatal record for history of previous pregnancies and outcomes, prenatal laboratory studies, pelvic measurements, allergies, weight gain, vital signs, last menstrual period, and EDB.	Provides information needed in formulating plan of care. Alerts nurse to the possibility of existing or developing problem(s).
Obtain history regarding insertion of laminaria tent or prostaglandin vaginal suppository preparations (e.g., p-gel).	Insertion of laminaria tent or prostaglandin preparations the evening before the induction softens the cervix and facilitates labor induction. Note: Development of adverse reactions, such as hypertonicity/hyperactivity of the uterus or nausea/vomiting, requires discontinuation/removal of the prostaglandin gel.
Perform sterile vaginal examination to determine readiness or ripeness of cervix and fetal station. Repeat as indicated by client's reaction and contraction pattern.	A soft, partially effaced (more than 50%) and/or dilated (at least 3 cm) "ripe" cervix is a good indication that induction will be successful. A firm, thick "unripe" cervix with little or no dilation may require two or three trials before induction is successful. Time of amniotomy (AROM) depends on fetal station. Repeat examinations determine labor progress, but to avoid infection, they should be limited as much as possible after membranes are ruptured.
Check BP and pulse per protocol after induction begins and before increasing oxytocin.	Assesses maternal well-being and detects development of hypotension/hypertension. With initiation of oxytocin infusion, BP may be decreased. As time passes, BP may increase up to 30% above baseline. Oxytocin is given slowly in increasing amounts based on maternal and fetal response. Approximately 40 min of infusion is necessary to reach therapeutic blood levels of oxytocin. It is rapidly metabolized and excreted by the kidneys, so constant infusion should be maintained in order to achieve regular, consistent contractions of good quality to dilate the cervix effectively.
Evaluate monitor tracing closely. Note rate and reactivity of FHR.	Careful monitoring is essential to determine client/fetal response to procedure, to identify adverse reactions, and to produce an effective labor pattern.
Palpate fundus to evaluate frequency and duration of contractions. Observe for overstimulation of uterus	External uterine monitoring indicates the frequency, not intensity, of contractions. Rapid

(tetanic contraction). Note intensity and resting tone between contractions per palpation or via IUPC, if used.

labor/delivery may occur, increasing risk of cervical and soft tissue trauma. Overstimulation causes fetal hypoxia, uterine rupture, and premature separation of placenta. If contraction lasts more than 90 sec, occurs more than 2–3 min apart, or if uterus is not completely relaxed between contractions, oxytocin should be discontinued.

Document vital signs, medications, oxytocin onset and dosage increases, change of position, oxygen administration, and times of sterile vaginal examinations on monitor tracing.

Monitor tracing is a legal document, showing progress of induction, fetal/maternal response, and actions taken by healthcare staff.

Monitor intake and output. Measure urine specific gravity as indicated. Palpate bladder.

Decreased output with increased specific gravity reflects fluid deficit. Urine retention may impede labor and fetal descent. In addition, oxytocin infusions of 20 ml/min or above may result in decreased urinary output because of antiduretic effect of medication.

Water intoxication may develop dependent on rate and type of fluid administration/oxytocin infusion above 20 ml/min.

Note reports of abdominal cramping, dizziness, headache, and nausea/vomiting; presence of lethargy, confusion, hypotension, tachycardia, and cardiac dysrhythmia (irregularities).

Provide perineal care, as indicated. Monitor temperature every 2 hr. Note color and odor of vaginal drainage.

Reduces risk of infection and/or provides early detection of developing infection. Presence of meconium staining indicates fetal distress.

Collaborative

Review prenatal laboratory work. Perform nitrazine paper or fern test, if indicated.

Evaluates maternal and fetal status, and determines whether membranes have ruptured.

Assist with application of prostaglandin preparations.

Facilitates cervical ripening; may stimulate labor and/or enhance effectiveness of oxytocin infusion.

Assist with amniotomy. Place client in low semi-Fowler's position with knees bent as for vaginal examination.

AROM may stimulate labor without need of drug infusion (successful in approximately 80% of clients at term), or it may be done in conjunction with oxytocin administration. Amniotomy is contraindicated if presenting part is high.

Start primary IV line with large-gauge indwelling catheter.

Large-gauge catheter is preferred in case of the need for surgical intervention, blood transfusion, or emergency fluid/drug administration.

Assist as necessary with insertion of IUPC, if used.

Internal monitoring accurately quantitates intensity and frequency of contractions and helps identify overstimulation and possible uterine rupture caused by overadministration of oxytocin.

Dilute and administer oxytocin (Pitocin) in electrolyte solution with a two-bottle IV system, piggybacking oxytocin close to IV site, according to unit policy and procedures.

The synthetic hormone oxytocin stimulates the uterine smooth muscle, increasing the excitability of the muscle cells, which increases the strength of contractions. Oxytocin can be discontinued if necessary, and the primary site can be quickly cleared and available for other infusions when solution is infused close to IV site. In addition, water intoxication can result from excessive or rapid fluid administration, especially when D_5W is used instead of electrolyte solutions (e.g., lactated Ringer's).

Observe safety precautions related to the use of infusion and to proper labeling of oxytocin solution.

Errors or fluctuations in rate of administration may cause undermedication or overmedication, resulting in inadequate contractions or uterine

269

Obtain/monitor electrolytes, as indicated.

Water retention may occur during oxytocin infusion resulting in hypochloremia or hyponatremia.

Discontinue oxytocin, as indicated, and increase infusion of plain IV solution. Notify physician.

Hyperstimulation of the uterus (intrauterine pressure greater than 75 mm Hg) can lead to abruptio placentae, uterine tetany, and possible rupture.

Administer 1–2 g $MgSO_4$ slowly, as necessary, or terbutaline (Brethaire) subcutaneously (SQ).

Although the circulatory half-life of oxytocin is 3–9 min, uterine activity from effects of oxytocin administration may last 20–30 min after infusion is stopped. $MgSO_4$ or terbutaline may be indicated to relieve oxytocin-induced uterine tetany.

rupture. Drug delivery is verified by closely monitoring the pump and the decreasing level of fluid. Note: Confusing solutions in two-bottle system could result in drug overdose.

NURSING DIAGNOSIS:	Gas Exchange, risk for impaired fetal
Risk Factors May Include:	Altered blood flow to placenta or through umbilical cord (prolapse)
Possibly Evidenced By:	[Not applicable; presence of signs/symptoms establishes an *actual* diagnosis]
DESIRED OUTCOMES/EVALUATION CRITERIA—FETUS WILL:	Display FHR within normal limits, free of late decelerations.
CLIENT WILL:	Engage in behaviors that enhance fetal safety.

ACTIONS/INTERVENTIONS	RATIONALE

Independent

Note fetal maturity based on client's history, EDB, and uterine measurements.	Gestational age of fetus should be 36 wk or more for induction or augmentation of labor to be performed, unless maternal condition warrants intervention before this time.
Perform Leopold's maneuvers and sterile vaginal examination. Note presentation and station of fetus.	Determines whether fetus is in vertex presentation and rules out CPD. If presenting part is too high (22 cm), amniotomy may need to be postponed owing to risk of prolapsed cord.
Position client on back with head of bed elevated and a pillow or wedge placed under one hip, preferably the right, so that client tilts to side.	Aids in obtaining an adequate external fetal monitor strip to evaluate contraction pattern and FHTs. Wedge relieves pressure of fetus on vena cava and enhances placental circulation.
Apply electronic fetal monitor (EFM) 15–20 min before induction procedure.	Determines fetal well-being and provides baseline assessment of FHR and uterine activity.
Monitor FHR, as indicated, in conjunction with amniotomy.	Determining FHR prior to and following procedure provides information to ensure fetal well-being. Acceleration for a short period after amniotomy is normal; however, signs of distress may indicate fetal hypoxia from compression of cord or late decelerations.
Note time of rupture of membranes and character and consistency of fluid.	To reduce risk of ascending infection, a mature fetus should be delivered within 24 hr of rupture of

Have client void before administration of oxytocin and before application of fetal electrode.

A full bladder can interfere with fetal position and placement of monitor.

Assess reaction of FHR to contractions, via continuous EFM, noting bradycardia and late/variable decelerations; or sustained tachycardia.

membranes. Note: If fetus is not mature, measures may be taken to avoid delivery as long as possible unless signs of infection/distress are noted.

Proper assessment is needed to avoid hypoxia. Normal range for FHR is 120–160 bpm. To ensure fetal well-being, oxytocin may need to be discontinued and different measures taken, depending on interpretation of EFM tracing.

Collaborative

Review results of ultrasonography and amniocentesis, pelvimetry, and L/S ratio.

Determines fetal age and presentation; helps identify CPD and potential needs of fetus/neonate during and following delivery.

Apply fundal pressure, as indicated.

Procedure is controversial but may be tried for firm positioning of presenting part on cervix to prevent cord prolapse during amniotomy.

Assist as needed in application of internal fetal electrode.

Internal fetal electrode should be used for more accurate observation, especially if signs of fetal distress or meconium are present.

NURSING DIAGNOSIS:	Pain [acute]
May Be Related To:	Altered characteristics of chemically stimulated contractions, psychological concerns
Possibly Evidenced By:	Verbalizations, increased muscle tone, distraction behaviors (restlessness, moaning, crying), facial mask of pain
DESIRED OUTCOMES/EVALUATION CRITERIA—CLIENT WILL:	Participate in behaviors to diminish pain sensations and enhance comfort.
	Appear relaxed between contractions.
	Report pain is reduced/manageable.

ACTIONS/INTERVENTIONS	RATIONALE

Independent

Establish a rapport that enables client/partner to feel comfortable asking questions.

Answers to questions can alleviate fear and promote understanding.

Discuss anticipated changes/difference in labor pattern and contractions.

Helps prepare client because induction procedures and use of oxytocin can result in rapid onset of strong, frequent contractions, which often interfere negatively with the client's ability to use learned coping techniques, which a slower buildup in the contractile pattern would allow.

Review/provide instruction in simple breathing techniques.

Encourages relaxation and gives client a means of coping with, and controlling the level of, discomfort.

Encourage client to use relaxation techniques. Provide instruction as necessary.

Relaxation can aid in reducing tension and fear, which magnify pain and hamper labor progress.

271

Provide comfort measures (e.g., effleurage, back rub, propping with pillows, applying cool washcloths, offering ice chips/lip balm).

Promotes relaxation, reduces tension and anxiety, and enhances client's coping and sense of control.

Encourage and assist client with change of position, and readjust EFM.

Prevents/limits muscle fatigue; enhances circulation.

Review analgesics that are available and appropriate for client, and explain their time factors and restrictions.

Enhances client's control of situation and provides information necessary for making an informed choice. If client is medicated before she is 5 cm dilated, labor progress may be slowed; if delivery is imminent (within 2–4 hr), medication may depress the newborn, although use of naloxone (Narcan) at time of delivery improves neonates' respiratory function.

Give encouragement; keep client informed of progress.

Reassures client/couple. Provides positive reinforcement for efforts and promotes focus on the future.

Collaborative

Administer analgesic medications once dilation and contractions are established.

Relieves pain; promotes relaxation and coping with contractions, allowing client to remain focused on work of labor.

Cesarean Birth

Cesarean birth is an alternative to vaginal birth only when the safety of the mother and/or fetus is compromised.

CLIENT ASSESSMENT DATA BASE

Activity/Rest

Fatigue may be present.

Circulation

Hypertension (escalating PIH)
Hypotension, ashen color, cool/clammy skin (uterine rupture)

Ego Integrity

May view anticipated procedure as a sign of failure and/or as a negative reflection on abilities
    as a female
May actually fear intervention/view surgery as life-threatening
Irritable/emotional tension, (emotional response to prolonged labor; physiological response to
    PIH)

Food/Fluid

Excessive weight gain, nausea/vomiting, generalized edema (PIH)

Pain/Discomfort

Prolonged/dysfunctional contractile pattern (dystocia).
Uterine tenderness may be present; severe abdominal pain (uterine rupture).
Right upper quadrant (RUQ)/epigastric pain (PIH).
Headache (PIH).

Neurosensory

Visual disturbance/scotomata (spots in visual field) (PIH)
Seizure activity (eclampsia)
Hyperreflexia, clonus (PIH)

Safety

Elevated temperature (infectious process/dehydration).
Active STD (e.g., herpes).
Severe Rh incompatibility.
Prolapsed cord.
Fetal distress.
Impending delivery of premature fetus.
Fetal macrosomia (estimated >4000 g).
Unsuccessful external cephalic version to rotate breech presentation, or transverse lie.
Membranes may have been ruptured for 24 hr or longer.

Sexuality

CPD; tumor/neoplasm obstructing the pelvis/birth canal
Multiple pregnancies or gestations (overdistended uterus)
Substantial vaginal bleeding (placenta previa/abruptio placentae)
Previous cesarean delivery with classical incision; previous uterine or cervical surgery

Teaching/Learning

Presence of maternal complication/risk factors, such as severe PIH, diabetes, renal or cardiac
    disease, or ascending infection; prenatal abdominal trauma; maternal age >35 yr.

Procedure may or may not be planned, affecting client's preparation and understanding of procedure.
Failed induction.
Maternal age.

DIAGNOSTIC STUDIES

Complete Blood Count (CBC), Blood Typing (ABO) and Cross-match, Coombs' test: Preoperative screening tests.
Urinalysis: Determines albumin/glucose levels.
Cultures: Identify presence of herpes simplex virus type II.
X-ray Pelvimetry: Determines CPD, flexion of head in breech position.
Amniocentesis: Assesses fetal lung maturity.
Ultrasonography: Locates placenta; determines fetal growth, lie, and presentation, as well as fetal anomalies/malformations favoring cesarean delivery.
Nonstress Test (NST) or Contraction Stress Test (CST): Assesses fetal response to movement/stress of uterine contractions.
Continuous Electronic Monitoring: Validates fetal status/uterine activity.

NURSING PRIORITIES

1. Promote maternal/fetal well-being.
2. Provide client/couple with necessary information.
3. Support client's/couple's desires to participate actively in birth experience.
4. Prepare client for surgical procedure.
5. Prevent complications.

NURSING DIAGNOSIS:	Knowledge deficit [Learning Need], regarding surgical procedure, expectations, postoperative regimen
May Be Related To:	Lack of exposure/unfamiliarity with information, misinterpretation
Possibly Evidenced By:	Request for information, statement of misconception, exaggerated behaviors
DESIRED OUTCOMES/EVALUATION CRITERIA—CLIENT WILL:	Verbalize understanding of indications for cesarean birth.
	Recognize this as an alternative childbirth method to obtain healthiest outcome possible.

ACTIONS/INTERVENTIONS	RATIONALE

Independent

Assess learning needs.	This birth method is discussed in prepared childbirth classes, but many clients fail to retain the information because it has no personal significance at the time. Clients having a repeat cesarean delivery may not clearly remember or understand the details of their previous delivery. Note: Some facilities provide cesarean preparation classes for those undergoing planned procedure.
Note stress level and whether procedure was planned or unplanned.	Identifies client's/couple's readiness to incorporate information.

Provide accurate information in simple terms, clarify misconceptions. Encourage couple to ask questions and verbalize their understanding.

Stress of the situation can interfere with client's ability to take in/comprehend information needed to make informed decisions. Provides an opportunity to evaluate client's/couple's understanding of situation. Note: Native Americans may fear procedure based on history of unwanted sterilization associated with consent for surgery.

Review indications necessitating alternative birth method.

Currently approximately one in five or six deliveries is a cesarean birth; and although one of CDC's goals for Healthy America 2000 is to reduce the rate to 15% or less, the procedure should be viewed as an alternative, not an abnormal situation, to enhance maternal/fetal safety and well-being.

Describe preoperative procedures in advance, and provide rationale as appropriate.

Information allows client to anticipate events and understand reasons for interventions/actions.

Provide postoperative teaching; including demonstration of leg exercises, coughing/deep breathing; splinting technique; and abdominal tightening exercises.

Provides techniques to prevent complications related to venous stasis and hypostatic pneumonia, and to decrease stress on operative site. Abdominal tightening decreases discomfort associated with gas formation and abdominal distension.

Discuss anticipated sensations during delivery and recovery period.

Knowing what to expect and what is "normal" helps prevent unnecessary concern.

NURSING DIAGNOSIS:	Anxiety [specify level]
May Be Related To:	Situational crisis, threat to self-concept, perceived/actual threat of maternal and fetal well-being, interpersonal transmission
Possibly Evidenced By:	Increased tension, distress, apprehension, feelings of inadequacy, sympathetic stimulation, restlessness
DESIRED OUTCOMES/EVALUATION CRITERIA—CLIENT/COUPLE WILL:	Verbalize fears for the safety of client and infant.
	Discuss feelings about cesarean birth.
	Appear appropriately relaxed.
	Use resources/support system effectively.

ACTIONS/INTERVENTIONS

RATIONALE

Independent

Assess psychological response to event and availability of support system(s).

The greater the client perceives the threat, the greater the level of her anxiety.

Note cultural influences/expectations.

Some cultures (e.g., Latin, Mexican/Arab-American) may view surgical intervention as detrimental to the client's well-being or may believe client will be stigmatized as a "weak woman" (e.g., Puerto Rican).

Ascertain whether procedure is planned or unplanned.

With unplanned cesarean birth, the client/couple usually has no time for physiological or psychological preparation. Even when planned, cesarean birth can create apprehension in the

275

ACTIONS/INTERVENTIONS	RATIONALE
	client/couple owing to an actual or perceived physical threat to the mother and infant related to the condition necessitating the procedure and to the surgery itself.
Stay with client, and remain calm. Speak slowly. Convey empathy.	Helps to limit interpersonal transmission of anxiety, and demonstrates caring for the client/couple.
Reinforce positive aspects of maternal and fetal condition.	Focuses on likelihood of successful outcome and helps to bring perceived/actual threat into perspective.
Encourage client/couple to verbalize and/or express feelings (cry).	Helps to identify negative feelings/concerns and provides opportunity to cope with ambivalent or unresolved feelings/grief. The client may also feel an emotional threat to her self-esteem, owing to her feelings that she has failed, that she is weak as a woman, and that her expectations have not been met. Partner may question own abilities in assisting client and providing needed support.
Support/redirect expressed coping mechanisms.	Enhances basic and automatic coping mechanisms, increases self-confidence and acceptance, and reduces anxiety. Note: Some client actions may be viewed as ineffective (e.g., screaming and throwing things) and need to be redirected to enhance client's sense of control.
Discuss past childbirth experience/expectations, as appropriate.	Client may have distorted memories of past delivery or unrealistic perceptions of abnormality of cesarean birth that will increase anxiety.
Provide period of privacy, if possible. Reduce environmental stimuli, such as the number of people present, as indicated by client's desires.	Allows client/couple opportunity to internalize information, marshal resources, and cope effectively.

NURSING DIAGNOSIS:	**Self Esteem, risk for situational low**
Risk Factors May Include:	Perceived "failure" at a life event
Possibly Evidenced By:	[Not applicable; presence of signs/symptoms establishes an *actual* diagnosis]
DESIRED OUTCOMES/EVALUATION CRITERIA—CLIENT WILL:	Identify and discuss negative feelings.
	Verbalize confidence in herself and in her abilities.

ACTIONS/INTERVENTIONS

RATIONALE

Independent

Determine client's usual feelings about self and pregnancy. Note cultural influences.	Diagnosis of a change in self-concept is based on knowledge of past perceptions and experiences. Cesarean birth, whether planned or unplanned, has the potential to alter the way the client feels about herself. The client sees that the birth plan has been altered and that surgical intervention is needed to

	deliver the infant, whereas most women are able to deliver without any such intervention.
Encourage verbalization of feelings.	Identifies areas to be addressed. Clients' reactions vary and may be difficult to diagnose in the preoperative period. Feelings of negative self-image related to disappointment in the birth experience may interfere with postpartal activities related to successful breastfeeding and infant care.
Encourage questions and provide information/reinforce previous learning.	Enhances understanding and clarifies misconceptions.
Refer to cesarean birth as an alternative method of childbirth.	Terms such as "C-section" and "normal delivery" may reinforce client's perception that the cesarean birth is different and unnatural, and client may view self as inadequate/flawed or weak.
Provide verbal communication of assessment and interventions. Written information can be provided at a later time.	When a problem of self-esteem arises for the client, it may become more severe in the postpartal period. During the preoperative period, client is focusing on the here and now and may not be ready to read or deal with additional information.
Identify other couples/resources to be referred to after delivery.	At this crucial time, the nature of the situation usually does not allow opportunity to talk with others who have shared the same experience. However, these activities may be beneficial in the future to help with resolution of feelings/perceptions.

Collaborative

Encourage partner's presence at the delivery as desired.	Provides support for the client, promotes parental bonding, and provides additional input to the client's recall of the birth experience, because memory lapses are more common during periods of crisis. Note: Cultural expectations may prevent participation of father in birth process, necessitating attendance by a female family member.
Encourage the client/couple to participate in delivery-room bonding activities (e.g., breastfeeding and holding the infant) as able.	Provides reinforcement of the birth experience and deemphasizes the surgical nature of the delivery.

NURSING DIAGNOSIS:	**Powerlessness**
May Be Related To:	Interpersonal interaction, perception of illness-related regimen, lifestyle of helplessness
Possibly Evidenced By:	Verbalization of lack of control, lack of participation in care or decision making, passivity
DESIRED OUTCOMES/EVALUATION CRITERIA—CLIENT/COUPLE WILL:	Verbalize fears and feelings of vulnerability.
	Express individual needs/desires.
	Participate in decision-making process whenever possible.

ACTIONS/INTERVENTIONS	RATIONALE

Independent

Assess factors contributing to sense of powerlessness.	Unplanned (and sometimes planned) cesarean birth may be characterized by the client's/couple's sense of loss of control over the birth experience. The client becomes subjected to the procedures and equipment used in illness. For those clients experiencing their first hospitalization, which involves fear of the unknown, powerlessness becomes a major stress factor.
Present options in care when possible (e.g., choice of anesthesia, IV placement, and use of mirror).	Allows the client/couple to have some sense of input/control over the situation.
Identify client's/couple's expectations and desires regarding the delivery experience.	Provides opportunity to accommodate needs and promote positive experience.
Provide personal space and time alone for the couple prior to surgery, if possible. Remain with client if partner is absent.	Creates sense of control and lets couple have time to talk about their situation. Leaving client alone may result in feelings of abandonment and increased level of anxiety.
Provide information, and discuss client's/couple's perceptions.	Reduces stress caused by misconceptions/ unfounded fears as well as fear of the unknown.

NURSING DIAGNOSIS:	**Pain [acute], risk for**
Risk Factors May Include:	Increased/prolonged muscle contractions, psychological reactions
Possibly Evidenced By:	[Not applicable; presence of signs/symptoms establishes an *actual* diagnosis]
DESIRED OUTCOMES/EVALUATION CRITERIA—CLIENT WILL:	Verbalize reduced discomfort/pain.

ACTIONS/INTERVENTIONS	RATIONALE

Independent

Assess location, nature, and duration of pain, especially as it relates to the indication for cesarean birth.	Indicates the appropriate choice of treatment. The client awaiting imminent cesarean birth may experience varying degrees of discomfort, depending on the indication for the procedure, e.g., failed induction, dystocia.
Eliminate anxiety-producing factors (e.g., loss of control), provide accurate information, and encourage presence of partner.	Levels of pain tolerance are individual and are affected by various factors. Excessive anxiety in response to the emergency situation may enhance discomfort because fear, tension, and pain are interrelated and impact client's ability to cope.
Instruct in relaxation techniques; position for comfort as possible. Use Therapeutic Touch, as appropriate.	May assist in reduction of anxiety and tension, promote comfort and enhance sense of well-being.

278

Collaborative

Administer sedative, narcotics, or preoperative medication as indicated.

Promotes comfort by blocking pain impulses. Potentiates the action of anesthetic agents.

NURSING DIAGNOSIS:	Infection, risk for
Risk Factors May Include:	Invasive procedures, rupture of amniotic membranes, break in the skin, decreased Hb, exposure to pathogens
Possibly Evidenced By:	[Not applicable; presence of signs/symptoms establishes an *actual* diagnosis]
DESIRED OUTCOMES/EVALUATION CRITERIA—CLIENT WILL:	Be free of infection.
	Achieve timely wound healing without complications.

ACTIONS/INTERVENTIONS	RATIONALE

Independent

Review history for preexisting conditions/risk factors. Note time of rupture of membranes.

Underlying maternal conditions, such as diabetes or hemorrhage, potentiate the risk of infection or poor wound healing. Risk of chorioamnionitis increases with the passage of time, placing mother and fetus at risk. Presence of infectious process may increase fetal risk of contamination.

Assess for signs/symptoms of infection (e.g., elevated temperature, pulse, WBC; abnormal odor/color of vaginal discharge, or fetal tachycardia).

Rupture of membranes occurring 24 hr prior to surgery may result in chorioamnionitis prior to surgical intervention and may impair wound healing.

Provide perineal care per protocol, especially once membranes have ruptured.

Reduces risk of ascending infection.

Collaborative

Carry out preoperative skin preparation; scrub according to protocol.

Reduces risk of skin contaminants entering the incision, reducing risk of postoperative infection.

Obtain blood, vaginal, and placental cultures, as indicated.

Identifies infecting organism and degree of involvement.

Note Hb and Hct, and estimated blood loss during surgical procedure.

Risk of postdelivery infection and poor healing is increased if Hb levels are low and blood loss is excessive. Note: Greater blood loss is associated with classic incision than with lower uterine segment incision.

Administer parenteral broad-spectrum antibiotic preoperatively.

Prophylactic antibiotic may be ordered to prevent development of an infectious process, or as treatment for an identified infection, especially if the client has had prolonged rupture of membranes. Note: Research suggests administration of antibiotic up to 2 hr before start of procedure provides the most protection from infection.

(Refer to CP: Labor: Stage I—Latent Phase; ND: Infection, risk for maternal.)

ACTIONS/INTERVENTIONS	RATIONALE
Independent	
Note presence of maternal factors that negatively affect placental circulation and fetal oxygenation.	Reduced circulating volume or vasospasms within the placenta reduce oxygen available for fetal uptake.
Continue monitoring FHR, noting beat-to-beat changes or decelerations during and following contractions.	Owing to hypoxia, fetal distress may occur; may be manifested by reduced variability, late decelerations, and tachycardia followed by bradycardia. Note: Infection from prolonged rupture of membranes also increases FHR.
Note presence of variable decelerations; change client's position from side to side.	Compression of cord between birth canal and presenting part may be relieved by position changes.
Note color and amount of amniotic fluid when membranes rupture.	Fetal distress in vertex presentation is manifested by meconium staining, which is the result of a vagal response to hypoxia.
Auscultate FHR when membranes rupture.	In the absence of full cervical dilation, occult or visible prolapse of the umbilical cord may necessitate cesarean birth.
Monitor fetal heart response to preoperative medications or regional anesthesia.	Narcotics usually reduce FHR variability and may require administration of naloxone (Narcan) following delivery to reverse narcotic-induced respiratory depression. Maternal hypotension in response to anesthesia commonly causes transient fetal bradycardia, reduced variability, and sleep.
Collaborative	
Apply internal lead, and monitor fetus electronically as indicated.	Provides more accurate measurement of fetal response and condition.
Provide supplemental oxygen to mother via mask.	Maximizes oxygen available for placental uptake.
Administer IV fluid bolus prior to initiation of epidural/spinal anesthesia.	Optimizes uteroplacental perfusion, helps prevent hypotensive response.
Assist physician with elevation of vertex, if required.	Position changes may relieve pressure on cord.
Arrange for presence of pediatrician and neonatal intensive care nurse in delivery room for both scheduled and emergency cesarean births.	Owing to underlying maternal condition(s) and/or alternative birth process, infant may be preterm or may experience altered responses, necessitating immediate care/resuscitation.

NURSING DIAGNOSIS:	Injury, risk for maternal
Risk Factors May Include:	Traumatized tissue, delayed gastric motility, altered mobility, effects of medication/decreased sensation
Possibly Evidenced By:	[Not applicable; presence of signs/symptoms establishes an *actual* diagnosis]
DESIRED OUTCOMES/EVALUATION CRITERIA—CLIENT WILL:	Be free of injury.

ACTIONS/INTERVENTIONS	RATIONALE

Independent

Remove prosthetic devices (e.g., contact lenses, dentures/bridges) and jewelry.	Reduces risk of accidental injury.
Determine time and content of last meal. Report information to anesthesiologist. Ensure availability and functioning of resuscitation equipment.	If client has eaten just before surgical procedure, risks of vomiting and aspiration increase, and general anesthesia may be contraindicated.
Restrict oral intake once decision for cesarean birth is made.	Reduces possibility of aspiration from vomiting.
Review labor record, noting voiding frequency, output, appearance, and time of last voiding.	May indicate urine retention or reflect fluid imbalance or dehydration in client who has been in prolonged labor.
Monitor urine output and color following insertion of indwelling catheter. Note any blood-tinged urine.	Reflects hydration level, circulatory status, and possible bladder trauma associated with surgical procedure.
Assist with positioning for anesthesia; support legs in postoperative transfer to stretcher. Note client's response during and after anesthesia. (Refer to CP: Care Following Cesarean Birth [4 Hours to 4 Days].)	Essential for placement of anesthesia. Client with epidural or spinal anesthesia may incur weakness/decreased sensation of lower extremities. Idiosyncratic responses to anesthesia can occur, such as anaphylaxis or respiratory paralysis if anesthetic block rises too high.
Keep accurate instrument and sponge counts at critical times during closure, according to hospital protocol.	Ensures that all equipment and sponges are accounted for and not accidentally left in client's body.

Collaborative

Obtain urine specimen for routine analysis, protein, and specific gravity. Ensure that laboratory results are available before surgery is started.	Client is at increased risk if infectious process or hypertensive state is present.
Insert indwelling catheter to continuous gravity drainage system either just before surgical procedure or in the operating room, as indicated.	Reduces risk of bladder injury during surgical procedure.
Administer preprocedural medication (e.g., atropine).	Reduces oral secretions, limiting risk of aspiration.

NURSING DIAGNOSIS:	Cardiac Output, risk for decreased
Risk Factors May Include:	Decreased venous return, alteration in systemic vascular resistance
Possibly Evidenced By:	[Not applicable; presence of signs/symptoms establishes an *actual* diagnosis]

DESIRED OUTCOMES/EVALUATION CRITERIA—CLIENT WILL:	Remain normotensive, with blood loss less than 800 ml.

ACTIONS/INTERVENTIONS	RATIONALE

Independent

ACTIONS/INTERVENTIONS	RATIONALE
Note length of labor, if applicable. Assess for dehydration or excess intrapartal fluid losses.	Decreased intake and/or increased fluid losses lead to reduced circulating volume and cardiac output.
Remove nail polish on fingernails/toenails.	Allows clear visualization of nailbeds for assessing circulatory status.
Monitor respirations, BP, and pulse before, during, and after administration of anesthesia.	Hypotension is an anticipated side effect of regional anesthesia (e.g., epidural or spinal anesthesia) because such anesthesia relaxes smooth muscles within vascular walls, affecting circulating volume and reducing placental perfusion.
Place towel or wedge under client's hip.	Shifts uterus off inferior vena cava and increases venous return. Compression caused by obstruction of the inferior vena cava and aorta by the gravid uterus in a supine position may cause as much as a 50% decrease in cardiac output.
Note change in behavior or mental status, cyanosis of mucous membranes.	Oxygen deficits are manifested first by changes in mental status, later by cyanosis.

Collaborative

ACTIONS/INTERVENTIONS	RATIONALE
Administer supplemental oxygen via mask, as indicated.	Increases oxygen available for maternal and fetal uptake. Note: Nasal cannula is not recommended because of excessive oxygen loss to environment.
Initiate IV infusion of electrolyte solution. Administer bolus, as indicated.	Expands circulatory volume, especially prior to administration of epidural/spinal anesthesia; provides route for emergency medication in the event of a complication.
Note alteration in vital signs; assist anesthetist as needed. Estimate and record blood losses.	Excess fluid losses and hemorrhage during labor and the intraoperative period may reduce cardiac output and promote vasoconstriction with shunting of blood to major organs. Diminished cardiac output and shock are manifested by decreased BP, increased or thready pulse, and cool/clammy skin.
Administer whole blood, plasma expanders, cryoprecipitate, platelets, or packed cells as indicated. (Refer to CP: Postpartal Hemorrhage; ND: Fluid Volume deficit [isotonic].)	Replaces fluid losses, increases circulating blood volume, and increases oxygen-carrying capacity.
Prepare and administer oxytocin (Pitocin) infusion.	Once delivery of infant and placenta is completed, Pitocin aids myometrium contraction and reduces blood loss from exposed endometrial blood vessels.

NURSING DIAGNOSIS:	*Sensory/Perceptual alterations, [overload]*
May Be Related To:	*Multiple environmental stimuli, increased number of personnel, excessive noise level, psychological stress*

Possibly Evidenced By:	Exaggerated emotional response, irritability, muscle tension
DESIRED OUTCOMES/EVALUATION CRITERIA—CLIENT WILL:	Verbalize understanding of need for increased level of activity.
	Appear appropriately relaxed.
	Maintain focus, tuning out extraneous distractions.

ACTIONS/INTERVENTIONS	RATIONALE

Independent

Assess environment for factors causing sensory overload.	Identifies factors, which may or may not be controllable. Cesarean birth necessitates many medical and nursing activities necessary to ensure the health of mother and infant. Client tends to focus on the procedures being performed and the conversations going on in the room. The birth experience may be compromised by invasive technology, tending to shift the focus from the birth of the infant to the surgical procedure.
Provide information about the surgical routine, including sounds, lights, dress, and instruments.	Knowledge about procedures, instruments, and alarms can help decrease anxiety, puts perceived "chaos" in perspective.
Decrease noise levels, limit conversations, and use equipment/alarms judiciously.	Client may be keenly aware of sounds. Conversation, noise from equipment, and alarms may confuse client/cause unnecessary anxiety.
Maintain eye contact, especially when wearing mask.	Acknowledges presence of client/couple, conveys feeling of caring.
Include client/couple in operating room conversation or silence, using concerned communication.	Ignoring the client can increase fear, which detracts from a positive birth experience.
Eliminate unnecessary personnel from the environment.	Avoids intrusions into personal space, which could increase anxiety. Individuals who are not involved in care of the client may detract from the intimacy of the birth experience.

Precipitous Labor/Delivery or Unplanned/Out-of-Hospital Delivery

Rapid progression of labor, lasting less than 3 hr from onset to delivery, and out-of-hospital delivery are emergency situations that place the client/fetus at increased risk for complications and/or untoward outcomes. The attending nurse may have primary responsibility for the safety of the mother and fetus.

CLIENT ASSESSMENT DATA BASE

Ego Integrity

Irritability

Food/Fluid

Nausea/vomiting

Pain/Discomfort

May have an unusually high pain threshold or not be aware of abdominal contractions
Possible absence of palpable contractions, as occurs with maternal obesity
Low back discomfort (may not be recognized as a sign of progressing labor)
Intense/prolonged uterine contractions; inadequate uterine relaxation between contractions
Involuntary urge to bear down

Safety

Accelerated cervical dilation and fetal descent
Preterm or small-for-gestational age infant (increases potential for rapid labor/delivery)
Rectal/perineal bulging
Increased vaginal show

Sexuality

History of short or rapid labor
Young maternal age; large pelvis
Multiparity or previous vaginal surgery (decreases soft-tissue resistance)

NURSING PRIORITIES

1. Promote maternal and fetal/newborn well-being.
2. Provide a physiologically and psychologically safe experience for client and newborn.
3. Prevent complications.

NURSING DIAGNOSIS:	Anxiety [specify level]
May Be Related To:	Situational crisis, threat to self/fetus, interpersonal transmission
Possibly Evidenced By:	Increased tension; scared, fearful, restless/jittery; sympathetic stimulation
DESIRED OUTCOMES/EVALUATION CRITERIA—CLIENT WILL:	Use breathing and relaxation techniques effectively.
	Cooperate with necessary preparations for a rapid delivery.
	Follow directions and/or actively participate in delivery process.

ACTIONS/INTERVENTIONS	RATIONALE

Independent

Maintain calm, deliberate manner. Offer clear, concise instructions and explanations.

An emergency or extremely rapid delivery occurring out of the hospital or in a hospital setting without the presence of a clinician (physician or nurse midwife) can be extremely anxiety-provoking for the client/couple, who had anticipated an orderly progression through labor and delivery. When the actual birth event is not in keeping with their expectations, reactions may include hostility, fear, and disappointment. Composure of nurse reassures client and prevents transmission of undue concern and anxiety.

Provide a quiet environment and privacy within parameters of the situation. Position client for optimal comfort.

Reduces distractions/discomfort, allowing client to focus attention. May reduce "contagious" anxiety of onlookers in out-of-hospital delivery and support modesty.

Encourage partner/support person to remain with client, provide support, and assist as needed.

Allowing full participation by a support person enhances self-esteem, furthers cohesion of family unit, reduces anxiety, and provides assistance for the professional.

Remain with client. Provide ongoing information regarding labor progress and anticipated delivery.

Reduces anxiety, fosters positive coping and cooperation, and reduces fear associated with the unknown.

Support appropriate coping/relaxation techniques.

Enhances sense of control; optimizes participation in the birth process.

Arrange for services of medical/nursing staff as soon as possible. Inform client that help has been requested.

The arrival of assistance helps the client/couple to feel less anxious and more secure.

Conduct delivery in a calm manner; provide ongoing explanations.

Helps client/couple remain calm and cooperate with instructions.

Place newborn on maternal abdomen once newborn respirations are established. Allow partner to hold infant.

Helps promote bonding and establishes a positive feeling about the experience.

Collaborative

Administer sedation as appropriate.

May help slow labor progress and allow client to regain control.

NURSING DIAGNOSIS:	Skin/Tissue Integrity, risk for impaired maternal
Risk Factors May Include:	Rapid progress of labor, lack of necessary equipment
Possibly Evidenced By:	[Not applicable; presence of signs/symptoms establishes an *actual* diagnosis]
DESIRED OUTCOMES/EVALUATION CRITERIA—CLIENT WILL:	Be free of lacerations/tears.

ACTIONS/INTERVENTIONS	RATIONALE

Independent

Assess level of preparedness and knowledge. Provide information as necessary regarding the labor process and breathing/relaxation techniques.	Information helps nurse to manage the situation effectively, promotes client cooperation with necessary emergency measures, and reduces risk of injury.
Perform Leopold's maneuvers to determine fetal position. If abnormal presentation or position is detected, arrange for immediate transfer, as appropriate.	If presentation and position are other than vertex/occiput anterior, complications could arise, so that transportation to hospital or delivery setting is imperative.
Perform vaginal examination, as appropriate and situation permits.	Determines cervical effacement, dilatation, fetal station, and imminence of delivery.
Stay with client continuously. Send for help in hospital setting, or enlist the aid of the most competent bystander or significant other in out-of-hospital setting.	Constant monitoring ensures nurse will be present should delivery occur.
Discontinue oxytocin, if being administered.	Reduces uterine stimulation; may enhance uterine relaxation between contractions.
Observe client for rectal distension, fecal discharge, or increased vaginal flow.	These signs indicate labor progress as descending; presenting part compresses sigmoid and rectum.
Encourage client to pant, rather than push, when crowning occurs.	Decreases urge to push and helps reduce likelihood/degree of lacerations and perineal trauma.
Gently massage perineum ("ironing") with index finger on inside of vagina and thumb on outer portion.	Aids in stretching perineal tissue, reducing risk of tearing.
Apply gentle pressure against fetal head; support perineum with other hand. Facilitate delivery of the shoulders with gentle upward traction.	Helps prevent fetal head from delivering too rapidly, which can contribute to lacerations of the birth canal.

NURSING DIAGNOSIS:	**Fluid Volume risk for deficit**
Risk Factors May Include:	Presence of nausea/vomiting, lack of intake, excessive vascular loss
Possibly Evidenced By:	[Not applicable; presence of signs/symptoms establishes an *actual* diagnosis]
DESIRED OUTCOMES/EVALUATION CRITERIA—CLIENT WILL:	Maintain adequate level of hydration, as evidenced by palpable pulses, prompt capillary refill, moist mucous membranes.

ACTIONS/INTERVENTIONS	RATIONALE

Independent

Note characteristics of labor pattern and uterine tone. Monitor uterine activity manually or electronically. Assess for any abnormal vaginal bleeding or uterine rigidity.	Abruptio placentae can be a complication of emergency childbirth.
Place newborn on client's abdomen following delivery, once respiratory pattern is well established.	Weight of newborn stimulates uterine contractions and aids in placental separation.

ACTIONS/INTERVENTIONS	RATIONALE

Observe for signs of placental separation; avoid exerting force on umbilical cord. Save placenta for inspection by physician or nurse midwife. If out-of-hospital setting, wrap up placenta to be sent with client on transfer to hospital.

A complete inspection of the placenta can be carried out later to ensure that no tissue remains in utero.

Monitor degree of uterine contractility and the color and amount of vaginal flow. Massage fundus gently; place infant to breast.

Stimulates uterine contractility, reducing vaginal flow, and helps to prevent hemorrhage caused by uterine atony. Potential for abruptio placentae exists in the presence of rapid, severe uterine contractions without a sufficient period of relaxation between them.

Inspect perineum for lacerations. If they are present, press clean perineal pad against perineum. Instruct client to keep thighs together.

Pressure limits bleeding until help is available to make needed repairs.

Arrange for transportation to acute-care setting in out-of-hospital birth.

Examination of client by physician or nurse midwife is necessary to rule out retained placental tissue, and possibly to repair perineal or vaginal lacerations.

Record time/method of placental expulsion, appearance of intactness of placenta, client's condition, and any medications administered.

Accurate record aids in identification of potential for complications.

NURSING DIAGNOSIS: **Infection, risk for**

Risk Factors May Include: Broken *skin*/traumatized tissue, increased environmental exposure, rupture of amniotic membranes

Possibly Evidenced By: [Not applicable; presence of *signs/symptoms* establishes an *actual* diagnosis]

DESIRED OUTCOMES/EVALUATION CRITERIA—CLIENT WILL: Be free of infection.

ACTIONS/INTERVENTIONS

RATIONALE

Independent

Provide as much privacy as possible in cases of unplanned out-of-hospital delivery. Prepare clean delivery surface using clean towels, clothes turned inside out, or unread newspapers placed under the client's buttocks.

Reduces possibility of contamination.

Scrub hands, don sterile gloves, place sterile towels under buttocks, and clean perineum with soap/water solution if time permits in hospital setting.

Reduces likelihood of postdelivery infection.

Remove undergarments/newspapers when soiled.

Removes media that would support growth of pathogens.

Record time of rupture of membranes. Note amount, color, and odor of drainage, and whether there is particulate present.

Rupture of membranes increases risk of ascending infection. Characteristics of drainage may indicate presence of infection.

287

NURSING DIAGNOSIS:	Pain [acute]
May Be Related To:	Occurrence of rapid, strong muscle contractions; psychological issues
Possibly Evidenced By:	Verbalizations of inability to use learned pain-management techniques, sympathetic stimulation, distraction behaviors (moaning, restlessness)
DESIRED OUTCOMES/EVALUATION CRITERIA—CLIENT WILL:	Relax between contractions.
	Report discomfort/pain is reduced.

ACTIONS/INTERVENTIONS

RATIONALE

Independent

Note character and location of pain. Evaluate strength and intensity of contractions and duration of relaxation period.	Contractions may be of unexpected severity. Excess myometrial hypoxia may result from a tumultuous labor, intensifying discomfort.
Initiate breathing and relaxation techniques. Have partner/support person provide effleurage and sacral back rub. Encourage client to assume position of comfort, preferably left lateral or semiupright.	In accordance with gate control theory, cutaneous stimulation and counter-pressure helps reduce discomfort. Positioning can increase circulation to myometrium.
Remove excess or constrictive clothing. Provide cool/comfortable environment, if possible. Change underpad/linens, as needed.	Promotes relaxation and comfort; enhances sense of well-being. Reduces discomfort.
Use physical restraint cautiously, using verbal commands, or have significant other(s) hold gently, if necessary.	Provides safety in an "uncontrolled" setting.
Monitor bladder distension; encourage voiding.	Urine retention and consequent bladder distension may increase discomfort, impede labor, and result in bladder trauma.

NURSING DIAGNOSIS:	Injury, risk for fetal
Risk Factors May Include:	Rapid descent/pressure changes, compromised circulation, environmental exposure
Possibly Evidenced By:	[Not applicable; presence of signs/symptoms establishes an *actual* diagnosis]
DESIRED OUTCOMES/EVALUATION CRITERIA—NEWBORN WILL:	Display Apgar score of 7 or better at 1 min and at 5 min.
	Be free of injury.

ACTIONS/INTERVENTIONS

RATIONALE

Independent

Assess fundal height and uterine size. If possible, obtain information from client interview or chart regarding prior testing to determine or confirm gestational age. Ascertain expected birth date.	Helps predict size and potential needs of infant at birth.

Monitor FHR electronically or with fetoscope in hospital setting. In any setting, assess fetal activity level.

Provides data regarding condition of fetus.

Remain with client. In hospital setting, send for emergency delivery kit. Have staff person notify attending physician or nurse midwife of imminent delivery.

Kit contains equipment necessary for management of newborn in precipitate labor and delivery.

Place client in left or right lateral position.

Helps promote adequate placental perfusion; prevents supine hypotensive syndrome.

Encourage client to pant rather than push as crowning occurs.

Helps prevent dural or subdural tears during rapid descent and delivery.

Assess for nuchal cord. If present, loop cord over newborn's head before delivery of body. In hospital setting, if cord is too tight, place two clamps on cord and cut cord before delivery of body. In out-of-hospital setting, clean shoelaces or cloth strips can be used.

Nuchal/short cord may cause hypoxia/anoxia to newborn during delivery process.

Rupture membranes if they are intact following delivery of head; suction (if available) mouth, throat, and then nasal passages.

Prevents aspiration of amniotic fluid. Removes secretions and facilitates initial respiration efforts.

Support newborn during delivery of body.

Vernix and amniotic fluid covering the body may make newborn difficult to grasp.

Hold newborn at the level of, or slightly lower than, the uterus.

While controversial, it is believed to facilitate blood flow through the umbilical cord, thereby providing an additional amount of blood to the newborn. Note: Holding the newborn above the uterus causes blood to flow from the cord by force of gravity.

Suction or clear oropharynx again. Place infant on client's abdomen, with infant's head slightly lower than body if respirations adequate.

Helps clear airway; facilitates drainage of mucus.

Dry newborn immediately (especially head); wrap infant in blanket, coat, or unused plastic food wrap; and give to client to hold next to her own body or place at client's breast. Without unwrapping infant, reassess temperature by feeling infant's stomach with back of fingers.

Reduces likelihood of cold stress. Mother's body warmth helps warm the newborn. Early feedings, help prevent hypoglycemia.

Determine infant's condition at birth, noting Apgar score at 1 min and at 5 min. Keep accurate record of time of delivery, position of fetus at birth, presence of nuchal cord, sex, and condition of newborn (including Apgar scores), any medications given to mother/newborn, and resuscitative measures used.

Provides information that is needed by medical personnel for later evaluation of the newborn.

Prepare for transfer to hospital setting. Placenta can be left attached to newborn during the transfer (wrapped in newspaper or towel).

Client and newborn need to be evaluated by medical personnel.

(Refer to CP: The First Hour of Life.)

Intrapartal Hypertension

PIH may have been diagnosed during the prenatal period, necessitating induction of labor/cesarean birth, or onset of symptoms may occur during labor (or early postpartum). Early recognition and prompt intervention promote optimal outcomes for client and fetus.

This plan of care is to be used in conjunction with the first five care plans in this chapter, which concern the three stages of labor, or with CPs: Induced/Augmented Labor Cesarean Birth, as indicated.

CLIENT ASSESSMENT DATA BASE

(Refer to CP: Pregnancy-Induced Hypertension and to the intrapartal assessment tool at the beginning of this chapter.)

Circulation

May have been monitored/treated for prenatal hypertension either at home or in hospital setting, or may have been normotensive throughout the pregnancy.
Blood pressure may be elevated at the onset of labor.
Progressive fluid retention may be present.

Safety

May be receiving an oxytocin infusion for induction or to offset tocolytic effects of $MgSO_4$.

Sexuality

May be scheduled for induction (if cervix is favorable) or cesarean birth (preferably after 36 weeks' gestation) because of deteriorating maternal and placental status.
Pregnancy may or may not be full term (with uterus at xiphoid process).

DIAGNOSTIC STUDIES

Kidney, liver, and coagulation studies may show altered function.
(Refer to CP: Pregnancy-Induced Hypertension.

NURSING PRIORITIES

1. Reduce/alleviate maternal hypertension.
2. Monitor client and fetal status.
3. Maintain/optimize placental circulation.
4. Prevent eclamptic state.

NURSING DIAGNOSIS:	**Fluid Volume excess/[circulating deficit]**
May Be Related To:	Compromised regulatory mechanism (pathological state with fluid shifts), excessive fluid intake, effects of drug therapy (oxytocin infusion)
Possibly Evidenced By:	Blood pressure changes, edema, weight gain, changes in mentation
DESIRED OUTCOMES/EVALUATION CRITERIA—CLIENT WILL:	Display usual mentation; BP, pulse, urine output, and specific gravity WNL; deep tendon reflexes (DTRs) 2+ (normal); free of headache and visual disturbances, absence of clonus.

ACTIONS/INTERVENTIONS	RATIONALE
Independent	
Assess location and extent of edema. Note Hb and Hct levels.	Helps determine degree of fluid retention and possible shifts to extracellular tissues. If the pathological state is excessive, involving vasospasms and hypertension, fluid that has shifted from the intravascular space to extracellular tissue may begin to reenter the circulatory system, contributing to fluid overload and significant increase in BP.
Assess BP and pulse as indicated, especially if client is receiving oxytocin.	Preexisting elevated BP may rise even higher in the intrapartal period, or a normotensive client may become hypertensive during labor in response to increased basal metabolic rate, anxiety, and/or sodium and water retention from oxytocin infusion.
Assess ankle clonus, DTRs, lung sounds, visual acuity, presence of RUQ/epigastric pain.	Progressive edema may be manifested by hyperreflexia or by cerebral, liver, or lung involvement. (Refer to CP: Pregnancy-Induced Hypertension; ND: Fluid Volume deficit [isotonic].)
Monitor urine output. Measure specific gravity; check albumin by dipstick test.	Kidney function is directly correlated to circulatory fluid volume, so that if fluid is trapped in third spaces, output decreases and specific gravity increases.
Position client on left or right side during stage I and II labor, or place wedge underneath right buttock.	Prevents compression of aorta and inferior vena cava; increases venous return, placental circulation, and kidney perfusion.
Collaborative	
Administer antihypertensives (e.g., hydralazine [Apresoline], sodium nitroprusside [Nipride]) IV by infusion pump, if diastolic readings are greater than 110 mm Hg.	Vasodilator drugs relax smooth muscle of blood vessels, thereby reducing BP immediately. In emergency situations, sodium nitroprusside acts within 30 sec, providing a rapid decline in blood pressure.
Insert indwelling urinary catheter.	Provides accurate hourly totals of urine output, and monitors client for developing renal problems or oliguria. (Refer to CP: Pregnancy-Induced Hypertension; ND: Tissue Perfusion, altered renal.)
Administer PO/IV fluids as ordered.	Controversy exists as to whether these individuals should receive approximately 125 ml/hr to correct circulatory deficits, or have fluids restricted at approximately 75 ml/hr to reduce risk of pulmonary edema. Note: Fluid restriction increases client's sensitivity to vasodilators with risk of fetal distress, and inability to use epidural anesthesia safely.
Administer furosemide (Lasix) if indicated.	On occasion, circulatory overload/failure may cause pulmonary edema requiring aggressive therapy. Otherwise, it is contraindicated as it may cause dehydration.

NURSING DIAGNOSIS:	**Gas Exchange, risk for impaired fetal**
Risk Factors May Include:	Altered blood flow, vasospasms, and/or prolonged uterine contractions

Possibly Evidenced By:	[Not applicable; presence of signs/symptoms establishes an *actual* diagnosis]
DESIRED OUTCOMES/EVALUATION CRITERIA—FETUS WILL:	Be free of late deceleration.
	Manifest good variability.
	Demonstrate a baseline heart rate of 120–150 bpm.

ACTIONS/INTERVENTIONS	RATIONALE

Independent

Assess FHR; note periodic changes (accelerations and decelerations) and patterns of short- or long-term variability. Report reduced variability and late decelerations, if present.	Recurrent or late decelerations combined with reduced variability or tachycardia and then bradycardia may indicate uteroplacental insufficiency or potential fetal compromise/demise.
Position client on side; use wedge under right buttock if client is supine.	Prevents supine hypotensive syndrome; increases placental perfusion, which is especially critical in the hypertensive client who has low fetal reserve manifested as late decelerations.

Collaborative

Note findings of prenatal testing, especially amniocentesis, nonstress test, contraction stress test, gestational age of fetus, and fetal lung maturity.	Helps in predicting fetal response to labor and in evaluating newborn's ability to establish respiratory function in the early neonatal period.
Apply internal electrode to presenting part.	Accurately monitors fetal response and variability.
Note administration of $MgSO_4$ or diazepam (Valium) to client.	May reduce beat-to-beat variability and depress newborn. Note: Valium use is generally restricted to treatment of severe eclampsia/seizure control.
In the event of late decelerations:	Continuation of pattern for more than 30 min markedly increases risk of negative effects of fetal hypoxia, acidosis, and asphyxia.
Increase plain IV fluid and discontinue oxytocin infusion. Notify physician immediately, especially if sinusoidal pattern is present.	Stopping oxytocin and increasing plain IV fluid may increase placental circulating volume/oxygenation. (Oxytocin infusion may reduce periods of maternal uterine relaxation between contractions, thereby reducing oxygen levels.) Note: A sinusoidal pattern with minimal to absent short- and long-term variability may occur just prior to death in a severely hypoxic fetus.
Elevate client's legs; administer oxygen via mask at 8–10 L/min.	Increases venous return, circulating blood volume, and oxygen available for fetal uptake.
Assist as necessary with obtaining fetal scalp sample.	Fetal scalp pH should range between 7.30 and 7.35. A preacidotic value of 7.20–7.24 should be repeated in 15 min, with expeditious delivery carried out if values are less than 7.20. Note: Normal values may vary, e.g., effects of altitude.
Arrange for presence of pediatrician or neonatal/pediatric intensive care unit nurse at delivery.	May be needed to provide resuscitation or immediate care of the newborn.
Prepare for vaginal delivery or cesarean birth, depending on fetal status and cervical dilation.	Intervention may be necessary to prevent fetal/neonatal compromise caused by asphyxia.

NURSING DIAGNOSIS:	Urinary Elimination, altered
May Be Related To:	Fluid shifts, hormonal changes, effects of medication
Possibly Evidenced By:	Changes in amount/frequency of voiding; bladder distension, changes in urine specific gravity, presence of albumin
DESIRED OUTCOMES/EVALUATION CRITERIA—CLIENT WILL:	Display individually adequate urine output with specific gravity WNL and urinary albumin not greater than 1+.

ACTIONS/INTERVENTIONS	RATIONALE
Independent	
Monitor intake and output.	Increased diuresis may occur, resulting in loss of 4 lb or more of retained fluid in a 24-hr period owing to bedrest, which reduces adrenal functioning.
Note color, amount, specific gravity, and albumin levels in each voiding.	Increasing urine output is reflected in less concentrated urine with decreasing specific gravity. Albumin greater than 2+ indicates glomerular spasms.
Assess bladder fullness; assist as necessary in emptying. (Refer to CP: Labor: Stage I—Active Phase; ND: Urinary Elimination, altered.)	A full bladder may impede fetal descent and increases risk of maternal injury.
Collaborative	
Insert indwelling urinary catheter for continuous drainage.	In severe PIH, there may be extensive kidney involvement requiring close and accurate monitoring of renal function. In many cases, the client with severe PIH requires a cesarean delivery because of deteriorating maternal, fetal, and placental status and usually has an indwelling catheter inserted prior to surgery to prevent bladder trauma.

(Refer to CP: Pregnancy-Induced Hypertension; ND: Tissue Perfusion, altered renal.)

NURSING DIAGNOSIS:	Injury, risk for maternal
Risk Factors May Include:	Tonic-clonic convulsions, altered clotting factors (release of thromboplastin from the placenta)
Possibly Evidenced By:	[Not applicable; presence of signs/symptoms establishes an *actual* diagnosis]
DESIRED OUTCOMES/EVALUATION CRITERIA—CLIENT WILL:	Restrict activities as indicated.
	Be free of seizure activity and related complications.

ACTIONS/INTERVENTIONS	RATIONALE

Independent

Assess for CNS involvement (i.e., headache, irritability, visual disturbances) and presence of RUQ/epigastric pain.	Suggestive of cerebral edema and vasoconstriction, indicating progression of condition. Multiorgan involvement (e.g., liver distension, creating epigastric pain) reflects the HELLP syndrome, increasing mortality and morbidity.
Provide quiet environment, limit visitors, reduce room lighting, and maintain bedrest.	Helps reduce stimuli that might precipitate a seizure.
Measure urine output prior to and during administration of $MgSO_4$.	Output of at least 30 ml/hr is required for administration of $MgSO_4$.
Elicit DTRs (brachial, wrist, knee); note ankle clonus. Note signs of hyperactivity, convulsion, or coma. Discontinue $MgSO_4$ in absence of patellar reflex.	Labor may precipitate eclamptic state, with hyperreflexia and progressive edema occurring just prior to the convulsion. Reduced DTRs suggest toxic levels of $MgSO_4$, which is administered to depress CNS.
Monitor respiratory rate/depth during $MgSO_4$ administration. Stop administration if respirations are fewer than 12/min.	Therapeutic range of drug is narrow, and elevated serum concentrations may depress respirations
Evaluate uterine activity and response to $MgSO_4$.	$MgSO_4$ has tocolytic properties that may reduce myometrial contractility, possibly necessitating oxytocin augmentation. (Refer to CP: Labor: Induced/Augmented.)
Give client nothing by mouth if seizure activity is suspected.	Reduces risk of aspiration.
Obtain emergency equipment (suction, oxygen, medications, emergency delivery pack).	May be needed in the event of a seizure or precipitious delivery.
Implement seizure precautions per protocol.	Reduces risk of injury if seizure activity occurs. An eclamptic episode may initiate the onset of labor, or labor may need to be artificially induced following an eclamptic seizure.
Palpate for uterine tenderness/rigidity; check for vaginal bleeding. Note history of concurrent medical conditions.	Client is at increased risk for abruptio placentae, especially if there is a preexisting medical problem such as diabetes mellitus, or renal or cardiac conditions causing vascular involvement.
Monitor for signs of disseminated intravasculaar coagulation (DIC): easy/spontaneous bruising, prolonged bleeding.	Abruptio placentae with release of thromboplastin predisposes client to DIC.

Collaborative

Administer $MgSO_4$ by infusion pump or intra-muscularly. Have calcium gluconate (10%) available. (Refer to CP: Pregnancy-Induced Hypertension; ND: Injury, risk for maternal.)	Acts on myoneural junction to depress CNS activity; helps prevent seizure intrapartally. Calcium gluconate is an antidote to $MgSO_4$.
Initiate oxytocin infusion using piggyback setup with isotonic solution, as indicated.	May be necessary for labor induction or augmentation to overcome tocolytic effects of $MgSO_4$. Note: May cause additional elevation of BP owing to sodium/water retention, thereby increasing risk of seizure activity.
Review laboratory studies, e.g.:	
Liver enzymes (AST, ALT);	Determines progression of condition, development of HELLP syndrome.

Platelet count, clotting factors.
(Refer to CP: Prenatal Hemorrhage.)
Administer pentobarbital (Nembutal), diazepam (Valium) IV, as indicated.

Release of thromboplastin from abruptio placentae may initiate DIC.
Although rarely used, these drugs depress the thalamus and hypothalamus and effectively manages eclamptic convulsions uncontrolled by MgSO4 therapy.

NURSING DIAGNOSIS:	Knowledge deficit [Learning Need], regarding condition, prognosis, treatment needs
May Be Related To:	Lack of exposure/unfamiliarity with information resources, misinterpretation
Possibly Evidenced By:	Request for information, statement of misconception, inappropriate behaviors, development of preventable complications
DESIRED OUTCOMES/EVALUATION CRITERIA—CLIENT WILL:	Verbalize understanding of situation and treatment plan.

ACTIONS/INTERVENTIONS	RATIONALE

Independent

Assess client's level of knowledge and degree of anxiety.	Determines specific information needs and readiness to learn.
Explain the impact of procedures, nursing activities, and medications on client and fetus. Clarify misconceptions and elicit questions.	Reduces fear associated with the unknown; even those who have had problems previously may benefit from review of information throughout the labor and delivery process.
Provide simple explanations about actual and potential physiological changes associated with prenatal and intrapartal hypertension.	Increases client awareness of the seriousness of her condition, and allows her to make informed decisions about her care.
Discuss impact of labor progress on condition.	Allows client to recognize that her hypertensive state may escalate during labor, requiring more intense interventions and possibly a rapid delivery (either vaginal or cesarean).

(Refer to CPs: Labor: Stage I—Latent Phase; Labor: Stage II (Expulsion); Labor: Stage III (Placental Expulsion); ND: Knowledge deficit [Learning Need].)

NURSING DIAGNOSIS:	Anxiety [specify level]
May Be Related To:	Situational crisis, interpersonal transmission/contagion, threat of death
Possibly Evidenced By:	Increased tension, apprehension, uncertainty, restlessness, sympathetic stimulation
DESIRED OUTCOMES/EVALUATION CRITERIA—CLIENT WILL:	Verbalize awareness of feelings of anxiety.
	Report reduction in level of anxiety.
	Appear relaxed between contractions.

295

ACTIONS/INTERVENTIONS	RATIONALE

Independent

Assess client's/couple's source and level of anxiety.	All clients approach labor and delivery with a certain degree of anxiety, which becomes even greater in a high-risk situation. Such anxiety is directly related to fear of the unknown and lack of predictable outcomes for the client and her fetus.
Encourage verbalization of feelings; provide appropriate emotional support.	Aids client/couple in identifying specific concerns and helps relieve tension.
Inform client that pediatrician will be present at delivery; if possible, introduce client to pediatrician prior to delivery.	Assures client/couple that at delivery, the infant will be in competent hands and receive appropriate care.

(Refer to CPs: Labor: Stage I—Latent Phase; Labor: Stage I—Active Phase; ND: Anxiety, risk for.)

NURSING DIAGNOSIS:	**Pain [acute]**
May Be Related To:	Intensification of uterine activity, discomfort associated with hypertension or oxytocin infusion; myometrial hypoxia (abruptio placentae) and anxiety
Possibly Evidenced By:	Verbalizations, altered muscle tone, distraction behaviors (restlessness, moaning, crying), facial mask of pain, autonomic responses
DESIRED OUTCOMES/EVALUATION CRITERIA—CLIENT WILL:	Use appropriate breathing and relaxation techniques.
	Report reduction of pain/discomfort.

ACTIONS/INTERVENTIONS	RATIONALE

Independent

Assess source and nature of pain/discomfort.	Helps in determining appropriate nursing responses. Discomfort levels associated with uterine activity may be intensified in the client with hypertension, owing to high anxiety level; myometrial hypoxia, which may be associated with placental separation (abruptio placentae), and/or intense onset of labor associated with oxytocin infusion, which has a negative impact on client's ability to cope with contractions.
Review/encourage use of relaxation techniques and controlled breathing.	Client may not have completed/participated in childbirth preparation classes, or stress of situation may interfere with her ability to recall/perform these activities.
Provide comfort measures; e.g., cool cloth, dry linens, back/sacral rub.	Promotes relaxation and may enhance ability to cope with contractions.
Discuss available anesthesia and analgesia.	Knowledge enables client to make informed choices and maintain a sense of control.
Investigate report of acute abdominal pain. Note	Client with hypertension is more prone to

increased vaginal bleeding. (Refer to CP: Prenatal Hemorrhage.)

Collaborative

Assess uterine response to labor using intrauterine catheter, if available, in place of tocotransducer.

Reduce/discontinue oxytocin infusion in presence of hyperactive uterine response or reduced relaxation between contractions.

Provide/assist with administration of meperidine hydrochloride (Demerol), fentanyl (Sublimaze), or local anesthetic.

abruptio placentae because of vasospasm and fibrin deposits.

Accurately measures intensity and resting tone of contractions and detects hyperstimulation caused by oxytocin induction.

Helps to terminate hypersensitive response. Tetanic contraction may cause uterine rupture.

Demerol administered in stage I labor and or local anesthetic (or possibly a pudendal block) administered in stage II labor are recommended; epidural anesthesia may be contraindicated because of its known hypotensive effect, which further reduces placental perfusion.

Intrapartal Diabetes Mellitus

Although most diabetic clients go to term with spontaneous labor, close management of the intrapartal period is necessary for optimal outcome.

This plan of care is to be used in conjunction with the first five plans of care in this chapter, concerning the three stages of labor, or with CP: Cesarean Birth, as indicated.

CLIENT ASSESSMENT DATA BASE

(Refer to CP: Diabetes Mellitus, Prepregnancy/Gestational and to the intrapartal assessment tool at the beginning of this chapter.)

Circulation

BP may be elevated.
History of ankle/leg edema.
Rapid pulse, pallor, diaphoresis (hypoglycemia).

Ego Integrity

Reports concerns regarding labor, impending delivery, and possible effects of diabetes on outcome
Anxious, irritable, increased tension

Elimination

Polyuria

Food/Fluid

May report episodes of hypoglycemia, glycosuria
Polydipsia, hunger (hyperglycemia)
Dependent edema
Ketonuria, elevated serum glucose

Sexuality

Large amount of amniotic fluid on rupture of membranes (suggests hydramnios)

Teaching/Learning

May have been hospitalized during the prenatal period for complications such as poor diabetic control, PIH, and preterm labor due to polyhydramnios

DIAGNOSTIC STUDIES

Serum Glucose: May or may not be elevated.
Glycosylated Hemoglobin (HbA$_{1c}$): Reflects diabetic control during the preceding 5 wk.
Urinalysis: Reveals presence of glucose and ketones (hyperglycemia, ketoacidosis, and nutritional status) and albumin (PIH).
Ultrasonography and Pelvimetry: Evaluates fetal size, and risk of macrosomia and shoulder dystocia.
Amniocentesis for lecithin to sphingomyelin (L/S) Ratio and Saturated Phosphatidyl Choline (SPC): Determines fetal lung maturity. SPG levels are better predictors of lung maturity than L/S ratio.

NURSING PRIORITIES

1. Monitor client/fetal status and progress of labor.
2. Maintain normoglycemia (euglycemia).
3. Provide emotional support to the client/couple.
4. Promote successful delivery of an appropriate-for-gestational-age (AGA) infant.

NURSING DIAGNOSIS:	Trauma, risk for/Gas Exchange, risk for impaired fetal
Risk Factors May Include:	Inadequate maternal diabetic control, presence of macrosomia or IUGR
Possibly Evidenced By:	[Not applicable; presence of signs/symptoms establishes an *actual* diagnosis]
DESIRED OUTCOMES/EVALUATION CRITERIA—NEONATE WILL:	Be full-term, AGA, free of injury.
	Display normal levels of serum glucose, free of signs of hypoglycemia.

ACTIONS/INTERVENTIONS	RATIONALE

Independent

Review prenatal course and maternal diabetic control.	Maternal hyperglycemia in the prenatal period promotes macrosomia, placing the fetus at risk for birth injury caused by shoulder dystocia or CPD. If the client has severe vascular involvement associated with diabetes (class C to F), the fetus often suffers IUGR and is at risk for hypoxia during the stress of labor, owing to uteroplacental ischemia. In addition, a high maternal glucose level at delivery stimulates the fetal pancreas, resulting in hyperinsulinemia, which can result in potentially severe neonatal hypoglycemia when the fetus is delivered and removed from the hyperglycemic environment.
Check maternal urine at each voiding for glucose/ketones, and albumin. Monitor blood pressure. (Refer to CP: Pregnancy-Induced Hypertension.)	Elevated glucose and ketone levels indicate maternal ketoacidosis, which can result in fetal acidosis and potential CNS injury. Elevated ketone levels alone suggest malnutrition/starvation affecting fetal growth. Elevated protein levels may indicate maternal vascular changes associated with PIH (occurs in 12%–13% of pregnant diabetics), which may reduce oxygen transfer to the fetus.
Monitor temperature as indicated. Note character of vaginal discharge.	There is increased risk of ascending infection in diabetic clients, which may result in neonatal sepsis.
Encourage lateral recumbent position for client during labor.	Promotes placental perfusion and increases oxygen available for fetal uptake.
Perform or assist with vaginal examination to determine progress of labor.	Prolonged labor may increase risk of fetal distress. Also with prolonged labor, diabetic control may deteriorate, resulting in negative effects on the fetus. In addition, a slowing of fetal descent and prolonged stage II may suggest macrosomia of fetus requiring additional assessment/intervention.

Collaborative

Review results of prenatal tests, such as biophysical profile (BPP), NST, CST, and estimation of fetal size.	Provides information about placental reserve for fetal oxygenation during intrapartal period, and identifies potential LGA/macrosomic fetus with risk of CPD/shoulder dystocia.
Obtain or review results from amniocentesis and ultrasonography.	Provides information about fetal lung maturity; helps predict intensity of medical support needed in delivery room. Because fetal hyperinsulinemia

interferes with surfactant production, the L/S ratio is not a good predictor of fetal maturity in the diabetic client; the presence of SPG is considered a reliable indicator.

Actions/Interventions	Rationale
Monitor maternal serum glucose level via fingerstick per protocol.	Levels vary during labor, owing to increased energy needs, depletion of glycogen levels, and a medically induced fasting state.
Monitor FHR with continuous fetal monitoring device, preferably with an internal electrode.	Tachycardia, bradycardia, or late decelerations with reduced variability indicate fetal hypoxia possibly related to diabetic vascular changes, which reduce uteroplacental perfusion.
Initiate IV infusion of 5% dextrose solution, as indicated.	It may be possible to maintain euglycemia without administering glucose until active labor starts. Glucose needs vary in the active phase, and some sources recommend dextrose infusion to equal 2.55 mg/kg/min. (Refer to ND: Injury, risk for maternal.)
Prepare for induction of labor using oxytocin (Pitocin) or for cesarean birth, if medically indicated as a result of complications.	Delivery is indicated when medical evidence supports belief that intrauterine environment is potentially more harmful to the fetus than the extrauterine environment, e.g., presence of hypertension, poor metabolic control. Cesarean birth may be indicated in presence of macrosomia/CPD or rapidly deteriorating fetal status. (Refer to CP: The Preterm Infant, for discussion of newborn complications.)
Assist with McRoberts maneuver, apply suprapubic pressure as appropriate.	Shoulder dystocia may occur following delivery of fetal head, especially when fetus weighs more than 4000 g, with incidence ranging from 13%–31%. Having client sharply flex thighs against her abdomen changes the angle of the maternal pelvis and may facilitate delivery of the anterior shoulder and decrease risk of brachial plexus stretching and clavicular fracture.
Arrange for pediatrician, neonatologist, or neonatal intensive care unit nurse to be present in delivery room, as indicated.	Helps ensure that the best-qualified professionals are available for assisting with or carrying out any necessary emergency measures.

NURSING DIAGNOSIS:	**Injury, risk for maternal**
Risk Factors May Include:	Inadequate diabetic control (hypertension, severe edema, ketoacidosis, uterine atony/overdistension and dystocia)
Possibly Evidenced By:	[Not applicable; presence of signs/symptoms establishes an *actual* diagnosis]
DESIRED OUTCOMES/EVALUATION CRITERIA—CLIENT WILL:	Maintain serum glucose levels below 100 mg/dL.
	Display stable vital signs.
	Be free of injury/complications.

ACTIONS/INTERVENTIONS

RATIONALE

Independent

Note time/content of last meal; amount/type/time of last dose of insulin. Ascertain recent serum	Useful in predicting client's needs. As client progresses into active labor, her metabolism

glucose levels and any fluctuations. Observe for signs and symptoms of hypoglycemia.

Check urine at each voiding for glucose, ketones, and protein.

Monitor vital signs every hour during induction. Monitor BP every 15 min.

Assess quality, duration, and frequency of contractions.

Evaluate skin turgor, pulse and temperature, and condition of mucous membranes.

Note presence, quality, and consistency of bloody show. If excess bleeding is present, notify physician.

Have glucagon available at the bedside.

Collaborative

Review results of ultrasonography and pelvimetry.

Monitor serum glucose level every hour until stable, then every 2–4 hr. Use client's own glucose reflectance meter, if available.

Maintain glucose level between 60 and 100 mg/dL:

   Initiate intravenous infusion of 5% dextrose
      solutions as indicated;
   Administer subcutaneous or IV regular insulin
      infusion as appropriate;

   Double rate of infusing dextrose for subsequent
      hour if blood glucose levels fall below 60 mg/dL;
   Use Biostator Glucose Controller (Miles Laboratories),
      if available.

Prepare for induction of labor by administration of oxytocin (Pitocin), or cesarean birth, if indicated. (Refer to CPs: Labor Induced/Augmented; Cesarean Birth.)

increases, making her more prone to a hypoglycemic episode.

Elevated ketone levels alone indicate a state of starvation. Elevated glucose and ketones reflect ketoacidosis. Elevated protein levels accompanied by edema and elevated BP suggest PIH.

Clients with diabetes mellitus are at risk for developing PIH. Pitocin increases sodium/water reabsorption from the kidney tubules, possibly elevating BP readings.

Dystocia may occur as a result of CPD related to macrosomia.

If serum glucose is initially elevated, dehydration may occur as a result of osmotic diuresis (glycosuria) and restriction of oral intake.

Clients with diabetes are prone to hemorrhage, owing to abruptio placentae or overdistension of the uterus resulting from polyhydramnios or macrosomia.

If serum glucose falls rapidly below 60 mg/dL, administration of glucagon may be necessary to trigger conversion of glycogen to glucose.

Macrosomic infant may cause prolonged labor and necessitate operative vaginal or cesarean birth.

Levels vary during labor, owing to increased energy needs, depletion of glycogen levels, and medically induced state of fasting. Self-monitoring promotes involvement/sense of control, is more economical and faster than laboratory testing.

Intrapartal glucose levels play a crucial role in outcome of pregnancy.

IV infusion prevents dehydration and maintains serum glucose, avoiding depletion of glycogen stores. Labor increases sensitivity to insulin, often reducing insulin requirements. Therefore, low doses (up to 2.0 units/hr) are usually sufficient to maintain normoglycemia. Additional insulin may not be required during stage II labor and immediately after delivery; IV infusion of insulin is discontinued at the end of stage III labor. Note: Long-acting insulin, if part of client's normal regimen, is discontinued at onset of labor/day before planned induction. Provides glucose to counteract hypoglycemia.

This is a closed-loop system that delivers insulin or dextrose, depending on the individual's needs, and eliminates need for repeated serum glucose sampling.

May be necessary to ensure maternal and newborn well-being.

Obtain CBC, blood type, and cross-match, if surgical procedure is planned.

Ensures availability of blood products in the event that replacement is needed as a result of hemorrhage.

Avoid use of solutions that contain glucose to expand the maternal plasma volume prior to regional block anesthesia or if cesarean birth is indicated.

Solutions containing glucose rapidly elevate serum glucose levels beyond normoglycemia.

NURSING DIAGNOSIS:	Anxiety [specify level]
May Be Related To:	Situational "crisis"/threat to health status (maternal or fetal)
Possibly Evidenced By:	Increased tension, apprehension, fear of unspecific consequences, sympathetic stimulation
DESIRED OUTCOMES/EVALUATION CRITERIA—CLIENT/COUPLE WILL:	Verbalize awareness of feelings concerning diabetes and labor. Use appropriate coping strategies.

ACTIONS/INTERVENTIONS

RATIONALE

Independent

Arrange for continued presence of primary nurse or other support person (e.g., doula) during labor. Position call light for easy access if primary nurse out of the room, and inform them summons will be answered promptly. Notify couple of substitute personnel and introduce them.

Enhances continuity of care. Client/couple needs to know they are not alone and that immediate help is available, especially who will respond in absence of primary nurse.

Ascertain present response to labor and to medical management; assess effectiveness of support systems.

Provides baseline assessment for future comparisons; identifies strengths to use and potential problems.

Involve couple in activities as much as possible. Encourage use of relaxation and breathing techniques.

Provides a feeling of control over situation.

Explain all procedures; reinforce information from other healthcare providers.

Knowledge of what is occurring helps to decrease fears.

Encourage questions and verbalization of concerns.

An open and encouraging atmosphere decreases intimidation by procedures or equipment, allowing concerns to be expressed and dealt with.

Keep couple informed concerning progress of labor. Be positive, providing accurate information.

Information on labor progress, given in a straightforward, open manner, can be helpful in diminishing concerns about the unknown. Provides reinforcement for efforts.

Keep couple informed of fetal status.

Helps to alleviate/minimize concerns and fosters trust.

CHAPTER 6

POSTPARTAL CONCEPTS

Postpartal Assessment Tool (Continuation of Intrapartal Assessment Tool)

ACTIVITY/REST

Subjective

Activity/sleep prior to onset of labor: _____
Length of labor: _____
Energy level: _____

Objective

Mental status (e.g., euphoric, withdrawn, lethargic): _____

CIRCULATION

Objective

(BP): _____ Pulse: _____
Extremities: Temperature: _____
    Color: _____ Homans' sign: _____
Blood loss during delivery: _____

EGO INTEGRITY

Subjective

Reality of labor/delivery experience
    compared with expectations of self: _____
    Support person: _____
    Primary nurse: _____
    Physician/midwife: _____

Objective

Emotional reaction: _____

ELIMINATION

Subjective

Time of last void: _____
Last bowel movement: _____

Objective

Presence of hemorrhoids: _____
Bladder palpable: _____
Presence of catheter: _____
    Color of urine: _____
Bowel sounds: _____

FOOD/FLUID

Subjective

Recent oral intake: _____
Specific requests: _____
Nausea/vomiting: _____

Objective

Skin turgor: _____
Edema: Legs: _____ Sacrum: _____
    Hands: _____ Face: _____
Appearance of tongue: _____
    Mucous membranes: _____

NEUROSENSORY

Subjective

Sensation of lower extremities: _____

Objective

Movement of lower extremities: _____
Deep tendon reflexes: _____

PAIN/DISCOMFORT

Subjective

Location: _____ Intensity: _____
Frequency: _____ Quality: _____
Duration: _____ Radiation: _____
Precipitating factors: _____

Objective

Facial expression: _____
Body movement: _____

SAFETY

Subjective

Time of ROM: _____
Intrapartal obstetric problems/treatment:
  PIH: _____ Hemorrhage: _____
Blood transfusion: _____

Objective

Temperature: _____
Condition of perineum: _____
Surgical repair: Episiotomy: _____
  Lacerations: _____

SEXUALITY

Subjective

Expression of feelings: _____

Objective

Fundus: Position: _____ Firm: _____
  Boggy: _____
Lochia: Color: _____ Flow: _____
  Presence of clots: _____
Breasts: Soft: _____ Firm: _____
  Presence of colostrum: _____

SOCIAL INTERACTIONS

Subjective

Perceptions regarding neonate: _____

Objective

Family interaction: _____
Presence of attachment behaviors (specify): _____

TEACHING/LEARNING

Subjective

Choice of infant feeding: _____
Response to initial feeding interaction: _____
Infant care class: _____

Discharge Considerations

(As noted in intrapartal history.)

STAGE IV (FIRST 4 HOURS FOLLOWING DELIVERY OF THE PLACENTA)

CLIENT ASSESSMENT DATA BASE

Activity/Rest

May appear "energized" or fatigued/exhausted, sleepy

Circulation

Pulse usually slow (50–70 beats per minute [bpm], owing to vagal hypersensitivity).
Blood pressure (BP) variable; may be lower in response to analgesia/anesthesia, or elevated in response to oxytocin administration or pregnancy-induced hypertension (PIH).
Edema, if present, may be dependent (e.g., confined to lower extremities); or may include upper extremities and facies, or may be generalized (signs of PIH).
Blood loss during labor and delivery up to 400–500 ml for vaginal delivery or 600–800 ml for cesarean birth.

Ego Integrity

Emotional reactions regarding birth experience varied and changeable, e.g., excitation, disinterest (exhausted), or disappointment
May express concern or apologize for intrapartal behavior or loss of control; may express fears regarding condition of newborn and immediate neonatal care

Elimination

Hemorrhoids often present and protruding.
Bladder may be palpable over symphysis pubis, or urinary catheter may be in place.
Diuresis may occur if pressure of presenting part obstructs urinary flow, and/or intravenous (IV) fluids are administered during labor and delivery.

Flood/Fluid

May report thirst, hunger, or nausea

Neurosensory

Sensation and movement of lower extremities decreased in presence of spinal anesthesia or caudal/epidural analgesia.
Hyperreflexia may be present (suggests developing or persistent hypertension, especially in diabetic, adolescent, or primiparous client).

Pain/Discomfort

May report discomfort from various sources; e.g., afterpains, tissue trauma/episiotomy repair, bladder fullness, or feeling cold/muscle tremors with "chills"

Safety

Slight temperature elevation initially (exertion, dehydration).
Episiotomy/laceration repair intact, with tissue edges closely approximated.
Perineum free of redness, edema, ecchymosis, or discharge.
Striae may be present on abdomen, thighs, and breasts.

Sexuality

Fundus firmly contracted, midline, and located at the level of the umbilicus
Moderate amount of vaginal drainage or lochia, dark red, with only a few small clots at most (up to small plum size)
Breasts soft, with nipples erect

Social Interaction

Varied response to infant based on individual expectations, energy level, response of others, and condition of infant

Teaching/Learning

Various medications may have been administered during intrapartal period (note time and amount).
Questions or concerns voiced regarding self/infant care.

DIAGNOSTIC STUDIES

Hemoglobin/Hematocrit (Hb/Hct), Complete Blood Count (CBC), Urinalysis (UA), Other Studies: May be done as indicated by physical findings.

NURSING PRIORITIES

1. Promote family unity and bonding.
2. Prevent or control bleeding.
3. Enhance comfort.

DISCHARGE CRITERIA (FROM RECOVERY SETTING)

1. Physiologically stable
2. Ambulating/appropriate movement of lower extremities

NURSING DIAGNOSIS:	FAMILY PROCESSES, altered (bonding process)
May Be Related To:	Developmental transition/gain of a family member
Possibly Evidenced By:	Hesitance to hold/interact with infant, verbalization of concerns
DESIRED OUTCOMES/EVALUATION CRITERIA—CLIENT/COUPLE WILL:	Hold infant, as maternal and neonatal conditions permit.
	Demonstrate culturally appropriate attachment and bonding behaviors.

ACTIONS/INTERVENTIONS	RATIONALE

Independent

Encourage client to hold, touch, and examine the infant, preferably touching skin to skin.	The first hours after delivery offer a unique opportunity for family bonding to occur, because both mother and infant are emotionally receptive to cues from each other, which initiates the attachment and acquaintance. Close physical contact soon after birth facilitates the bonding process and capitalizes on infant's receptivity during the first period of reactivity, which coincides with a maternal period of heightened awareness ("ecstasy") in the 1st hour postpartum. Note: Even if the client has chosen to relinquish her child, interacting with the newborn may facilitate the grieving process.
Encourage father to touch and hold infant and assist with infant care, as allowed by the situation.	Helps facilitate bonding/attachment between father and infant. Fathers who actively participate in

Observe and record family-infant interactions, noting behaviors thought to indicate bonding and attachment within specific culture.

the birth process and early infant interactional activities commonly report feeling a special bond with the infant.

Eye-to-eye contact, use of en face position, talking in a high-pitched voice, and holding infant closely are associated with attachment in American culture. On first contact with the infant, a mother manifests a progressive pattern of behaviors whereby she initially uses fingertips to explore the infant's extremities and progresses to use of the palm before enfolding the infant with whole hand and arms.

Note verbalizations/behaviors suggesting disappointment or lack of interest/attachment.

The arrival of a new family member, even when wanted and anticipated, creates a transient period of disequilibrium, requiring incorporation of the new child into the existing family.

Welcome family and siblings during recovery period, if desired by client and if allowed by maternal/neonatal condition and setting.

Promotes family unit, and helps siblings to begin process of positive adaptation to new roles and incorporation of new member into family structure.

Ensure family privacy between examinations during initial interaction with the newborn, as conditions of mother and infant permit.

Client, father, siblings, and infant need time to become acquainted with one another.

Encourage and assist with breastfeeding, dependent on client's choice and cultural beliefs/practices.

Early contact has a positive effect on duration of breastfeedings; skin-to-skin contact and initiation of maternal tasks promotes bonding. Some cultures (e.g., Hispanic, Navajo, Filipino, Vietnamese) may refrain from breastfeeding until the milk flow is established.

Answer client's questions regarding protocol of care during postdelivery period.

Information relieves anxiety that may interfere with bonding or result in self-absorption rather than in attention to newborn.

Collaborative

Notify appropriate healthcare team members (e.g., nursery staff or postpartal nurse) of observations, as indicated.

Inadequate bonding behaviors or poor interaction between client/couple and infant necessitates support and further evaluation. (Refer to CP: The Client at 4 Hours to 3 Days Postpartum; NDs: Parenting, risk for altered; Family Coping: potential for growth.)

NURSING DIAGNOSIS:	**FLUID VOLUME, risk for deficit**
Risk Factors May Include:	Myometrial fatigue/failure of homeostatic mechanisms (e.g., continued uteroplacental circulation, incomplete vasoconstriction, inadequate fluid shifts, effects of PIH)
Possibly Evidenced By:	[Not applicable; presence of signs/symptoms establishes an actual diagnosis]
DESIRED OUTCOMES EVALUATION CRITERIA—CLIENT WILL:	Display stable vital signs within normal limits.
	Demonstrate uterus firmly contracted at the umbilicus, lochial flow moderate and free of clots.
	Display episiotomy repair or cesarean incision approximated and surgical dressing dry and intact.

ACTIONS/INTERVENTIONS	RATIONALE

Independent

Place client in recumbent position.	Optimizes cerebral blood flow, and facilitates monitoring of fundus and vaginal flow.
Assess contributing intrapartal events, especially induced/augmented labor or prolonged labor.	In many cases, oxytocin-stimulated labor requires increased amounts of oxytocin in the postpartal period to maintain myometrial contractility. Prolonged labor results in myometrial fatigue, increasing risk of uterine atony.
Note type of delivery and anesthesia, blood loss at delivery, and length of stage III labor.	Excess uterine manipulation, operative delivery, anesthesia, or problems with placental separation may contribute to blood loss and myometrial fatigue. The postdelivery client may incur loss of as much as 300–400 ml of blood during a vaginal birth, and twice that amount in a cesarean birth, with no negative effects. Blood loss during delivery is quickly replaced by mobilization of extravascular fluid (physiological edema), so that total blood volume changes are minimal unless losses exceed normal fluid shifts.
Palpate location and consistency of the fundus every 15 min (advance per protocol/client's condition), and record findings.	Uterine myometrial activity contributes to hemostasis by compressing the endometrial blood vessels. The fundus should be firm and located at the umbilicus. Displacement may indicate a full bladder, retained blood clots, or uterine relaxation.
Gently massage fundus if it is soft (boggy). Hold or support uterus with one hand just above the symphysis pubis while massaging the fundus with the other hand. Use a firm, steady, downward pressure on the fundus. Record results of intervention.	Fundal massage stimulates uterine contractions and controls bleeding. Overstimulation can cause uterine relaxation owing to muscle exhaustion. Downward pressure enhances expulsion of clots that may have interfered with uterine contractility.
Place infant at client's breast if client has chosen to breastfeed, respecting cultural beliefs.	Infant suckling stimulates posterior pituitary release of oxytocin, which promotes myometrial contractility. Some clients may choose to postpone breastfeeding until milk production begins.
Assess for bladder fullness above symphysis pubis. Notify physician if distension is noted and client is unable to void. (Refer to CP: The Client at 4 Hours to 2 Days Postpartum; ND: Urinary Elimination, altered.)	A full bladder displaces the fundus and interferes with uterine contractility.
Assess amount (using a predetermined scale), color, and nature of lochial flow every 15 min (advance per protocol and client's condition).	Helps identify potential lacerations of vagina and cervix, which could result in excessive, bright red flow. (Saturation of a perineal pad in a 15-min period is considered excessive flow and requires prompt evaluation.) Uterine atony increases lochial flow.
Assess BP and pulse every 15 min.	As fluid shifts occur and blood is redistributed into the venous bed, a moderate drop in the systolic and diastolic BP and mild tachycardia may be noted. More marked changes may occur in response to anesthesia, magnesium sulfate ($MgSO_4$), or shock, or may be elevated in response to oxytocin or PIH. Bradycardia may occur normally in response to increased cardiac output and increased stroke volume, and vagal hypersensitivity following delivery. Sustained tachycardia may accompany shock.

Examine perineum every 15 min per protocol, noting condition of episiotomy/laceration repair, excess edema, ecchymosis, or intense internal pressure.

Excess edema may cause loss of approximation of wound edges. Ecchymosis, excess perineal edema,signs or symptoms of shock in presence of well-contracted uterus, and no visible vaginal blood loss may indicate hematoma formation. Note: Continuous trickle of blood in presence of firm fundus may reflect missed lacerations of the vagina/cervix or unligated vessel in episiotomy.

Notify physician or healthcare provider if blood loss is excessive and/or vital signs are unstable. Prepare for transfer to acute-care facility if client is in a home setting, or free-standing birth center as indicated.

Medical intervention may be needed to identify or treat underlying problems. Although freestanding birth center can provide basic care if problem is severe, more advanced care may be required.

Collaborative

Review initial Hb and Hct levels. Obtain stat levels as indicated. (Refer to CP: Postpartal Hemorrhage; ND: Tissue Perfusion, altered.)

Aids in estimating amount of blood loss. Pregnancy-induced hypervolemia acts as a safeguard against hemorrhage. Client with lower-than-normal Hb (10 mg or less) or Hct (30% or less) is less able to tolerate blood loss. Usually, as much as 10% of total blood volume can be lost with no negative effects.

Start/maintain IV infusion of isotonic solution or insert saline lock, as indicated.

Increases blood volume and provides open vein for administration of emergency medication, if needed.

Administer oxytocin or ergot preparation. Increase rate of IV oxytocin infusion per protocol if uterine bleeding persists.

Stimulates contractility of myometrium, closing off exposed blood vessels at former placental site, and reduces blood loss.

Obtain platelet count, levels of fibrinogen and fibrin split products, prothrombin time (PT), and activated partial thromboplastin time (APTT).

Alterations may suggest developing coagulation disorders.

Replace fluid losses with plasma, packed cells, or whole blood as indicated.

Replacement of fluid losses may be needed to increase circulating volume and prevent shock.

Assist in preparation, as necessary, for further treatment such as dilation and curettage (D&C), laparotomy, evacuation of hematoma, repair of birth canal lacerations, or hysterectomy.

If bleeding does not respond to conservative measures/oxytocin administration, surgery may be indicated.

NURSING DIAGNOSIS:	PAIN [acute]
May Be Related To:	Effects of hormones/medications, mechanical trauma/tissue edema, physical and psychological exhaustion, anxiety
Possibly Evidenced By:	Reports of cramping (afterpains), muscle tremors, guarding/distraction behaviors, facial mask of pain
DESIRED OUTCOMES/EVALUATION CRITERIA—CLIENT WILL:	Verbalize reduction of level of discomfort/pain.
	Display relaxed posture and facial expression.

ACTIONS/INTERVENTIONS	RATIONALE
Independent	
Assess nature and degree of discomfort, type of delivery, nature of intrapartal events, length of labor, and anesthesia or analgesia administered.	Helps identify factors that intensify discomfort/pain.
Congratulate the client/couple on birth of newborn. Provide opportunity for talking about childbirth experience.	Promotes a sense of accomplishment, positive self-esteem, and emotional well-being. Helps relieve tension. Allows client/couple opportunity to work through and accept intrapartal events.
Provide appropriate information about routine care during postpartal period.	Information may lessen anxiety associated with fear of the unknown, which could intensify perception of pain.
Inspect episiotomy/laceration repair. Evaluate approximation of wound repair; note presence of edema or hemorrhoids. Apply ice pack.	Trauma and edema increase degree of discomfort and may cause stress on suture line. Ice provides local anesthesia, promotes vasoconstriction, and reduces edema formation.
Assess for leg or body tremors or uncontrollable shaking. Place warm blankets on client.	Postdelivery tremors (chills) may be due to sudden release of pressure on pelvic nerves or may possibly be related to fetus-to-mother transfusion occurring with placental separation. Warm blankets may promote muscle relaxation and a feeling of well-being.
Institute comfort measures (e.g., mouth care, partial bath; clean, dry linen; periodic perineal care).	Promotes comfort, feeling of cleanliness, and well-being. Higher-level psychological needs can be met only after basic physical needs are satisfied.
Offer clear fluids, as appropriate.	Relieves thirst associated with fluid losses in delivery, side effects of anesthesia, and breathing through mouth.
Assess for bladder fullness by palpating above symphysis pubis. Determine time of last voiding; note prenatal fluid retention.	Intrapartal bedrest, postdelivery mobilization of fluids, and IV fluid support may result in diuresis and discomfort associated with a full bladder.
Massage uterus gently as indicated. Note presence of factors that intensify the severity and frequency of afterpains.	Gentle massage promotes contractility but should not cause excessive discomfort. Multiparity, uterine overdistension, oxytocin stimulation, and breastfeeding increase degree of afterpains associated with myometrial contractions.
Encourage use of breathing/relaxation techniques.	Enhances sense of control and may reduce severity of discomfort associated with afterpains (contractions) and fundal massage.
Position or reposition client as needed. Assess for combined effects of anesthesia.	Sensation and movement of lower extremities may still be affected by subarachnoid or peridural block, which interferes with client's ability to assume a comfortable position.
Provide quiet environment; encourage rest between assessments.	Labor and delivery are exhausting processes. Although client may be "too excited to sleep," quiet and rest may prevent undue fatigue.
Collaborative	
Administer analgesic as needed.	Analgesics act on higher brain centers to reduce perception of pain, promoting relaxation, facilitating rest and sense of well-being.

THE CLIENT AT 4 HOURS TO 2 DAYS POSTPARTUM

CLIENT ASSESSMENT DATA BASE

Progressive continuation of data base for stage IV.

Activity/Rest

Extreme fatigue and decreased energy level may be noted.
Insomnia may be noted.

Circulation

Diaphoretic episodes occur more often during night.

Ego Integrity

Irritability, tearful/crying ("postpartum blues" often noted about day 3 following delivery)

Elimination

Diuresis between day 2 and 5.
Constipation may occur.

Food/Fluid

Loss of appetite may be reported at about day 3.

Pain/Discomfort

Perineal soreness from stretching, and sutures if episiotomy performed/laceration occurred
Uterine contractions strong and regular in first 24-hr period, diminishing daily in frequency and
    intensity

Safety

Headache may be reported (subarachnoid/spinal block).

Sexuality

Uterus between one finger breadth above to two finger breadths below umbilicus at 12 hr
    following delivery, descending approximately one finger breadth daily thereafter
Lochia rubra continues for 2–3 days, progressing to lochia serosa with flow dependent on
    position (e.g., recumbent versus up and ambulating) and activity (e.g., breastfeeding or
    exercise).
Breasts: Production of colostrum first 48 hr progressing to mature milk, usually by day 3; may
    be earlier, depending on when breastfeeding is begun and how frequently mother nurses
    infant

NURSING PRIORITIES

1. Promote comfort and general well-being.
2. Prevent complications.
3. Support family bonding.
4. Provide information and anticipatory guidance.

DISCHARGE GOALS

1. Physiological/psychological needs being met
2. Complications prevented/resolving
3. Family bonding initiated
4. Postpartal needs understood

NURSING DIAGNOSIS:	PAIN [acute]/[DISCOMFORT]
May Be Related To:	Mechanical trauma, tissue edema/engorgement or distension, hormonal effects
Possibly Evidenced By:	Reports of cramping (afterpains), headache, perineal discomfort, and breast tenderness; guarding/distraction behaviors, facial mask of pain
DESIRED OUTCOMES/EVALUATION CRITERIA—CLIENT WILL:	Identify and use appropriate interventions to manage discomfort. Verbalize lessening of levels of discomfort.

ACTIONS/INTERVENTIONS	RATIONALE
Independent	
Determine presence, location, and nature of discomfort. Review labor and delivery record.	Identifies specific needs and appropriate interventions.
Inspect perineum and episiotomy repair. Note edema, ecchymosis, localized tenderness, purulent exudate, or loss of approximation of suture line. (Refer to ND: Infection, risk for.)	May reflect excess trauma to perineal tissue and/or developing complications requiring further evaluation/intervention.
Apply ice pack to perineum, especially during the first 24 hr following delivery.	Provides localized anesthesia, promotes vasoconstriction, and reduces edema and vasodilation.
Encourage use of moist heat (e.g., sitz/tub bath) between 100°F and 105°F (38.0°C–43.2°C) for 20 min, 3–4 times daily, after the first 24 hr.	Increases circulation to perineum, enhances oxygenation and nutrition of tissues, reduces edema, and promotes healing.
Recommend sitting with gluteal muscles contracted over episiotomy repair.	Use of gluteal tightening while sitting reduces stress and direct pressure on perineum.
Inspect perineum for hemorrhoids. Suggest application of ice for 20 min every 4 hr, use of witch hazel compresses, and elevation of pelvis on pillow. (Refer to ND: Constipation, risk for.)	Aids in regression of hemorrhoids and vulvar varicosities by promoting localized vasoconstriction; reduces discomfort and itching, enhancing return to normal bowel function.
Assess uterine tenderness; determine presence and frequency/intensity of afterpains. Note contributing factors.	During the first 12 hr postpartum, uterine contractions are strong and regular, and they continue for the next 2–3 days, although their frequency and intensity are reduced. Factors intensifying afterpains include multiparity, uterine overdistension, breastfeeding, and administration of oxytocin/ergot preparations.
Suggest client lie prone with pillow under abdomen. Encourage use of visualization techniques or diversional activities.	Promotes comfort, enhances sense of control, and refocuses attention.
Inspect breast and nipple tissue; assess for presence of engorgement and/or cracked nipples.	At 24 hr postpartum, breasts should be soft and nontender, and nipples should be free of cracks or reddened areas. Breast engorgement, nipple tenderness, or presence of cracks on nipple (if client is lactating) may occur at 2 or 3 days postpartum. Note: Presence of flat or inverted nipples may prevent infant from "latching on," resulting in engorgement/nipple soreness.

Encourage wearing of supportive bra.

Provide information regarding increasing the frequency of feedings, applying heat to breasts before feedings, positioning the infant properly, and expressing milk manually.

Suggest client initiate feedings on nontender nipple for several feedings in succession if only one nipple is sore or cracked.

Apply ice to axillary area of breasts if the client is not planning to breastfeed. Provide tight compression with binder for 72 hr or use of well-fitting supportive bra. Avoid excess exposure of breasts to heat or stimulation of breasts by infant, sexual partner, or client until suppression process is completed (approximately 1 wk).

Assess client for bladder fullness; implement measures to facilitate voiding. Instruct client in use of Kegel exercise after anesthesia wears off. (Refer to ND: Urinary Elimination, risk for altered.)

Evaluate for headache, especially following subarachnoid anesthesia. Avoid medicating client before nature and cause of headache are determined. Note character of headache (e.g., deep location behind the eyes, with pain radiating to both temples and occipital area; relieved in supine position but increased in sitting or standing position) to distinguish from headache associated with anxiety or PIH. Encourage bedrest, increase oral fluids, and notify healthcare provider or anesthesiologist, as indicated.

Collaborative

Administer mild analgesic 30–60 min prior to breastfeeding. For nonlactating client, administer analgesics every 3–4 hr for breast engorgement and afterpains.

Provide anesthetic sprays, topical ointments, and witch hazel compresses for perineum, as appropriate.

Assist as needed with saline injection or administration of "blood patch" over site of dural puncture. Keep client in horizontal position following the procedure.

Lifts breasts inward and upward, creating a more comfortable position.

These measures can help the lactating client stimulate the flow of milk and relieve stasis and engorgement. (Refer to ND: Breastfeeding [specify].)

Initial suckling response is strong and may be painful. Starting feeding with unaffected breast and then proceeding to involved breast may be less painful and may enhance healing.

Binding and ice prevent lactation by mechanical means and are the preferred method for suppression of lactation. Discomfort lasts approximately 48–72 hr but eases or ceases with avoidance of nipple stimulation.

Return of normal bladder function may take 4–7 days, and overdistension of bladder may create feelings of urgency and discomfort. Kegel exercise aids in healing and recovery of tone of pubococcygeal muscle to limit/prevent urinary stress incontinence.

Leakage of cerebrospinal fluid (CSF) through the dura in the extradural space reduces volume needed to support brain tissue, causing the brain stem to fall onto the base of the skull when client is in an upright position, resulting in a headache on about the 2nd postpartal day. Fluids help stimulate production of CSF. PIH may result in cerebral edema, necessitating other interventions. (Refer to ND: Fluid Volume, risk for excess.)

Provides comfort, especially during lactation, when afterpains are most intense owing to the release of oxytocin. When client is free of discomfort, she can focus on care of herself and her infant, and on mastering mothering tasks.

Promotes localized comfort.

Effective for relief of severe spinal headache. The blood patch procedure has a 90%–100% success rate; creates a blood clot that produces pressure and seals the leak. Note: Postspinal headache may last several days to a week.

NURSING DIAGNOSIS:	BREASTFEEDING [specify] (depends on whether mother-infant dyad exhibits satisfaction or dissatisfaction with breastfeeding experience)
May Be Related To:	Level of knowledge, previous experiences, infant gestational age, level of support, physical structure/characteristics of the maternal breasts
Possibly Evidenced By:	Maternal verbalization regarding level of satisfaction, observations of breastfeeding process, infant response/weight gain
DESIRED OUTCOMES/EVALUATION CRITERIA—CLIENT WILL:	Verbalize understanding of breastfeeding process/situation.
	Demonstrate effective techniques for breastfeeding.
	Display mutually satisfactory breastfeeding regimen, with infant content after feedings.

ACTIONS/INTERVENTIONS	RATIONALE

Independent

Assess client's knowledge and previous experience with breastfeeding.	Helps in identifying current needs and developing plan of care.
Determine support systems available to client, and attitude of partner/family. Note cultural expectations.	Having sufficient support enhances opportunity for a successful breastfeeding experience. Negative attitudes and comments interfere with efforts and may cause client to abandon attempt to breastfeed. Some cultures may require client to postpone initiation of breastfeeding until milk comes in.
Provide information, verbal and written, regarding physiology and benefits of breastfeeding, nipple and breast care, special dietary needs, factors that facilitate or interfere with successful breastfeeding, use of breast pump/appropriate suppliers.	Helps ensure adequate milk supply, prevents nipple cracking and soreness, facilitates comfort, and establishes role of breastfeeding mother. Benefits include providing comfort for infant, stimulation of hormones to contract uterus after birth, decrease risk of hemorrhage, and facilitate client's return to pregravid weight. Pamphlets and books provide resources that client can refer to as needed.
Demonstrate and review breastfeeding techniques, including latching on and removal from breast. Note positioning of infant during feeding and length of feedings.	Proper positioning usually prevents sore nipples, regardless of the length of feedings.
Assess client's nipples; recommend that client inspect nipples after each feeding.	Early identification and intervention may prevent/limit development of nipple soreness or cracking, which could impair breastfeeding process.
Encourage client to air-dry nipples for 20–30 min after feedings (after first expressing some breast milk on sore nipples) and to apply lanolin preparation after feedings, or to use heat lamp with 40-W bulb placed 18 in from breast for 20 min. Instruct client to avoid the use of soaps or the use of plastic liners inside bra pads, and to change nursing pad when wet or moist.	Exposure to air or heat helps toughen nipples, whereas soaps may cause drying. Keeping nipples in a wet medium promotes bacterial growth and skin breakdown. Note: Studies suggest that applying a small amount of breast milk to the nipple area may be useful for treating cracked nipples by keeping the area soft and pliable and allowing live antibodies in the milk to facilitate healing.

314

Instruct client to avoid use of nipple shield, unless specifically indicated.

These have been found to contribute to lactation failures. Shields prevent the infant's mouth from coming into contact with the mother's nipple, which is necessary for continued release of prolactin (promoting milk production), and can interfere with or prevent establishment of adequate milk supply. Note: Temporary use of shield may be beneficial in the presence of severe nipple cracking.

Provide special nipple breast shields (e.g., Eschmann shields) for lactating client with flat, inverted nipple. Suggest application of ice prior to feedings and exercise of nipple by rolling between thumb and forefinger and using Hoffman's technique.

Lacted cups/breast shields, exercises, and ice help make nipple more erect; Hoffman technique breaks adhesions, which cause inversion of nipple.

Collaborative

Refer client to support groups; (e.g., La Leche League International, Lact-Aid) or lactation consultant.

Provides ongoing help to promote a successful outcome.

Identify available community resources as indicated, e.g., Women, Infants, and Children (WIC) program.

WIC and other federal programs support breastfeeding through client education and enhanced nutritional intake.

NURSING DIAGNOSIS:	INJURY, risk for
Risk Factors May Include:	Biochemical, regulatory function (e.g., orthostatic hypotension, development of PIH or eclampsia); effects of anesthesia; thromboembolism; abnormal blood profile (anemia, rubella sensitivity, Rh incompatibility)
Possibly Evidenced By:	[Not applicable; presence of signs/symptoms establishes an *actual* diagnosis]
DESIRED OUTCOMES/EVALUATION CRITERIA—CLIENT WILL:	Demonstrate behaviors to reduce risk factors/protect self.
	Be free of complications.

ACTIONS/INTERVENTIONS

RATIONALE

Independent

Review Hb level and blood loss at delivery. Note signs of anemia (e.g., fatigue, dizziness, pallor).

Anemia or excessive blood loss predisposes client to syncope or fainting spells, owing to inadequate delivery of oxygen to the brain.

Encourage early ambulation and exercise except in client who has received subarachnoid anesthesia, who may remain flat for 6–8 hr, without use of pillow or raising head, as indicated by protocol and return of sensation/muscle control. (Refer to ND: Pain [acute]/[Discomfort].)

Enhances circulation and venous return of lower extremities, reducing risk of thrombus formation, which is associated with stasis. Although recumbent position after subarachnoid anesthesia is debatable, it may aid in prevention of CSF leakage and resultant headache.

Assist client with initial ambulation. Provide

Orthostatic hypotension may occur when

adequate supervision in shower or sitz bath. Leave call bell within client's reach.

changing from supine to upright position on initial ambulation, or it may result from vasodilation caused by the heat of the shower or sitz bath.

Have client sit on floor or chair with head between legs, or have her lie down in a flat position, if she feels faint. Use ammonia capsule (smelling salts).

Helps maintain or enhances circulation and delivery of oxygen to brain.

Assess client for hyperreflexia, right upper quadrant (RUQ)/epigastric pain, headache, or visual disturbances. Maintain seizure precautions, and provide quiet environment, as indicated. (Refer to ND: Fluid Volume, risk for excess; CP: Pregnancy-Induced Hypertension; ND: Injury, risk for maternal.)

Danger of eclampsia caused by PIH exists for up to 72 hr postpartum, although literature suggests that the convulsive state has occurred as late as the 5th day postpartum.

Note effects of MgSO$_4$, if administered. Assess patellar response, and monitor respiratory rate.

Absence of patellar reflex and respiratory rate below 12/min indicate toxicity and a need to reduce or discontinue drug therapy.

Inspect lower extremities for signs of thrombophlebitis (e.g., redness, warmth, pain/tenderness). Note presence or absence of Homans' sign. (Refer to CP: Postpartal Thrombophlebitis.)

Elevated fibrin split products (possibly released from placental site), reduced mobility, trauma, sepsis, and extensive activation of blood clotting following delivery predispose the client to the development of thromboembolism. Homans' sign may be present with deep venous thrombus, but may be absent with superficial phlebitis.

Apply local heat; promote bedrest with affected limb elevated.

Stimulates circulation and decreases venous pooling in lower extremities, reducing edema and promoting healing.

Evaluate rubella status on prenatal chart (less than 1:10 titer indicates susceptibility). Assess client for allergies to eggs or feathers; if present, withhold vaccine. Provide written and oral information, and obtain informed consent for vaccination after reviewing side effects, risks, and the necessity to prevent conception for 2–3 mo following the vaccination.

Helps prevent teratogenic effects in subsequent pregnancies. Administration of vaccine in the immediate postpartal period may cause side effects of transient arthralgia, rash, and cold symptoms during incubation period of 14–21 days. Allergic anaphylactic or hypersensitivity response may occur, necessitating administration of epinephrine.

Collaborative

Administer MgSO$_4$ by infusion pump, as indicated.

Helps reduce cerebral irritability in presence of PIH or eclampsia. (Refer to ND: Fluid Volume risk for excess.)

Apply support hose or elastic wrap to legs when risk or symptoms of phlebitis are present.

Reduces venous stasis, enhancing venous return.

Administer anticoagulant; evaluate coagulation factors, and note signs of failure to clot. (Refer to CP: Postpartal Thrombophlebitis.)

Although usually not required, anticoagulant may help prevent further development of thrombus.

Administer Rh$_0$(D) immune globulin (RhIgG) intramuscularly (IM), within 72 hours' postpartum, as indicated, for Rh-negative mother who has not been previously sensitized and who delivers an Rh-positive infant whose direct Coombs' test on cord blood is negative. Obtain Betke-Kleihauer smear if significant fetal-maternal transfusion is suspected at delivery.

Dose of 300 mg is usually sufficient to promote lysis of fetal Rh-positive red blood cells (RBCs) that may have entered maternal circulation during delivery, and that may potentially cause sensitization and problems of Rh incompatibility in subsequent pregnancies. Presence of 20 ml or more of Rh-positive fetal blood in maternal circulation necessitates higher dose of RhIgG. Note: If drug is not administered within 72 hr of delivery, a window of opportunity exists for up to 2 wk, although the degree of effectiveness may be reduced.

NURSING DIAGNOSIS:	INFECTION, risk for
Risk Factors May Include:	Tissue trauma and/or broken skin, decreased Hb, invasive procedures and/or increased environmental exposure, prolonged rupture of amniotic membranes, malnutrition
Possibly Evidenced By:	[Not applicable; presence of signs/symptoms establishes an *actual* diagnosis]
DESIRED OUTCOMES/EVALUATION CRITERIA—CLIENT WILL:	Demonstrate techniques to reduce risks/promote healing.
	Display wound free of purulent drainage.
	Be free of infection, be afebrile, and have normal lochial flow and character.

ACTIONS/INTERVENTIONS	RATIONALE

Independent

Assess prenatal and intrapartal records, noting frequency of vaginal examinations and complications such as premature rupture of membranes (PROM), prolonged labor, lacerations, hemorrhage, or retained placenta.	Helps identify risk factors that may impair healing and/or retard epithelial growth of endometrial tissue and predispose client to infection.
Monitor temperature and pulse routinely and as indicated; note signs of chills, anorexia, or malaise.	Elevation of temperature to 101°F (38.3°C) within the first 24 hr is highly indicative of infection; an elevation to 100.4°F (38.0°C) on any 2 of the first 10 days postpartum is also significant. Note: Research suggests epidural anesthesia during labor is associated with postpartal fever (100.4°F [40.0°C] or greater) in some clients, with rate of occurrence rising in proportion to length of labor. However, actual infection is rare.
Assess location and contractility of uterus; note involutional changes or presence of extreme uterine tenderness.	The fundus, which is initially 2 cm below the umbilicus, rises to the level of the umbilicus and involutes at the rate of 1–2 cm/day (one finger breadth per day). Failure of the myometrium to involute at this rate, or development of extreme tenderness, signals possible retained placental tissue or infection. Note: Size of the uterus is influenced by the size of the infant just delivered. (Refer to CP: Puerperal Infection.)
Note amount and odor of lochial discharge or change in normal progression from rubra to serosa.	Lochia normally has a fleshy odor; however, in endometritis, the discharge may be purulent and foul-smelling and may fail to demonstrate normal progression from rubra to serosa to alba.
Evaluate condition of nipples, noting presence of cracks, redness, or tenderness. Recommend routine examination of breasts. Review proper care and infant feeding techniques. (Refer to ND: Pain [acute]/[Discomfort].)	The development of nipple fissures/cracks potentiates risk of mastitis. Note: Use of soap is not recommended for nipple care because it is drying and increases risk of cracking.
Inspect site of episiotomy/laceration repair every 8 hr. Note excessive tenderness, redness, purulent exudate, edema, gapping at suture line (loss of approximation).	Early diagnosis of localized infection may prevent spread to uterine tissue. Note: Presence of third- to fourth-degree lacerations increases risk of infection.

317

Note frequency/amount of voidings.

Assess for signs of urinary tract infection (UTI) or cystitis (e.g., increased frequency, urgency, or dysuria, cloudy/foul-smelling urine, visible hematuria, and presence of suprapubic pain).

Encourage perineal care using perineal bottle or sitz bath 3–4 times daily or after voiding/defecation. Recommend that client shower daily and change perineal pads at least every 4 hr, applying pad from front to back.

Demonstrate and encourage use of careful handwashing technique and appropriate disposal of soiled underpads, perineal pads, and contaminated linen. Discuss with client the importance of continuing these measures after discharge.

Assess client's nutritional status. Note appearance of hair, fingernails, skin, and so forth. Review prepregnancy weight and prenatal weight gain.

Provide information about selecting foods high in protein, vitamin C, and iron. Encourage client to increase fluid intake to 2000 ml/day.

Promote sleep and rest.

Collaborative

Assess white blood cell (WBC) count.

Note Hb and Hct. Administer iron preparations and supplemental vitamins, as necessary.

Administer methylergonovine maleate (Methergine) or ergonovine maleate (Ergotrate) every 3–4 hr, as appropriate.

Assist with, or obtain cultures from, vagina, serum, and site of episiotomy repair, as indicated.

Encourage client to apply antibiotic creams to perineum, as indicated.

Obtain clean catch (midstream) urine specimen for analysis as needed.

Urinary stasis increases the risk of infection.

Symptoms of UTI may appear on days 2–3 postpartum owing to ascending tract infection from urethra to bladder and possibly to kidney.

Frequent cleaning from front to back (symphysis pubis to anal area) helps prevent rectal contaminants from entering vagina or urethra. Sitz or tub baths stimulate perineal circulation and promote healing. Note: Some cultures (e.g., African- or Arab-American) may abstain from tub/shower bath or even washing hair until after cessation of lochial flow, or possibly longer. Other cultures (e.g., Haitian) may engage in ritual baths for several days following delivery.

Helps prevent or retard spread of infection.

Client who is 20% below normal weight, or who is anemic or malnourished is more susceptible to postpartal infection and may have special dietary needs for protein, iron, and calories.

Protein helps promote healing and regeneration of new tissue and overcomes delivery losses. Iron is necessary for hemoglobin synthesis. Vitamin C facilitates iron absorption and is necessary for cell wall synthesis. Increased fluid helps prevent urinary stasis and kidney problems.

Reduces metabolic rate and allows nutrition and oxygen to be used for healing process rather than for energy needs.

An increase in WBC count the first 10–12 days postpartum normally occurs as a protective mechanism and is associated with an increase in neutrophils and a shift to the left, which may interfere initially with identification of infection.

Determines whether anemic state is present. Helps correct deficiencies.

Fosters myometrial contraction and uterine involution in nonlactating client, reducing risk of infection. Note: May be contraindicated in presence of elevated BP.

To identify causative organism, if present, and determine appropriate antibiotic.

Eradicates local infectious organisms.

Urine retention, bacteria introduced by catheterization, and/or bladder trauma during delivery combine to create an excellent environment

Administer antipyretic after cultures are obtained.

When administered before identification of infectious process, antipyretics may mask signs and symptoms necessary for a differential diagnosis.

Administer broad-spectrum antibiotic until culture/sensitivity report is returned; then alter therapy as indicated. (Note: Parenteral route via saline lock is preferred for treatment of endometritis and sepsis.)

Prevents infection from spreading to surrounding tissues or bloodstream. Choice of antibiotic depends on sensitivity of infecting organism.

Contact appropriate community agencies, such as visiting nurse/homecare services, for follow-up on diet, antibiotic course, possible complications, and return medical examination.

Any postpartal infection places the client in a debilitated state that requires more rest, closer monitoring, and assistance with home maintenance and self/infant care.

NURSING DIAGNOSIS:	URINARY ELIMINATION, altered
May Be Related To:	Hormonal effects (fluid shifts/increased renal plasma flow), mechanical trauma, tissue edema, effects of anesthesia
Possibly Evidenced By:	Increased bladder filling/distension, changes in amount/frequency of voiding
DESIRED OUTCOMES/EVALUATION CRITERIA—CLIENT WILL:	Void unassisted within 6–8 hr after delivery.
	Empty bladder with each void.

ACTIONS/INTERVENTIONS	RATIONALE

Independent

Assess current fluid intake and urine output. Note intrapartal I/O and length of labor.

In the early postpartal period, approximately 5 lb of fluid is lost through urine output and insensible losses, including diaphoresis. Prolonged labor and ineffective fluid replacement may result in dehydration and reduced urine output.

Palpate bladder. Monitor fundal height and location, and amount of lochial flow.

Renal plasma flow, which increases by 25%–50% during the prenatal period, remains elevated in the first week postpartum, resulting in increased bladder filling. Bladder distension, which can be assessed by degree of uterine displacement, causes increased uterine relaxation and lochial flow.

Note presence of edema or lacerations/episiotomy, and type of anesthesia used.

Trauma to bladder or urethra, or edema, may hinder voiding; anesthesia may interfere with sensation of fullness.

Test urine for albumin and acetone. Distinguish between proteinuria associated with PIH and that associated with normal processes. (Refer to ND: Fluid Volume, risk for excess.)

Catalytic process associated with uterine involution may result in normal proteinuria (1+) for the first 2 days postpartum. Acetone may indicate dehydration associated with prolonged labor/delivery.

Encourage voiding within 6–8 hr postpartum, and every 4 hr thereafter. If condition permits, have client walk to bathroom. Pour warm water

A variety of nursing interventions may be necessary to stimulate or facilitate voiding. A full bladder interferes with uterine motility and

319

over the perineum, run water from the faucet, add spirits of peppermint to bedpan, or have client sit in sitz bath or take a warm shower, as indicated.

involution, and increases lochial flow. Prolonged bladder overdistension can damage the bladder wall and result in atony.

Instruct client to use Kegel exercise daily after effects of anesthesia subside.

Performing Kegel exercise 100 times per day increases circulation to perineum, aids in healing and recovery of tone of pubococcygeal muscle, and prevents or reduces stress incontinence.

Encourage drinking 6–8 glasses of fluid per day.

Helps prevent stasis and dehydration, and replaces fluid lost at delivery.

Assess for signs of UTI (e.g., burning on urination, increased frequency, cloudy urine).

Stasis, poor hygiene, and introduction of bacteria may predispose client to UTI. (Refer to ND: Infection, risk for.)

Collaborative

Catheterize, using straight or indwelling catheter, as indicated.

May be necessary to reduce bladder distension, allow for uterine involution, and prevent bladder atony associated with bladder overdistension.

Obtain urine specimen, using clean catch technique or catheterization, if client has symptoms of UTI.

Presence of bacteria or positive culture and sensitivity are diagnostic for UTI.

Monitor laboratory test results, such as blood urea nitrogen (BUN) and 24-hr urine for total protein, creatinine clearance, and uric acid as indicated.

In the client who has had PIH, kidney or vascular involvement may persist, or it may appear for the first time during the postpartal period. As steroid levels decrease following delivery, renal function, reflected by BUN and creatinine clearance, begins to return to normal within 1 wk; anatomic changes (e.g., dilation of ureters and renal pelvis) may take up to 1 mo to return to normal.

NURSING DIAGNOSIS:	FLUID VOLUME, risk for deficit
Risk Factors May Include:	Reduced intake/inadequate replacement, excessive losses (vomiting, diaphoresis, increased urine output and insensible losses, hemorrhage)
Possibly Evidenced By:	[Not applicable; presence of signs/symptoms establishes an *actual* diagnosis]
DESIRED OUTCOMES/EVALUATION CRITERIA—CLIENT WILL:	Remain normotensive with fluid intake and urine output appropriately balanced, and Hb/Hct within normal levels.

ACTIONS/INTERVENTIONS	RATIONALE

(Refer to CP: Stage IV [First 4 Hours Following Delivery of Placenta].)

Independent

Note fluid losses at delivery; review intrapartal history. (Refer to CP: Postpartal Hemorrhage.)

Potential hemorrhage or excess blood loss at delivery that continues into the postpartum period may result from prolonged labor, oxytocin stimulation, retained tissue, uterine overdistension, or general anesthesia.

Evaluate location and contractility of uterine fundus, amount of vaginal lochia, and condition of perineum every 2 hr for the first 8 hr, as appropriate, then every 8 hr for the remainder of hospitalization. Note administration of medication, such as $MgSO_4$, that would cause uterine relaxation.

Differential diagnosis may be needed to determine cause of fluid deficit and protocol of care. A relaxed or boggy uterus with increased lochial flow may result from myometrial fatigue or retained placental tissue. Immediately after delivery, the fundus should be firm and located at the umbilicus, and then involute approximately one finger breadth per day.

Gently massage fundus if uterus is boggy.

Stimulates uterine contraction; may control bleeding.

Note presence of thirst; provide liquids as tolerated.

Thirst may be a homeostatic means of replacing fluid losses through increased oral intake.

Evaluate status of bladder; promote emptying if bladder is full. (Refer to ND: Urinary Elimination, altered.)

A full bladder interferes with uterine contractility and causes displacement and relaxation of fundus.

Monitor temperature, pulse, BP, as indicated.

Increased temperature may signify dehydration, or infection. (Refer to CP: Puerperal Infection.) Tachycardia may occur to maximize fluid circulation in the event of dehydration or hemorrhage, whereas elevation of BP may be due to the effects of oxytocin vasopressor drugs, or to preexisting or newly developed PIH. Falling BP may be a late sign of excess fluid loss, especially if accompanied by other signs or symptoms of shock.

Evaluate fluid intake and urine output during IV infusion, or until normal voiding patterns are re-established.

Helps in analyzing fluid balance and degree of deficit.

Monitor filling of breasts and milk supply if lactating.

The dehydrated client is unable to produce sufficient milk supply.

Collaborative

Replace fluid losses with IV infusion containing electrolytes.

Helps re-establish circulating blood volume and replace losses from delivery and diaphoresis.

Administer ergot products such as ergonovine maleate (Ergotrate) or methylergonovine maleate (Methergine) parenterally or orally, or administer IM/IV synthetic oxytocin preparations (Syntocinon, Pitocin). Assess BP before administering ergot preparations; withhold medication and notify healthcare provider if BP is elevated.

These products act directly on the myometrium to promote uterine contraction. Ergot, a vasoconstrictor, may cause hypertension and should be withheld if BP is 140/90 mm Hg or greater.

Initiate or increase rate of IV fluid such as lactated Ringer's solution with 10–20 units of oxytocin.

Oxytocin (Pitocin) may be needed to stimulate the myometrium if excess bleeding persists and if uterus fails to contract. Persistent bleeding in presence of firm fundus may indicate lacerations and the need for further investigation. (Refer to CP: Postpartal Hemorrhage.)

Review prenatal Hb/Hct levels; note blood loss at delivery. Obtain postpartal Hb/Hct as indicated.

Hb/Hct usually return to normal within 3 days. Hb should not drop more than 2 g/100 ml unless blood loss is excessive. Elevation of Hct levels occurs normally by the 3rd–7th day postpartum, owing to plasma loss in excess of blood cell decreases that occurs during the first 72 hr. However, such elevation may also indicate excess shift of intravascular fluids to extracellular spaces.

ACTIONS/INTERVENTIONS

RATIONALE

Independent

Review prenatal and intrapartal history for PIH,
noting elevated BP, proteinuria, and edema.

Helps determine likelihood of similar
complications persisting/developing in postpartal
period.

Monitor BP and pulse. Auscultate breath sounds,
noting moist cough, rales, or rhonchi. Note
presence of dyspnea or stridor.

Circulatory overload is manifested by increases in
BP and pulse, and by fluid accumulation in the
lungs. Elevated BP may also be related to PIH and
fluid retention associated with oxytocin infusion.

Monitor fluid intake and urine output; measure
urine-specific gravity.

Indicates fluid needs/adequacy of therapy.

Note dosage of oxytocin (Pitocin) when it is
administered parenterally.

Oxytocin increases sodium/water resorption from
the kidney tubules and may result in elevated BP.

Assess presence, location, and extent of edema.
Monitor for signs of progressive edema (e.g., visual
disturbances, hyperreflexia, clonus, RUQ/epigastric
pain, and headache). (Note: Assess for headache
prior to administering any analgesics.)

Danger of eclampsia or convulsive state exists for
72 hr, but can actually occur as late as 5 days after
delivery. Medication may mask signs of headache
caused by cerebral edema.

Using a dipstick, test for presence of proteinuria
every 4 hr.

Postpartal proteinuria of 1+ is normal, owing to
catalytic process of uterine involution. Levels of 2+
or greater may be associated with glomerular spasms
of PIH.

Evaluate client's neurological status. Note
hyperreflexia, irritability, or personality changes.

Cerebral intoxication is an early indicator of excess
fluid retention.

Have client monitor weight daily, especially if
postpartal toxemia is present.

At delivery, client should lose approximately
10–12 lb, attributable to infant, products of
conception, urine, and insensible losses, and 5 lb
more in the early postpartal period through fluid and
electrolyte shifts.

Collaborative

Note test results for uric acid, 24-hr protein and
creatinine clearance, and serum creatinine levels.

Abnormal results, such as increasing uric acid (> 7
mg/100 ml) and elevated creatinine levels, indicate
deterioration of renal function.

Insert indwelling catheter, as indicated.

May be needed to monitor urine output on hourly
basis if warranted by client's condition (e.g., severe
PIH or oliguria).

Evaluate for HELLP syndrome (i.e., *h*emolisis
of RBC, *e*levated *l*iver enzymes, and *l*ow *p*latelet
count).

HELLP syndrome is a potential postpartal
consequence of PIH with liver involvement or
with hemorrhage of hepatic vessels.

Administer medications as indicated, e.g.:

MgSO$_4$ per infusion pump (refer to CP: Pregnancy-Induced Hypertension; ND: Injury, risk for maternal);

Hydralazine (Apresoline) or methyldopa (Aldomet) per protocol (e.g., if diastolic readings are 110 mm Hg or greater);

Furosemide (Lasix);

Mannitol (Osmitrol).

MgSO$_4$ acts at myoneural junction and may have transient effects of lowering BP and increasing urine output.

Hydralazine relaxes peripheral arterioles and promotes vasodilation to lower BP, whereas methyldopa acts on postganglionic nerve endings, interfering with chemical neurotransmission to reduce peripheral vascular resistance.

Lasix acts on loop of Henle to increase urine output and relieve pulmonary edema.

For client with PIH, impending renal failure, or oliguria, mannitol acts as osmotic diuretic to draw fluids into vascular bed and increase renal plasma flow and urine output.

NURSING DIAGNOSIS:	CONSTIPATION
May Be Related To:	Decreased muscle tone (diastasis recti), effects of progesterone, dehydration, excess analgesia or anesthesia, prelabor diarrhea, lack of intake, perineal/rectal pain
Possibly Evidenced By:	Reported abdominal/rectal fullness or pressure, nausea, less than usual amount of stool, straining at stool, decreased bowel sounds
DESIRED OUTCOMES/EVALUATION CRITERIA—CLIENT WILL:	Resume usual/optimal bowel habits within 4 days after delivery.

ACTIONS/INTERVENTIONS	RATIONALE

Independent

Auscultate for presence of bowel sounds; palpate for diastasis recti, determine normal evacuation habits.

Evaluates bowel function, identifies deviation from client's "normal" or usual routine. Presence of severe diastasis recti (separation of the two rectus muscles along the median line of the abdominal wall) reduces abdominal muscle tone needed for efforts to bear down during evacuation.

Assess for presence of hemorrhoids. Provide information about reinserting hemorrhoid into anorectal canal with lubricated finger cot or rubber glove, and applying ice or witch hazel compresses or local anesthetic creams.

Promotes localized vasoconstriction, reducing size of hemorrhoids, relieving itching and discomfort.

Provide appropriate dietary information regarding importance of roughage, increased fluids, and the attempt to establish normal evacuation pattern.

Roughage (e.g., fruits and vegetables, especially with seeds and skins) and increased fluids provide bulk, improve consistency of stool, and stimulate elimination.

Encourage increase in activity level and ambulation, as tolerated.

Helps promote gastrointestinal peristalsis.

Assess episiotomy; note presence of laceration and degree of tissue involvement.

Excess edema or perineal trauma with third- and fourth-degree lacerations may cause discomfort and prevent client from relaxing perineum during evacuation for fear of further injury.

323

Collaborative

Administer stool softeners, suppositories, enemas, laxatives as indicated.

May be necessary to promote return to normal bowel habits and to prevent straining or perineal stress during evacuation. Note: Administration of suppositories or enemas in presence of third- or fourth-degree perineal laceration may be contraindicated because further trauma may occur. In addition, laxatives are contraindicated for the lactating client.

NURSING DIAGNOSIS:	PARENT/INFANT ATTACHMENT; PARENTING, risk for altered
Risk Factors May Include:	Lack of support between/from significant other(s), lack of knowledge, ineffective and/or no available role model, anxiety associated with the parent role, unrealistic expectations for self/infant/partner, unmet social/emotional maturation needs of client/partner, presence of stressors (e.g., financial, housing, employment)
Possibly Evidenced By:	[Not applicable; presence of signs/symptoms establishes an *actual* diagnosis]
DESIRED OUTCOMES/EVALUATION CRITERIA—CLIENT/COUPLE WILL:	Engage in mutually satisfying interactions with infant.
	Verbalize concerns and questions about parenting.
	Discuss parenting role realistically.
	Identify available resources to meet needs of family members.

ACTIONS/INTERVENTIONS	RATIONALE

Independent

Assess strengths, needs, age, marital status, available sources of support, and cultural background.	Identifies potential risk factors and sources of support, which influence the client's/couple's ability to take on the challenging role of parenthood. For example, the adolescent may still be formulating goals and an identity. She may have difficulty accepting the infant as a person and coping with full-time parenting responsibility. The single parent who lacks support systems may have difficulty assuming sole responsibility for parenting. Cultures in which the extended family members live together may provide more emotional and physical support, facilitating adoption of the new role.
Note client's/partner's response to birth and to parenting role.	Client's ability to adapt positively to parenting may be strongly influenced by the father's reaction.
Initiate primary nursing care for mother and baby as a unit.	Promotes family-centered care, continuity, and individualization of care, and may facilitate development of positive family bonds.
Evaluate nature of emotional and physical parenting that client/couple received during childhood.	Parenting role is learned, and individuals use their own parents as role models. Those who experienced a negative upbringing or poor parenting

324

Assess partners' interpersonal communication skills and their relationship to one another.

Review intrapartal record for length of labor, presence of complications, and role of partner in labor.

Evaluate past and present physical status and occurrence of prenatal, intrapartal, or postpartal complications.

Determine infant's condition; communicate with nursery staff, as indicated. Note any special problems or concerns.

Administer the Neonatal Perception Inventory (NPI), part I, within the first 2 days postpartum when indicated. Arrange for the follow-up inventory, part II, to be administered at 1 mo postpartum.

Monitor and document the client's/couple's interactions with infant. Note presence of bonding (acquaintance) behaviors, e.g.: making eye contact, using high-pitched voice and en face (face-to-face) position, calling infant by name, and holding infant closely. Determine family cultural background.

Encourage "rooming-in" or provide physical space and privacy for contact between mother, father, and infant.

Encourage couple/siblings to visit and hold the infant and to participate in infant care activities, as permitted. Provide telephone number of special care nursery if baby remains in the hospital for observation or special procedures; take pictures of the infant for the couple.

Assess client's readiness and motivation to learn.

Provide formal and informal educational opportunities followed by staff demonstration,

are at greater risk for failing to meet the challenge than those who received positive parenting.

A strong relationship characterized by honest communication and good interpersonal and listening skills fosters growth.

Long, difficult labor may temporarily deplete the physical and emotional energy necessary for learning the mothering role and may negatively affect lactation. Note: It often takes 24 hr following delivery for the mother to progress beyond her own "taking-in" phase.

Events such as preterm labor, hemorrhage, infection, or any maternal complication may influence client's psychological status, reducing her ability to learn new parenting skills and undermining her attachment to, and ability to care for, the newborn.

Mothers often undergo grief for the loss of the idealized perfect infant in contrast with their own infant. Emotional problems and the inability to adjust positively to parenting may result from the infant's temporary birth disfigurement, the birth of a high-risk infant, or the mother's inability to reconcile differences between prenatal fantasies and postnatal reality.

The NPI may be used to assess adaptive potential of mother-infant pair by evaluating the mother's perceptions of average baby versus her own. This tool is particularly helpful in assessing the mothering potential of the adolescent, who often fantasizes about the infant's behaviors and capabilities, and who may not cope positively with stressor of caring for a newborn. This inventory provides a statistically significant relationship between its indications at 1 mo and the emotional development of children at age $4\frac{1}{2}$ yr and later at age 10–11 yr.

Few mothers or fathers experience significant love at first; instead, they become acquainted with the infant gradually. Infant and parent who do not develop positive attachment are at risk for physical or emotional abuse. Cultural background often determines type of bonding and acquaintance behaviors.

Facilitates attachment behaviors; fosters acquaintance process.

Helps promote bonding and prevent feelings of helplessness. Emphasizes the reality of baby's existence.

Many factors influence individual learning (e.g., understanding of need for information, anxiety, postdelivery euphoria).

Helps parents learn the fundamentals of infant care, promotes discussion and mutual problem staff assistance, and educational videotapes on infant care, infant feeding, and parenting.

Have client demonstrate learned behaviors associated with infant feeding and care. Provide written information and telephone number of contact person for client to take home.

Initiate follow-up telephone call or home visit by primary nurse, if possible, at 1 wk, and at 4–6 wk postpartum.

Collaborative

Refer to community support groups, such as visiting-nurse/home-care services, social services, parenting groups, or adolescent clinics.

Refer to counseling if family is at high risk for parenting problems or if positive bonding between client/couple and infant is not occurring.

solving, and provides group support. Helps parents to become more comfortable and gain skills and comfort in handling and caring for infant prior to discharge.

Helps reinforce teaching program and prevent anxiety related to unanswered questions, especially if family is part of early discharge program or if delivery took place in an alternative birth setting.

Some maternity centers now include such follow-up, especially for the adolescent or for the family at high risk for parenting problems.

Helps promote positive parenting through group support and mutual problem-solving experience. Adolescents, particularly, may benefit from such support.

Negative parenting behaviors and ineffective coping may need to be corrected through counseling, nurturing, or even lengthy psychotherapy, and new behaviors and role models incorporated, to avoid repetition of parenting mistakes and child abuse.

NURSING DIAGNOSIS:	COPING, INDIVIDUAL, risk for ineffective
Risk Factors May Include:	Maturational crisis of pregnancy/childbearing and assuming the role of motherhood and parenting (or relinquishing for adoption), personal vulnerability, inadequate support systems, unrealistic perceptions
Possibly Evidenced By:	[Not applicable; presence of signs/symptoms establishes an *actual* diagnosis]
DESIRED OUTCOMES/EVALUATION CRITERIA—CLIENT WILL:	Verbalize anxieties and emotional responses.
	Identify individual strengths and own coping abilities.
	Seek appropriate resources as needed.

ACTIONS/INTERVENTIONS	RATIONALE

Independent

Observe client's emotional response during prenatal and intrapartal periods and ascertain client's perception of her performance during labor. (Refer to CP: First Trimester; ND: Role Performance, risk for altered.)

Encourage discussion by client/couple of perceptions of birth experience.

Discuss for symptoms of transitory depression (postpartal "blues"), which may occur on about

There is a direct correlation between positive acceptance of the feminine role and uniquely feminine functions on the one hand, and positive adaptation to childbirth, mothering, and lactation on the other. In addition, the client who is relinquishing her child encounters these issues in a different context and needs support for her decisions.

Assists client/couple to work through process and clarify reality from fantasized experience.

As many as 80% of mothers experience a transitory depression or a feeling of emotional let-down

3rd day postpartum (e.g., anxiety, tearfulness, despondency, poor concentration, and mild or severe depression). Provide information about the normalcy of this condition and associated mood swings and emotional lability.

following delivery, perhaps related to genetics, social or environmental factors, or physiological endocrine responses. These symptoms usually resolve spontaneously within a week or so following discharge. For some, however, initial feelings of discouragement may be replaced by excessive depression caused by a cycle of anxiety, anorexia, and excessive fatigue beginning soon after discharge.

Identify client's past coping abilities, cultural background, support systems, and plans for domestic help on discharge.

Helps in assessing client's ability to handle stress. The ability to cope positively is also influenced by father's reaction. The emotional and physical support offered by extended families or other home assistance may facilitate coping.

Provide emotional support and anticipatory guidance to help client learn new roles and strategies for coping with newborn. Discuss the normal emotional responses that occur after discharge.

Mothering/parenting skills are not instinctive but must be learned. Coping with interrupted sleep and meeting the infant's needs on a 24-hr basis may be difficult, and coping strategies must be developed.

Evaluate and document client-infant interaction. Note presence or absence of bonding (attachment) behaviors. (Refer to ND: Parenting, risk for altered.)

Mother and infant are equal participants in the attachment process, and both must receive rewarding responses during the interaction. A lack of maternal attachment or absence of maternal behaviors evident in the postpartal period can lead to serious long-term consequences.

Encourage verbalization of negative thoughts, feelings of guilt, personal failure, or doubt about individual parenting abilities, especially if family is at high risk for problems with parenting. (Refer to CP: The Parents of a Child with Special Needs.)

Helps couple to evaluate strengths and problem areas realistically and recognize the need for appropriate professional help.

Provide opportunity for client to review decision to relinquish child, when appropriate.

Following delivery, the normal emotional responses are compounded by the previous decision to have child adopted. The client may experience conflict and require nonjudgmental support to facilitate coping at this time.

Collaborative

Refer client/couple to parenting, classes/support group, social services, community groups, or visiting nurse/homecare services.

Support and role modeling enhances coping and facilitates assumption of parenting role. However, approximately 40% of women with mild postpartal depression have symptoms that persist for up to 1 yr and may require further follow-up.

NURSING DIAGNOSIS:	SLEEP PATTERN disturbance
May Be Related To:	Hormonal and psychological responses (intense exhilaration, anxiety, excitement), pain/discomfort, exhausting process of labor and delivery
Possibly Evidenced By:	Verbal reports of difficulty falling asleep/not feeling well rested, irritability, dark circles under eyes, frequent yawning
DESIRED OUTCOMES/EVALUATION CRITERIA—CLIENT WILL:	Identify adjustments to accommodate changes required by demands of new family member.
	Report increased sense of well-being and feeling rested.

ACTIONS/INTERVENTIONS	RATIONALE

Independent

Assess level of fatigue and need for rest. Note length of labor and type of delivery.

Long, difficult labor or delivery, especially when it occurs during the night, increases the level of fatigue.

Determine factors, if any, interfering with rest. Organize care to allow minimum disturbances and extra resting or sleeping periods. Encourage verbalization about birth experience. Provide quiet environment.

Helps promote rest, sleep, and relaxation. If mother does not get needed sleep, "sleep hunger" may result, prolonging the restorative processes of the postpartal period.

Provide information about needs for sleep/rest following discharge.

Creative planning to allow retiring early with the baby and napping during the day helps meet bodily needs and overcome excess fatigue.

Provide information about effects of fatigue and anxiety on milk supply.

May negatively affect psychological adjustment, milk supply, and let-down reflex.

Assess home environment, availability of assistance, and presence of siblings and other family members.

The multipara with children at home may need more sleep to overcome sleep deficits and meet her needs and the needs of her family.

Collaborative

Administer analgesics as indicated.

May be needed to promote relaxation and sleep.

NURSING DIAGNOSIS:	KNOWLEDGE deficit [LEARNING NEED], regarding self and infant care
May Be Related To:	Lack of exposure/recall, misinterpretation, unfamiliarity with resources
Possibly Evidenced By:	Verbalizations of concerns/misconceptions; hesitancy in, or inadequate performance of, activities; inappropriate behaviors (e.g., apathy)
DESIRED OUTCOMES/EVALUATION CRITERIA—CLIENT WILL:	Verbalize understanding of physiological changes, individual needs, expected outcomes.
	Perform necessary activities/procedures correctly and explain reasons for the actions.

ACTIONS/INTERVENTIONS	RATIONALE

Independent

Ascertain client's perception of labor and delivery, length of labor, and client's fatigue level.

There is a correlation between length of labor and the ability of some clients to assume responsibility for self-care/infant care tasks and activities. The longer the labor is, the more negative the client's perception tends to be of her performance in labor, and the longer it may take her to refocus and assume responsibility for her own care and to synthesize new information and learn new roles.

Assess client's readiness and motivation for learning. Assist client/couple in identifying needs.

The postpartal period can be a positive experience if opportune teaching is provided to foster maternal growth, maturation, and competence. However, the client needs time to move from a

Initiate written teaching plan using standardized format, checklist, or clinical pathway. Document information given and client's response.

Provide information about role of a progressive postpartal exercise program.

Provide information about self-care, including perineal care and hygiene; physiological changes, including normal progression of lochial discharge; needs for sleep and rest; role changes; and emotional changes. Have client demonstrate the material learned, when appropriate.

Discuss sexuality needs and plans for contraception. Provide information about available methods, including advantages and disadvantages. (Refer to CP: One Week Following Discharge; ND: Knowledge deficit [Learning Need].)

Reinforce importance of 4- to 6-wk postpartal examination by healthcare provider and interim follow-up, as appropriate.

Identify potential problems necessitating medical evaluation prior to the scheduled 4- to 6-wk visit (e.g., a return to bright red vaginal bleeding, foul-smelling lochia, elevated temperature, malaise, prolonged feelings of anxiety/depression).

Discuss normal physical and psychological changes and needs associated with the postpartal period.

Identify available resources; e.g., visiting nurse services, Public Health Service, WIC program, La Leche League International.

"taking in" to a "taking hold" phase, in which her receptiveness and readiness is heightened and she is emotionally and physically ready for learning new information to facilitate mastery of her new role.

Helps standardize the information parents receive from staff members, and reduces client confusion caused by dissemination of conflicting advice or information.

Exercise helps tone musculature, increases circulation, produces a trimmer figure, and enhances feelings of general well-being.

Helps prevent infection, fosters healing and recuperation, and contributes to positive adaptation to physical and emotional changes.

Couple may need clarification regarding available contraceptive methods and the fact that pregnancy could occur even prior to the 4- to 6-wk visit.

Follow-up visit is necessary to evaluate recovery of reproductive organs, healing of episiotomy/laceration repair, general well-being, and adaptation to life changes.

Further intervention or treatment may be needed before the 4- to 6-wk visit to prevent or minimize potential complications.

Client's emotional state may be somewhat labile at this time and often is influenced by physical well-being. Anticipating such changes may reduce the stress associated with this transition period that necessitates learning new roles and taking on new responsibilities.

Promotes independence and provides support for adaptation to multiple changes.

NURSING DIAGNOSIS:	**FAMILY COPING: potential for growth**
May Be Related To:	Sufficiently meeting individual needs and adaptive tasks, enabling goals of self-actualization to surface
	Family member(s) moving in direction of health-promoting and enriching lifestyle
Possibly Evidenced By:	
DESIRED OUTCOMES/EVALUATION CRITERIA—CLIENT/FAMILY WILL:	Verbalize desire to undertake tasks leading to incorporation of new family member.
	Express feelings of self-confidence and satisfaction with progress and adaptation being made.

ACTIONS/INTERVENTIONS	RATIONALE

Independent

Assess relationship of family members to one another; establish primary nurse.

The nurse can help to provide a positive hospital experience and prepare the family for growth through the developmental stages that accompany acquisition of a new family member.

Provide for unlimited participation for father and siblings. Ascertain whether siblings attended an orientation program.

Facilitates family development and ongoing process of acquaintance and attachment. Helps family members feel comfortable caring for newborn.

Initiate parent support group and individual or group instruction in breastfeeding, infant care, and the physical and emotional changes during the postpartal period.

Verbalization and discussion in group setting fosters sharing of ideas, opportunities for problem solving, and group support. Aids development of positive self-esteem, mastery, comfort, and understanding of new role.

Encourage equal participation of parents in infant care.

Flexibility and sensitization to family needs help foster self-esteem and sense of competence in caring for newborn following discharge.

Provide anticipatory guidance regarding the normal emotional changes associated with postpartal period.

Helps prepare couple for possible changes they may experience; reduces stress associated with the unknown or with unexpected events, and may promote positive coping.

Provide written information regarding suggested books for children (siblings) about the new baby. Encourage siblings to verbalize feelings of replacement or abandonment. Recommend that parents spend extra time with older children.

Helps children to identify and cope with new feelings/fears. Parents should know that feelings of jealousy are normal.

Suggest that friends include older children in activities outside of the home.

School-age children probably adjust more easily to a new baby when their horizons are already expanded to include attachment activities outside of the home.

Collaborative

Refer client/couple to postpartal parent groups in community.

Increases parents' knowledge of child rearing and child development, and provides supportive atmosphere while parents incorporate new roles.

CARE FOLLOWING CESAREAN BIRTH (4 HOURS TO 3 DAYS POSTPARTUM)

CLIENT ASSESSMENT DATA BASE

Review prenatal and intraoperative record, and the indication(s) for cesarean delivery.

Circulation

Blood loss during surgical procedure approximately 600–800 ml

Ego Integrity

May display emotional lability, from excitation, to apprehension, anger, or withdrawal.
Client/couple may have questions or misgivings about role in birth experience.
May express inability to deal with current situation.

Elimination

Indwelling urinary catheter may be in place; urine clear amber.
Bowel sounds absent, faint, or distinct.

Food/Fluid

Abdomen soft with no distension initially.
Mouth may be dry.

Neurosensory

Impaired movement and sensation below level of spinal epidural anesthesia

Pain/Discomfort

May report discomfort from various sources, e.g., surgical trauma/incision, afterpains, bladder/abdominal distension, effects of anesthesia

Respiratory

Lung sounds clear and vesicular

Safety

Abdominal dressing may have scant staining or may be dry and intact.
Parenteral line/saline lock when used, is patent, and site is free of erythema, swelling, and tenderness.

Sexuality

Fundus firmly contracted and located at the umbilicus.
Lochia flow moderate and free of excessive/large clots.

DIAGNOSTIC STUDIES

CBC, Hb/Hct: Assesses changes from preoperative levels and evaluates effect of blood loss in surgery.
Urinalysis (UA); Urine, Blood, Vaginal, and Lochial Cultures: Additional studies are based on individual need.

NURSING PRIORITIES

1. Promote family unity and bonding.
2. Enhance comfort and general well-being.

3. Prevent/minimize postoperative complications.
4. Promote a positive emotional response to birth experience and parenting role.
5. Provide information regarding postpartal needs.

DISCHARGE GOALS

1. Family bonding initiated
2. Pain/discomfort easing
3. Physical/psychological needs being met
4. Complications prevented/resolving
5. Positive self-appraisal regarding birth and parenting roles expressed
6. Postpartal care understood and plan in place to meet needs after discharge

NURSING DIAGNOSIS:	PARENT/INFANT ATTACHMENT, altered
May Be Related To:	Developmental transition/gain of a family member, situational crisis (e.g., surgical intervention, physical complications interfering with initial acquaintance/interaction, negative self-appraisal)
Possibly Evidenced By:	Hesitancy to hold/interact with infant, verbalization of concerns/difficulty coping with situation, not dealing with traumatic experience constructively
DESIRED OUTCOMES/EVALUATION CRITERIA—CLIENT WILL:	Hold infant, as maternal and neonatal conditions permit.
	Demonstrate appropriate attachment and bonding behaviors.
	Begin to actively engage in newborn care tasks, as appropriate.

ACTIONS/INTERVENTIONS	RATIONALE
Independent	
Encourage client to hold, touch, and examine the infant, depending on condition of client and the newborn. Assist as needed.	The first hours after birth offer a unique opportunity for family bonding to occur because both mother and infant are emotionally receptive to cues from each other, which initiate the attachment and acquaintance process. Assistance in first few interactions or until IV line is removed helps client avoid feelings of discouragement or inadequacy. Note: Even if client has chosen to relinquish her child, interacting with the newborn may facilitate the grieving process.
Provide opportunity for father/partner to touch and hold infant and assist with infant care as allowed by situation.	Helps facilitate bonding/attachment between father and infant. Provides a resource for the mother, validating the reality of the situation and the newborn at a time when procedures and her physical needs may limit her ability to interact.
Observe and record family-infant interactions, noting behaviors indicative of bonding and attachment within specific culture.	Eye-to-eye contact, use of en face position, talking in a high-pitched voice, and holding infant closely are associated with attachment in American culture. On first contact with the infant, a mother manifests a progressive pattern of behaviors, whereby she initially uses fingertips to explore the infant's

Discuss need for usual progression and interactive nature of bonding. Reinforce normalcy of variation of response from one time to another and among different children.

Note verbalizations/behaviors suggesting disappointment or lack of interest/attachment.

Allow parents the opportunity to verbalize negative feelings about themselves and the infant.

Note circumstances surrounding cesarean birth, parents' self-appraisal and perception of birth experience, their initial reaction to infant, and their participation in birth experience.

Encourage and assist with breastfeeding, dependent on client's choice and cultural beliefs/practices.

Welcome family and siblings for brief visit as soon as maternal/newborn condition permits. (Refer to CP: The Client at 4 Hours to 2 Days Postpartum; ND: Family Coping: potential for growth.)

Provide information, as desired, about infant's safety and condition. Support couple as needed.

Initiate contact between client/couple and infant as soon as possible. If infant is sent to neonatal intensive care unit, establish line of communication between nursery staff and client/couple. Take pictures of neonate and allow for visits when client's physical status permits. (Refer to CP: The Parents of a Child with Special Needs.)

Answer client's questions regarding protocol of care during early postdelivery period.

Collaborative

Notify appropriate healthcare team members (e.g., nursery staff or postpartal nurse) of observations as indicated.

Prepare for ongoing support/follow-up after discharge, e.g., visiting nurse services, community agencies, and parent support group.

extremities and progresses to using the palm before enfolding the infant with her whole hand and arms.

Helps client/couple understand significance and importance of the process and provides reassurance that differences are to be expected.

The arrival of a new family member, even when wanted and anticipated, creates a transient period of disequilibrium, requiring incorporation of the new child into the existing family.

Unresolved conflicts during the early parent-infant acquaintance process may have long-term negative effects on the future parent-child relationship.

Parents need to work through meaning attributed to stressful events surrounding childbirth and orient themselves to reality before they can focus on infant. Effects of anesthesia, anxiety, and pain can alter the client's perceptual abilities during and following surgical intervention.

Early contact has a positive effect on duration of breastfeedings; skin-to-skin contact and initiation of maternal tasks promotes bonding. Some cultures (e.g., Hispanic, Navajo, Filipino, Vietnamese) may refrain from breastfeeding until the milk flow is established.

Promotes family unity, and helps siblings begin process of positive adaptation to new roles and incorporation of new member into family structure.

Helps couple to process and evaluate necessary information, especially if initial acquaintance period has been delayed.

Reduces anxiety that may be associated with handling infant, fear of unknown, and/or assuming the worst regarding infant status.

Information relieves anxiety that may interfere with bonding or result in self-absorption rather than inattention to newborn.

Inadequate bonding behaviors or poor interaction between client/couple and infant necessitates support and further evaluation. Note: In some cultures, e.g., Native American, the father may practice a period of ritual avoidance beginning immediately after the birth. (Refer to CP: The Client at 4 Hours to 2 Days Postpartum; ND: Parenting, risk for altered.)

Many couples have unresolved conflicts regarding initial parent-infant acquaintance process that may require resolution after discharge.

333

NURSING DIAGNOSIS:	PAIN [acute]/[DISCOMFORT]
May Be Related To:	Surgical trauma, effects of anesthesia, hormonal effects, bladder/abdominal distension
Possibly Evidenced By:	Reports of incisional pain, cramping (afterpains), headache, abdominal bloating, breast tenderness; guarding/distraction behaviors, facial mask of pain
DESIRED OUTCOMES/EVALUATION CRITERIA—CLIENT WILL:	Identify and use appropriate interventions to manage pain/discomfort.
	Verbalize lessening of level of pain.
	Appear relaxed, able to sleep/rest appropriately.

ACTIONS/INTERVENTIONS	RATIONALE

Independent

Determine characteristics and location of discomfort. Rate severity on a 0–10 scale. Note verbal and nonverbal cues, such as grimacing, rigidity, and guarding or restricted movement.	Client may not verbally report pain and discomfort directly. Comparing specific characteristics of pain aids in differentiating postoperative pain from developing complications (e.g., ileus, bladder retention or infection, wound dehiscence).
Provide information and anticipatory guidance regarding causes of discomfort and appropriate interventions.	Promotes problem solving, helps reduce pain associated with anxiety and fear of the unknown, and provides sense of control.
Evaluate BP, pulse, and behavior changes (e.g., distinguish between restlessness associated with excessive blood loss from that resulting from pain).	In many clients pain may cause restlessness and an increase in BP and pulse. Administration of analgesics may lower BP.
Note uterine tenderness and presence/characteristics of afterpains; postoperative infusion of oxytocin.	During the first 12 hr postpartum, uterine contractions are strong and regular, and they continue for the next 2–3 days, although their frequency and intensity are reduced. Factors intensifying afterpains include multiparity, uterine overdistension, breastfeeding, and administration of ergot and oxytocin preparations.
Reposition client, reduce noxious stimuli, and offer comfort measures, e.g., back rubs. Encourage use of breathing and relaxation techniques and distraction (stimulation of cutaneous tissue) as learned in childbirth preparation classes. Encourage presence and participation of partner as appropriate.	Relaxes muscles, and redirects attention away from painful sensations. Promotes comfort, and reduces unpleasant distractions, enhancing sense of well-being.
Initiate deep-breathing exercises, incentive spirometry, and coughing using splinting procedures, as appropriate, 30 min after administration of analgesics.	Deep breathing enhances respiratory effort. Splinting reduces strain and stretching of incisional area and lessens pain and discomfort associated with movement of abdominal muscles. Coughing is indicated when secretions or rhonchi are auscultated.
Encourage early ambulation, use of rocking chair or left side-lying position, as appropriate. Recommend avoidance of gas-forming foods or fluids, e.g., beans, cabbage, carbonated beverages, whole milk, very hot or very cold beverages, or use of straws for drinking. (Refer to ND: Constipation.)	Decreases gas formation and promotes peristalsis to relieve discomfort of gas accumulation, which often peaks on 3rd day after cesarean birth.

334

Recommend use of left lateral recumbent position.

Allows gas to rise from descending to sigmoid colon, facilitating expulsion.

Inspect perineum for hemorrhoids. Suggest application of ice for 20 min every 4 hr, use of witch hazel compresses, and elevation of pelvis on pillow, as appropriate.

Aids in regression of hemorrhoids and vulvar varicosities by promoting venous return and localized vasoconstriction, reducing associated edema, discomfort, and itching.

Palpate bladder, noting fullness. Facilitate periodic voiding after removal of indwelling catheter.

Return of normal bladder function may take 4–7 days, and overdistension of bladder may create feelings of urgency and discomfort.

Investigate reports of headache, especially following subarachnoid anesthesia. Avoid medicating client before nature and cause of headache are determined. Note character of headache (e.g., deep location behind the eyes, with pain radiating to both temples and occipital area; relieved in supine position but increased in sitting or standing position) to distinguish from headache associated with anxiety or PIH.

Leakage of CSF through the dura mater into the extradural space reduces volume needed to support brain tissue, causing the brain stem to fall onto the base of the skull when client is in an upright position. PIH may result in cerebral edema, necessitating other interventions. (Refer to CP: The Client at 4 Hours to 2 Days Postpartum; ND: Fluid Volume, risk for excess.)

Encourage bedrest in flat-lying position, increase fluids, offer caffeinated beverage, assist as needed with client and infant care, and apply abdominal binder when client is upright, in presence of postspinal headache. Notify physician or anesthesiologist, as indicated.

Reduces severity of headache by increasing fluid available for production of CSF and limiting position shifts of the brain. Severe headache may interfere with client's ability to carry out self/infant care. Ongoing headache may require more aggressive therapy.

Inspect breast and nipple tissue; assess for presence of engorgement and/or cracked nipples.

At 24 hr postpartum, breasts should be soft and nontender, with nipples free of cracks or reddened areas. Breast engorgement, nipple tenderness, or presence of cracks on nipple (if client is lactating) may occur 2–3 days postpartum and require prompt intervention to facilitate continuation of breastfeeding and prevent more serious complications.

Encourage wearing of supportive bra.

Lifts breasts inward and upward, resulting in a more comfortable position and decreasing muscle fatigue.

Provide information to the lactating client about increasing the frequency of feedings, applying heat to breasts before feedings, proper positioning of the infant, and expressing milk manually. (Refer to CP: The Client at 4 Hours to 2 Days Postpartum; ND: Breastfeeding [specify].)

These measures can help the lactating client stimulate the flow of milk and relieve stasis and engorgement. Use of "football hold" directs infant's feet away from abdomen. Pillow helps support infant and protects incision in sitting or side-lying position.

Suggest that client initiate feedings on nontender nipple for several feedings in succession if only one nipple is sore or cracked.

Initial suckling response is strong and may be painful. Starting feeding with unaffected breast and then proceeding to involved breast may be less painful and enhance healing.

Apply ice to axillary area of breasts if the client is not planning to breastfeed. Recommend use of well-fitting supportive bra, and avoidance of excess exposure of breasts to heat, or stimulation of breasts by infant, sexual partner, or client until suppression process is completed (approximately 1 wk).

Use of supportive bra and ice suppresses lactation by mechanical means and are the preferred method for cessation of lactation. Discomfort lasts approximately 48–72 hr but eases or ceases with avoidance of nipple stimulation.

Collaborative

Assist with bolus dose of morphine sulfate (Duramorph) via epidural prior to removal of epidural catheter.

Provides approximately 24-hr period of pain control, at the end of which oral medications are usually appropriate.

335

Administer analgesics every 3–4 hr, progressing from IV/IM (e.g., meperidine [Demerol], butorphanol [Stadol], nalbuphine [Nubain]) to oral route (e.g., oxycodone-acetaminophen [Percocet], oxycodone-aspirin [Percodan]). Medicate lactating client 45–60 min before breastfeeding.

Promotes comfort, which improves psychological status and enhances mobility. Use of medication with limited ability to cross into milk allows lactating mother to enjoy feeding without adverse effects on infant.

Review/monitor use of patient-controlled analgesia (PCAs) as indicated.

PCA using meperidine or morphine may be used to provide rapid pain relief without excessive side effects/oversedation. Enhances sense of control, general well-being, and independence.

Administer antiflatulent, e.g., Mylicon. Provide rectal/nasogastric (NG) tube as indicated.

Occasionally necessary to relieve gas buildup.

Assist as needed with saline injection or administration of "blood patch" over site of dural puncture. Keep client in horizontal position following the procedure.

Effective for relief of severe spinal headache. The blood patch procedure, which has a 90%–100% success rate, creates a blood clot, which produces pressure and seals the leak.

NURSING DIAGNOSIS:	SELF ESTEEM, situational low
May Be Related To:	Perceived failure at a life event, maturational transition, perceived loss of control in current situation
Possibly Evidenced By:	Verbalization of negative feelings about self in situation (e.g., helplessness, shame/guilt), evaluates self as unable to handle situation, difficulty making decisions
DESIRED OUTCOMES/EVALUATION CRITERIA—CLIENT/COUPLE WILL:	Discuss concerns related to her/his role in and perception of the birth experience.
	Verbalize understanding of individual factors that precipitated current situation.
	Express positive self-appraisal.

ACTIONS/INTERVENTIONS	RATIONALE

Independent

Determine client's/couple's emotional response to cesarean birth.

Both members of the couple may have a negative emotional reaction to the surgical intervention. An unplanned cesarean birth may have a negative effect on the client's self-esteem, leaving her feeling that she is inadequate and has failed as a woman. The father or partner, especially if he was unable/unwilling to be present at the cesarean delivery, may feel that he abandoned his partner and did not fulfill his anticipated role as emotional supporter during the childbirth process. Even though a healthy baby may be the outcome, parents often grieve and feel a sense of loss at missing out on the anticipated vaginal birth.

Determine client's level of anxiety and source of concern. Encourage client/couple to verbalize unmet needs and expectations. Provide information regarding the normalcy of such feelings.

Cesarean birth may be viewed by the client/couple as a failure at a life event, and this may have a negative impact on the bonding/parenting process. Note: Emergency cesarean birth may create

Review client's/couple's participation and role in birth experience. Identify positive behaviors during prenatal and antepartal process.

Encourage presence/participation of partner in all that is going on.

Emphasize similarities between vaginal and cesarean birth. Convey positive attitude, and manage postpartal care as close as possible to care provided to clients following vaginal birth.

Assist client/couple in identifying usual coping mechanisms and developing new coping strategies if needed. (Refer to CP: The Client at 4 Hours to 2 Days Postpartum; ND: Coping, Individual, risk for ineffective.)

Provide accurate information about client/infant status.

Collaborative

Refer client/couple for professional counseling if reactions are maladaptive.

---

problems for care of siblings because of unexpected prolonged hospital stay. Father may encounter conflicts in spending time with client/infant and meeting needs of siblings.

Refocuses client's/couple's attention to help them view pregnancy in its totality and to see that their actions have contributed to an optimal outcome. May help to avoid guilt/placing of blame. Note: Grief response may be lessened if both mother and father were able to share in experience of delivery.

Provides emotional support; may encourage verbalization of concerns.

Client may alter her perception of cesarean birth experience as well as her perception of her own wellness or illness based on the professional's attitudes. Similar care conveys the message that cesarean birth is a necessary alternative to vaginal delivery, focusing on the optimal outcome rather than on the birth process.

Helps facilitate positive adaptation to new role; reduces feelings of inadequacy.

Fantasies caused by lack of information or misunderstanding may increase sense of helplessness/loss of control.

Client who is unable to resolve grief or negative feelings may need further professional help.

NURSING DIAGNOSIS:	INJURY, risk for
Risk Factors May Include:	Biochemical or regulatory functions (e.g., orthostatic hypotension, development of PIH or eclampsia), effects of anesthesia, thromboembolism, abnormal blood profile (anemia/excessive blood loss, rubella sensitivity, Rh incompatibility), tissue trauma
Possibly Evidenced By:	[Not applicable; presence of signs/symptoms establishes an *actual* diagnosis]
DESIRED OUTCOMES/EVALUATION CRITERIA—CLIENT WILL:	Demonstrate behaviors to reduce risk factors and/or protect self.
	Be free of avoidable complications.

ACTIONS/INTERVENTIONS

RATIONALE

Independent

Review prenatal and intrapartal record for factors that predispose client to complications. Note Hb level and operative blood loss.

Presence of risk factors, such as myometrial fatigue, uterine overdistension, prolonged oxytocin stimulation, general anesthesia,

337

Monitor BP, pulse, and temperature. Note cool, clammy skin; weak, thready pulse; behavior changes; delayed capillary refill; or cyanosis. (Refer to CP: Postpartal Hemorrhage.)

Encourage early ambulation and exercise, except in client who received subarachnoid anesthesia who may remain flat for 6–8 hr without use of pillow or raising head, as indicated by protocol and return of sensation/muscle control. (Refer to ND: Pain [acute]/[Discomfort].)

Assist client with initial ambulation. Provide adequate supervision in shower or sitz bath. Leave call bell within client's reach.

Have client sit on floor or chair with head between legs, or have her lie down in a flat position, if she feels faint. Use ammonia capsule ("smelling salts").

Assess for hyperreflexia, RUQ/epigastric pain, headache, or visual disturbances. Maintain seizure precautions, and provide quiet environment as indicated. (Refer to CP: The Client at 4 Hours to 2 Days Postpartum; ND: Fluid Volume, risk for excess; CP: Pregnancy-Induced Hypertension; ND: Injury, risk for.)

Note effects of $MgSO_4$, if administered. Assess patellar response and monitor respiratory rate.

Inspect incision regularly; note signs of delayed or altered healing (e.g., lack of approximation).

Inspect lower extremities for signs of thrombophlebitis (e.g., redness, warmth, pain/tenderness). Note presence or absence of Homans' sign. (Refer to CP: Postpartal Thrombophlebitis.)

Encourage leg/ankle exercises and early ambulation.

Evaluate client's rubella status on prenatal chart (>1:10 titer indicates susceptibility). Assess client for allergies to eggs or feathers; if present, vaccine is contraindicated. Provide written and oral information, and obtain informed consent for vaccination after reviewing side effects, risks, and the necessity to prevent conception for 2–3 mo following the vaccination.

anemia/excessive blood loss, or prenatal thrombophlebitis renders the client more susceptible to postoperative complications.

Elevated BP may indicate developing or continuing hypertension, necessitating $MgSO_4$ or other antihypertensive treatment. Hypotension and tachycardia may reflect dehydration and hypovolemia. Pyrexia may indicate infection.

Enhances circulation and venous return of lower extremities, reducing risk of thrombus formation, which is associated with stasis. Although recumbent position after subarachnoid anesthesia is debatable (no research to date supports effectiveness), it may aid in prevention of CSF leakage and resultant headache.

Orthostatic hypotension may occur when changing from supine to upright position on initial ambulation, or it may result from vasodilation caused by the heat of the shower or sitz bath.

Helps maintain or enhance circulation and delivery of oxygen to brain.

Danger of eclampsia due to PIH exists for up to 72 hr postpartum, although literature suggests the convulsive state has occurred as late as the 5th day postpartum.

Absence of patellar reflex and respiratory rate below 12/min indicates toxicity and a need to reduce or discontinue drug therapy.

Excessive strain on the incision or delayed healing may render client prone to tissue separation and possible hemorrhage.

Elevated fibrin split products (possibly released from placental site), reduced mobility, trauma, sepsis, and extensive activation of blood clotting following delivery predispose the client to the development of thromboembolism. Homans' sign may be present with deep venous thrombus, but may be absent with superficial phlebitis. In addition, plasma losses, elevated platelet counts, and relaxation of blood vessels from anesthesia increase risk for thrombophlebitis.

Promotes venous return; prevents stasis/pooling in lower extremities, reducing risk of phlebitis.

Vaccination helps prevent teratogenic effects in subsequent pregnancies. Administration of vaccine in the immediate postpartal period may cause side effects of transient arthralgia, rash, and cold symptoms during incubation period of 14–21 days. Allergic anaphylactic or hypersensitivity response may occur, necessitating administration of epinephrine.

Collaborative

Administer MgSO₄ by infusion pump, as indicated.

Helps reduce cerebral irritability in presence of PIH or eclampsia. (Refer to CP: The Client at 4 Hours to 2 Days Postpartum; ND: Fluid Volume, risk for excess.)

Apply support hose or elastic wrap to legs when risk or symptoms of phlebitis are present.

Reduces venous stasis, enhancing venous return and reducing risk of thrombus formation.

Administer anticoagulant; evaluate coagulation factors, and note signs of failure to clot. (Refer to CP: Postpartal Thrombophlebitis.)

Although usually not required, may help prevent further development of thrombus.

Administer RhIgG IM within 72 hr postpartum, as indicated for Rh-negative mother who has not been previously sensitized and who delivers an Rh-positive infant with negative result on direct Coombs' test on cord blood. Obtain Betke-Kleihauer smear if significant fetal-maternal transfusion is suspected at delivery.

Dose of 300 mg is usually sufficient to promote lysis of fetal Rh-positive RBCs that may have entered maternal circulation during delivery and that may potentially cause sensitization and problems of Rh incompatibility in subsequent pregnancies. Presence of 20 ml or more of Rh-positive fetal blood in maternal circulation necessitates higher dose of RhIgG. Note: If drug is not administered within 72 hr of delivery, a window of opportunity exists for up to 2 wk, although the degree of effectiveness may be reduced.

NURSING DIAGNOSIS:	INFECTION, risk for
Risk Factors May Include:	Tissue trauma/broken skin, decreased Hb, invasive procedures and/or increased environmental exposure, prolonged rupture of amniotic membranes, malnutrition
Possibly Evidenced By:	[Not applicable; presence of signs/symptoms establishes an *actual* diagnosis]
DESIRED OUTCOMES/EVALUATION CRITERIA—CLIENT WILL:	Demonstrate techniques to reduce risks and/or promote healing.
	Display wound free of purulent drainage with initial signs of healing (i.e., approximation of wound edges), uterus soft/nontender, with normal lochial flow and character.
	Be free of infection, be afebrile, have no adventitious breath sounds, and void clear amber urine.

ACTIONS/INTERVENTIONS	RATIONALE

Independent

Encourage and use careful hand washing technique and appropriate disposal of soiled underpads, perineal pads, and contaminated linen. Discuss with client the importance of continuing these measures after discharge.

Helps prevent or retard spread of infection.

Review prenatal Hb/Hct; note presence of conditions/risk factors that predispose client to postoperative infection.

Anemia, obesity, diabetes, prolonged labor (especially with membranes ruptured) prior to cesarean delivery, corticosteroid therapy, malnutrition, smoking, and chronic lung disease increase the risk of infection and delayed healing.

339

Assess client's nutritional status. Note appearance of hair, fingernails, skin, and so forth. Determine prepregnancy weight and prenatal weight gain.

Client who is 20% below normal weight, or who is anemic or malnourished, is more susceptible to postpartal infection and may have special dietary needs.

Encourage oral fluids and diet high in protein, vitamin C, and iron.

Prevents dehydration; maximizes circulation and urine flow. Protein and vitamin C are needed for collagen formation; iron is needed for Hb synthesis.

Inspect abdominal dressing for exudate or oozing. Remove dressing, as indicated.

A sterile dressing covering the wound in the first 24 hr following cesarean birth helps protect it from injury or contamination. Oozing may indicate hematoma, loss of suture approximation, or wound dehiscence, requiring further intervention. Removing the dressing allows incision to dry and promotes healing.

Note operative record for use of drain and nature of incision. Clean wound and change dressing when wet.

Moist environment is an excellent medium for bacterial growth; bacteria can travel by capillary action through the wet dressing to the wound. Note: Incision into the lower uterine segment heals more rapidly than classic incision and is less likely to rupture in subsequent pregnancies.

Inspect incision, evaluate healing process, noting localized redness, edema, pain, exudate, or loss of approximation of wound edges.

These signs indicate wound infection, usually caused by streptococci, staphylococci, or *Pseudomonas* species. Note: Wound infections are usually clinically apparent 3–8 days after the procedure.

Assist as needed with removal of skin sutures or clips.

Incision is usually sufficiently healed to remove sutures on the 4th or 5th day following surgical procedure.

Encourage client to take warm showers daily.

Showers, usually allowed after the 2nd postoperative day, promote hygiene and may stimulate circulation and healing of wound. Note: In some cultures, showers/tub baths are avoided until lochial flow ceases or longer, as dictated.

Assess temperature, pulse, and WBC count.

Fever after the 3rd postoperative day, leukocytosis, and tachycardia suggest infection. Elevation of temperature to 101°F (38.3°C) within the first 24 hr is highly indicative of infection; an elevation to 100.4°F (38.0°C) on any 2 of the 1st 10 days postpartum is significant.

Assess location and contractility of uterus; note involutional changes or presence of extreme uterine tenderness.

Following cesarean birth, the fundus remains at the level of the umbilicus for up to 5 days, when involution begins, accompanied by an increase in lochial flow. Delayed involution increases the risk of endometritis. Development of extreme tenderness signals possible retained placental tissue or infection.

Note amount and odor of lochial discharge or change in normal progression from rubra to serosa.

Lochia normally has a fleshy odor; however, in endometritis, the discharge may be purulent and foul-smelling, and may fail to demonstrate normal progression from rubra to serosa to alba.

Maintain sterile, closed injury drainage system with drainage bag in dependent position.

Prevents introduction of bacteria when indwelling catheter is used and avoids urinary reflux, reducing risk of infection.

Provide perineal and catheter care, per protocol.

Helps eliminate medium of bacterial growth; promotes hygiene.

Note frequency/amount and characteristics of urine.	Urinary stasis increases the risk of infection. Cloudy or malodorus urine indicates presence of bacteria.
Promote rest and encourage use of semi-Fowler's position once anesthesia precautions are completed.	Rest reduces metabolic process, allowing oxygen and nutrients to be used for healing. Semi-Fowler's position promotes flow of lochia and reduces pooling in uterus, and maximizes respiratory function.
Inspect IV site for signs of erythema or tenderness.	Indicates local infection, requiring removal of catheter and possibly restarting the IV line in another site.
Evaluate condition of nipples, noting presence of cracks, redness, or tenderness. Recommend routine examination of breasts. Review proper care and infant feeding techniques. (Refer to ND: Pain [acute]/[Discomfort].)	The development of nipple fissures/cracks potentiates risk of mastitis.
Assess lung sounds and respiratory ease or effort. Note crackles/rhonchi, dyspnea, chest pain, fever, or mucopurulent sputum.	Rhonchi indicative of retained secretions should not be present, yet breath sounds may be diminished for the first 24 hr after surgery. Absence of lung sounds indicates consolidation or lack of air exchange, suggesting atelectasis or possibly pneumonia. Note: Atelectasis usually occurs in the first 72 hr after the procedure, whereas pneumonia typically develops after 72 hr.
Institute turning, coughing, and deep-breathing routines with splinting of incision every 2–4 hr while awake. Note productive cough.	Improves depth of respirations and alveolar expansion; clears secretions that could block bronchioles. Productive cough indicates client is clearing bronchial secretions effectively. Splinting prevents excessive strain on incision, reducing discomfort and enhancing client's participation in activity.

Collaborative

Administer oxytocin or ergot preparation. (Note: Oxytocin infusion is often ordered routinely for 4 hr following surgery.)	Maintains myometrial contractility, thereby retarding bacterial spread through walls of uterus; aids in expulsion of clots/membranes.
Monitor laboratory test results, such as BUN and 24-hr urine, for total protein, creatinine clearance, and uric acid, as indicated.	In the client who has had PIH, kidney or vascular involvement may persist, or it may appear for the first time during the postpartal period. As steroid levels decrease following delivery, renal function, evidenced by BUN and creatinine clearance, begins to return to normal within 1 wk; anatomic changes (e.g., dilation of ureters and renal pelvis) may take up to 1 mo to return to normal.
Administer prophylactic antibiotic infusion, with first dose usually administered immediately after cord clamping and two more doses 6 hr apart.	Decreases likelihood of postpartal endometritis as well as complications such as incisional abscesses or pelvic thrombophlebitis.
Demonstrate/encourage use of incentive spirometer.	Promotes sustained maximal respiration, inflates alveoli, and prevents atelectasis.
Obtain sputum specimen as indicated by changes in color or odor of sputum, presence of congestion, and temperature elevation.	Identifies specific pathogens and appropriate therapy.
Review chest x-rays, as indicated.	Confirms presence of infiltrate(s) or atelectasis.
Obtain blood, vaginal, and urine cultures, if infection is suspected.	Bacteremia is more frequent in client whose membranes were ruptured for 6 hr or longer than in client whose membranes remained intact prior to cesarean birth.

341

Administer specific antibiotic for identified infectious process.

Necessary to effectively eradicate organism.

NURSING DIAGNOSIS:	FLUID VOLUME, risk for deficit
Risk Factors May Include:	Period of restricted oral intake, presence of nausea/vomiting, excessive blood loss during surgery
Possibly Evidenced By:	[Not applicable; presence of signs/symptoms establishes an *actual* diagnosis]
DESIRED OUTCOMES/EVALUATION CRITERIA—CLIENT WILL:	Maintain fluid volume at a functional level as evidenced by individually adequate urinary output, stable vital signs, moist mucous membranes, and Hb/Hct within normal limits.

ACTIONS/INTERVENTIONS	RATIONALE

Independent

Review prenatal and intrapartal/surgical records for Hb level, operative blood loss, fluid replacement, presence of edema.	Data helpful in evaluating current fluid status and potential for diuresis.
Monitor BP, pulse, status of mucous membranes, capillary refill; note presence of cyanosis.	Hypotension, tachycardia, and dry mouth may reflect dehydration and hypovolemia but may not occur until circulating blood volume has decreased by 30%–50%, at which time signs of peripheral vasoconstriction may be noted.
Inspect dressing for excessive bleeding. Outline, date drainage on dressings (if not changed). Notify physician of continued oozing.	Surgical wounds with a drain may saturate a dressing; however, oozing is usually not expected and may suggest developing complications.
Note character and amount of lochial flow and consistency of fundus. Gently massage fundus as indicated.	Lochial flow should not be heavy or contain clots; fundus should remain firmly contracted at the umbilicus. A boggy uterus results in increased flow and blood loss. Note: As a rule, lochial flow is usually decreased by second postoperative day, thus "normal" amount of flow expected after vaginal delivery would be suspect for this client.
Monitor fluid intake and urine output. Note appearance, color, concentration, and specific gravity of urine.	Kidney function is a key index to circulating blood volume. As output decreases, specific gravity increases, and vice versa. Bloody urine or urine containing clots signifies possible bladder trauma associated with surgical intervention.
Encourage adequate oral fluids (e.g., 6–8 glasses/day).	Preferred route for replacement once nausea is resolved/peristalsis returns. Adequate intake allows for timely removal of IV.

Collaborative

Replace fluid losses intravenously, as indicated.	Average blood loss is usually 600–800 ml, but prenatal physiological edema, which mobilizes postpartum, alleviates need for large fluid volume replacement. A total of 3 L of fluid infused intravenously in the intraoperative and early

postoperative (24-hr) period is recommended. Note: If epidural anesthesia is used, more fluids are usually required.

Monitor postoperative Hb/Hct; compare with preoperative levels.

Client with Hct of 33% or greater and increased plasma associated with pregnancy can usually tolerate actual blood loss of up to 1500 ml without difficulty. A significant change in volume may necessitate replacement with blood products, although iron replacement may be preferred.

Increase oxytocin infusion if uterus is relaxed and/or lochia is heavy.

Stimulates myometrial contractility and reduces blood loss. Oxytocin is usually added to infusion intraoperatively after delivery of the infant's shoulders and is maintained into the early postoperative period.

NURSING DIAGNOSIS:	CONSTIPATION
May Be Related To:	Decreased muscle tone (diastasis recti, excess analgesia or anesthesia), effects of progesterone, dehydration, prelabor diarrhea, lack of intake, perineal/rectal pain
Possibly Evidenced By:	Reported abdominal/rectal fullness or pressure, nausea, less than usual amount of stool, straining at stool, decreased bowel sounds
DESIRED OUTCOMES/EVALUATION CRITERIA—CLIENT WILL:	Demonstrate return of intestinal motility, as evidenced by active bowel sounds and the passing of flatus.
	Resume usual/optimal elimination pattern within 4 days postpartum.

ACTIONS/INTERVENTIONS	RATIONALE

Independent

Auscultate for presence of bowel sounds in all four quadrants every 4 hr following cesarean birth.

Determines readiness for oral feedings, and possible developing complication, e.g., ileus. Usually, bowel sounds are not heard on the 1st day after surgical procedure, are faint on the 2nd day, and are active by the 3rd day.

Palpate abdomen, noting distension or discomfort.

Indicates gas formation and accumulation or possible paralytic ileus.

Note passing of flatus or belching.

Indicates return of motility.

Encourage adequate oral fluids (e.g., 6–8 glasses/day) once oral intake resumes. Recommend increased dietary roughage and fruits and vegetables.

Roughage (e.g., fruits and vegetables, especially with seeds and skins) and increased fluids provide bulk, stimulate elimination, and prevent constipated stool. Note: Food or fluid offered before return of peristalsis may contribute to paralytic ileus.

Encourage leg exercises and abdominal tightening; promote early ambulation.

Leg exercises tighten abdominal muscles and improve abdominal motility. Progressive ambulation after 24 hr promotes peristalsis and gas expulsion, and alleviates or prevents gas pains.

343

Identify those activities that client can use at home to stimulate bowel action.

Helps in re-establishing normal evacuation pattern and promotes independence.

Collaborative

Administer analgesics 30 min before ambulation.

Facilitates ability to ambulate; however, narcotics, if used, may reduce bowel activity.

Provide stool softener or mild cathartic.

Softens stool, stimulates peristalsis, and helps re-establish bowel function.

Administer hypertonic or small soap suds enema.

Promotes bowel evacuation and relieves gaseous distension.

Insert or maintain NG tube as indicated.

May be necessary to decompress the stomach and relieve distension associated with paralytic ileus.

NURSING DIAGNOSIS:	KNOWLEDGE deficit [LEARNING NEED], regarding physiological changes, recovery period, self care, and infant care needs
May Be Related To:	Lack of exposure/recall, misinterpretation, unfamiliarity with resources
Possibly Evidenced By:	Verbalized concerns/misconceptions, hesitancy in or inadequate performance of activities, inappropriate behaviors (e.g., apathy)
DESIRED OUTCOMES/EVALUATION CRITERIA—CLIENT WILL:	Verbalize understanding of physiological changes, individual needs, expected outcomes.
	Perform necessary activities/procedures correctly and explain reasons for the actions.

ACTIONS/INTERVENTIONS

RATIONALE

Independent

Assess client's readiness and motivation for learning. Assist client/couple in identifying needs.

The postpartal period can be a positive experience if opportune teaching is provided to foster maternal growth, maturation, and competence. However, the client needs time to move from a "taking in" to a "taking hold" phase, in which her receptiveness and readiness is heightened and she is emotionally and physically ready for learning new information to facilitate mastery of her new role. Although basic information may be provided/reviewed the 1st day, the client is usually receptive to learning more in-depth material by the 2nd or 3rd day postpartum.

Initiate written teaching plan using standardized format, checklist, or clinical pathway. Document information given and client's response.

Helps assure completeness of information parents receive from staff members and reduces client confusion caused by dissemination of conflicting advice or information.

Assess client's physical status. Plan group or individual sessions following administration of medication or when client is comfortable and rested.

Discomfort associated with incision or afterpains, or bowel/bladder discomfort, is usually less severe by the 2nd or 3rd postoperative day, allowing the client to concentrate more fully and be more receptive to learning.

344

Note psychological state and response to cesarean birth and mothering role. (Refer to ND: Self Esteem, situational low.)

Anxiety related to ability to care for herself and her child, possible disappointment over the birth experience, or concerns regarding her separation from the infant may have a negative impact on client's learning abilities and readiness.

Provide information related to normal physiological and psychological changes associated with cesarean birth and needs associated with the postpartal period.

Helps client to recognize normal changes from abnormal responses that may require treatment. Client's emotional state may be somewhat labile at this time and often is influenced by physical well-being. Anticipating such changes may reduce the stress associated with this transition period that necessitates learning new roles and taking on new responsibilities. Note: Client has had a major abdominal surgical procedure requiring at least 6–8 wk for physiological recovery, but client may not feel fully recovered for up to 6 mo.

Stress importance of adequate rest, fluid/dietary intake, and necessity for specific activity limitations (e.g., avoidance of lifting and driving).

Promotes healing, facilitates recovery, protects incision—reducing risk of dehiscence.

Review self-care needs (e.g., perineal care, incisional care, hygiene, voiding). Encourage participation in self-care, as client is able. Demonstrate method of getting out of a flat bed without the use of siderails.

Facilitates autonomy, helps prevent infection, and promotes healing. By turning on her side, using her arms to lift herself to a sitting position, and pushing with her hands to lift buttocks off the bed to a standing position, client can continue to ease stress on incision after discharge.

Discuss prescribed exercise program.

A progressive exercise program can usually be started once abdominal discomfort has eased (by approximately 3–4 wk postpartum). Helps tone musculature, increases circulation, produces a trimmer figure, and enhances feelings of general well-being. Client should be advised not to lift objects heavier than the infant for approximately 2 wk, and to bend at knees when lifting baby.

Identify signs/symptoms requiring notification of healthcare provider (e.g., fever, dysuria, increase in amount of lochial flow or return to bright red lochial exudate, or separation of suture line).

Prompt evaluation and intervention may prevent/limit development of complications (e.g., hemorrhage, infection, delayed healing).

Demonstrate techniques of infant care. Observe return demonstration by client/couple. (Refer to CP: The Neonate at 2 Hours to 2 Days of Age; ND: Knowledge deficit [Learning Need].)

Assists parents in mastery of new tasks.

Review information regarding appropriate choice for infant feeding (e.g., physiology of breastfeeding, diet, positioning, breast and nipple care, and removal of infant from breast; formula types/preparation, infant position during bottle feeding, burping techniques).

Promotes independence and optimal feeding experience. When bottle feeding, it is important to feed the infant alternately on the right and left side to promote eye development. Slight dehydration or physical or emotional trauma may delay onset of lactation for the client who has undergone a cesarean birth.

Discuss plans for home management: assistance with housework, physical layout of house, infant sleeping arrangements.

Client who has undergone cesarean birth may need more assistance when first home than the client who has given birth vaginally. Stairs and the use of low cradles or bassinets may cause difficulties for the postoperative client.

Determine availability of support system(s), plans after discharge.

Helps to identify individual needs, necessity of home visitation, and provides opportunity to correct

Provide numbers for appropriate telephone contacts. Identify available community resources; e.g., visiting nurse/home care services, Public Health Service, WIC program, La Leche League, Mothers of Twins.

misconceptions/unrealistic expectations. Promotes problem solving.

Provides ready resources to answer questions. Promotes independence and provides support for adaptation to multiple changes.

Discuss resumption of sexual intercourse and plans for contraception. Provide information about available methods, including advantages and disadvantages. (Refer to CP: 1 Week Following Discharge; ND: Knowledge deficit [Learning Need].)

Intercourse may be resumed as soon as it is comfortable for the client and healing has progressed, generally 4–6 wk postpartum. Couple may need clarification regarding available contraceptive methods and the fact that pregnancy could occur even prior to the 4–6-wk visit.

Provide or reinforce information related to follow-up postpartal examination.

Postpartum evaluations for the client who has undergone cesarean delivery may be scheduled at 3 wk rather than 6 wk because of increased risk of infection and delayed healing.

NURSING DIAGNOSIS:	URINARY ELIMINATION, altered
May Be Related To:	Mechanical trauma/diversion, hormonal effects (fluid shifts and/or increased renal plasma flow), effects of anesthesia
Possibly Evidenced By:	Increased bladder filling/distension, changes in amount/frequency of voiding
DESIRED OUTCOMES/EVALUATION CRITERIA—CLIENT WILL:	Resume usual/optimal voiding patterns following catheter removal. Empty bladder with each void.

ACTIONS/INTERVENTIONS

RATIONALE

Independent

Note and record amount, color, and concentration of urinary drainage.

Oliguria (output less than 30 ml/hr) may be caused by excess fluid loss, inadequate fluid replacement, or antidiuretic effects of infused oxytocin.

Test urine for albumin and acetone. Distinguish between proteinuria associated with PIH and that associated with normal processes (Refer to CP: The Client at 4 Hours to 2 Days Postpartum; ND: Fluid Volume, risk for excess.)

Catalytic process associated with uterine involution may result in normal proteinuria (1+) for the first 2 days postpartum. Acetone may indicate dehydration associated with prolonged labor and/or delivery.

Provide oral fluid, e.g., 6–8 glasses per day, as appropriate.

Fluids promote hydration and renal function, and help prevent bladder stasis.

Palpate bladder. Monitor fundal height and location and amount of lochial flow.

Renal plasma flow, which increases by 25%–50% during the prenatal period, remains elevated in the 1st wk postpartum, resulting in increased bladder filling. Bladder distension can be assessed by degree of uterine displacement; causes increased uterine relaxation and lochial flow.

Note signs and symptoms of UTI (e.g., cloudy color,

Presence of indwelling catheter predisposes client

foul odor, burning sensation, or frequency) following catheter removal.

Use methods to facilitate voiding after catheter removal (e.g., run water in sink, pour warm water over perineum).

Instruct client to perform Kegel exercise daily after effects of anesthesia have subsided.

to introduction of bacteria and UTI. (Refer to ND: Infection, risk for.)

Client should void within 6–8 hr following catheter removal, yet may have difficulty emptying bladder completely.

Performing Kegel exercise 100 times/day increases circulation to perineum, aids in healing and recovery of tone of pubococcygeal muscle, and prevents or reduces stress incontinence.

Collaborative

Maintain IV infusion for 24 hr following surgery, as indicated. Increase infusion rate if output is 30 ml/hr or less.

Remove catheter per protocol/as indicated.

Monitor laboratory test results, such as BUN and 24-hr urine for total protein, creatinine clearance, and uric acid, as indicated.

Usually, 3 L of fluid, including lactated Ringer's solution, is adequate to replace losses and maintain renal flow/urine output.

Generally, catheter may be safely removed between 6–12 hr postpartum; but for convenience it may remain in client until the morning after surgery.

In the client who has had PIH, kidney or vascular involvement may persist, or it may appear for the first time during the postpartal period. As steroid levels decrease following delivery, renal function, evidenced by BUN and creatinine clearance, begins to return to normal within 1 wk; anatomic changes (e.g., dilation of ureters and renal pelvis) may take up to 1 mo to return to normal.

NURSING DIAGNOSIS:	SELF CARE deficit [specify type/level]
May Be Related To:	Effects of anesthesia, decreased strength and endurance, physical discomfort
Possibly Evidenced By:	Verbalization of inability to participate at level desired
DESIRED OUTCOMES/EVALUATION CRITERIA—CLIENT WILL:	Demonstrate techniques to meet self-care needs.
	Identify/use available resources.

ACTIONS/INTERVENTIONS

RATIONALE

Independent

Ascertain severity/duration of discomfort. Note presence of postspinal headache.

Intense pain affects emotional and behavioral responses, so that the client may be unable to focus on self-care activities until her physical needs for comfort are met. Intense headache associated with upright position requires modification of activities and additional assistance to meet individual needs.

Assess client's psychological status.

Physical pain experience may be compounded by mental pain that interferes with client's desire and motivation to assume autonomy.

Note cultural expectations/practices.

Some cultures, (e.g., Mexican/Arab-American, Haitian, Russian) require the new mother to observe a specified period of bed rest/activity restrictions

Determine type of anesthesia, and associated orders or protocol regarding positioning/ambulation.

during which other female members of her family may provide care.

Epidural anesthesia (especially following bolus dose of duramorph) may cause generalized weakness, creating safety concerns, and requires careful assessment before sitting upright/getting out of bed. Clients who have undergone spinal anesthesia may be directed to lie flat and without pillow for several hours following administration of anesthesia.

Reposition client every 1–2 hr; assist with pulmonary exercises, ambulation, and leg exercises.

Helps prevent surgical complications such as phlebitis or pneumonia, which may occur when discomfort levels interfere with client's normal repositioning/activity.

Offer assistance as needed with hygiene (e.g., mouth care, bathing, back rubs, and perineal care).

Improves self-esteem; increases feelings of well-being.

Offer choices when possible (e.g., selection of juices, scheduling of bath, destination during ambulation).

Allows some autonomy, even though client depends on professional assistance. Note: Some cultures restrict bathing/showers for a predetermined length of time after delivery or until cessation of lochial flow.

Collaborative

Administer analgesic agent every 3–4 hr, as needed.

Reduces discomfort, which could interfere with ability to engage in self-care.

Convert IV line to saline lock, as appropriate.

Permits unrestricted movement of extremities, thereby allowing client to function more independently, regardless of ongoing intermittent IV therapy (e.g., antibiotics).

THE CLIENT AT 24 TO 48 HOURS FOLLOWING EARLY DISCHARGE

This plan of care focuses on the client who is discharged within 30 hr of delivery. It is to be used in conjunction with CP: The Client at 4 Hours to 2 Days Postpartum.

CLIENT ASSESSMENT DATA BASE

Circulation

BP remains at same level as pregnant readings (slightly below baseline).
Pulse between 60 and 90 bpm.
Superficial varicosities may be visible in lower extremities.

Ego Integrity

May feel isolated, anxious, depressed, or fatigued, even though early discharge had been desired by client
May report stressors (e.g., employment, financial, living situation), concerns about personal abilities and assumption of mothering role

Elimination

Voiding 100 ml or greater in amount, without suprapubic tenderness or retention.
Probably has not experienced a return of normal bowel habits.
Hemorrhoids varying in size and number may be present.
Abdominal musculature may be weak and of "bread dough" consistency.

Food/Fluid

Weight reduced by 10–12 lb following delivery.
Physiological edema may still be present.

Pain/Discomfort

Discomforts associated with episiotomy, perineal trauma, hemorrhoids, or afterpains.
Breast tenderness/engorgement may occur between days 3–5 postpartum.
Uterine contractions diminishing daily in frequency and intensity.

Safety

Lochia rubra moderate in amount with fleshy odor; may increase during breastfeeding.
Striae may be present on abdomen, breasts, and thighs.
Perineum or site of episiotomy repair may be edematous with good approximation of wound edges.

Sexuality

Breasts soft, nontender, and free of masses
Nipples soft and free of fissures or lesions
Uterus firm, midline, and located at or just below the umbilicus (uterus is larger in multipara or in client with overdistension)

Social Interactions

May now report lack of/or inadequate support systems; concerns regarding roles of individual family members, role mastery, or disequilibrium (especially in blended family)

DIAGNOSTIC STUDIES

Routine assessment may include CBC or Hb/Hct and UA, and culture and sensitivity, as indicated by physical findings.

349

NURSING PRIORITIES

1. Determine postpartum status of client.
2. Promote optimal physical and emotional well-being.
3. Facilitate client's/couple's positive adaptation to parenting roles, family growth, and autonomy.

NURSING DIAGNOSIS:	PAIN [acute]/[DISCOMFORT]
May Be Related To:	Mechanical trauma, tissue edema/engorgement or distension, hormonal effects, excessive fatigue
Possibly Evidenced By:	Reports of cramping (afterpains) and perineal discomfort, guarding/distraction behaviors
DESIRED OUTCOMES/EVALUATION CRITERIA—CLIENT WILL:	Identify sources of discomfort.
	Take appropriate measures to reduce discomfort.

ACTIONS/INTERVENTIONS	RATIONALE
Independent	
Inspect breast and nipple tissue; note presence of engorgement and/or cracked nipples.	Breast engorgement, nipple tenderness, or presence of cracks on nipple (in lactating client) may occur 2–3 days postpartum and result in severe discomfort.
Review appropriate interventions specific to lactating/nonlactating client. (Refer to CP: The Client at 4 Hours to 2 Days Postpartum; ND: Pain, [acute]/[Discomfort].)	Reduces level of discomfort/pain, enhancing self-care ability and sense of control.
Assess uterine tenderness; determine presence and frequency/intensity of afterpains.	Afterpains may continue for 2–3 days postpartum, although their frequency and intensity lessen with time. Factors intensifying afterpains include multiparity, uterine overdistension, and breastfeeding.
Ascertain frequency/amount of voidings. Instruct client in use of Kegel exercise. (Refer to ND: Urinary Elimination, risk for altered.)	Return of normal bladder function may take 4–7 days, and overdistension of bladder may create feelings of urgency and discomfort. Kegel exercise aids in healing and recovery of tone of pubococcygeal muscle to limit urinary stress incontinence.
Inspect condition of perineum or site of episiotomy repair. Note swelling, ecchymosis, lacerations, or discomfort. Recommend that client inspect area daily to evaluate healing process.	Identifies potential sources of pain and discomfort. Routine monitoring may prevent or lessen development of complications.
Recommend use of ice, topical sprays, ointments, creams; sitting with gluteal muscles contracted over site of episiotomy repair, and warm sitz (tub) baths.	Ice or other cold application is useful in the first 24 hr postpartum to reduce edema and provide localized anesthesia. After that, use of heat promotes vasodilation and perineal healing. Topical medications contain local anesthetics and reduce discomfort. Use of gluteal tightening while sitting reduces stress and direct pressure on perineum.
Inspect perineum for hemorrhoids. Suggest reinsertion of hemorrhoid with lubricated finger cot or rubber glove.	Aids in regression of hemorrhoids, reduces vulvar varicosities, and promotes return to normal bowel functioning.

Discuss continuing increased intake of fluid/dietary fiber, and regular exercise program.

Prevention of constipation helps limit discomfort of defecation/hemorrhoids.

Provide information about needs for sleep and rest; assess emotional state and well-being.

Overwhelming fatigue and negative feelings may magnify discomfort associated with normal healing and regeneration in the postpartal period.

Encourage client to adopt progressive level of ambulation and activity. Assess cultural impact on activity.

Early, progressive ambulation facilitates bladder and bowel functioning and enhances circulation, thereby reducing edema and promoting healing. Various cultural groups believe in restricting activity (e.g., some Southeast Asians may believe that the mother should remain in bed close to a fireplace for 30 days after delivery; some Latin cultures adhere to both dietary and rest restrictions for specific periods of time; some Native-American mothers may remain indoors with their infant for 20 days or until the umbilical cord drops off).

Collaborative

Suggest use of mild analgesics as recommended or prescribed by healthcare provider. Emphasize need to avoid products containing aspirin. For lactating client, medications should be taken 30–60 min prior to breastfeeding.

Promotes comfort without side effects of acetylsalicylic acid (reduced prothrombin synthesis may possibly increase lochial discharge). Analgesics given early enough to allow onset of action can reduce discomfort associated with oxytocin stimulation of myometrium during lactation.

Suggest use of bulk additives, such as Metamucil, or use of stool softeners, as indicated.

Enhances bowel elimination, reducing discomfort of constipation and associated hemorrhoids. (Refer to CP: The Client at 4 Hours to 2 Days Postpartum; ND: Constipation.)

NURSING DIAGNOSIS:	KNOWLEDGE deficit [LEARNING NEED], regarding progression of condition, self care needs, and possible complications
May Be Related To:	Unfamiliarity with information resources, lack of recall/incomplete information presented, misinterpretation
Possibly Evidenced By:	Verbalizations of concerns/misconceptions, hesitancy in or inadequate performance of activities
DESIRED OUTCOMES/EVALUATION CRITERIA—CLIENT WILL:	Verbalize understanding of physiological changes, individual needs, expected outcomes. Perform necessary activities/procedures correctly and explain reasons for actions.

ACTIONS/INTERVENTIONS

RATIONALE

Independent

Assess client's knowledge, understanding, and ability to apply concepts related to self-care.

Usually, some information is presented during hospitalization; however, fatigue, anxiety, or time limitations may have a negative impact on learning at that time. Additional teaching and/or reinforcement may therefore be needed.

351

Identify client's perception of learning needs regarding self-care and of needs related to anticipated physical and emotional changes.	Collaborative plan based on client's perceived needs reduces anxiety, promotes self-responsibility, and optimizes learning.
Provide information related to normal uterine involution, lochial changes, and the benefits of fundal massage.	Self-massage stimulates uterine contractility, reduces lochial flow, and promotes involution.
Review nutritional status; note prenatal Hb/Hct levels and estimated blood loss during delivery. Provide appropriate information about dietary and fluid needs. (Refer to CP: The Client at 1 Week Following Discharge; ND: Nutrition: altered, risk for less than body requirements)	Healthy dietary intake is essential to facilitate recuperation, and promote lactation as desired.
Provide information about breast care for nonlactating client, including discussion of the need for support, application of ice, decreased nipple stimulation, and only minimal expression of breast milk to relieve pressure.	Mechanical means of lactation suppression through use of binder and ice are recommended over lactation suppressants, which have fallen out of favor because of the high rate of rebound engorgement.
Provide information for lactating client, including nipple and breast care, physiology of lactation, concept of demand feedings, infant positioning, dietary and fluid needs, and the need to avoid taking medications without first consulting healthcare provider.	Helps promote successful lactation, enhances milk supply, and reduces possible trauma to nipples. Some drugs are contraindicated and should be used with caution during lactation because of possible effects on newborn.
Discuss need for adequate sleep and rest. (Refer to ND: Sleep Pattern disturbance).	Extra sleep and rest are needed to overcome sleep deficit and fatigue, and to facilitate coping.
Provide information regarding hygiene and perineal care.	Helps facilitate autonomy, prevent infection, and aid healing.
Discuss importance of progressive postpartal exercise program.	Beneficial in toning musculature; increases circulation, and enhances feelings of general well-being.
Review importance of preventing venous stasis and signs/symptoms of complications (e.g., warmth, redness, tenderness, presence of positive Homans' sign).	Plasma losses, increased platelets, and persistent vasodilation from progesterone increase likelihood of venous stasis (e.g., visible varicosities) and thrombophlebitis.
Discuss relationship between parenting role, use of effective coping mechanisms, and physical and emotional factors (e.g., adequate rest, nutrition, and support).	Provides information to assist client in making decisions regarding routine activities that foster positive physical and emotional adaptation.
Review symptoms/normalcy of transitory depression (postpartal blues).	As many as 80% of mothers experience a transitory depression, which usually resolves spontaneously within a week or so. Persistence of mood swings and emotional lability indicates need for further evaluation.
Provide number of 24-hr telephone resource contact.	Promotes reassurance that assistance is available if needed.
Reinforce importance of 4- to 6-wk postpartal examination by healthcare provider.	Follow-up visit is necessary to evaluate recovery of reproductive organs, healing of incision/episiotomy repair, general well-being, and adaptation to life changes.
Refer family to community resource groups or for follow-up with social services or home healthcare agency as indicated.	Provides information and emotional support; reduces possibility of negative outcome for infant and family.

NURSING DIAGNOSIS:	SLEEP PATTERN disturbance
May Be Related To:	Hormonal and psychological responses (intense exhilaration, anxiety, excitement), pain/discomfort, exhausting process of labor and delivery, needs/demands of family members
Possibly Evidenced By:	Verbal reports of difficulty falling asleep/not feeling well rested, irritability, dark circles under eyes, frequent yawning
DESIRED OUTCOMES/EVALUATION CRITERIA—CLIENT WILL:	Identify adjustments to accommodate changes required by demands of new family member.
	Attain at least 8 hr of sleep per night and nap daily.
	Report feeling rested.

ACTIONS/INTERVENTIONS	RATIONALE

Independent

Assess client's perception of fatigue, needs for sleep, and sleep deficits.	Identifies client's perception of the severity of the problem.
Assess home environment, family size and situation, routine, and available help including whether client's partner can take paternity leave.	The client who is discharged early may believe that she has to take on sole responsibility for infant care tasks, as well as immediately assuming her former roles associated with household management and mother tasks. Such a situation results in excess fatigue, intensifying a sleep deficit.
Assist client in planning rest/sleep periods during day (especially when infant is napping), being realistic within the schedule of family members. Discuss need to retire earlier than usual while infant is waking for night feedings.	Examination of household pattern allows realistic appraisal of available times for resting and sleeping, and how family schedule can be revised.
Provide information related to positive aspects of sleep and rest.	Sleep and inactivity reduce basal metabolic rate and allow oxygen and nutrients to be used for healing.
Encourage client to take a vitamin and iron tablet daily, and to select appropriate diet.	Helps restore Hb levels needed to transport oxygen and promote healing; helps overcome nutritional deficiencies, which contribute to feelings of excess fatigue and inadequate energy levels.
Encourage limitation of number and length of visiting sessions/use of visitors to assist with childcare, homemaker activities.	Overexhaustion may result from time spent with frequent visitors and well-meaning friends. Involving friends in providing meaningful assistance can be rewarding for the client and her support group.
Note prenatal Hb/Hct levels and estimated blood loss.	Low Hb/Hct levels increase feelings of fatigue, weakness, and faintness necessitating further evaluation/intervention.

NURSING DIAGNOSIS:	SELF CARE risk for deficit
Risk Factors May Include:	Fatigue, decreased endurance, pain/discomfort
Possibly Evidenced By:	[Not applicable; presence of signs/symptoms establishes an *actual* diagnosis]

353

ACTIONS/INTERVENTIONS	RATIONALE
Independent	
Assess client's physical and psychological well-being.	Any alteration in physical or emotional well-being may retard assumption of autonomous role in self-care. Until client moves from a "taking in" to a "taking hold" phase, she may require assistance with self-care and infant care.
Determine client's fatigue level, length of labor, time of delivery (i.e., day or night), and sleep deficit before and since delivery. (Refer to ND: Sleep Pattern disturbance.)	Physical need for sleep must be met before client can begin to assume self-care.
Note degree of autonomy and self-responsibility. Determine cultural influence.	Client begins to assume increasing responsibility for her own care as her condition improves. However, some cultures require specific periods of bedrest for the new mother following delivery and may even restrict personal hygiene activities (e.g., some Arab- or African-Americans may be reluctant to shower or bathe until after cessation of lochial flow, and some Mexican-Americans believe the new mother should care for her infant while other family members take responsibility for her care).
Evaluate client's understanding of postpartal needs and self-responsibility. Provide information as needed.	Knowledge base determines amount of information necessary to facilitate assuming self-care role.
Review plans for home assistance during recovery period.	Help in home, especially for the first several days following discharge, is critical to assist the client and her family with household management and meal preparation, and to provide care as needed for client and infant.
Discuss available community resources (e.g., additional discharge visit by hospital/health maintenance organization [HMO] nurse, visiting nurse services, home care aide).	Visiting nurse can assess health status of client. Home care aide, now an integral part of many hospital early-discharge programs, assists in home management and provides specific infant/client care as necessary. Note: Some doulas may provide services to mother during early-discharge period.

NURSING DIAGNOSIS:	**INFECTION, risk for**
Risk Factors May Include:	Tissue trauma and/or broken skin, decreased Hb, invasive procedures, and/or increased environmental exposure
Possibly Evidenced By:	[Not applicable; presence of signs/symptoms establishes an *actual* diagnosis]
DESIRED OUTCOMES/EVALUATION CRITERIA—CLIENT WILL:	Identify techniques to reduce risks and/or promote healing.
	Display wound free of purulent drainage.
	Be free of infection, be afebrile, and have normal lochial flow and character.

ACTIONS/INTERVENTIONS	RATIONALE

Independent

Assess client's temperature, pulse, and respirations.

Reinforce medical asepsis for pad changes, and application of topical sprays, ointments, or witch hazel compresses.

Encourage client to take warm sitz baths 3–4 times daily for 20 min, especially if signs of localized congestion/infection are present.

Reiterate instructions regarding fundal massage (i.e., gently 4–5 times, several times per day, with cupped hand, using second hand for support above symphysis pubis).

Note amount and odor of lochial discharge. Review normal progression from rubra to serosa to alba.

Evaluate condition of nipples.

Recommended routine examination of breasts and perineum.

Provide information about UTI and evaluate client for signs and symptoms, including dysuria, frequency, urgency, and pain. Note any tenderness of suprapubic or costovertebral angle.

Review importance of nutrition, fluid intake, and adequate test.

Rationale:

Elevation of vital signs may reflect developing infection.

Helps prevent rectal contaminants from entering vagina or urethra.

Promotes localized vasodilation, and increased oxygenation of tissues, enhancing healing.

Enhances uterine contractility. Uterus involutes approximately 1–2 cm (1 finger breadth) per day from the level of the umbilicus. Delayed involution may suggest infection.

Lochia normally has a fleshy odor; however, in endometritis, the discharge may be purulent and foul-smelling, and may fail to demonstrate normal progression.

The development of nipple fissures/cracks potentiates risk of mastitis.

Early detection of developing problems allows for timely intervention, thereby reducing the risk of serious complications.

Stasis, poor hygiene, overdistension, or bacteria introduced during labor and delivery may predispose client to development of UTI.

Promotes healing and general well-being, reducing risk of infection.

Collaborative

Obtain "clean catch" urine specimen for culture, if signs or symptoms present. Notify healthcare provider.

Discuss rationale and protocol for administration of antibiotic therapy if UTI is present.

Discuss findings suggestive of endometritis with physician or nurse midwife. Help family arrange for transportation to health center or hospital emergency room for further assessment.

Initiate use of home IV service or visiting nurse services if antibiotic by parenteral infusion is ordered. (Refer to CP: Puerperal Infection.)

Rationale:

Verifies presence and type of infection, and appropriate treatment needs.

Antibiotic therapy eradicates pathogenic organisms.

Findings need to be confirmed by healthcare provider and laboratory culture.

Allows client to remain at home while receiving treatment to eradicate infection. Note: Obstetric department may provide follow-up/home visit services during initial recovery period.

NURSING DIAGNOSIS:	FLUID VOLUME, risk for deficit
Risk Factors May Include:	Reduced intake and/or inadequate replacement, increased urine output, excessive bleeding at delivery/early postpartum

355

ACTIONS/INTERVENTIONS	RATIONALE
Independent	
Assess BP and pulse.	Risk of postpartal hemorrhage exists up to 28 days following delivery. Possible causes of hemorrhage include inadequate myometrial contractions (uterine atony), retention of placental tissue, and birth canal lacerations. Hypotension and tachycardia may reflect hypovolemia.
Reinforce the use of uterine massage and fundal monitoring.	Promotes uterine contractility, reducing risk of atony and hemorrhage.
Discuss normal involutionary changes and signs of subinvolution.	Client should be able to identify signs of hemorrhage and institute appropriate interventions if excessive bleeding occurs. (Refer to CP: Postpartal Hemorrhage.)
Assess client's understanding of normal lochial changes.	Briskly flowing, bright red lochia with clots is abnormal and indicates possible hemorrhage. Multiparas or clients with overdistension of the uterus tend to have more lochia than primiparas. Breastfeeding clients have an increased amount of lochia during or just after feedings.
Assist client using a mirror to assess own episiotomy/laceration repair.	Lacerations of the birth canal constitute the second leading cause of postdelivery hemorrhage.
Discuss needs for fluid replacement and signs of dehydration, especially in lactating client.	Client should consume at least eight glasses or more of fluid per day to replace losses and to provide sufficient fluid for milk production.
Assess voiding frequency and amounts.	Kidney function is an indicator of circulating blood volume.
Collaborative	
Notify healthcare provider if fundus remains boggy or fails to contract with massage.	Oxytocin (Pitocin) or methylergonovine (Methergine) may be required to correct uterine atony/reduce bleeding. Client may need to be evaluated by healthcare provider for possible readmission to acute-care setting or administration of medication in outpatient clinic.
Prepare client and her family for transfer to clinic or hospital setting, if necessary.	Situation may warrant additional evaluation/intervention, use of hospital emergency equipment, or treatment for stabilization purposes.

NURSING DIAGNOSIS:	**URINARY ELIMINATION, risk for altered**
Risk Factors May Include:	Hormonal effects (fluid shifts and/or increased renal plasma flow), mechanical trauma, tissue edema

Possibly Evidenced By:	[Not applicable; presence of signs/symptoms establishes an *actual* diagnosis]
DESIRED OUTCOMES/EVALUATION CRITERIA—CLIENT WILL:	Empty bladder with each void.

ACTIONS/INTERVENTIONS	RATIONALE
Independent	
Assess urinary functioning, noting frequency and amount of voidings per day, and feelings of urine retention or bladder fullness.	Voidings should be moderate in amount (at least 100 ml) to be considered sufficient, although client usually does not measure them at home. Client should empty her bladder 5–7 times per day, depending on amount of prenatal fluid retention and degree of diuresis. Retention may occur, possibly leading to infection or overdistension, which may cause nerve damage.
Assess fundal height and location before and after voiding. Note displacement to the right of umbilicus.	A full bladder displaces the fundus and may interfere with contraction or involution of uterus.
Discuss normal fluid needs and replacement.	Six to eight glasses of fluid per day help prevent stasis and dehydration, replacing fluid lost at delivery.
Note prenatal and intrapartal history of episodes of UTI, catheterizations, or bladder trauma.	These factors may contribute to infection, with consequent alteration in pattern of elimination.
Instruct client to do 50–100 Kegel exercises daily.	Increases circulation to perineum and helps treat stress incontinence.
Encourage client to sit in warm bath or take a warm shower if she has difficulty voiding.	Warm water running over the body enhances relaxation of the perineum and urethra, facilitating voiding.

THE CLIENT AT 1 WEEK FOLLOWING DISCHARGE

CLIENT ASSESSMENT DATA BASE

Circulation

Vital signs within normal limits

Ego Integrity

Emotional tone and responses may vary from one of delight to a sense of overwhelming disorganization or anxiety, especially in first-time mother. Irritability, crying, "postpartum blues."

Elimination

May report voiding difficulty or stress incontinence
May report difficulty with bowel evacuation, with decreased frequency, hard-formed stool

Pain/Discomfort

May report continued discomfort associated with afterpains.
Engorgement may be present in lactating client.

Safety

Episiotomy or cesarean incision free of edema, indurated areas, redness, and exudate; tissue edges approximated

Sexuality

Uterus nontender, palpable at symphysis pubis.
Lochial flow scant and pinkish-brown in color (serosa) and of 4–10 days' duration.
Breasts in lactating client increased in size with increased milk supply.
Nipples free of redness, cracks, and fissures.
Engorgement may be present in lactating client, subsiding in nonlactating client.

DIAGNOSTIC STUDIES

Urine: Negative for albumin/glucose.
Additional testing as indicated; e.g., UA, culture and sensitivity, Hb/Hct or CBC to include WBC count.

NURSING PRIORITIES

1. Promote maternal/infant well-being.
2. Foster optimal adaptation to physical emotional changes.
3. Provide anticipatory guidance for optimal integration of new family member and adaptation to role changes.

NURSING DIAGNOSIS:	FATIGUE, risk for
Risk Factors May Include:	Physical and emotional demands of infant and other family members, psychological stressors, continued discomfort
Possibly Evidenced By:	[Not applicable; presence of signs/symptoms establishes an *actual* diagnosis]
DESIRED OUTCOMES/EVALUATION CRITERIA—CLIENT WILL:	Identify basis of fatigue and individual areas of control. Report improved sense of energy.

ACTIONS/INTERVENTIONS	RATIONALE
Independent	
Discuss signs of excess physical and emotional fatigue.	Lack of energy, deep circles under the eyes, and statements suggesting extreme fatigue indicate inadequate sleep and rest. Self-monitoring and awareness of developing problem allow for timely intervention.
Review intrapartal and early postpartal events.	Cumulative sleep loss must be overcome as soon as possible to facilitate psychological and physiological recuperation.
Determine infant's sleep-wake cycles. Suggest ongoing efforts to modify the infant's behaviors to promote more wakeful periods during the daytime and recommend that mother naps when infant does.	Helps infant to maintain progressively longer wakeful periods during the day and to sleep longer stretches at night. Note: Approximately 5 wk are needed to regulate the infant's cycle.
Encourage restriction or lessening of outside activities. Limit number of visitors.	Helps prevent overexhaustion.
Provide information about daily iron and vitamin intake and the need for a balanced diet.	Helps restore Hb levels needed for oxygen transport, promotes healing, and overcomes nutritional deficiencies, which may contribute to feelings of excess fatigue and inadequate energy levels.
Determine family structure and number of members. Assess work capabilities and responsibilities of each member.	Household tasks should be shared so that division of labor reduces amount of responsibility that client assumes and allows client to conserve energy.
Review family's daily routine.	Assists client in creative problem solving to identify times available for resting and napping throughout the day.
Assess availability/use of support systems (including doulas, as appropriate).	Identifies needs and means of physical and emotional assistance.
Encourage client to establish a quiet, relaxing routine prior to retiring (e.g., reading a book or having a glass of warm milk or wine).	Aids in relaxation; promotes sleep.

NURSING DIAGNOSIS:	**KNOWLEDGE deficit [LEARNING NEED], regarding self care and infant care**
May Be Related To:	Lack of exposure/recall, misinterpretation, unfamiliarity with resources
Possibly Evidenced By:	Verbalization of concerns/misconceptions, hesitancy in or inadequate performance of activities, inappropriate behaviors (e.g., excessive crying)
DESIRED OUTCOMES/EVALUATION CRITERIA—CLIENT WILL:	Identify individual learning needs.
	Perform necessary activities/procedures correctly and explain reasons for the actions.
	Verbalize understanding of physiological changes, individual and infant needs.
	Modify behaviors, when appropriate.

359

ACTIONS/INTERVENTIONS	RATIONALE

Independent

Determine client's perception of problems and needs.	Establishes individual needs and promotes problem solving.
Ascertain understanding of normal physical changes at 1 wk following discharge. Provide information about appropriate measures to take, should a problem arise.	Identifies normal and abnormal physical findings, and encourages anticipatory planning, enhancing independence.
Identify emotional concerns at this time, and discuss normalcy of these feelings. Note reports of depressed mood/tearfulness, emotional lability, with insomnia, poor concentration, headaches.	Most mothers, especially first-time mothers, verbalize a sense of disorganization and feeling of an emotional letdown in the early postpartal period. Such feelings are intensified by fatigue and crying infant. In addition, postpartal or "baby" blues occur in 50%–80% of clients. Symptoms are usually transient, beginning about day 3 postpartum and often resolve without therapeutic intervention in 1–2 wk.
Provide information as needed about signs and symptoms associated with endometritis, mastitis, incisional infection, and UTI, and the need to notify healthcare provider.	Identifies potential problems necessitating prompt evaluation/intervention.
Provide information regarding resumption of menstrual cycle/ovulation and sexual intercourse.	Among nonlactating women, 40% menstruate by 2 wk postpartum; of these, 50% do not ovulate during the first menstrual cycle. Among lactating women, 15% resume menstrual cycle by 6 wk postpartum, and 80% of the first menstrual cycles are anovulatory. Couple can resume sexual activity when client is comfortable and lochial flow has ceased (usually 3–4 wk after vaginal delivery). Client who underwent cesarean delivery should delay intercourse until 6 wk postpartum.
Discuss plans for contraceptive usage.	Conception could occur prior to the 4- to 6-wk checkup, and studies indicate increased risk of complications or untoward outcomes for pregnancies spaced close together. Couple needs to select and use a temporary or permanent method of family planning that meets their individual needs.
Provide information about physiological changes in sexual response postpartum. (Refer to CP: The Client at 4 to 6 Weeks Following Delivery; ND: Sexuality Patterns, altered.)	Reduction in rapidity and intensity of sexual response is normal. Continued low estrogen levels result in vaginal dryness, possibly necessitating use of water-soluble jelly, cocoa butter, or contraceptive creams or jellies for lubrication. Size of orgasmic platform and strength of orgasmic contraction are reduced, and vasoconstriction of labia minora and labia majora is delayed.
Reinforce information, as appropriate, for lactating client regarding physiology of lactation, dietary concerns, measures to reduce discomfort of engorgement, and nipple/breast care. Recommend books and other written materials, videos, and related support groups.	Facilitates positive adaptation to breast feeding role.
Review nutritional needs for lactating or nonlactating client; include information on caloric needs, protein, iron, and vitamin C. (Refer to ND: Nutrition: altered, less than body requirements.)	Helps client meet nutritional needs necessary for recuperation, restoration, and healing in postpartal period.

Emphasize need to prevent venous stasis, and review signs of phlebitis formation, e.g. warmth, redness, tenderness, calf pain.

Instruct client in appropriate perineal muscle-tightening exercises, e.g., Kegel exercise.

Discuss/evaluate ongoing exercise program. Provide information about importance of adhering to prescribed program.

Provide information for client with cesarean birth regarding activity level and exercise and the need to avoid strenuous lifting/stretching.

Reinforce need for evaluation by healthcare provider at 4–6 weeks after delivery.

Identify community resources, e.g., breastfeeding support groups, parenting classes, Family Effectiveness Training (FET).

Changes in circulating volume or cellular components and alterations in mobility increase risk of thrombophlebitis.

Helps strengthen and tone perineal urethral muscles to improve control of urine flow.

Exercise helps tone muscles and restore body contours.

Lifting any object heavier than the baby for 2 wk after delivery may contribute to stress on healing tissues and result in wound dehiscence.

Necessary to ensure that physiological/emotional homeostasis has been re-established.

Helps meet continued educational and developmental needs of client/couple.

NURSING DIAGNOSIS:	PARENT/INFANT ATTACHMENT; PARENTING, risk for altered
Risk Factors May Include:	Lack of support between/from significant others, multiple demands of home/family, excess fatigue, unrealistic expectations for self/infant/partner, presence of stressors (e.g., financial, housing, employment, use of outside helper/extended family members)
Possibly Evidenced By:	[Not applicable; presence of signs/symptoms establishes an *actual* diagnosis]
DESIRED OUTCOMES/EVALUATION CRITERIA—CLIENT/COUPLE WILL:	Demonstrate appropriate bonding behaviors. Identify concerns related to parenting. Discuss parenting role realistically. Identify available resources.

ACTIONS/INTERVENTIONS

RATIONALE

Independent

Assess client's/couple's interaction with infant. Document verbal and nonverbal responses and presence of positive or negative behaviors.

Note impact of culture on interaction.

Assess client's/couple's strengths and weaknesses, maturity level, reaction to conception, and preparation for parenting.

Determine client's/couple's perception of infant behaviors.

In American culture, attachment is considered positive if the parent makes eye contact with the infant, calls the infant by name, uses an en face position, talks in a high-pitched voice, and holds the baby close. Lack of culturally appropriate attachment behaviors places infant at risk for abuse.

Different cultures have different values/beliefs about what constitutes positive attachment behaviors.

Directly impacts on ability/desire to gain comfort/skill in parenting.

Client/couple with unrealistic perception of infant behaviors or who voices displeasure with specific

361

Develop plan for subsequent visits, highlighting areas of particular concern.

caretaking tasks (e.g., diapering/feeding) will need closer monitoring and more extensive support.

Helps promote positive adaptation to new role; helps client focus on possible problems.

Collaborative

Refer family to social services, home healthcare agency, volunteer support program (e.g., Bright Beginnings, First Visitor), or to community resource groups.

Provides support and reduces possible negative outcomes for infant/family. Volunteer support programs provide home visitation, ongoing follow-up as indicated, and role modeling of parenting skills.

NURSING DIAGNOSIS:	PAIN/[DISCOMFORT], risk for
Risk Factors May Include:	Tissue edema/engorgement, mechanical trauma, excessive fatigue
Possibly Evidenced By:	[Not applicable; presence of signs/symptoms establishes an *actual* diagnosis]
DESIRED OUTCOMES/EVALUATION CRITERIA—CLIENT WILL:	Use appropriate measures to promote comfort. Verbalize relief of pain/discomfort.

ACTIONS/INTERVENTIONS	RATIONALE

Independent

Determine location/nature of discomfort.

Identifies individual needs.

Review sleep/rest pattern; note feelings of excess fatigue.

Fatigue can negatively affect lactation and increase discomforts associated with engorgement, as well as impair coping and client's response to pain.

Inspect breasts for degree of engorgement.

Helps determine severity of problem. Engorgement is usually more severe in primipara than in multipara.

Encourage use of supportive bra.

Supports and uplifts, alleviating pain and tenderness caused by heavy, engorged breasts.

Recommend application of ice or cool compresses for 20–30 min 3–4 times daily, for nonlactating client; apply breast binder. Advise client to avoid breast stimulation or milk expression.

Provides vasoconstriction of blood vessels; promotes local anesthesia and comfort. Prevents or reduces milk production and engorgement.

Encourage use of creams, air drying of nipples for 20 min after feedings, avoidance of soaps, and avoidance of plastic liners inside nursing pads. Instruct client to change pads when wet or moist.

Helps toughen nipples and prevent cracking. By allowing nipples to remain in a moist environment, plastic liners promote bacterial growth and may cause skin breakdown.

Note frequency and length of feedings in lactating client.

Engorgement may interfere with breastfeeding, because it makes the breast and nipple hard, making it difficult for the infant to suckle. Increasing frequency of feedings during engorgement promotes comfort and helps to empty breasts to ensure an adequate milk supply.

Suggest warm compresses/shower before feedings for lactating client.

Aids in let-down reflex to promote easier emptying during feeding.

Instruct lactating client in removal of milk through manual expression or use of breast pump.

Removal of milk from breast often provides relief from engorgement; however, removal of too much

Inspect nipples for any areas of indurated masses, cracks, fissures, or redness.

milk increases the milk supply, possibly causing further engorgement.

Sore or cracked nipples can create intense discomfort during lactation, especially at the beginning of the feeding when the infant is most hungry and sucking is most intense.

Limit feedings to 5 min on each breast when nipple is cracked, gradually increasing feedings by 2 min each day. Initiate feeding on nontender/less tender nipple for several feedings in succession if only one nipple is sore or cracked.

Helps limit exposure to trauma; however, limiting sucking for too long reduces milk supply and promotes engorgement. Baby suckles most intensely in the first 5 min of the feeding, creating greater pressure on the initial breast.

Note fundal height; assess for rigidity or guarding on examination. Note presence of foul-smelling lochia.

Uterine discomfort should have disappeared by 1 wk following discharge. Continued tenderness may signify infection.

Inspect site of episiotomy repair or cesarean incision.

Continued discomfort, tenderness, edema, or loss of tissue approximation indicates need for further evaluation by healthcare provider.

Suggest continued sitz baths 3–4 times daily for 20 min if site of episiotomy is uncomfortable, or if third- to fourth-degree lacerations were present at delivery.

Promotes vasodilation and increased tissue oxygenation/nutrition, enhancing healing.

Collaborative

Suggest use of mild, nonaspirin analgesics if necessary, especially 30–60 min before breastfeeding.

Reduces discomfort and promotes relaxation during feeding; facilitates the let-down reflex in lactating client.

Refer to healthcare provider if uterine or wound discomfort is excessive.

Further evaluation is needed to determine the cause of discomfort and appropriate interventions.

NURSING DIAGNOSIS:	**FAMILY COPING: potential for growth**
May Be Related To:	Sufficiently meeting individual needs and adaptive tasks, enabling goals of self-actualization to surface
Possibly Evidenced By:	Family member(s) moving in direction of health-promoting and enriching lifestyle
DESIRED OUTCOMES/EVALUATION CRITERIA—CLIENT/FAMILY WILL:	Verbalize gradual improvement and smooth transition of new family member into home situation.
	Identify tasks leading to desired changes.
	Express feelings of self-confidence and satisfaction with progress and adaptation being made.

ACTIONS/INTERVENTIONS

RATIONALE

Independent

Evaluate situational support and home assistance used (e.g., husband, relatives, friends, private duty nurses, home care service).

Home assistance is an essential element in facilitating postpartal adaptation.

Determine past successful coping mechanisms.

Building on strengths promotes self-esteem and enhances ability to deal with current situation.

Encourage client to rest and to assume only the responsibilities directly related to care of herself and of the newborn. Encourage client to allow others to take on responsibilities related to upkeep of the house and meals.

Allows client to focus energy on interaction between infant and herself; allows client to conserve energy for physical and emotional recuperation.

Discuss client's/couple's perceptions of adjustment to the infant and to parenting roles and responsibilities. Provide information about normalcy of feelings of inadequacy, stress, and disequilibrium associated with role transition, especially for first-time parents. Document areas of concern for future assessments.

First-time parents have been known to experience varying degrees of stress and crisis associated with adjustment to their child and integration of this child into the family. The challenge of the crisis can serve as a catalyst to growth and enhanced adaptive capacity.

Evaluate family structure and situation, relationships of individual members to one another, and cultural background.

Blended family resulting from remarriage may require a longer period of adaptation and present a more complex situation than a nuclear family. Extended families may provide added physical and emotional support if available, especially for adjustment to single parent. Note: Folk beliefs/rituals/customs may dictate who provides assistance for client/family.

Provide anticipatory guidance related to the time needed to adjust to the new situation and family member.

Period of stress associated with adjustment to the birth of a newborn is often resolved in 4–6 wk. However, because of the potentially overwhelming transition required, this period may last as long as 3 mo.

Collaborative

Refer to parent support group.
Discuss need for family counseling; make appropriate referrals, when indicated.

May be necessary to help members resolve changes and to continue positive adjustment to new roles.

NURSING DIAGNOSIS:	NUTRITION: altered, risk for less than body requirements
Risk Factors May Include:	Intake insufficient to meet metabolic demands/correct existing deficiencies (e.g., lactation, anemia/excessive blood loss, infection/excessive tissue trauma, desire to regain prenatal weight)
Possibly Evidenced By:	[Not applicable; presence of signs/symptoms establishes an *actual* diagnosis]
DESIRED OUTCOMES/EVALUATION CRITERIA—CLIENT WILL:	Report dietary intake that meets needs for lactation (as appropriate) and tissue healing/general physical restoration. Continue to take daily vitamin preparation as indicated.

ACTIONS/INTERVENTIONS	RATIONALE

Independent

Determine dietary intake for past 24 hr, history of dietary habits prior to and during pregnancy, and cultural beliefs/background.

Identifies usual eating habits/deficiencies and individual needs. Cultural practices may dictate intake of special foods (e.g., Hmong people eat only chicken and white rice for 30 days postpartum).

Provide information regarding the basic food groups. Stress need for increased amounts (and food sources) of dietary protein, calories, and vitamin C while considering constraints of family budget and cultural preferences.	Helps correct deficiencies and inadequacies. Protein is needed to promote tissue growth, healing, and regeneration and to offset catabolic process. Calories are necessary for normal metabolic processes, especially for the underweight client; vitamin C is necessary for cell wall synthesis. Financial needs may necessitate use of protein sources other than meat.
Review prenatal Hb and Hct and the amount of blood loss at delivery. Note signs of anemia (e.g., dizziness, excess fatigue, and pallor).	Preexisting anemic state or excessive blood loss may result in pallor and listlessness. Reduced Hb levels may retard healing process.
Provide information about need for daily intake of vitamin and iron preparation, as indicated.	Iron and vitamin intake for 4–6 wk postpartum can overcome dietary deficiencies, ensure nutritious milk supply (as desired), and aid in tissue healing.
Suggest temporary use of ready-made convenience foods or having meals prepared by relatives, friends, or significant other(s).	Demands of caring for newborn leave little time for preparation of balanced meals.
Weigh client. Establish desired weight, and compare with prepregnancy and initial postpartum weight.	Average weight loss at delivery is 10–12 lb, mainly attributable to infant and products of conception. An additional loss of approximately 5 lb usually follows over the next 2 wk.
Determine caloric requirements for nonlactating client and possible weight reduction diet.	Caloric requirements return to prepregnancy levels, unless client was severely underweight. Desired weight can be obtained by reducing caloric intake by 300 kcal/day and establishing an appropriate exercise program.
Discuss dietary needs for the lactating client. Identify foods that may have risk of allergic or other adverse effects on infant. Identify ways of assessing infant's discomfort.	Intake needs to be increased by 500–800 kcal/day to provide adequate milk production and infant nourishment. Protein needs are 10 g less than they were during pregnancy. Needs for iron, calcium, thiamine, ascorbic acid, and vitamin D are similar to those during pregnancy; the need for vitamin A, niacin, and riboflavin increases. Some foods are passed through the mother's milk and may cause discomfort or allergic reaction in the infant.
Review importance of fluid intake of 2500–3000 ml/day for lactating client.	Necessary to support adequate milk production to meet infant's needs as well as client's own bodily needs.
Provide information regarding progressive postpartal exercise program. Provide illustrations/demonstration as needed.	Exercise increases metabolic rate and improves utilization of calories while enhancing muscle tone.

Collaborative

Consult with dietitian, as needed.	May be necessary to plan and restructure diet to meet individual needs/restrictions.

NURSING DIAGNOSIS:	**INFECTION, risk for**
Risk Factors May Include:	Tissue trauma and/or broken skin, decreased Hb, invasive procedures and/or increased environmental exposure, malnutrition
Possibly Evidenced By:	[Not applicable; presence of signs/symptoms establishes an actual diagnosis]

DESIRED OUTCOMES/EVALUATION CRITERIA—CLIENT WILL:	Relate techniques to reduce risks and promote healing.
	Display signs of wound healing and be free of purulent drainage.
	Be free of infection.

ACTIONS/INTERVENTIONS	RATIONALE

Independent

Check vital signs; assess client's general physical status.	Temperature greater than 100.4°F (38°C), general malaise, anorexia, and chills suggest infection.
Review intrapartal and postpartal events, noting prolonged labor, premature rupture of membranes, excessive blood loss, or retained/adherent placenta.	These factors increase risk of endometritis or other infectious process.
Determine whether infant was colonized with staphylococci in the nursery.	Increases risk of cross-contamination, especially to lactating clients.
Evaluate client's hygiene practices. Stress need for washing hands before and after perineal pad changes and before handling breasts or infant.	Identifies practices that could contribute to development of infection.
Assess height of fundus. Note color, amount, and character of lochial flow.	Endometritis may be associated with subinvolution or with presence of foul-smelling or purulent lochial flow.
Inspect site of episiotomy repair or cesarean incision. Note redness, exudate, or loss of tissue approximation.	These signs indicate presence of infectious process, requiring further evaluation/intervention.
Assess nipples for cracks or fissures. Provide or reinforce information regarding breast and nipple care. Discuss use of creams, air drying of nipples, and need to avoid use of plastic-lined nursing pads.	Identifies potential source of infection. Breast care measures help toughen nipples, prevent skin breakdown and cracking, and limit presence of moisture, reducing risk of irritation/infection.
Discuss dietary practices. Stress need for increased amounts of food rich in protein, carbohydrates, iron, zinc and vitamins A, B-complex, and C.	Protein helps in tissue growth and healing; carbohydrates are necessary to spare proteins. Iron is used for Hb synthesis; zinc strengthens cell membranes; vitamin A supports differentiation and cell proliferation, and stimulates epithelialization; vitamin B enhances metabolism of proteins, carbohydrates, and lipids; vitamin C is needed for cell wall synthesis.
Note presence of risk factors such as delivery trauma, malnutrition, diabetes, previous UTI/renal problems, or use of indwelling catheter during hospital stay.	These factors may predispose the client to UTI following delivery.
Assess for, and review signs and symptoms of, UTI (e.g., dysuria, hematuria, frequency, urgency, retention, fever, and pain in suprapubic region or costovertebral angle).	UTI requires prompt evaluation and intervention to prevent further involvement and complications.
Note reports of stress incontinence.	May indicate cystocele and the need for further evaluation or surgical repair.
Instruct in use of appropriate muscle-tightening exercises (e.g., Kegel exercise).	Exercise strengthens and tones perineal and urethral muscles to improve control of urine flow and reduce risk of infection.

Test urine pH.

Alkaline urine increases potential for bacterial growth.

Encourage client to increase fluid intake, especially with cranberry or orange juice.

Helps prevent urinary stasis; produces more acidic urine reducing adherence of bacteria to bladder wall.

Collaborative

Assess laboratory results, especially WBC count.

Leukocytosis during initial 10–12 days postpartum is a normal protective mechanism associated with an increase in neutrophils and a shift to the left and must be distinguished from an abnormal finding indicating infection.

Obtain cultures of lochia, nipple discharge, wound drainage, or urine as indicated.

Confirms presence of infection and identifies type.

Discuss antibiotic administration, as appropriate.

Antimicrobial agent whose selection is based on culture and sensitivity findings helps eradicate pathogenic bacteria.

Refer for urologic consultation, as indicated.

May be needed for persistent symptoms, cystocele, or failure to respond to antimicrobial agents.

NURSING DIAGNOSIS:	ROLE PERFORMANCE, altered
May Be Related To:	Situational crisis (addition and demands of new family member, changes in responsibilities of family members)
Possibly Evidenced By:	Change in usual patterns or responsibility, conflict in roles
DESIRED OUTCOMES/EVALUATION CRITERIA—CLIENT WILL:	Verbalize awareness of role expectations and potential problems.
	Begin to set realistic goals.
	Talk with family members about situation and changes that have occurred.

ACTIONS/INTERVENTIONS

RATIONALE

Independent

Determine family structure and individual expectations.

The ease with which each family member adapts to the new role and accommodates the new member may be influenced by the size, stability, and complexity of the family. For example, the blended family may create special concerns, whereby the newborn is a half-brother or half-sister. Although all members of the family are to some extent influenced by the transition, the client herself often suffers the greatest impact in terms of personal and professional responsibilities and must make the most significant accommodations and sacrifices in terms of her time and energy.

Evaluate individual and family goals and client's perception of new family situation. Encourage open communication and sharing of feelings and concerns among family members.

Client who feels cheated, disappointed, or unfulfilled with the mothering role may have difficulty adapting, as may the mother who is forced to return to work for economic reasons but

367

Aid client in setting realistic goals and expectations for herself.

Assist client in acquiring skill and comfort in feeding and bathing infant.

Reinforce client's successes at mothering and specific accomplishments of individual family members.

Discuss concerns; provide information about potential sources and ways of evaluating child care providers.

Collaborative

Refer client to visiting nurse services or community support groups (e.g., La Leche League, step-family organizations).

Refer for professional counseling.

would prefer to remain at home. Identification of problems can be helpful in reaching solutions that are compatible for all concerned.

Too much activity and unrealistic goals compound fatigue and reduce energy levels needed for coping and role integration.

Client who is having difficulty or feels awkward providing care may believe that she is failing in her mothering skills.

Client's self-confidence may be tenuous; she may need constant assurance that she is performing well. Recognition of efforts of those involved supports ongoing change and participation in problem solving.

Sufficient time is required to select safe and appropriate resources that will meet individual needs and allow client to return to personal and professional activities.

Client may need additional assistance in home adjustment. Four weeks may be required for families to integrate infant care into their patterns of daily living.

Further intervention may be needed to promote positive individual and family adjustment.

NURSING DIAGNOSIS:	BODY IMAGE disturbance
May Be Related To:	Unrealistic expectations of postpartum recovery, permanency of some changes
Possibly Evidenced By:	Verbalization of negative feelings about body, feelings of helplessness, preoccupation with change, focus on past appearance, fear of rejection/reaction by others
DESIRED OUTCOMES/EVALUATION CRITERIA—CLIENT WILL:	Verbalize realistic perceptions of new body contours.
	Report acceptance of self as she is at this moment.
	Dress comfortably.
	Set realistic goals for change.
	Initiate progressive, ongoing prescribed exercise program.

ACTIONS/INTERVENTIONS	RATIONALE

Independent

Determine perception of new body image and of actual or imagined changes that pregnancy and childbirth created.	Client's self-esteem and adaptation to body image are influenced by her perceptions. The client who has fantasized or imagined that she would resume

Provide information honestly regarding integumentary and musculoskeletal changes.

her pregravid appearance and body contours following delivery may be depressed or disappointed when this has not occurred. The client may actually grieve the loss of her prepregnancy appearance. A potential crisis exists, particularly for the emotionally immature client who places much emphasis on appearance. The adolescent, whose primary focus may be dating or reentry into a heterosexual relationship, may experience even greater difficulty adapting to, and coping with, a new body image.

Chloasma, nevi, palmar erythema, fine hair growth, changes in condition of hair and fingernails, and joint hypermobility usually disappear or return to pregravid state. Coarse hair, areolar hyperpigmentation, linea nigra, increased foot growth, and spider nevi may not regress completely postpartum. Approximately 6 wk is required for abdominal wall and uterus to return to prepregnancy state.

Discuss ways of dressing attractively and the importance of taking time for personal appearance with application of cosmetics, trips to the hairdresser, and so forth.

Attractive, loose-fitting, nonmaternity clothes and new hairstyle enhance self-esteem and feelings of attractiveness.

Evaluate client's normal physical activity level and participation in sports or exercise program.

Involvement in physical activities aids client in regaining both a positive self-image and her pregravid shape.

Provide information about postpartal exercises (e.g., lifting hips off bed) or sleeping on abdomen.

Regular exercise program that is specific for each day up to 1 wk postpartum is continued thereafter, as indicated, to trim figure and increase muscle tone.

Weigh client, review ideal weight, and discuss proper nutrition as the key to losing weight. Discourage dieting in the lactating client until she stops breastfeeding.

The client retains approximately 60% of weight gained in excess of 24 lb (11 kg), which must be lost through proper diet and exercise. Restriction of calories in the lactating mother results in inadequate milk production.

Ascertain male partner's perception of client's physical appearance. Recommend avoidance of jokes or negative comments regarding her weight and appearance. Encourage male to express caring through increased time and attention or small gifts such as flowers and cards.

Helping male partner become aware of the client's emotional feelings may prevent him from making comments about her body that could reinforce negative feelings. Client may misinterpret the male's focus on the newborn as lack of interest in her, which may enhance her feelings of unattractiveness.

Collaborative

Refer to support groups, follow-up with community resources, or for counseling as needed.

May be necessary to resolve conflicts of self-esteem and poor body image.

NURSING DIAGNOSIS:	CONSTIPATION, risk for
Risk Factors May Include:	Inadequate fluid/fiber intake, decreased physical activity, pain on defecation
Possibly Evidenced By:	[Not applicable; presence of signs/symptoms establishes an *actual* diagnosis]
DESIRED OUTCOMES/EVALUATION CRITERIA—CLIENT WILL:	Re-establish usual/optimal evacuation pattern.

ACTIONS/INTERVENTIONS	RATIONALE

Independent

Discuss normal evacuation pattern. Determine presence of hemorrhoids, perineal trauma, or third-degree lacerations.

A history of problems with evacuation or constipation may contribute to problems following delivery, especially after the dilating and relaxing effects of progesterone experienced during the prenatal period.

Review role of client's current intake and the role of fluid and diet in stool formation and evacuation.

Lack of roughage and inadequate fluid intake reduce peristaltic motion of fecal matter through intestine, thereby increasing water reabsorption, resulting in dry, hard stools.

Encourage adequate fluid intake (including lactation needs, as appropriate) and diet high in roughage, fruits, and vegetables.

Use of warm beverages (hot water, coffee, tea), fruits/juices, and roughage promotes soft formed stool, eases evacuation, and supports client self-care.

Assess healing of episiotomy or lacerations. Provide information regarding the use of sitz baths 3–4 times daily.

Warmth from sitz bath helps relax anal sphincter, promotes healing, encourages general relaxation, and reduces discomfort associated with evacuation.

Recommend regular exercise, including daily walking program.

Activity enhances muscle tone, stimulates peristalsis, and enhances sense of well-being. Note: Some cultures limit activity following delivery for a prescribed period of time.

Collaborative

Encourage continued use of stool softener, if appropriate.

Helps prevent straining and reduces pain associated with evacuation.

Provide information regarding use of laxatives, enemas, or suppositories.

May be necessary to stimulate peristalsis, promote evacuation, and prevent fecal impaction. Note: Laxatives are not recommended for lactating clients.

NURSING DIAGNOSIS:	**FLUID VOLUME, risk for deficit**
Risk Factors May Include:	Increased fluid needs/inadequate intake, active vascular loss (retained placental fragments)
Possibly Evidenced By:	[Not applicable; presence of signs/symptoms establishes an *actual* diagnosis]
DESIRED OUTCOMES/EVALUATION CRITERIA—CLIENT WILL:	Demonstrate fluid balance as evidenced by adequate urine output, moist mucous membranes, good skin turgor, vital signs within normal limits.
	Display scant lochial flow that is brownish pink in color (serosa) and is free of clots following vaginal delivery.

ACTIONS/INTERVENTIONS	RATIONALE

Independent

Ascertain frequency of voiding and character of urine. Note condition of skin, lips, and mucous membranes.

Declining frequency/amount, presence of dark/strong urine, dry lips/mucous membranes, and poor skin turgor suggest inadequate fluid intake in relation to fluid needs.

ACTIONS/INTERVENTIONS	RATIONALE

Note reports of excessive fatigue or dizziness.

Assess BP and pulse.

Determine fundal height and note character and amount of lochial flow.

Review client's activity level.

Assess condition of perineum or cesarean incision; note healing.

Hypovolemia may result in orthostatic changes.

Decrease in BP and increase in pulse may reflect hypovolemia.

Failure of the fundus to involute properly (should be located at the symphysis pubis) is associated with increased vaginal flow. A return to bright red bleeding is abnormal. Brisk, heavy flow indicates late postpartal hemorrhage secondary to retained placental fragments. (Refer to CP: Postpartal Hemorrhage.)

Slight increase in flow may be secondary to inadequate rest associated with periods of increased activity.

To identify delayed healing and the potential for hemorrhage or dehiscence.

Collaborative

Obtain screening Hb/Hct and compare with levels obtained prior to discharge (if done), or with prenatal levels.

Notify healthcare provider and prepare client for additional evaluation/intervention, as necessary.

Provide information regarding medications such as methylergonovine (Methergine) 0.2 mg PO every 3–4 hr for 1–2 days, as needed.

Provides comparative readings to assess severity of blood loss. Hb/Hct should return to normal within 3 days postpartum. Hb should not drop more than 2 g/100 ml unless blood loss is excessive. (Each milliliter of blood lost contains 0.5 mg of Hb.)

Repeat laboratory studies or more invasive procedure such as surgical D & C may be necessary to determine severity of condition, or to diagnose/correct problem.

Used to promote uterine contractility, which may foster passage of retained placental tissue if BP is below 140/90.

NURSING DIAGNOSIS:	FAMILY COPING: ineffective, risk for compromised
Risk factors May Include:	Situational/developmental changes, temporary family disorganization and role changes, little support provided by client for partner/family members
Possibly Evidenced By:	[Not applicable; presence of signs/symptoms establishes an *actual* diagnosis]
DESIRED OUTCOMES/EVALUATION CRITERIA—CLIENT/FAMILY WILL:	Identify individual stressors. Set realistic goals and expectations. Verbalize resources within themselves to deal with the transition. Recognize need for and use outside support appropriately.

ACTIONS/INTERVENTIONS	RATIONALE

Independent

Evaluate client's actual and perceived physiological state.

Negative feelings, especially in the primipara, may be manifested by real or imagined physiological

	symptoms. Perhaps owing to unrealistic perceptions, first-time parents tend to experience the greatest degree of crisis, disintegration, and problems with adjustment.
Assess psychological status and discuss normalcy of negative feelings in the client/couple.	The fourth trimester, a transitional period lasting approximately 3 mo following birth, is a difficult period, because the client is vulnerable to negative feelings during crisis resolution and adaptation to stress. Negative feelings of anxiety, depression, and isolation are common, and awareness of the normalcy of these feelings may offset excessive self-concern or self-preoccupation.
Determine individual stressors for client/couple. Note strengths, weaknesses, coping mechanisms, and presence of realistic problem-solving capabilities.	The degree of individual and family stress depends on realistic perception of events, available coping mechanisms, and situational support. Crisis "balancing" factors help facilitate quick resolution of problems, positive adaptation, and growth for client/couple and family. Lack of balancing factors results in continued state of disorganization and persistence of crisis state.
Assist couple with identification of anticipated and unanticipated stressors and formulation of realistic problem solving.	Emotional disorganization associated with crisis is often accompanied by distortion of cognitive perceptions and the ability to respond appropriately to stressors.
Assess available means of assistance with housework and meal preparation.	Assistance with physical labor needed for household maintenance frees the client to devote her psychological energies to herself and infant.
Assess for maladaptive behaviors or ineffective coping.	Potential for maladaptation, disequilibrium, and continued crisis exists, necessitating immediate intervention, especially if existing support systems are inadequate for the postpartal mother.
Provide telephone contact number for 24-hr access.	New mothers (regardless whether first or fifth child) need access to healthcare resources early in the postpartal period and thereafter to facilitate adaptation.

Collaborative

Refer client to appropriate community agency, counselor, or social services.	May need additional assistance if existing support systems are inadequate or not available.

THE CLIENT AT 4 TO 6 WEEKS FOLLOWING DELIVERY

CLIENT ASSESSMENT DATA BASE

Activity/Rest

Lack of energy, fatigue, inability to maintain usual/expected routines

Circulation

Vital signs have returned to normal prepregnancy levels.

Ego Integrity

Emotional response may include irritability, anxiety, or feeling emotionally overwhelmed.

Elimination

Bowel sounds are active in all quadrants; usual elimination pattern resumes.
Abdominal muscle tone improving; flaccidity may persist.
Dipstick urinalysis for albumin, ketones, and glucose negative.

Food/Fluid

Return to prepregnancy weight, with retention of approximately 60% of weight gain in excess of 24 lb

Safety

Perineal episiotomy/laceration repair, cesarean incision should be healed.
Striae and linea nigra beginning to fade.

Sexuality

Lochial flow is absent.
Menstruation may resume beginning 4–5 wk postpartum, especially in nonlactating client.
Libido may be decreased.
Intercourse may be painful initially (dyspareunia).
Breasts in nonlactating client are soft, nontender, and of pregravid size; breasts in lactating client are full, free of nipple cracks and fissures, and lactation is well established.
Uterus not palpable, having returned to near pregravid size.
Pelvic examination, if performed, shows restored muscle tone, with cervix healed and closed, appearing as transverse slit.

Social Interaction

Comfort with parenting role; infant integrating into family unit
May be planning on returning to/seeking employment, or involvement in activities outside the home

DIAGNOSTIC STUDIES

Dependent on assessment findings, and individual client needs.
Hb/Hct: return to normal levels ± 5%, e.g., 12 g and 37%
Papanicolaou Smear: negative

NURSING PRIORITIES

1. Promote maternal/infant well-being.
2. Provide/reinforce health teaching.
3. Foster positive client and family adaptation to newborn.

DISCHARGE GOALS

1. Maternal/infant physiological/psychological needs being met.
2. Current health care behaviors and ongoing needs understood.
3. Satisfactory adaptation to parenting roles reported/observed.

NURSING DIAGNOSIS:	FAMILY COPING: potential for growth
May Be Related To:	Sufficiently meeting individual needs and adaptive tasks, enabling goals of self-actualization to surface
	Family member(s) moving in direction of health-promoting and enriching lifestyle
Possibly Evidenced By:	
DESIRED OUTCOMES/EVALUATION CRITERIA—CLIENT/COUPLE WILL:	Verbalize continued improvement with transition of new family member into home situation.
	Undertake tasks leading to change.
	Express feelings of self-confidence and satisfaction with progress and adaptation being made.

ACTIONS/INTERVENTIONS	RATIONALE
Independent	
Assess client's/couple's self-esteem and adaptation to parenting.	Parents need to learn to be flexible and adapt positively to changing circumstances rather than adhere to rigid schedules.
Determine parents' perception of family growth, mastery of infant care activities, and satisfaction or dissatisfaction with maternal/paternal role.	Parents should recognize that required skills change with the child's mental and physical growth. Increased self-esteem is associated with mastery of infant care tasks and satisfaction with parental role.
Discuss client's/couple's ability to modify or accept infant's behaviors. Provide appropriate anticipatory guidance.	Helps foster mutual capacity for behavior modification in parents and infant. To facilitate growth, parents need to learn to respond to the infant's needs while not neglecting the needs of other family members, to accept both successes and failures in attempts to modify the infant's behavior, and to make necessary adaptations based on needs of individual family members.
Evaluate ongoing educational and maturational progress and adjustment in sibling(s). Assess quality of interaction of sibling(s) with other children.	Helps identify actual or potential problems with family integration. Hostile-aggressive interaction of sibling(s) with other children signals inappropriate method of coping.
Provide bibliography (including audio, video, and electronic resources) list for parents and children. Encourage client/couple to spend time alone with each child, and allow opportunity for ongoing verbalization of feelings.	Helps parents to assist siblings with positive role adaptation; allows incorporation of newborn into family structure.
Assess parental response to positive or negative feedback from spouse or others (e.g., mother, mother-in-law, other family member, healthcare providers).	Mastery of parental tasks and growing self-esteem fosters independence, continued growth, and reduces excessive need for support of others.
Collaborative	
Refer to parenting classes, social services, visiting nurse services, or professional counselor, as appropriate.	May be needed to support desires for learning new tasks/roles and continued growth.

NURSING DIAGNOSIS:	NUTRITION: altered, risk for less than body requirements
Risk Factors May Include:	Inadequate caloric intake/increased caloric needs (lactation)
Possibly Evidenced By:	[Not applicable; presence of signs/symptoms establishes an *actual* diagnosis]
DESIRED OUTCOMES/EVALUATION CRITERIA—CLIENT WILL:	Identify individual needs and appropriate goal weight.
	Eat a well-balanced diet.
	Maintain/demonstrate progress toward desired weight.

ACTIONS/INTERVENTIONS	RATIONALE

Independent

Weigh client. Compare current weight with pregravid and ideal weight. Evaluate weight changes since delivery.	Weight generally returns to prepregnancy level by 6 wk postpartum, with approximately 60% retention of weight gain in excess of 24 lb.
Determine dietary habits using 24 hr recall. Provide information and encourage use of all food groups for a balanced diet.	Helps identify and correct inadequacies of protein, vitamin, or mineral intake.
Review Hb and Hct. Note behaviors associated with low Hb (e.g., fatigue, dizziness). Discuss dietary intake/use of sources rich in iron, if Hb levels are low.	Hb levels should be 12 g/100 ml; Hct 37% (plus or minus 5%). Reduction of activity may be necessary if Hb is low. Ingestion of iron-rich or fortified foods helps restore low iron levels, but supplements (such as prenatal vitamins with iron) may be needed for as long as 2 mo to correct iron deficiency.
Reinforce individual dietary needs in relation to type of infant feeding (i.e., breast or bottle).	Lactating client requires 500–800 cal/day more than the usual 2000 cal/day for the nonlactating client. Fluid intake should be increased by 500 ml/day for adequate milk production. Lactating client should not begin weight reduction diet while breastfeeding. Note: Continuation of vitamin supplements with iron is indicated for duration of lactation.
Provide information regarding iron and vitamin supplements and appropriate measures to facilitate absorption of iron (e.g., taking iron tablets between meals with fruit juice) as indicated.	Supplements may be required to correct vitamin and iron deficiencies/support recuperative process. Iron is best absorbed in acidic medium; taking iron with milk or meals impedes absorption.

NURSING DIAGNOSIS:	KNOWLEDGE deficit [LEARNING NEED], regarding recuperation, self care, infant needs
May Be Related To:	Information misinterpretation, lack of recall
Possibly Evidenced By:	Verbalization of concerns/misconceptions, inaccurate follow-through of instructions, development of preventable complications

375

ACTIONS/INTERVENTIONS	RATIONALE

Independent

ACTIONS/INTERVENTIONS	RATIONALE
Review client's understanding of physiological recovery for this time period.	By the end of the puerperium, involution should be complete (with the uterus returning to normal size and cessation of lochia) and incisions should be healed. However, the body may not have resumed its pregravid state. The client may still be 10 lb or more over her usual weight; she may note sore nipples and contour changes such as widening of her hips, breast enlargement/sagging, and decreased abdominal muscle tone with protruding stomach.
Review client's understanding of information received during prenatal, intrapartal, and postpartal periods and provide information and/or clarify misconceptions as necessary.	In many cases, material presented throughout the pregnancy is not incorporated or valued and/or is misinterpreted because of such other factors as pain and fatigue. Repetition of information is helpful at this time and provides an opportunity for discussion of ideas and concerns.
Reinforce information regarding infant care, immunization needs, feeding, and normal/anticipated growth and development. Provide pamphlets and identify other resources such as videos, electronic home pages.	Aids in meeting physical, psychological, and nutritional needs of infant. Availability of written materials and other resources increases likelihood that client can find answers to questions in home setting as they arise, enhancing independence and responsibility.
Discuss client's expectations regarding employment, family, and her own needs.	Balancing multiple demands may be overwhelming, especially if the client's/family's expectations are unrealistic.
Assist in developing realistic plans, identifying resources, and setting goals.	Sharing duties and responsibilities helps reduce individual fatigue, enhances adaptation to changes, and promotes general well-being.
Encourage client to involve other family members in this process.	Involvement in the problem-solving process promotes willingness to follow through on solutions. In addition, changes in sexual response, family demands, and ongoing fatigue affect the client's level of functioning and well-being.
Determine client's/couple's plans for contraceptive use. Provide information and review options as indicated.	Helps prevent unwanted or unplanned pregnancies; fosters adoption of family planning method. Studies suggest that closely spaced pregnancies (<9 mo apart) have increased risks for both mother and infant. Note: Based on personal/religious/cultural beliefs, client may choose not to use contraceptives.
Assess client's understanding and practice of breast self-examination. Provide information/visual aids as needed.	Helps client understand the importance of health promotion and of early detection of abnormalities.
Provide/reinforce information to lactating client regarding breastfeeding in relation to professional or working demands. Review options of using breast pump, manual expression, or gradual weaning.	Assists client with identifying problems and making decisions to meet infant's and her own needs during times of separation. Note: Using electric pump with double collection system allows emptying of both breasts simultaneously in a shorter time frame.

Encourage client to "anticipate" needs,
>   e.g., once breastfeeding is well established, begin
>   to familiarize infant with bottle;
>
>   practice use of breast pump in home several
>   weeks before returning to work; or,
>
>   gradually taper off breastfeeding during projected
>   hours of work several weeks before returning
>   to work, then breastfeed before and after work,
>   using formula during work hours.

Less traumatic for infant, facilitates eventual transfer to bottle feeding during client's absence. Provides opportunity to "master" new skill and stockpile milk for future use.

Allows for continuation of breastfeeding without the need to routinely pump breasts while at work. Note: Milk supply will diminish with this option.

Discuss proper handling/storage of expressed milk.

Washing hands, using sterile collection bottles, storage in refrigerator/freezer as appropriate helps assure safety of milk. Note: Refrigerated milk should be stored in plastic container to prevent loss of protective effect of WBCs, which will adhere to glass.

Provide information about need for follow-up medical care.

Reevaluation at 6 mo postpartum provides opportunity to assess client's well-being and identify any unresolved/developing problems.

NURSING DIAGNOSIS:	SEXUALITY PATTERNS, altered
May Be Related To:	Individual response to health-related transition, altered body functioning (including lactation), lack of privacy, fear of pregnancy
Possibly Evidenced By:	Reported difficulties, changes in sexual behaviors/activities
DESIRED OUTCOMES/EVALUATION CRITERIA—CLIENT/COUPLE WILL:	Discuss nature of current sexual relationship in comparison to before and during pregnancy.
	Identify potential problems during the early postpartal period.
	Resume sexual relationship as mutually desired.
	Adopt a mutually agreeable method of contraception if appropriate.

ACTIONS/INTERVENTIONS

RATIONALE

Independent

Discuss client's/couple's sexual relationship prior to pregnancy and the effects that newborn has had on client's/couple's physiological and psychological energy levels.

Nature of sexual relationship prior to pregnancy affects resumption of sexual activity more than any other factor. However, fatigue, physical discomforts, stress of new roles/responsibilities, depression, and individual self-perceptions may delay this process. In addition, presence of baby may have negative influence on lovemaking, leaving one or both members of the couple frustrated and unsatisfied.

Determine client's body image and her feelings of physical attractiveness following delivery. Note views of significant other(s).

Much of sexual response and desire is psychologically based, so that a negative body image may reduce sexual urges. Partner may not find mate as sexually attractive if she is lactating or has not regained her pregravid weight and body contours; or partner may be more attracted and client may not share same level of desire.

377

Provide information about physiological changes in sexual response for first 3 mo following delivery.

Reduction in rapidity/intensity of response is normal. Continued low estrogen levels result in vaginal dryness. Size of orgasmic platform and strength of orgasmic contraction are reduced; vasoconstriction of labia minora and labia majora is delayed.

Prepare couple for possibility of a temporary difficulty with achieving erection or arousal.

Fatigue and heightened expectations may increase or decrease libido, altering sexual response.

Ascertain whether couple has resumed sexual relationship.

Most couples can safely resume intercourse 3–4 wk after vaginal delivery or following 4- to 6-wk checkup after cesarean delivery.

Assess degree of pleasure or displeasure associated with resumption of sexual activity. Suggest use of water-soluble jelly/lubricant (cocoa butter), or contraceptive creams or jellies, and side-by-side or female-superior positions.

Vaginal dryness may cause pain/dyspareunia, necessitating use of lubrication. Female-superior or side-by-side position allows client to control the rate and degree of penile penetration, thereby gradually distending tissues and reducing discomfort.

Discuss alternatives to penile penetration to achieve orgasm (e.g., masturbation, lubricated stroking of genital area, or cunnilingus).

Helps client achieve sexual gratification while avoiding possible discomfort associated with penile penetration. Note: Some couples might not find such alternatives mutually/culturally acceptable.

Encourage verbalization of concerns.

May stimulate identification of problems and foster creative problem solving.

Encourage couple to share intimate thoughts.

Helps create open communication; increases psychological readiness for sexual relationship.

Discuss effects of lactation on sexual response and interest level. Suggest planning lovemaking so that it occurs just after or midway between feedings.

Lactating women often have a greater interest in resuming sexual activity than nonlactating women and may report higher levels of postdelivery eroticism. Orgasm may stimulate the let-down reflex, causing milk leakage; breastfeeding itself may evoke sexual arousal, possibly to the point of reaching plateau/orgasmic levels. Intercourse may be more enjoyable just after or midway between feedings, when breasts are not as full or leaking and infant is not likely to be hungry.

Discuss client's/couple's choice of contraception method within cultural/religious beliefs. Reinforce information and provide oral/video and written information as needed regarding method, effectiveness, proper usage, expense, availability, advantages/disadvantages, and contraindications. Assess plan for future offspring and desired family size.

Pregnancy is possible before onset of regular menses. Cooperation with contraceptive method is enhanced if client/couple participates in decision-making process. Couple may elect to abstain from intercourse, engage in rhythm method, adopt temporary means of contraception (foams, condom, or gel) until postpartal examination by healthcare provider, or couple may elect surgical method (vasectomy or tubal ligation). Although oral contraceptives may be the most practical and effective method for the sexually active adolescent, they are contraindicated for breastfeeding clients and for clients with diabetes, hypertension, kidney or cardiac problems, or history of phlebitis. Because of the risk of infection, intrauterine device is not usually advised for the diabetic client. Note: Client should be refitted for a diaphragm following birth of infant or a weight change of 10 lb or more.

Collaborative

Refer for counseling as indicated.

Couple unable to achieve mutual sexual satisfaction may need help in analyzing causative factors and in initiating open communication and problem solving with each other.

NURSING DIAGNOSIS:	PARENTING, risk for altered
Risk Factors May Include:	Lack of/or ineffective role model, lack of support between/from significant other(s), unrealistic expectation for self/infant/partner, presence of stress (addition of new family member, financial concerns)
Possibly Evidenced By:	[Not applicable; presence of signs/symptoms establishes an *actual* diagnosis]
DESIRED OUTCOMES/EVALUATION CRITERIA—CLIENT/COUPLE WILL:	Demonstrate responsiveness to infant cues.
	Verbalize positive resolution of feelings regarding change in lifestyle, addition of new family member.
	Report satisfaction with parenting roles.

ACTIONS/INTERVENTIONS	RATIONALE

Independent

Assess strength of parent-infant attachment.	Attachment bond should be strong 4–6 wk postpartum. Little or no reciprocal interaction requires immediate intervention.
Review cultural factors and expectations.	Cultural beliefs affect parent-child interaction (e.g., types of behaviors observed and the degree of attachment noted).
Note progress toward recovery and stabilization of lifestyle.	Failure to progress and/or continuation of postpartal depression have a negative impact on attachment and indicate need for further evaluation/intervention.
Assess resolution of grief associated with assumption of new role and loss of former lifestyle.	Adaptation to the new parenting role and integration of the infant into the family involve some grieving over the loss of former life patterns and the need to reduce or alter career pursuits or social roles.
Discuss client's use and adequacy of current/available resources.	Without effective support, the difficult process of integrating a new member into the family may be more difficult.
Discuss client's/couple's concerns regarding infant behaviors and parenting skills. Reinforce previous information.	Assists in relieving anxiety, provides opportunity for positive reinforcement for efforts, and promotes growth.
Administer NPI, as indicated.	Assesses adaptive potential of mother-infant pair and provides a statistically significant relationship between the findings at 1 mo and the emotional development of the child at age $4^{1}/_{2}$, and later at age 10–11.
Note presence of problems and evidence of possible neglect or abuse. Notify authorities as indicated.	Index of suspicion requires further evaluation to determine necessary interventions.

Collaborative

Refer client/couple to peer support group, postpartal parenting group, or classes, such as Parent Effectiveness Training.	Sharing concerns may increase parent's knowledge of childrearing and child development and provide supportive atmosphere during role acquisition and transition.
Refer to community health nurse, social services, or professional counselor.	May be necessary to assist parents in adopting effective parenting skills.

379

ACTIONS/INTERVENTIONS	RATIONALE
Independent	
Review type of delivery and prenatal or intrapartal events that might have predisposed client to infection or excessive trauma.	Provides clues to increased risk for postpartal complications.
Assess client for any vaginal discharge or persistence/return of lochial flow. Note odor of drainage.	Although lochial flow should have ceased by this time, the client may have resumed her menstrual cycle or may have failed to complete involution. The presence of foul-smelling discharge is indicative of infection and requires further evaluation.
Note status of perineum, incisions/lacerations, uterus, and cervix.	Wound should be well approximated and without inflammation or drainage. Uterus should return to near prepregnancy state by 4–6 wk postpartum, with closure of the cervix completed. Relaxed or tender uterus, and opening of the cervix suggests infection.
Note reports of fever, chills, headache, malaise, vomiting, diarrhea, presence of tachycardia, and abdominal tenderness.	These general signs and symptoms suggest endometritis, requiring further evaluation and intervention.
Inspect nipples for redness, cracks, or fissures. If present, suggest use of localized heat, starting feedings on unaffected nipple, limiting infant suckling, and air drying nipples for 20–30 min after each feeding.	Helps prevent clogged nipples and lobes, which can lead to mastitis. Limiting feeding on affected breast and initiating feeding on unaffected breast help reduce trauma to nipple and allow healing to occur.
Encourage breast support and application of local heat.	Facilitates circulation/lymph drainage and increases oxygen/nutrients to affected area to promote healing.
Palpate breasts for marked tenderness, palpable mass(es), note redness or areas of induration. Suggest increased rest and fluids, localized heat, and frequent emptying of breasts if inflammation is present. Instruct in use of manual expression or breast pump.	Induration or mass(es) may indicate full milk duct, possible tumor, or mastitis. Rest, fluids, heat, and frequent emptying of breasts help reduce discomfort associated with full breasts and relieve stasis and engorgement, especially if breastfeeding is contraindicated during antibiotic therapy for mastitis.
Instruct client to discontinue breastfeeding if fever is present prior to antibiotic administration or if indicated by antibiotic therapy selected.	Breast milk may become purulent; antibiotic may cross into the breast milk.
Note reports of dysuria, frequency, foul/cloudy urine, dragging back pain.	Indicative of urinary tract infection, which requires further evaluation to rule out cystocele.

Recommend increased fluid intake.

Promotes urine output, reducing urinary stasis and risk of infection or reinfection.

Collaborative

Refer to healthcare provider, as indicated.

Promotes diagnosis/treatment; may prevent progression and/or limit severity of problem.

Culture lochia/drainage, as indicated.

Identifies infectious organism and appropriate treatment.

Review appropriate use of analgesics/antipyretics.

Analgesics promote comfort; antipyretics reduce/control fever. Note: Drugs may be contraindicated until diagnosis is made.

Initiate/provide information about antibiotic therapy.

Combination therapy such as penicillin and an aminoglycoside (e.g., gentamicin) may be required for endometritis following vaginal birth, or clindamycin and aminoglycoside for postcesarean endometritis. For mastitis, dicloxacillin or a cephalosporin.

Assist as needed with incision/drainage/care of wound. Carry out sterile dressing changes as needed.

May be necessary if abscess develops, although such progression can usually be prevented with prompt diagnosis and treatment.

Prepare client/family for follow-up procedures such as D & C, as indicated.

Surgical removal of placental fragments through D & C may be necessary.

NURSING DIAGNOSIS:	COPING, INDIVIDUAL/FAMILY, risk for ineffective (specify)
Risk Factors May Include:	Situational/developmental changes, temporary family disorganization and role changes, little support provided for client by partner/family members
Possibly Evidenced By:	[Not applicable; presence of signs/symptoms establishes an *actual* diagnosis.]
DESIRED OUTCOMES/EVALUATION CRITERIA—CLIENT WILL:	Report assistance from significant other(s) and effective use of resources.
	Verbalize sense of competence and not feeling overwhelmed with infant care.
	Plan activities outside of house for client/couple, the baby, and siblings.
	Demonstrate initial progress toward realistic goals.

ACTIONS/INTERVENTIONS

RATIONALE

Independent

Assess past and present coping skills; explore available coping strategies, relationships between individual and family members, and support systems.

Past coping skills may be effective in the current situation, or client may need to develop new coping strategies. Positive coping mechanisms involve open communication of fears and wishes among family members, empathy, competency in role playing and role reversal, and negotiation within

Determine client's perception of stressors and events of past 4–6 wk and of her own adaptability. Note competency in organizing activities associated with infant care and parental responsibilities.	the family structure to the mutual satisfaction of each member.
	Accurate perception of problems and adaptability to changing or new situations are factors that promote positive coping during times of increased stress/crisis. Persistent feelings of being overwhelmed by activities associated with child care, persistent depression or exhaustion, or persistent low self-esteem indicate negative coping.
Allow client opportunity to cry or to express her concerns freely. Use "self-disclosure," if appropriate.	Provides opportunity for emotional catharsis and relief of tension. Self-disclosure (i.e., the sharing of one's own experiences with client) may be effective in stimulating client to talk, providing that the disclosure is client- rather than nurse-centered.
Identify and discuss apparent strengths of client/couple. Avoid criticism.	Promotes self-awareness and fosters positive self-esteem and coping.
Assess response of siblings to new baby. Provide anticipatory guidance regarding typical sibling reactions. Recommend age-appropriate children's videos, books, and other reading matter.	All siblings are somewhat resentful of the diminished parental attention that occurs when the new baby arrives, and acting-out behaviors may reflect normal feelings of frustration. Helps parents/child(ren) understand normalcy of feeling/reactions, and provides opportunities to share and reaffirm family ties with addition of a new member.
Encourage client to develop creative solutions and to rearrange schedule to spend time alone with her other child(ren).	Individual attention to sibling(s) reduces feelings of threat that the new baby creates, allows sibling(s) to feel secure in the child-parent relationship, and helps foster coping.
Suggest that client plan activities outside of home with baby and sibling(s).	Provides stimulation and change of daily routine for mother, baby, and sibling(s).
Help client/couple set priorities for tasks and to accept help from friends and relatives for tasks related to housework and cooking.	Allows client to focus on her infant and family. Excessive concerns about household tasks such as cooking detract from time and energy devoted to the baby and family.
Provide information about increased needs for sleep and rest.	Excessive fatigue can have a negative effect on coping skills, especially those needed for 24-hr responsibility associated with infant care.
Determine client's opportunities for recreation and relaxation. Encourage client to participate in appropriate activities.	Provides positive outlet for release of stress, and enhances feelings of wellness and self-esteem.
Encourage client/couple to arrange for time together away from newborn.	Allows time for needed growth/reflection; helps achieve a sense of equilibrium.
Assess amount of support client receives from significant other(s) or family members, and the demands placed on her by each individual.	Lack of effective support and assistance may impair client's ability to cope and increase risk of postpartal depression, especially if partner expects to receive the same amount of attention following delivery as before delivery.
Discuss client's/couple's plans for the future, especially if client expects to return to work. Review plans for child care.	Return to employment and/or addition of outside responsibilities will affect all family members and requires sharing of duties/household tasks. Confidence in child care arrangements eases or reduces parent's anxiety/guilt regarding separation from infant.

Investigate reports of excessive crying, despondency, insomnia, unexpected weight loss, social withdrawal. Ascertain whether client has suicidal/homicidal (infanticidal) ideation.

Postpartal depression may be noted 2 wk to 6 mo after delivery, requiring further evaluation and therapeutic intervention. Postpartal psychosis is rarer and can occur as late as 12 mo after delivery, possibly requiring hospitalization of the client as well as close monitoring of client/infant interactions.

Collaborative

Recommend peer support group or parenting group.

Mutual sharing of successes and failures associated with parenting helps foster coping and helps client to recognize normalcy of her situation and feelings.

Reinforce availability of healthcare resources.

Relieves parents of feeling solely responsible for health of new baby; provides needed information regarding sources of healthcare.

Refer to community health nurse, social service, or professional counselor, as appropriate.

Postpartum depression affects, in varying degrees, an estimated 70% of women. Negative coping, manifested by excessive feelings of failure, depression, self-accusatory thoughts, excess use of drugs (such as alcohol), or a sense of being overwhelmed with child care, suggests postpartal psychosis, which tends to peak at 6 wk postpartum and indicates need for aggressive evaluation and follow-up. Note: Clients suffering from severe postpartal depression and necessitating hospitalization for psychoses such as affective disorders (e.g., depression or depression with manic episode) and schizophrenia range from 1%–2%.

Administer/instruct in use of diazepam (Valium), promethazine (Phenergan), nortriptyline (Pamelor), sertraline hydrochloride (Zoloft), or lithium carbonate, as indicated.

Severe, prolonged difficulties may require additional intervention. Selection of drug therapy depends on whether short- or long-term control is needed, whether client is lactating, and whether the sedative effect of dosage prescribed may impair client's ability to hear/respond to baby's cries. Note: Fluoxetine (Prozac) is not recommended during lactation because slow metabolism of drug may cause higher levels in breast milk. Lithium is contraindicated because it can cause lethargy and lowered body temperature in nursing infant.

NURSING DIAGNOSIS:	CONSTIPATION/BOWEL INCONTINENCE, risk for
Risk Factors May Include:	Decreased muscle tone, inadequate fluid/dietary intake, reduced physical activity, pain on defecation
Possibly Evidenced By:	[Not applicable; presence of signs/symptoms establishes an actual diagnosis]
DESIRED OUTCOMES/EVALUATION CRITERIA—CLIENT WILL:	Identify/use appropriate interventions related to specific situation.
	Re-establish optimal bowel pattern.

ACTIONS/INTERVENTIONS	RATIONALE
Independent	
Review usual pregravid evacuation patterns.	Provides useful information for setting goals. Problems may be new, or they may be long-standing and aggravated by pregnancy.
Evaluate nature and severity of problems associated with evacuation.	Helps in determining individual needs and selecting specific interventions.
Determine methods used to correct constipation.	Every effort should be made to use diet and exercise to promote bowel functioning and to reduce dependence on laxatives, if used.
Review dietary and fluid intake and exercise level. Recommend increased intake of fluids, whole grains, fruits, and vegetables, as well as daily exercise, as appropriate.	Stimulates peristalsis, reducing excessive water absorption from fecal matter, thus promoting a softer stool.
Note presence of hemorrhoids/bleeding. Suggest reinsertion of hemorrhoid with lubricated glove or finger cot.	Painful or bleeding hemorrhoids may increase likelihood that client will postpone evacuation, which would contribute to further constipation and dry stool as more fluid is absorbed from the stool.
Assess intrapartal record for possible third- or fourth-degree laceration.	Lacerations extending into the anal sphincter may cause client to postpone evacuation, thus increasing constipation.
Collaborative	
Refer to evaluation of rectocele or fecal incontinence.	May require surgical intervention. Incontinence may be associated with nerve damage to anal sphincter occurring with fourth-degree laceration.

POSTPARTAL HEMORRHAGE

Postpartal hemorrhage is usually defined as the loss of more than 500 ml of blood during or after delivery. It is one of the leading causes of maternal mortality. Hemorrhage may occur early, within the first 24 hr after delivery, or late, up to 28 days postpartum (the end of the puerperium).

CLIENT ASSESSMENT DATA BASE

General Findings

Activity/Rest

May report excessive fatigue

Circulation

Blood loss at delivery generally 400–500 ml (vaginal delivery), 600–800 ml (cesarean delivery), although research suggests that blood loss is often underestimated
History of chronic anemia, congenital/incidental coagulation defects, idiopathic thrombocytopenia purpura

Ego Integrity

May be anxious, fearful, apprehensive

Sexuality

Labor may have been prolonged/augmented or induced, precipitous/traumatic; use of forceps/vacuum extractor, general anesthesia, tocolytic therapy.
Difficult or manual delivery of placenta.
Examination of placenta following birth may have revealed missing placental fragments, tears, or evidence of torn blood vessels.
Vaginal birth after cesarean (VABC).

Teaching/Learning

Previous postpartal hemorrhage, PIH, uterine or cervical tumors, grand multiparity
Ongoing/excess aspirin ingestion

Early Postpartal Hemorrhage (Up to 24 Hr Following Delivery)

Circulation

Changes in BP and pulse (may not occur until blood loss is significant)
Delayed capillary refill
Pallor; cold/clammy skin
Dark, venous bleeding from uterus externally evident (retained placenta)
May have excessive vaginal bleeding, or oozing from cesarean incision or episiotomy; oozing from IV catheter, sites of intramuscular injections, or urinary catheter; bleeding gums (signs of disseminated intravascular coagulation [DIC])
Profuse hemorrhage or symptoms of shock out of proportion to the amount of blood lost (inversion of uterus)

Elimination

Difficulty voiding may reflect hematoma of the upper portion of the vagina.
Bladder distension (urinary retention).

Pain/Discomfort

Painful burning/tearing sensations (lacerations), severe vulvar/vaginal/pelvic/back pain (hematoma formation), lateral uterine pain, flank pain (hematoma into the broad ligament), abdominal tenderness (uterine atony, retained placental fragments), severe uterine and abdominal pain (uterine inversion)

Safety

Lacerations of the birth canal: Persistent trickle of bright red blood (may be profuse) with firm, well-contracted uterus; visible tears in labia majora/labia minora, from vaginal introitus to perineum; extended tears from episiotomy, extension of episiotomy into vaginal vault, or tears in cervix

Hematomas: Unilateral, tense, fluctuant, bulging mass at vaginal introitus or encompassing labia majora; firm, painful to touch; unilateral bluish or reddish discoloration of skin of perineum or buttocks; (abdominal hematoma following cesarean delivery may be asymptomatic except for changes in vital signs)

Sexuality

Uterus: Soft, boggy, or enlarging, difficult to palpate; bright red bleeding from vagina (slow or profuse); large clots expressed on massage of uterus (uterine atony)

Firm, well-contracted or partially contracted, and slightly boggy (retained placental fragments, which may necrose and over time form polyps)

Fundus of uterus inverted; comes into close contact with, or may protrude through, the external os (uterine inversion)

Current pregnancy may have involved uterine overdistension (multiple gestation, hydramnios, macrosomia), abruptio placentae, placenta previa

Late Postpartal Hemorrhage (24 to 28 Days Following Delivery)

Circulation

Continued oozing or sudden bleeding
May appear pale, anemic

Pain/Discomfort

Uterine tenderness (retained placental fragments)
Vaginal/pelvic discomfort, backache (hematoma)

Safety

Foul-smelling lochial discharge (infection)
Reported premature rupture of membranes (risk for infection)

Sexuality

Fundal height or uterine body fails to return to prepregnancy size and function (subinvolution).
Leukorrhea may be present.
Continues to pass tissue.

DIAGNOSTIC STUDIES

Blood Typing: Determines Rh, ABO group, and cross-match.
CBC: Reveals decreased Hb/Hct and/or elevated WBC count (shift to the left, and increased sedimentation rate suggests infection).
Platelet Count: Levels below 50,000/μL can lead to spontaneous bleeding.
Uterine and Vaginal Culture: Rules out/identifies specific postpartal infection.
Urinalysis: Ascertains damage to bladder.
Coagulation Profile: Elevated fibrin degradation product/fibrin split product (FDP/FSP) levels, decreased fibrinogen levels; activated partial thromboplastin time/partial thromboplastin time (APTT/PTT), prothrombin time (PT) prolonged in presence of DIC.
Sonography: Determines presence of retained placental tissue.

NURSING PRIORITIES

1. Maintain or restore circulating volume/tissue perfusion.
2. Prevent complications.
3. Provide information and appropriate support for client/couple.
4. Have plan in place to meet needs after discharge.

DISCHARGE GOALS

1. Tissue perfusion/organ function WNL
2. Complications prevented/resolving
3. Clinical situation and treatment needs understood

NURSING DIAGNOSIS:	**FLUID VOLUME deficit [isotonic]**
May Be Related To:	Excessive vascular loss
Possibly Evidenced By:	Hypotension, tachycardia, changes in mentation, decreased/concentrated urine, dry skin/mucous membranes, delayed capillary refill
DESIRED OUTCOMES/EVALUATION CRITERIA—CLIENT WILL:	Demonstrate stabilization/improvement in fluid balance as evidenced by stable vital signs, prompt capillary refill, appropriate sensorium, and individually adequate urine output and specific gravity.

ACTIONS/INTERVENTIONS	RATIONALE
Independent	
Review records of pregnancy and labor/delivery, noting causative factors or those contributing to hemorrhagic situation (e.g., lacerations, retained placental fragments, sepsis, abruptio placentae, amniotic fluid emboli, or retention of dead fetus for more than 5 wk).	Aids in establishing appropriate plan of care and provides opportunity to prevent or limit developing complications. Note: Approximately 20% of early postpartal hemorrhage is related to lacerations of the perineum, vagina, or cervix. Late postpartal hemorrhage is usually caused by abnormal involution of the uterus or retained placental fragments.
Assess and record amount, type, and site of bleeding; weigh and count pads; save clots and tissue for evaluation by physician.	Estimate of blood loss, venous versus arterial, and presence of clots helps to make a differential diagnosis and determines replacement needs. Note: One gram of increased pad weight is equal to approximately 1 ml of blood loss. Blood losses of more than 1000 ml lead to shock state and increase risk of other complications, e.g., infection, extensive pelvic thrombophlebitis.
Assess location of uterus and degree of uterine contractility. Massage boggy uterus with one hand while placing second hand just above the symphysis pubis.	Degree of uterine contractility aids in differential diagnosis. Increasing myometrial contractility may decrease blood loss. Placing one hand above symphysis pubis prevents possible uterine inversion during massage.
Note presence of vulvar hematoma; apply ice pack as indicated and observe periodically.	Small hematomas may be controlled by ice and rest.
Monitor BP, pulse; observe capillary refill, nail beds, and mucous membranes.	Hypotension, tachycardia, delayed capillary refill; cyanosis of nail beds, mucous membranes, and lips

387

Measure hemodynamic parameters, such as central venous pressure (CVP) or pulmonary artery wedge pressure (PAWP), if available.	reflects severe hypovolemia and developing shock. Changes in BP are not detectable until fluid volume has decreased by 30%–50%. Cyanosis is a late sign of hypoxia. (Refer to ND: Tissue Perfusion, altered.) Note: Reports of fatigue, headache, thirst, presence of pallor, orthostatic hypotension may be signs of slow moderate blood loss that may be reported during follow-up visit.

Measure hemodynamic parameters, such as central venous pressure (CVP) or pulmonary artery wedge pressure (PAWP), if available.

Provides more direct measurement of circulating volume, replacement needs, and response to therapy in severe/life-threatening situations.

Institute bedrest with legs elevated 20–30 degrees and trunk horizontal.

Bleeding may decrease or cease with reduction in activity. Proper positioning increases venous return, ensuring greater availability of blood to brain and other vital organs.

Maintain nothing-by-mouth (NPO) regimen while determining client status/needs.

Prevents aspiration of gastric contents in the event that sensorium is altered and/or surgical intervention is required.

Measure intake and output, and urine specific gravity, as indicated. Investigate reports of difficulty voiding/emptying bladder.

Useful in estimating extent/significance of fluid loss. Adequate perfusion/circulating volume is reflected by output 30–50 ml/hr or greater. Note: Difficulty voiding may occur with hematomas in the upper portion of the vagina causing pressure on the urethra or meatus.

Avoid repeat/use caution when performing vaginal and/or rectal examinations.

May increase hemorrhage if cervical, vaginal, or perineal lacerations or hematomas are present. Note: Careful examination may be required to monitor status of hematomas.

Provide quiet environment and psychological support.

Promotes relaxation; reduces anxiety and metabolic demand.

Investigate reports of persistent perineal pain or feeling of vaginal fullness. Apply counterpressure on labial or perineal lacerations.

Hematomas often result from continued bleeding from lacerations of the birth canal.

Monitor clients with placenta accreta (slight penetration of myometrium by placental tissue), PIH, or abruptio placentae for signs of DIC. (Refer to CP: Prenatal Hemorrhage; ND: Injury, risk for maternal.)

Thromboplastin released during attempts at manual removal of the placenta may result in coagulopathy as manifested by continued vaginal bleeding; expistaxis; oozing from incisions, mucous membranes, gums, IV site.

Collaborative

Start 1 or 2 IV infusion(s) of isotonic or electrolyte fluids with 18-gauge catheter or via central venous line. Administer whole blood or blood products (e.g., plasma, cryoprecipitate, platelets), as indicated.

Necessary for rapid or multiple infusions of fluid or blood products to increase circulating volume and enhance clotting. Note: Each unit of whole blood raises the Hct by 3 percentage points.

Administer medications as indicated, e.g.:
  Oxytocin (Pitocin), methylergonovine maleate (Methergine), prostaglandin F_2a (Prostin 15M);

  $MgSO_4$;

  Heparin;

  Antibiotic therapy (based on culture and sensitivity of lochia).

Increases contractility of boggy uterus and myometrium, closes off exposed venous sinuses, and stops hemorrhage in presence of atony. Some studies report use of $MgSO_4$ to facilitate uterine relaxation during manual examination. While controversial, if other means fail, heparin may be used cautiously to stop the clotting cycle in DIC. Antibiotics act prophylactically to prevent infection or may be needed for infection that

Monitor laboratory studies as indicated, e.g.: Hb and Hct;	caused or contributed to uterine subinvolution or hemorrhage. Helps in determining amount of blood loss. Each milliliter of blood carries 0.5 mg of Hb. Hct levels below 30% require red cell replacement.
Platelets, FDP, fibrinogen and APTT.	Measures severity of DIC; determines replacement needs and effects of therapy.
Insert indwelling urinary catheter.	Provides more accurate assessment of renal function and perfusion relative to fluid volume. Note: If vaginal packing has been inserted, pressure on urethra may obstruct urine flow/cause bladder distension.
Assist with procedures as indicated, e.g.: Manual separation and removal of placenta;	Hemorrhage stops once placental fragments are removed and uterus contracts, closing venous sinuses.
Insertion of large indwelling catheter into cervical canal;	Some studies have reported success in controlling hemorrhage caused by implantation of placenta into noncontractile cervical segment by placing an indwelling catheter in the cervical canal and filling the balloon with 60 ml of saline solution to act as a tamponade.
Uterine replacement or packing if inversion seems about to recur.	Replacement of uterus allows uterus to contract, closing venous sinuses and controlling bleeding.
Prepare for surgical intervention as indicated; e.g., exploration/repair to close tear, laceration, or episiotomy extension; evacuation of hematoma and ligation of bleeding point; D & C; bilateral ligation of hypogastric arteries, supracervical hysterectomy, or immediate abdominal hysterectomy.	Surgical repair of lacerations/episiotomy, incision/evacuation of hematomas, and removal of retained tissues will stop bleeding. Immediate abdominal hysterectomy is indicated for abnormally adherent placenta. Note: D & C may be contraindicated if there is concern that the procedure may traumatize the implantation site and increase bleeding.

NURSING DIAGNOSIS:	**TISSUE PERFUSION, altered**
May Be Related To:	Hypovolemia
Possibly Evidenced By:	Diminished arterial pulsations, cold extremities, changes in vital signs, delayed capillary refill, changes in sensorium, decreased milk production
DESIRED OUTCOMES/EVALUATION CRITERIA—CLIENT WILL:	Display BP, pulse, arterial blood gases (ABGs), and Hb/Hct WNL.
	Demonstrate normal hormonal functioning by adequate milk supply for lactation (as appropriate) and resumption of normal menses.

ACTIONS/INTERVENTIONS	RATIONALE
Independent	
Note Hb/Hct prior to and following blood loss. Assess nutritional state, height, and weight.	Comparative values help determine severity of blood losses. Preexisting state of poor health increases extent of injury from oxygen deficits.

389

ACTIONS/INTERVENTIONS	RATIONALE
Monitor vital signs; record degree and duration of hypovolemic episode.	Extent of pituitary involvement may be related to degree and duration of hypotension. Increased respiratory rate may reflect an effort to combat metabolic acidosis.
Note level of consciousness and any behavior changes.	Changes in sensorium are early indicators of hypoxia. Cyanosis, a later sign, may not appear until PO_2 levels fall below 50 mm Hg.
Observe color of nail beds, buccal mucosa, gums, and tongue; note skin temperature.	With compensatory vasoconstriction and shunting to vital organs, circulation in peripheral blood vessels is reduced, with resulting cyanosis and cool skin temperatures.
Inspect breasts daily, noting presence or absence of lactation and changes in breast size.	Anterior pituitary damage or involvement (Sheehan's syndrome) reduces prolactin levels, resulting in absence of milk production and eventually a decrease in breast tissue.

Collaborative

Monitor ABGs and pH level.	Helps in diagnosing degree of tissue hypoxia or acidosis, reflecting lactic acid buildup from resulting anaerobic metabolism (prolonged shock).
Provide supplemental oxygen as needed.	Maximizes available oxygen for circulatory transport to tissues.
Insert airway; suction as indicated.	Facilitates oxygen administration in presence of retained secretions.
Administer sodium bicarbonate.	May be necessary to correct metabolic acidosis.

NURSING DIAGNOSIS:	ANXIETY [specify level]
May Be Related To:	Situational crisis, threat of change in health status or death, interpersonal transmission/contagion, physiological response (release of catecholamines)
Possibly Evidenced By:	Increased tension, apprehension, feelings of inadequacy/helplessness, sympathetic stimulation, focus on self, restlessness
DESIRED OUTCOMES/EVALUATION CRITERIA—CLIENT WILL:	Verbalize awareness of feelings and causes of anxiety (postpartal hemorrhage is perceived as a threat to her physical integrity). Identify healthy ways to deal with feelings. Report anxiety is lessened. Appear relaxed, able to sleep/rest appropriately.

ACTIONS/INTERVENTIONS	RATIONALE

Independent

Evaluate client's psychological response to postpartal hemorrhage and perception of events. Clarify misconceptions.	Aids in formulation of plan of care. Client's perception of the event may be distorted, intensifying her anxiety.
Evaluate physiological response to postpartal	Although changes in vital signs may be due to

hemorrhage, e.g., tachycardia, tachypnea, restlessness, or irritability.

Convey calm, empathic, supportive attitude.

Provide information about treatment modalities and effectiveness of interventions.

Encourage client to verbalize feelings. Assist client and family to identify feelings of anxiety.

Assess coping strategies and long-term implications of hemorrhagic episode. (Refer to ND: Parent/Infant Attachment, risk for altered.)

Collaborative

Refer client/couple to a community support group such as Coping with Overall Pregnancy/Parenting Experience (COPE) or for counseling, as indicated.

physiological responses, they may be intensified or complicated by psychological factors.

Can help client maintain emotional control in response to changing physiological status. Aids in reducing interpersonal transmission of anxiety.

Accurate information can reduce anxiety and fear of the unknown.

Verbalization provides an opportunity to clarify information, correct misconceptions, and gain perspective, facilitating the problem-solving process.

Prolonged or excessive anxiety may be anticipated if complications are permanent (such as with anterior pituitary necrosis).

Helps reduce anxiety through peer or professional support and interaction.

NURSING DIAGNOSIS:	FLUID VOLUME, risk for excess
Risk Factors May Include:	Excessive/rapid replacement of fluid losses, intravascular fluid shifts (PIH)
Possibly Evidenced By:	[Not applicable; presence of signs/symptoms establishes an *actual* diagnosis]
DESIRED OUTCOMES/EVALUATION CRITERIA—CLIENT WILL:	Display BP, pulse, urine specific gravity, and neurological signs WNL, without respiratory difficulties.

ACTIONS/INTERVENTIONS	RATIONALE

Independent

Monitor for increasing BP and pulse; note respiratory signs of dyspnea, stridor, moist crackles, or rhonchi.

Monitor infusion rate manually or electronically (preferable). Record intake/output. Measure urine specific gravity.

Assess neurological status, noting behavior changes and increasing irritability.

Collaborative

Monitor Hct level.

If fluid replacement is excessive, symptoms of circulatory overload and respiratory difficulties (e.g., pulmonary edema) may occur.

With stabilization of fluid levels, intake should approximate output. Specific gravity readings change inversely to output so that as kidney function improves, specific gravity readings decrease, and vice versa. Note: In the client with glomerular spasms caused by PIH, output may be diminished until extracellular fluids return to general circulation.

Changes in mentation/behavior may be an early sign of cerebral edema caused by fluid retention.

As plasma volume is restored, the Hct level drops.

391

ACTIONS/INTERVENTIONS	RATIONALE
Independent	
Demonstrate proper handwashing and self-care techniques. Review appropriate handling and disposal of contaminated materials (e.g., peripads, tissues, dressings).	Prevents cross-contamination/spread of infectious organisms.
Monitor vital signs.	Temperature elevations of 100.4°F (38°C) on 2 consecutive days (not counting the first 24 hr postpartum), tachycardia, suggest infection.
Observe perineum/episiotomy site, abdominal wound (cesarean birth).	Erythema, edema, induration, tenderness, separation of wound edges, purulent drainage suggest localized infectious process requiring prompt intervention to prevent systemic complications.
Note symptoms of malaise, chills, anorexia, uterine tenderness, or pelvic pain.	These symptoms indicate systemic involvement, possibly leading to bacteremia, shock, or death if not treated.
Monitor rate of uterine involution and nature and amount of lochial discharge. (Refer to CP: Puerperal Infection.)	Uterine infection delays involution and prolongs lochial flow.
Investigate other potential sources of infection, such as respiratory (changes in breath sounds, productive cough, purulent sputum), mastitis (swelling, erythema, pain), or urinary tract infection (cloudy, odoriferous urine; urgency, frequency, pain).	Differential diagnosis is critical for effective treatment.
Collaborative	
Review WBC count.	Leukocytosis with shift to the left signifies infection.
Assess Hb/Hct levels. Administer iron supplement, as indicated.	Anemia often accompanies infection, delays healing, and impairs the immune system.
Obtain Gram's stain or bacterial culture if lochia is foul-smelling or profuse/purulent wound drainage is present.	Gram's stain identifies type of infection, whereas cultures identify specific pathogen.
Administer IV antibiotics, as indicated.	Broad-spectrum antibiotic may be ordered until results from culture and sensitivity studies are available, at which time organism-specific antibiotic may be started.
Assist as necessary with surgical procedures (e.g., D & C, hysterectomy).	D & C may be necessary to remove any remaining placental fragments; hysterectomy may be necessary in septic shock.

NURSING DIAGNOSIS:	PAIN, risk for
Risk Factors May Include:	Tissue trauma/distension
Possibly Evidenced By:	[Not applicable; presence of signs/symptoms establishes an *actual* diagnosis]
DESIRED OUTCOMES/EVALUATION CRITERIA—CLIENT WILL:	Identify individually appropriate methods to promote comfort.
	Verbalize relief of pain and discomfort.

ACTIONS/INTERVENTIONS	RATIONALE

Independent

Determine characteristics, type, location, and duration of pain. Rate intensity on a 0–10 scale. Assess client for persistent perineal pain, feeling of fullness in vagina, uterine contractions, or abdominal tenderness.	Aids in differential diagnosis and selection of treatment methods. Discomfort associated with hematomas is caused by pressure from concealed hemorrhage into vaginal or perineal tissues. Abdominal tenderness may result from uterine atony or retained pieces of placenta. Severe pain, both uterine and abdominal, may occur with inversion of the uterus. Lacerations may result in painful burning or tearing sensations.
Assess possible psychological causes of discomfort.	Emergency situation may precipitate fear and anxiety, which intensify perception of discomfort. (Refer to ND: Anxiety [specify level].)
Instruct client in relaxation techniques; provide diversional activities as appropriate.	Educating client in physiological and psychological methods of pain control decreases anxiety and perception of discomfort.
Provide comfort measures, such as application of ice to perineum or heat lamp to episiotomy extension, use of sitz bath.	Cold applications minimize edema and reduce hematoma and pain sensation; heat (after first 24 hr) promotes vasodilation, which facilitates resorption of hematoma.

Collaborative

Administer analgesics, narcotics, or sedatives, as indicated.	Decreases pain and anxiety; promotes relaxation.

NURSING DIAGNOSIS:	KNOWLEDGE deficit [LEARNING NEED], regarding condition, prognosis, and treatment needs
May Be Related To:	Lack of exposure to, and unfamiliarity with, information resources
Possibly Evidenced By:	Request for information, statement of misconceptions, inappropriate or exaggerated behaviors
DESIRED OUTCOMES/EVALUATION CRITERIA—CLIENT WILL:	Verbalize in simple terms the pathophysiology and implications of her clinical situation.
	Identify behaviors to enhance recovery.
	Use resources effectively.

393

ACTIONS/INTERVENTIONS	RATIONALE

Independent

Explain predisposing or causative factors and treatment specific to the cause of hemorrhage.

Provides information to help client/couple understand and cope with situation.

Assess client's/couple's level of knowledge, readiness, and ability to learn. Listen, talk calmly, and allow time for questions and review of material.

Provides information necessary to develop individual plan of care and engage in problem-solving activities. Reduces anxiety and stress, which can block learning, and provides clarification and repetition to enhance understanding.

Discuss short-term implications of postpartal hemorrhage, such as delay or interruption in process of maternal-infant attachment, inability to assume care of self and infant as soon as desired.

Reduces anxiety and provides realistic time frame for resumption of bonding and infant/self-care activities. (Refer to ND: Parent/Infant Attachment, risk for altered.)

Discuss long-term implications of postpartal hemorrhage as appropriate; e.g., risk of postpartal hemorrhage in subsequent pregnancies, uterine atony, or the inability to bear children in the future if hysterectomy is performed.

Permits client to make informed decisions and to begin to resolve feelings about current and past events.

Instruct client to report failure to lactate, fatigue, loss of pubic or axillary hair, amenorrhea, genital atrophy, premature aging (cachexia).

These signs suggest Sheehan's syndrome, which occurs in 15% of survivors of severe postpartal hemorrhage; causes partial or total loss of thyroid, adrenocortical, and gonadal functions and requires long-term treatment with estrogen, thyroid, or cortisone replacement therapy. Note: Sheehan's syndrome often results in irreversible infertility, reduced resistance to infection, premature aging, and increased risk of shock.

Determine availability of personal resources/supports. Discuss necessity of adequate rest/sleep, healthy nutritional intake, and pacing of activities.

Fatigue associated with anemia/hemorrhage will delay client's resumption of normal activities, necessitating problem solving and reliance on others for a period of time. Note: This may be very frustrating for client (and her family).

Recommend client be seated when holding infant and to change position slowly when lying down or seated.

Orthostatic hypotension places client at risk for lightheadedness/falls.

Refer to support group(s) as appropriate.

Specific groups, such as a hysterectomy support group, may provide ongoing information and role models to facilitate positive adaptation.

NURSING DIAGNOSIS:	PARENT/INFANT ATTACHMENT, risk for altered
Risk Factors May Include:	Interruption in bonding process, physical condition, perceived threat to own survival
Possibly Evidenced By:	[Not applicable; presence of signs/symptoms establishes an *actual* diagnosis]
DESIRED OUTCOMES/EVALUATION CRITERIA—CLIENT WILL:	Demonstrate appropriate behaviors associated with positive attachment to infant.
	Assume responsibility for physical and emotional care of the newborn, as able.
	Express comfort with parenting role.

ACTIONS/INTERVENTIONS	RATIONALE

Independent

Explain factors resulting from postpartal hemorrhage that necessitate separation of mother and infant.

Provide opportunity for client/couple to express their fears and anger at the situation.

Discuss client's perceptions of infant care responsibilities and parenting role.

Encourage contact with infant (verbal reports, photos, information from significant other who has seen baby) until client can see and begin to care for the infant.

Evaluate attachment process, bonding behaviors, and parenting abilities once client assumes care of her infant.

Provide client/couple with information on community resources and with follow-up healthcare referrals, including parenting classes, child care facilities, and well-baby clinics.

Helps reduce anxiety and feelings of frustration and helplessness related to client's inability to assume caregiving role with infant.

Promotes acceptance of physiological and psychological constraints, which may help reduce anxiety associated with development of complications.

Provides information about how client views these role changes; identifies areas of learning need.

Reassures mother of infant's health status and of proper care being provided to the infant.

Provides information on psychological and physiological capabilities related to parenting; identifies client's needs.

Reinforces positive information previously given by health team. Reduces anxiety; promotes independence and personal growth.

395

POSTPARTAL DIABETES MELLITUS

(To be used in conjunction with customary postpartal plans of care.)

CLIENT ASSESSMENT DATA BASE

(Refer to CP: Diabetes Mellitus: Prepregnancy/Gestational; and CP: Intrapartal Diabetes Mellitus.)

Activity/Rest

Fatigue, especially when labor was long or difficult (increases glucose needs)

Circulation

May have elevated BP, edema (signs of PIH that developed during prenatal, intrapartal, or postpartal period
History of vascular changes associated with diabetes that impair circulation/kidney functioning; venous thrombosis

Elimination

Polyuria

Food/Fluid

Polydipsia, polyphagia
Nausea/vomiting
Ketonuria, elevated serum glucose
May report episodes of hypoglycemia, glycosuria

Safety

Healing of episiotomy or cesarean incision may be delayed.
May report visual disturbances.

Sexuality

Uterus may be relaxed/boggy, and lochia may be heavy with clots present.
Current pregnancy may have involved uterine overdistension (macrosomia or hydramnios).
Labor may have been prolonged/augmented or induced.
Preterm, large-for-gestational age, or low-birth-weight infant.

Teaching/Learning

Change in stability of diabetes, adjustment of insulin therapy.
Type of infant feeding planned affects caloric needs and insulin requirements.

DIAGNOSTIC STUDIES

Fasting (Daily) or Serum Glucose: Assesses control (increased risk of hypoglycemia).
Hb/Hct: Baseline studies.
Glycosylated Hemoglobin (HbA$_{1c}$): May be elevated (greater than 8.5%), indicating inadequate control of serum glucose levels.
Urinalysis: May show glucose, ketones, or protein.

NURSING PRIORITIES

1. Maintain normoglycemia.
2. Prevent or minimize complications.
3. Promote parent-infant bonding.
4. Provide information concerning postpartal changes and diabetic management.

DISCHARGE CRITERIA

Gestational Diabetes

1. Regains euglycemia without need of medication
2. Understands nature of condition and prognosis for future

Diabetes

Because this is a life-long condition, client's care will be transferred to primary care provider at completion of postpartum period.

NURSING DIAGNOSIS:	NUTRITION: altered, risk for less than body requirements
Risk Factors May Include:	Inability to ingest/utilize nutrients appropriately, increased metabolic demands (recuperation, lactation)
Possibly Evidenced By:	[Not applicable; presence of signs/symptoms establishes an *actual* diagnosis]
DESIRED OUTCOMES/EVALUATION CRITERIA—CLIENT WILL:	Maintain serum glucose levels within individually determined parameters, free of hypoglycemia/hyperglycemia.
	Verbalize understanding of, and participate in, self-monitoring and individual treatment regimen.

ACTIONS/INTERVENTIONS	RATIONALE

Independent

Review onset of diabetes (prepregnancy versus gestational) and type of infant feeding planned.	The client with gestational diabetes mellitus (GDM) usually requires no further insulin after delivery; the client with prepregnancy onset must be re-regulated based on fasting blood sugar and 1-hr postprandial serum glucose levels. In addition, breastfeeding has an antidiabetogenic effect because carbohydrates are used in milk production.
Assess for hypoglycemic or hyperglycemic reactions. Note changes in mentation and behavior, visual disturbances, nausea or vomiting, tachycardia, slurred speech, or Kussmaul's respirations.	Because the half-life of human placental lactogen is 20–30 min, most of this insulin antagonist has disappeared within 2–3 hr postpartum, rendering the client susceptible to hypoglycemia, if insulin dosages are not accurately recalculated.
Monitor urine for glucose and ketones.	The presence of ketones indicates inadequate carbohydrate intake and fat breakdown and may necessitate modifying diet or discontinuing breastfeeding.
Advise GDM client to avoid obesity and to lose weight during postpartal period if she is not lactating.	Helps reduce risk of developing insulin-dependent diabetes (type I), although 70% of individuals who develop GDM develop type 2 diabetes later in life, often within 10 yr.

Collaborative

Coordinate multi-specialty care conference as appropriate.	Provides opportunity to determine individual postpartal diabetic control based on client's specific needs (e.g., diabetic classification, lactation).

Monitor serum glucose levels by fingerstick per protocol and as indicated.

Following removal of the placenta with its anti-insulin hormones, insulin requirements decrease in the first 48–96 hr postpartum. Such a change results in a glucose-insulin imbalance. Frequent assessment (e.g., every 2 hr) is continued until serum glucose levels stabilize and carbohydrate hemostasis occurs. Whereas hypoglycemia is common during the first 24 hr after delivery, it may compromise wound healing, and poor control is associated with increased morbidity and infection.

Discontinue insulin infusion after vaginal delivery, as indicated; continue infusion of glucose until oral feedings are started.

Insulin requirements quickly decline after delivery of the placenta. Glucose infusion helps prevent hypoglycemic response. Note: IV infusion of 5% dextrose with insulin at 1 unit/hr via pump may be used to maintain normoglycemic control in early postpartal period.

Continue insulin infusion after cesarean birth until client has resumed eating.

Surgical procedure/stress may increase insulin needs.

Administer insulin subcutaneously or monitor self-administration of insulin for client with prepregnancy diabetes.

During first 1 or 2 days postpartum, insulin dosage is usually equal to one-half to two-thirds of prepregnancy levels with the resumption of a "regular" diet.

Adjust diet to increase calories by 500–800 kcal/day above pregravid requirements if client is breastfeeding.

Inadequate caloric intake with resulting hypoglycemia negatively affects milk supply and let-down reflex.

Reevaluate serum glucose levels at 4- to 6-wk checkup or when breastfeeding stops. Institute new dietary insulin control if fasting plasma glucose is greater than 120–140 mg/dl, or if 2-hr oral glucose tolerance test (GTT) is 140–200 mg/dl and at least one other value is greater than 200 mg/dl.

Although temporary remission of diabetes may occur, necessitating lowering insulin needs, return to prepregnancy doses is usually required to 6 wk postpartum, or when weaning occurs.

NURSING DIAGNOSIS:	**INJURY, risk for**
Risk Factors May Include:	Biochemical or regulatory complications (e.g., uterine atony/hemorrhage, hypertension [PIH], hyperglycemia)
Possibly Evidenced By:	[Not applicable; presence of signs/symptoms establishes an *actual* diagnosis]
DESIRED OUTCOMES/EVALUATION CRITERIA—CLIENT WILL:	Display vital signs, reflex response, lochial discharge, and WBC count WNL, with uterus well contracted.

ACTIONS/INTERVENTIONS	RATIONALE

Independent

Monitor contractility and location of uterus.	Uterine atony and hemorrhage may occur, owing to overdistension associated with a large (macrosomic) infant, hydramnios, or oxytocin stimulation.
Gently massage uterus, as indicated.	Increases uterine tone and myometrial contractility, reducing risk of hemorrhage.
Assess amount and type of lochial flow with each check of the fundus. (Refer to CP: Postpartal Hemorrhage; ND: Fluid Volume, risk for deficit.)	Increased or heavy flow may indicate developing complications.

Assess bladder fullness; encourage voiding within 6–8 hr following delivery. Monitor intake and output.

Polyuria (increased urine output) associated with diabetes occurs as a means of excreting excess glucose and retained fluids. A full bladder may interfere with uterine involution.

Monitor BP and pulse. Note location and extent of edema and presence of proteinuria, visual disturbances, hyperreflexia, or RUQ/epigastric pain. Institute seizure precautions. (Refer to CP: Pregnancy-Induced Hypertension.)

With hemorrhage, BP decreases and pulse increases. Elevated BP, proteinuria, and extensive edema may indicate PIH or potential eclampsia. Danger of eclampsia exists for up to 72 hr postpartum, but can actually occur for up to 1 wk postpartum, depending on severity of hypertension, fluid retention, and organ involvement.

Monitor temperature and WBC count. Assess lochia and episiotomy or abdominal incision. Note progressive rate of uterine involution.

Infection is indicated by elevated temperature and WBC count; redness, erythema, or exudate at site of episiotomy or abdominal incision; and foul-smelling lochia. Infection may occur in diabetic client owing to poor healing associated with vascular involvement and hyperglycemia. (Refer to CP: Puerperal Infection.)

NURSING DIAGNOSIS:	KNOWLEDGE deficit [LEARNING NEED], regarding condition, prognosis, and treatment needs
May Be Related To:	Lack of exposure/recall, misinterpretation, unfamiliarity with resources
Possibly Evidenced By:	Verbalization of concerns/misconceptions, inadequate performance of procedures, development of preventable complications
DESIRED OUTCOMES/EVALUATION CRITERIA—CLIENT/COUPLE WILL:	Verbalize understanding of physiological changes, individual needs, possible outcomes.
	Perform necessary activities/procedures correctly and explain reasons for actions.
	Select family planning method prior to discharge.

ACTIONS/INTERVENTIONS	RATIONALE

Independent

Discuss dietary needs based on individual weight gain and choice of infant feeding.

Calorie needs will be determined by desired weight goal and whether client is breastfeeding. (During lactation, glucose is used as energy in milk production, thus lowering glucose levels in client.)

Stress importance of home monitoring of condition and maintenance of log of dietary intake, medication, exercise, and signs/symptoms of serum glucose fluctuation.

Although the demands of pregnancy are concluded, postpartal demands of healing/return to nonpregnant state and needs of infant (including lactation) and family will affect diabetic control. Keeping a log provides insight to individual needs/responses to therapy. Note: Increased sensitivity to insulin during first few weeks following delivery places client at high risk for hypoglycemia.

Evaluate client's eyesight and ability to provide infant care in client with long-standing diabetes.

Approximately 15% of diabetic clients will incur an increase of retinopathy during the prenatal period,

399

| | negatively affecting client's independence and requiring additional teaching/support. |

Provide information for class A diabetic client (White's classification) about the need to return for a 3-hr GTT at 6–8 wk postpartum or at cessation of breastfeeding. If tests results are normal, annual follow-up testing is recommended.

About 18% of class A diabetic clients manifest carbohydrate intolerance at 6 wk postpartum. Greater than 70% of clients with GDM eventually develop type 2 diabetes, many within 10 yr following delivery.

Identify signs/symptoms requiring notification of healthcare provider; e.g., continued oozing or lack of progression of lochia, fever, or foul-smelling urine/vaginal drainage.

Prompt evaluation and intervention may prevent or limit development of complications such as hemorrhage and infection.

Discuss client's/couple's plans for future pregnancies and the impact of diabetes on fertility. Review the critical importance of obtaining metabolic control of diabetes prior to conception.

Diabetes, if well controlled, does not alter or reduce fertility rate. Uncontrolled diabetes and elevated HbA_{1c} levels during organogenesis greatly increase incidence of malformations. Good metabolic control started before conception and continued during these critical weeks may prevent such malformations.

Determine client's/couple's plans for selecting a contraceptive method.

Choosing a method of contraception involves some compromise between benefits and risks, especially with the diabetic client. Risk of using oral contraceptives or the intrauterine device (IUD) in diabetic clients must be weighed against the risk of pregnancy with other forms of contraception. Note: Cultural/religious beliefs may limit options.

Provide information and review side effects associated with contraceptive choices:

Oral contraceptives;

Side effects include elevated BP and acceleration of blood vessel disease (thrombophlebitis, vascular complications). Estrogen increases the production of cholesterol and triglycerides, and progesterone interferes with insulin activity, accelerating the subclinical diabetic process and creating deterioration in the diabetic state. Note: Progestin-only or triphasic products are considered safer than combined oral contraceptives.

IUD;

Some studies indicate an increased risk of pelvic salpingitis (especially during first 20 days after insertion).

Barrier methods (i.e., condom, diaphragm, cervical caps, sponges, or spermicidal creams);

No side effects or contraindications of these methods are specific for diabetic client, although these methods are not as effective in preventing unwanted pregnancies, in part because of inconsistent use. When a device such as the diaphragm is used in conjunction with a spermicidal cream, effectiveness is significantly increased.

Tubal ligation.

May be desirable for diabetic client with complications of nephropathy, retinopathy, or vascular disease, rather than risk the possibility of future pregnancies with negative maternal/fetal outcomes.

Provide information about effects of diabetes on future offspring.

Heredity contributes to the risk of diabetes. Type 1 (insulin-dependent) diabetes mellitus appears to be transmitted less frequently to offspring of diabetic women than to offspring of diabetic men, although this phenomenon may be caused by perinatal loss of affected offspring by diabetic mothers. If a parent develops type 2 diabetes mellitus, the children are at a greater risk than the general population for developing this type of diabetes.

(Refer to CP: The Client at 4 Hours to 2 Days Postpartum; ND: Knowledge deficit [Learning need], for additional actions.)

NURSING DIAGNOSIS:	PARENT/INFANT ATTACHMENT, risk for altered
Risk Factors May Include:	Interruption in bonding process, physical illness/changes in physical abilities
Possibly Evidenced By:	[Not applicable; presence of signs/symptoms establishes an *actual* diagnosis]
DESIRED OUTCOMES/EVALUATION CRITERIA—CLIENT/COUPLE WILL:	Demonstrate positive attachment behaviors.
	Verbalize fears and concerns about infant's condition.
	Participate optimally in infant contact and care.

ACTIONS/INTERVENTIONS	RATIONALE

Independent

Determine current status of infant.	The special needs of the infant of the diabetic mother include hypoglycemia, hypocalcemia, prematurity, and respiratory distress syndrome, possibly necessitating a short- or long-term stay in the neonatal intensive care unit (NICU). Such separation, with diminished physical contact coupled with excessive parental anxiety, may interfere with positive bonding and may create a high-risk parenting situation.
Provide information concerning condition of infant.	Information helps reduce fears and emphasizes the reality of the infant's presence.
Determine client's/couple's feelings concerning infant. Observe contact with infant. (Refer to CP: The Parents of a Child with Special Needs.)	Provides baseline for future comparison; identifies needs and potential concerns.
Assess effectiveness/use of support systems by client/couple.	Strong system of support from family/friends or community facilitates positive adaptation to stress.
Encourage frequent interaction with infant and participation in infant care tasks as client's/infant's condition allows.	Couple may be extremely anxious if infant is in NICU and may be fearful of touching or holding the infant.
Facilitate communication between couple and nursery staff. Point out normal and positive aspects of infant.	Staff can reduce fears, act as role models, and facilitate bonding, especially in caring for preterm infant.
Refer parents to other couples who have had	Increases parents' sense of support and helps them

401

similar experiences with their newborn infants or to the appropriate support groups. to feel that they are not alone. Provides opportunity for creative problem solving.

Collaborative

Refer to visiting nurse services or parenting classes, as indicated.

Client/couple may need additional assistance to promote family integration.

(Refer to CP: Maternal Assessment: 4 to 6 Weeks Following Delivery; ND: Parenting, risk for altered.)

PUERPERAL INFECTION

Puerperal infection is an infection of the reproductive tract occurring within 28 days following childbirth or abortion. It is one of the major causes of maternal death (ranking second behind postpartal hemorrhage) and includes localized infectious processes as well as more progressive processes that may result in endometritis/metritis (inflammation of endometrium), peritonitis, or parametritis/pelvic cellulitis (infection of connective tissue of broad ligament and possibly connective tissue of all pelvic structures).

(This plan of care is an adjunct to the regular postpartal plans of care.)

CLIENT ASSESSMENT DATA BASE

Activity/Rest

Malaise, lethargy
Exhaustion and/or ongoing fatigue (prolonged labor, multiple postpartal stressors)

Circulation

Tachycardia of varying severity

Elimination

Diarrhea may be present.
Bowel sounds may be absent if paralytic ileus occurs.

Ego Integrity

Marked anxiety (peritonitis)

Food/Fluid

Anorexia, nausea/vomiting
Thirst, dry mucous membranes
Abdominal distension, rigidity, rebound tenderness (peritonitis)

Hygiene

Lack of or inadequate perineal care

Neurosensory

Headache

Pain/Discomfort

Localized pain, dysuria, abdominal discomfort
Severe or prolonged afterpains, lower abdominal or uterine pain and tenderness with guarding (endometritis)
Unilateral/bilateral abdominal pain/rigidity (salpingitis/oophoritis, parametritis)

Respiration

Rapid/shallow respirations (severe/systemic process)

Safety

Temperature: 100.4°F (38.0°C) or higher, occurring on any 2 successive days but excluding the first 24 hr postpartum, is indicative of infection; however, temperature higher than 101°F (38.3°C) in the first 24 hr is highly indicative of ensuing infection (although persistent low-grade fever during this time may also reflect infectious process).

403

Low-grade fever of less than 101°F (38.3°C) suggests incisional infection; fever greater than 102°F (38.8°C) is indicative of more extensive infection (e.g., salpingitis, parametritis, peritonitis).

Chills may occur; severe/recurrent chills (often lasting 30–40 min), with temperature spikes to 104°F (40.0°C), suggest pelvic infections, thrombophlebitis, or peritonitis.

Reports of internal monitoring, frequent intrapartal vaginal examinations, lapses in aseptic technique, traumatic delivery and/or lacerations of reproductive tract, operative procedures/incisions.

Preexisting infections, including human immunodeficiency virus (HIV).

Environmental exposure.

Sexuality

Premature or prolonged rupture of membranes, prolonged labor (24 hr or more).

Retention of products of conception, uterine exploration/manual removal of placenta, or postpartal hemorrhage.

Incision edges may be reddened, edematous, firm, tender, or separated, with drainage of purulent or sanguineous liquid.

Uterine subinvolution may be present.

Lochia may be foul-smelling, odorless (as in beta-hemolytic streptococci infection), scant, or profuse.

Social Interaction

Low socioeconomic status with corresponding stressors (including homelessness)

Teaching/Learning

Lack of prenatal care/postpartal follow-up
Chronic conditions; e.g., malnutrition, anemia, diabetes

DIAGNOSTIC STUDIES

White Blood Cell Count (WBC): Normal or elevated with differential shifted to the left.

Erythrocyte Sedimentation Rate (ESR), and Red Blood Cell (RBC) Count: Markedly increased in presence of infection.

Hemoglobin/Hematocrit (Hb/Hct), RBC Count: Decreased in presence of anemia.

Cultures (Aerobic/Anaerobic) of Intrauerine or Intracervical Material or Wound Drainage, or Gram's Stain of Lochia, Cervix, and Uterus: Identify causative organism(s).

Urinalysis and Culture: Rule out UTI.

Ultrasonography: Determines presence of retained placental fragments; locates peritoneal abscess.

Bimanual Examination: Determines nature and location of pelvic pain, mass or abscess formation, or presence of thrombosed veins.

NURSING PRIORITIES

1. Control spread of infection.
2. Promote healing.
3. Support ongoing process of family acquaintance.

DISCHARGE GOALS

1. Infection resolving
2. Involution progressing, sense of well-being expressed
3. Attachment/bonding demonstrated and care of infant resumed

NURSING DIAGNOSIS:	INFECTION, risk for spread/sepsis
Risk Factors May Include:	Presence of infection, broken skin and/or traumatized tissues, high vascularity of involved area, invasive procedures and/or increased environmental exposure, chronic disease (e.g., diabetes), anemia, malnutrition, immunosuppression and/or untoward effect of medication (e.g., opportunistic/secondary infections)
Possibly Evidenced By:	[Not applicable: presence of signs/symptoms established an *actual* diagnosis]
DESIRED OUTCOMES/EVALUATION CRITERIA—CLIENT WILL:	Verbalize understanding of individual causative risk factors. Initiate behaviors to limit spread of infection, as appropriate, and reduce risk of complications. Achieve timely healing, free of additional complications.

ACTIONS/INTERVENTIONS	RATIONALE
Independent	
Review prenatal, intrapartal, and postpartal record.	Identifies factors that place client in high-risk category for development/spread of postpartal infection.
Demonstrate and maintain strict hand-washing policy for staff, client, and visitors.	Helps prevent cross-contamination.
Provide for, and instruct client in, proper disposal of contaminated linens, dressings, chux, and peripads. Initiate/maintain isolation, if indicated.	Prevents spread of infection.
Demonstrate/encourage correct perineal cleaning after voiding and defecation, and frequent changing of peripads.	Cleaning removes urinary/fecal contaminants. Changing pad removes moist medium that favors bacterial growth.
Demonstrate proper fundal massage. Review importance and timing of procedure.	Enhances uterine contractility; promotes involution and passage of any retained placental fragments.
Monitor temperature, pulse, and respirations. Note presence of chills or reports of anorexia or malaise.	Elevations in vital signs accompany infection; fluctuations, or changes in symptoms, suggest alterations in client status. Note: Persistent fever unresponsive to antibiotic therapy may indicate pelvic thrombophlebitis.
Observe perineum/incision for other signs of infection (e.g., redness, edema, ecchymosis, discharge and approximation [REEDA scale]). Note subinvolution of uterus, extreme uterine tenderness.	Allows early identification and treatment; promotes resolution of infection. Note: Although localized infections are usually not severe, occasional progression to necrotizing fasculitis can be life-threatening.
Monitor oral/parenteral intake, stressing the need for at least 2000 ml fluid per day. Note urine output, degree of hydration, and presence of nausea, vomiting, or diarrhea.	Increased intake replaces losses and enhances circulating volume, preventing dehydration and aiding in fever reduction.
Encourage semi-Fowler's position.	Enhances flow of lochia and uterine/pelvic drainage.

405

Promote early ambulation, balanced with adequate rest. Advance activity as appropriate.	Increases circulation; promotes clearing of respiratory secretions and lochial drainage; enhances healing and general well-being. Note: Presence of pelvic/femoral thrombophlebitis may require strict bedrest.
Investigate reports of leg or chest pain. Note pallor, swelling, or stiffness of lower extremity. (Refer to CP: Postpartal Thrombophlebitis.)	These signs and symptoms are suggestive of septic thrombus formation. Note: Embolic sequelae, especially pulmonary embolism, may be initial indicator of thrombophlebitis.
Recommend that breastfeeding mother periodically check infant's mouth for presence of white patches.	Oral thrush in the newborn is a common side effect of maternal antibiotic therapy.
Encourage client/couple to prioritize postdischarge responsibilities (e.g., homemaking tasks, child care).	Client will require additional rest to facilitate recuperation/healing. Household duties need to be reassigned or delayed as appropriate.
Instruct in proper medication use (e.g., take entire course of antibiotic, as prescribed).	Oral antibiotics may be continued after discharge. Failure to complete medication may lead to relapse.
Discuss importance of pelvic rest as appropriate (avoidance of douching, tampons, and intercourse).	Promotes healing and reduces risk of reinfection.

Collaborative

Encourage application of moist heat in the form of sitz baths and of dry heat in the form of perineal lights for 15 min 2–4 times daily.	Water promotes cleansing. Heat dilates perineal blood vessels, increasing localized blood flow and promotes healing.
Demonstrate perineal application of antibiotic creams, as appropriate.	Eradicates local infectious organisms, reducing risk of spreading infection.
Monitor laboratory studies, as indicated:	
Culture(s)/sensitivity;	Identifies infectious process/causative organism and appropriate antimicrobial agents.
CBC, WBC count, differential, and ESR;	Aids in tracking resolution of infectious or inflammatory process. Identifies degree of blood loss and determines presence of anemia.
Partial thromboplastin time/prothrombin time (PTT/PT), clotting times;	Helps in identifying alterations in clotting associated with development of emboli. Aids in determining effectiveness of anticoagulation therapy.
Renal/hepatic function studies.	Hepatic insufficiency and decreased renal function may develop, altering drug half-life and increasing risks of toxicity.
Administer medications as indicated:	
Antibiotics, initially broad-spectrum, then organism-specific, as indicated by results of cultures/sensitivity;	Combats pathogenic organisms, helping prevent infection from spreading to surrounding tissues and bloodstream. Note: Parenteral route is preferred for parametritis, peritonitis, and, on occasion, endometritis.
Oxytocics, such as pitocin and methylergonovine maleate (Methergine);	Promotes myometrial contractility to retard the spread of bacteria through the uterine walls, and aids in the expulsion of clots and retained placental fragments.
Anticoagulants (e.g., heparin).	In presence of pelvic thrombophlebitis, anticoagulants prevent or reduce additional thrombi formation and limit spread of septic emboli.

Assist with procedures, such as incision and drainage (I&D) or D & C, as necessary.	Draining the infected area, and possible insertion of iodoform gauze packing, promotes healing and reduces risk of rupture into peritoneal cavity. D & C may be needed to remove retained products of conception and/or placental fragments.
Administer whole blood/packed RBCs, if needed.	Replaces blood losses and increases oxygen-carrying capacity in presence of severe anemia/hemorrhage.
Provide supplemental oxygen when necessary.	Promotes healing and tissue regeneration, especially in presence of anemia; may enhance oxygenation when pulmonary emboli are present.
Arrange for transfer to intensive care setting as appropriate.	May be necessary for client with severe infection (e.g., peritonitis, sepsis) or pulmonary emboli to provide appropriate care leading to optimal recovery.

NURSING DIAGNOSIS:	**NUTRITION: altered, less than body requirements**
May Be Related To:	Intake insufficient to meet metabolic demands (anorexia, nausea/vomiting, medical restrictions)
Possibly Evidenced By:	Aversion to eating, decreased oral intake or lack of oral intake, unanticipated weight loss
DESIRED OUTCOMES/EVALUATION CRITERIA—CLIENT WILL:	Meet nutritional needs, as evidenced by timely wound healing, appropriate energy level, and Hb/Hct within normal postpartal expectations.

ACTIONS/INTERVENTIONS	RATIONALE

Independent

Encourage choice of foods high in protein, iron, and vitamin C when oral intake permitted.	Protein helps promote healing and regeneration of new tissue. Iron is necessary for Hb synthesis. Vitamin C facilitates iron absorption and is necessary for cell wall synthesis.
Promote intake of at least 2000 ml/day of juices, soups, and other nutritious fluids.	Provides calories and other nutrients to meet metabolic needs and replaces fluid losses, thereby increasing circulating fluid volume.
Encourage adequate sleep/rest.	Reduces metabolic rate, allowing nutrients and oxygen to be used for healing process.

Collaborative

Administer parenteral fluids/nutrition, as indicated.	May be necessary to combat dehydration, replace fluid losses, and provide necessary nutrients when oral intake is limited/restricted.
Administer iron preparations and/or vitamins, as indicated.	Useful in correcting anemia or deficiencies when present.
Assist with placement of nasogastric (NG) or Miller-Abbott tube.	May be necessary for gastrointestinal decompression in presence of abdominal distension or peritonitis.

407

NURSING DIAGNOSIS:	PAIN [acute]
May Be Related To:	Body response to infective agent, properties of infection (e.g., skin/tissue edema, erythema)
Possibly Evidenced By:	Verbalizations, restlessness, guarding behavior, self-focusing, autonomic responses
DESIRED OUTCOMES/EVALUATION CRITERIA—CLIENT WILL:	Identify/use individually appropriate comfort measures.
	Report decreased level of pain/discomfort.

ACTIONS/INTERVENTIONS	RATIONALE

Independent

Assess location and nature of discomfort or pain, rate pain on a 0–10 scale.	Aids in differential diagnosis of tissue involvement in infectious process.
Provide instruction regarding, and assist with, maintenance of cleanliness and warmth.	Promotes sense of general well-being and enhances healing. Alleviates discomfort associated with chills.
Change client's position frequently. Provide comfort measures; e.g., back rubs, linen changes.	Reduces muscle fatigue, promotes relaxation and comfort.
Instruct client in relaxation techniques; provide diversionary activities such as radio, television, or reading.	Refocuses client's attention, promotes positive attitude, and enhances comfort.
Encourage continuation of breastfeeding as client's condition permits. Otherwise suggest and provide instruction in use of manual or electric breast pump.	Prevents discomfort of engorgement; promotes adequacy of milk supply in breastfeeding client.

Collaborative

Administer analgesics or antipyretics.	Reduces associated discomforts of infection.
Apply local heat using heat lamp or sitz bath as indicated.	Heat promotes vasodilation, increasing circulation to the affected area and promoting localized comfort.

NURSING DIAGNOSIS:	PARENT/INFANT ATTACHMENT, risk for altered
Risk Factors May Include:	Interruption in bonding process, physical illness, perceived threat to own survival
Possibly Evidenced By:	[Not applicable; presence of signs/symptoms establishes an actual diagnosis]
DESIRED OUTCOMES/EVALUATION CRITERIA—CLIENT WILL:	Exhibit ongoing attachment behaviors during parent-infant interactions.
	Maintain/assume responsibility for physical and emotional care of the newborn, as able.
	Express comfort with parenting role.

ACTIONS/INTERVENTIONS	RATIONALE

Independent

Provide opportunities for maternal-infant contact whenever possible. Place pictures of infant at client's bedside (especially if nature of infection/client's condition or hospital policy requires separation of infant from mother during febrile period).

Facilitates attachment, prevents client from engaging in self-preoccupation to the exclusion of the infant.

Monitor client's emotional responses to illness and separation from infant, such as depression and anger. Encourage client to verbalize feelings and reinforce normalcy as appropriate.

Normal expectations are of an uncomplicated postpartal period with the family unit intact. Illness due to infection alters the situation and may result in separation of client from family or newborn, which can contribute to feelings of isolation and depression.

Encourage client to feed infant if possible and to increase her participation in infant care as the infection resolves/client is able.

Success in accomplishing infant care tasks enhances client's outlook and promotes her attachment with infant. Note: Dependent on type of infection, bottle-fed infants may need to be separated from mother for longer period because they do not receive protective advantages of breastfeeding.

Observe maternal-infant interactions.

Provides information regarding status of bonding process and client needs.

Encourage father/other family members to care for and interact with the infant.

May be encouraging to mother to know that family is caring for the infant and providing emotional support. Note: Unexpected/prolonged hospital stay may reduce father's ability to spend time with newborn because of other responsibilities, including care of siblings. Father may require additional support during this stressful time.

Discuss availability/effectiveness of support systems in home setting.

Client requires additional support to accomplish homemaker tasks, allowing client to obtain adequate rest and spend time with infant/other children.

Collaborative

Make arrangements for appropriate follow-up evaluation of mother-infant interactions/responses through home visit.

Provides resources and support to client; useful in identifying specific needs and facilitates problem-solving.

Identify individual support systems. Refer to visiting nurse services, home care agencies, as indicated.

Client may require assistance with home maintenance and activities of daily living while following discharge instructions for rest and recuperation.

POSTPARTAL THROMBOPHLEBITIS

Superficial thrombophlebitis is seen more often during the postpartal period than during pregnancy and is more common in women with preexisting varices. Postpartal deep vein thrombosis (DVT) and superficial thrombophlebitis have been attributed to trauma to pelvic veins from pressure of the presenting fetal part, sluggish circulation caused by mechanical edema, and alterations in coagulation related to the large amounts of estrogens produced during pregnancy. Thrombosis that involves only the superficial veins of the leg or thigh is unlikely to generate pulmonary emboli (PE). While approximately 50% of clients with DVT are asymptomatic, DVT is more serious in terms of potential complications, including PE, postphlebotic syndrome, chronic venous insufficiency, and vein valve destruction.

(This plan of care is an adjunct to the regular postpartal plans of care.)

CLIENT ASSESSMENT DATA BASE

Activity/Rest

History of prolonged sitting, either work-related or as a result of activity restrictions
Current immobility associated with bedrest and anesthesia
Activity/prolonged standing limited by pain
Fatigue/weakness of affected extremity, general malaise

Circulation

Varicose veins; thrombosis may be palpable, bumpy/knotty.
Slight elevation of pulse rate (superficial).
History of previous venous thrombosis, heart disease, hemorrhage, PIH, diabetes mellitus, hypercoagulability in early puerperium.
Peripheral pulses diminished, positive Homans' sign may or may not be noted (indicators of DVT).
Lower extremity (calf/thigh) may be warm and pinkish-red in color, or affected limb may be cool, pale, edematous.

Food/Fluid

Excessive weight gain/obesity.
Poor skin turgor, dry mucous membranes (dehydration predisposes to hypercoagulability).
Milk supply may occasionally be reduced in lactating client.
Edema of affected extremity (dependent on location of thrombus).

Pain/Discomfort

Throbbing, tenderness, aching pain in affected area (e.g., calf or thigh) aggravated by standing or movement
Lower abdominal pain (involvement of ovarian vein)
Guarding of affected extremity

Safety

Presence of postpartal endometritis or pelvic cellulitis.
Temperature may be slightly elevated; progression to marked elevation and chills (signs of DVT); high fever (septic pelvic thrombophlebitis).

Sexuality

Multiparity; hydramnios
Prolonged labor associated with fetal head pressure on pelvic veins, use of stirrups or faulty positioning of extremities during intrapartal phase/operative delivery

Teaching/Learning

Use of oral contraceptives
Use of estrogen for suppression of lactation

DIAGNOSTIC STUDIES

Hematocrit (Hct): Identify hemoconcentration.

Coagulation Studies: Reveals hypercoagulability.

Noninvasive Vascular Studies (Doppler Oscillometry, Exercise Tolerance, Impedance Plethysmography, and Real-Time [Duplex] Ultrasonography): Changes in blood flow and volume identify venous occlusion, vascular damage, and vascular insufficiency. Ultrasonography appears to be most accurate noninvasive method for diagnosing multiple proximal DVT (iliac, popliteal) but is less reliable in detecting isolated calf vein thrombi.

Trendelenburg Test: May demonstrate vessel valve incompetence.

Contrast Venography: Confirms diagnosis of DVT through changes in blood flow and/or size of channels.

NURSING PRIORITIES

1. Maintain/enhance tissue perfusion, facilitate resolution of thrombus.
2. Promote optimal comfort.
3. Prevent complications.
4. Provide information and emotional support.

DISCHARGE GOALS

1. Tissue perfusion improved in affected limb/area
2. Pain/discomfort relieved
3. Complications prevented/resolved
4. Disease process/prognosis and therapeutic needs understood
5. Plan in place to meet needs after discharge

NURSING DIAGNOSIS:	TISSUE PERFUSION, altered peripheral
May Be Related To:	Interruption of venous flow
Possibly Evidenced By:	Edema of affected extremity; erythema (superficial thrombophlebitis) or pallor and coolness (DVT), diminished peripheral pulses, pain
DESIRED OUTCOMES/EVALUATION CRITERIA—CLIENT WILL:	Demonstrate improved circulation of involved extremity with palpable peripheral pulses of good quality, timely capillary refill, and decreased edema and erythema. Engage in behaviors/activities to enhance tissue perfusion. Display increasing tolerance to activity.

ACTIONS/INTERVENTIONS	RATIONALE
Independent Encourage bedrest with elevation of feet and lower legs 6 in above heart level during acute phase.	Minimizes the possibility of dislodging thrombus and creating emboli. Rapidly empties superficial and tibial veins and keeps veins collapsed, thereby increasing venous return. Note: Caution is required in presence of leg ischemia.
Evaluate neurological function of extremity (both sensory and motor). Observe extremity for color; inspect from groin to foot for edema. Note	Symptoms help distinguish between superficial thrombophlebitis and DVT. Redness, heat, tenderness, and localized edema are characteristic

411

asymmetry; measure and record calf/thigh circumference of both legs as appropriate. Report proximal progression of inflammation, traveling pain.

of superficial involvement. Pallor and coolness of extremity are more characteristic of DVT. Calf vein involvement of DVT is usually associated with absence of edema; mild to moderate edema suggests femoral vein involvement, and severe edema is characteristic of ileofemoral vein thrombosis.

Assess capillary refill, and check for Homans' sign.

Diminished capillary refill usually present in DVT. Positive Homans' sign (deep calf pain in affected leg upon dorsiflexion of foot) is not as consistent a clinical manifestation as once thought and may or may not be present.

Instruct client to elevate legs when in bed or chair, as indicated. Periodically elevate feet and legs above heart level.

Reduces tissue swelling and rapidly empties superficial and tibial veins, preventing overdistension and, thereby, increasing venous return. Note: Some physicians believe that elevation may potentiate release of thrombus, thus increasing risk of embolization and decreasing circulation to the most distal portion of the extremity.

Caution client not to cross legs or wear constrictive clothing.

Physical restriction of circulation impairs blood flow, thus increasing venous stasis, pain, and trauma.

Instruct client to avoid rubbing and massaging the affected extremity.

Prevents fragmentation/dislodging thrombus, which could lead to embolism.

Initiate active or passive exercises while in bed (e.g., flex/extend/rotate foot periodically). Assist with gradual resumption of ambulation (e.g., walking 10 min/h) as soon as client is permitted out of bed.

These measures are designed to increase venous return from lower extremities and reduce venous stasis, as well as improve general muscle tone/strength. They also promote normal organ function and enhance general well-being.

Encourage deep-breathing exercises.

Produces increased negative pressure in thorax, which assists in emptying large veins.

Observe respiratory ease and auscultate lung sounds, noting crackles or friction rub. Investigate reports of chest pain or feelings of anxiety.

Pulmonary congestion, sharp substernal chest pain, sudden apprehension, dyspnea, tachypnea, and hemoptysis are indicative of pulmonary emboli, especially in DVT. Note: Client may remain symptom-free and undiagnosed until emboli develop.

Recommend increased fluid intake to 2000+ ml/day.

Dehydration increases blood viscosity and venous stasis, predisposing to thrombus formation.

Collaborative

Apply warm, moist compresses or heat cradle to affected extremity as indicated.

Increases circulation to area; promotes vasodilation, venous return, and resolution of edema.

Administer medication, e.g.:

Heparin (via continuous IV drip, intermittent administration using heparin lock, or subcutaneous administration) or coumarin derivatives;

Heparin is usually preferred initially, owing to its prompt and predictable antagonistic action toward thrombin formation and prevention of further clot formation. Because of its large molecular size, heparin does not pass through to breast milk as coumarin derivatives do; however, coumarin, which blocks formation of prothrombin from vitamin K, may be used for long-term therapy following discharge.

Thrombolytic agents (streptokinase, urokinase);

May be used for treatment of acute (less than 5 days old) or massive DVT to prevent valvular damage and development of chronic venous

Antibiotic agents.

Apply/regulate graduated compression stockings, intermittent pneumatic compression, if used.

Assist with/monitor application of elastic support hose. Stress need for care to avoid any tourniquet effect.

Monitor laboratory studies, e.g.:

PT, PTT/APTT; Hb/Hct;

Aspartate aminotransferase (AST), lactate dehydrogenase (LDH).

Prepare for surgical intervention when indicated.

insufficiency. Heparin is usually begun several hours after the completion of thrombolytic therapy.
Infections of reproductive tract may lead to septic pelvic thrombophlebitis.

Sequential compression devices may be used to improve blood flow velocity and emptying of vessels by providing artificial muscle-pumping action.

Following acute phase, useful in superficial thrombosis because they exert a sustained, evenly distributed pressure over the entire surface of calves and thighs, reducing caliber of superficial veins, increasing blood flow to deep veins, and reducing stasis.

Monitors effectiveness of anticoagulant therapy. Hemoconcentration and dehydration can potentiate clot formation.
Elevated levels may indicate emboli.

Thrombectomy (excision of thrombus) is occasionally necessary if inflammation extends proximally or circulation is severely restricted. Multiple/recurrent thrombotic episodes unresponsive to medical treatment (or when anticoagulant therapy is contraindicated) may require insertion of a vena caval screen/umbrella).

NURSING DIAGNOSIS:	PAIN [acute]/[DISCOMFORT]
May Be Related To:	Presence of inflammatory process, vascular spasms, accumulation of lactic acid
Possibly Evidenced By:	Verbalizations, restlessness, guarding behavior, self-focus, autonomic responses
DESIRED OUTCOMES/EVALUATION CRITERIA—CLIENT WILL:	Participate in behaviors/techniques to promote comfort.
	Report pain is relieved/controlled.
	Appear relaxed and sleep/rest appropriately.

ACTIONS/INTERVENTIONS

RATIONALE

Independent

Assess characteristics, and degree of discomfort or pain using 0–10 scale; palpate leg with caution. Note guarding of extremity.

Degree of pain is directly related to extent of arterial involvement, degree of hypoxia, and extent of edema associated with thrombus development in inflamed venous wall. Client may guard or immobilize affected extremity to decrease painful sensations associated with muscle movement. Changes in characteristics of pain may indicate progression of problem/development of complications.

413

ACTIONS/INTERVENTIONS	RATIONALE
Maintain bedrest during acute phase.	Reduces discomfort associated with muscle contraction and movement. Minimizes possibility of dislodging thrombus.
Monitor vital signs, noting elevated temperature or pulse.	Elevation of vital signs may indicate increasing pain, or occur in response to fever and inflammatory process. Fever may contribute to general discomfort.
Elevate affected extremity; provide foot cradle.	Encourages venous return, facilitates circulation. Foot cradle keeps pressure of bedclothes off the affected leg, thereby reducing pressure discomfort.
Encourage change of position, keeping extremity elevated.	Decreases or prevents fatigue, helps minimize muscle spasm, and increases venous return.
Explain procedures, treatments, and nursing interventions.	Involving the client in the nursing care increases her sense of control and decreases her level of anxiety. Note: Anxiety/fear can result in muscle tension and increased perceptions of pain.
Investigate reports of sudden and/or sharp chest pain, dyspnea, tachycardia, or apprehension.	These signs and symptoms suggest PE as a complication of DVT.

Collaborative

Administer medications as indicated:	
Analgesics (narcotic/nonnarcotic).	Relieves pain and decreases muscle tension, promoting relaxation/rest.
Antipyretics, anti-inflammatory agents (e.g., acetaminophen, phenylbutazone).	Reduces fever and inflammation. Note: Risk of bleeding may be increased by concurrent use of drugs that affect platelet function, e.g., acetylsalicylic acid (ASA) and nonsteroidal anti-inflammatory drugs (NSAIDs).
Apply moist heat to extremity.	Causes vasodilation, which increases circulation, relaxes muscles, and may stimulate release of endorphins.

NURSING DIAGNOSIS:	**ANXIETY [specify level]**
May Be Related To:	Change in health status, perceived or actual threat to self, situational crisis, interpersonal transmission of anxiety from family members
Possibly Evidenced By:	Increased tension, apprehension, restlessness, sympathetic stimulation
DESIRED OUTCOMES/EVALUATION CRITERIA—CLIENT WILL:	Verbalize awareness of feelings of anxiety.
	Report anxiety reduced to a manageable level.
	Exhibit a decrease in behavioral signs, such as restlessness and irritability.

ACTIONS/INTERVENTIONS	RATIONALE

Independent

ACTIONS/INTERVENTIONS	RATIONALE
Explain procedures, treatments, and nursing interventions.	Reduces fear of the unknown; promotes client's learning and involvement in treatment.

Demonstrate/encourage use of relaxation techniques. Provide opportunity to verbalize concerns.

Energy-release techniques and verbalization of concerns reduce emotional tension, lessening anxiety. Relaxation prevents muscle fatigue and allows client to rest.

Monitor vital signs and behavioral signs such as restlessness, irritability, and crying.

May reflect change in level of anxiety; may indicate decreasing ability to cope with events.

Assist client in caring for herself and infant.

Client's anxiety may lessen when she finds that her needs are met and that she is able to cope and engage in self-care and infant care tasks.

Involve client/significant other(s) in development of plan of care; review instructions and restrictions.

Provides information and helps the client and significant other understand the need for interventions and restrictions; provides them with a sense of control over the situation.

Encourage frequent contact, in person or by telephone, with spouse and children if client is hospitalized. Encourage regular contact/ "rooming in" with newborn as condition allows.

Helps to reduce feelings of separation and isolation. Facilitates transition to home.

Determine anticipated availability/effectiveness of supports following discharge. Prioritize responsibilities/household tasks.

Helps identify specific needs, encourages problem solving to meet needs of client/family before client is discharged.

Collaborative

Refer to social services, visiting nurse, homecare agency, as appropriate.

May require additional support to facilitate recovery/meet needs of family.

NURSING DIAGNOSIS:	KNOWLEDGE deficit [Learning Need], regarding condition, treatment needs, and prognosis
May Be Related To:	Lack of exposure/recall, misinterpretation
Possibly Evidenced By:	Verbalizations, inaccurate follow-through of instructions, development of preventable complications
DESIRED OUTCOMES/EVALUATION CRITERIA—CLIENT WILL:	Verbalize understanding of condition, treatment, and restrictions.
	Initiate necessary behavioral changes/correctly perform therapeutic procedures.
	Identify signs/symptoms requiring medical evaluation.

ACTIONS/INTERVENTIONS

RATIONALE

Independent

Assess client's knowledge and understanding of disease process. Correct misconceptions as needed

Helps in determining specific needs and clarifying previous information.

Provide information about management and diagnostic tests. Identify signs and symptoms requiring notification of healthcare provider;

Can increase understanding and decrease anxiety associated with condition and home management. Progression of condition and/or development of e.g., coolness or pallor of extremity, tenderness in affected area, or edema.

Explain purpose of bedrest/activity restrictions need for adequate rest.

Demonstrate application of antiembolic stocking, if worn. Encourage removal of elastic stockings for brief intervals at least twice daily.

Discuss purpose, dosage of anticoagulant. Emphasize importance of taking drug as prescribed.

Identify possible interactions between oral anticoagulant therapy and other medications (e.g., salicylates, vitamins, antibiotics, barbiturates, and alcohol). Stress need to read ingredient labels of over-the-counter (OTC) drugs.

Recommend safety measures to avoid trauma, such as use of a soft toothbrush, electric razors for shaving, walking barefoot.

Identify untoward anticoagulant effects requiring medical attention, e.g., bleeding from mucous membranes (nose, gums), continued oozing from cuts/punctures, severe bruising after minimal trauma, development of petechiae.

Stress importance of medical follow-up/ laboratory testing.

bleeding requires prompt evaluation and possible changes in therapy to prevent serious complications. Note: Up to 33% will experience a recurrence of DVT.

Rest reduces oxygen and nutrient needs of compromised tissues and decreases risk of fragmentation of thrombosis. Balancing rest with activity prevents exhaustion and further impairment of cellular perfusion.

Continuous constriction may alter or reduce surface perfusion, leading to muscle fatigue. Removal of elastic stockings allows for detection of further vascular involvement or inflammation.

Promotes client safety by reducing risk of inadequate therapeutic response/deleterious side effects.

Oral anticoagulant therapy may last 3–4 mo and may cause problems or require alterations in drug dosage if it is allowed to interact with other medications. Salicylates and excess alcohol decrease prothrombin activity; vitamin K in multivitamins increases prothrombin activity; antibiotics alter intestinal flora and may interfere with vitamin K synthesis; barbiturates increase metabolism of coumarin drugs.

Alterations in coagulation process may result in increased tendency to bleed, which may indicate a need to alter anticoagulant therapy.

Early detection of deleterious effects of therapy (prolongation of clotting time) allows for timely interventions and may prevent serious complications.

Understanding that close supervision of anticoagulant/therapy is necessary (therapeutic dosage range is narrow and complications may be deadly) promotes client participation/adherence to therapeutic regimen.

THE PARENTS OF A CHILD WITH SPECIAL NEEDS

The birth of a child with special needs, regardless of whether the condition is temporary or permanent, creates unique concerns for the family, who mourns the loss of a normal, healthy child. Conditions range from prematurity, growth deviations, and infections to gross anomalies. Although each case is individual and varies in degree of involvement, many similarities are observed in the parents' responses to their child.

(This plan of care is to be used in conjunction with the routine postpartal plans of care.)

CLIENT ASSESSMENT DATA BASE

(Refer to Client Assessment Data Base in CPs: The Client at 4 Hours to 2 Days Postpartum; Care Following Ceasarean Birth (4 Hours to 3 Days Postpartum); The Client at 24 Hours Following Early Discharge; The Client at 1 Week Following Discharge; and The Client at 4 to 6 Weeks Following Delivery.)

Ego Integrity

Varied emotional responses (e.g., calm, withdrawal, irritability, restlessness, weeping, anger)
History of postpartal depression or psychosis

Safety

History of exposure to teratogenic factors
Presence of infectious agents (including HIV), premature rupture of membranes

Sexuality

Unexpected intrapartal event (e.g., dysfunctional labor, hemorrhage)
History of birth of a child with special needs and/or perinatal loss

Teaching/Learning

History of substance use/abuse

DIAGNOSTIC STUDIES

Genetic Studies/Chromosomal Analysis: Helps determine presence of syndromes/inherited disorders, general prognosis, and future expectations.
Other Testing: Dependent on specific findings and individual risk factors.

NURSING PRIORITIES

1. Facilitate grieving and positive coping.
2. Provide appropriate information related to short- and long-term implications of child's illness or anomaly.
3. Facilitate learning of parenting role and participation in infant care tasks.

DISCHARGE CRITERIA

1. Demonstrate progress in dealing with grief at own pace.
2. Display appropriate attachment/bonding behaviors.
3. Participate in infant care; develop mastery of therapeutic regimen.
4. Have plan in place to meet needs after discharge.

NURSING DIAGNOSIS:	**GRIEVING [expected], related to**
May Be Related To:	Perceived loss of the perfect child/ pregnancy/delivery, alterations of future expectations

417

Possibly Evidenced By:	Expression of distress at loss, sorrow, guilt, anger; choked feelings; reliving of pregnancy events; interference with life activities; crying
DESIRED OUTCOMES/EVALUATION—CLIENT/COUPLE WILL:	Verbalize feelings freely/effectively.
	Demonstrate expected grief responses.
	Look forward/plan for future one day at a time.

ACTIONS/INTERVENTIONS

Independent

Promote trusting relationship with parents and significant other(s). Encourage verbalization of feelings through listening and an unhurried attitude.

Facilitate the grief process, even if the newborn's problem is temporary or surgically correctable.

Determine parents' religious orientation, and contact appropriate support, if they desire it.

Assess for usual grieving responses (e.g., initial shock, disbelief, and denial, then anger, guilt, sadness, and negative self-evaluation/questioning, followed by acceptance) based on cultural/religious practices. Let parents know that these responses are normal.

Note the stage of grief being expressed. Discuss the individual nature of movement through the stages of grief; let parents know that delays in the grief process or relapses of grief are normal.

Accept use of defense mechanisms (e.g., denial, anger, or silence). Encourage expression of angry feelings, setting limits on unacceptable acting-out behavior.

Provide information about extreme mood swings, which may be hormonally induced in the postpartal period.

Offer objective feedback, without judgment, on how behavior is being perceived.

Avoid "personalizing" statements made by the parents.

RATIONALE

Facilitates sharing of feelings, fears, and concerns. Helps parents to focus on reality of the situation and examine their emotional responses. Grieving for the loss of the perfect child must be completed before parents can establish a positive relationship with their offspring. Staff needs to remain available, even if client seems self-sufficient or withdrawn.

The amount of grief the parents experience is independent of the severity/permanency of the infant's problem.

Many couples lean heavily on their faith as a source of strength during crisis resolution. Note: Perception of situation/condition and individual's response will also be affected by religious beliefs.

Grief is the anticipated, healthy emotional response to the profound experience of giving birth to a special needs child, and it involves mourning the loss of the idealized perfect newborn.

The process of grieving is not usually a fluid progression through the stages to resolution; more often the individual fluctuates between the stages, possibly skipping one or more. Understanding that grieving is individual helps the couple let each other grieve at her or his own pace.

Use of defense mechanisms at this time may be the best way for parents to deal productively with the situation. However, continued use of defense mechanisms may impair resolution of grief. In addition, preventing destructive behavior is important to the maintenance of the client's self-esteem.

Usual hormonal adjustments of postpartal period can trigger labile responses and may require further evaluation/treatment.

When behavior is unacceptable, gentle statements about angry or withdrawn actions can help the individual cope more effectively with the situation.

Parents may use the nurse as a sounding board and means of ventilating their feelings. Their

Ascertain parents' perceptions of infant's special needs and condition.

statements, although spoken to the individual nurse, are usually directed at the situation in general.

The parents' emotional responses are associated with the perceived loss of the perfect child, in addition to concerns about the infant's well-being/life expectancy. They may occur regardless of whether the defect appears to healthcare professionals to be relatively minor and/or reparable, or major and life-threatening.

Ask parents what helps them most in dealing with the affected child. Observe nonverbal signals, such as anguished tone of voice, looking down, or crying.

Parents may have a hard time handling the crisis and may have difficulty identifying means of facilitating coping.

Encourage parents to see, hold, and help care for the child.

Interacting with the child as he/she is helps parents to work toward the acceptance phase of the grief process.

Instruct parents in caring for the infant. (Refer to ND: Knowledge deficit [Learning Need].)

Grieving may increase the parents' fear of caring for the child; in many cases, they feel overwhelmed initially.

Prepare parents for/role-play difficult situations such as discharge from the hospital and other people's thoughtless comments, questions, and stares.

Parents can develop plan of action to lessen discomfort before actual confrontation with difficult situations.

Evaluate parents for abnormal grief responses, such as inappropriate humor; lack of interest in infant; continued denial of, or failure to recognize, infant's problem; poor eye contact; continual crying, excessive or vague complaints; inability to carry out self-care activities; or use of distancing in interactions with child (e.g., holding child at arm's length instead of cuddling).

Inappropriate initial responses may result in long-term emotional dysfunction and lack of resolution of grief. Thus, the grief process may be left open-ended, and the parents' unresolved feelings continually resurface. Early identification of problems and prompt intervention facilitates individual growth and coping abilities. Note: Parents may be afraid of becoming emotionally attached if they believe that the child might die.

Collaborative

Refer for appropriate individual or family counseling.

Counseling may be necessary for resolution of grief and maintenance of family unity.

NURSING DIAGNOSIS:	PARENT/INFANT ATTACHMENT, risk for altered
Risk Factors May Include:	Delay/interruption in bonding process (separation, physical barriers), perceived threat to infant's survival, presence of stress (financial, family needs), lack of appropriate response of newborn, lack of support between/from significant other(s)
Possibly Evidenced By:	[Not applicable; presence of signs/symptoms establishes an *actual* diagnosis]
DESIRED OUTCOMES/EVALUATION CRITERIA—PARENT(S) WILL:	Demonstrate beginning attachment behaviors.
	Verbalize acceptance of situation.
	Develop realistic plans for care of the infant.

ACTIONS/INTERVENTIONS	RATIONALE

Independent

Provide information honestly about newborn's appearance and condition at birth, encouraging an optimistic perspective (e.g., let parents know the potential for survival or recovery) as appropriate. Describe appearance and show pictures of newborn if initial interaction is delayed and/or following surgery.

The child's appearance may be incongruent with the parents' idealized picture of the perfect infant. Helps prepare parents psychologically for interaction with newborn and reduces the shock associated with initial viewing of infant. Aids in developing parents' trust and in giving them accurate information with which to make decisions. Optimistic perspective helps encourage parents to develop an attachment, although the infant may be unable to participate actively in the interactional process because of illness and/or need for technologic assistance. Note: Based on severity of infant's condition, family may choose to engage in cultural rituals, e.g., Native-Americans may desire to conduct a naming ceremony.

Facilitate communication between parents and nursery staff through use of telephone and letters, especially if infant is transferred to a high-risk facility. Suggest that parents provide tapes, photographs, and personal items for use in infant's environment.

Maintains open channel for exchange of information and clarification of concerns. Fosters continued acquaintance process; helps parents to feel an integral part of infant care and growth. Parents can talk, sign, or tell stories into tape recorder, which can be played for infant, providing audio stimulation and voice recognition of parents.

Encourage verbalization of feelings regarding prenatal/intrapartal and postpartal periods and perceptions of the financial and emotional burdens created by the birth of special needs infant.

Unresolved anticipatory anger and excessive threats to self-esteem and to financial status may predispose parents to subconscious or overt rejection of infant.

Discuss normalcy of feelings related to the grief response (e.g., shock, disbelief, anger, guilt, and sadness).

Parents need to identify and cope with their own grief response before they can begin to bond emotionally with the newborn.

Provide anticipatory and ongoing emotional support to client/couple.

Helps couple whose infant's prognosis is grave to bond with, and then let go of, infant, if death ensues. Parental anticipatory grieving, which begins during the intrapartal period and lasts until the infant dies or shows signs of improvement, may result in a withdrawal from bonding as a protective mechanism. (Refer to CP: Perinatal Loss.)

Determine parents' understanding of infant's condition and needs. Review and clarify questions, and provide opportunity for discussion about the condition and its short- and long-term implications as early as possible after birth.

Initial denial, shock, and disbelief may interfere with understanding and processing of information. Parents may cling to unrealistic expectations or goals if they are not psychologically ready to accept the situation. Review of information helps dispel fantasies, initiate the grief process, and mobilize internal and external support.

Provide information regarding physical and personality characteristics appropriate for gestational age when child is preterm, rather than the characteristics of a full-term infant.

Allows appropriate comparisons for helping parents identify parenting behaviors and activities appropriate for their infant.

Assist parents in identifying familial characteristics, personality traits, positive attributes, and normal behaviors in the infant.

Emphasizes the infant's value as a person and facilitates recognition of individual capabilities and personality traits. Initiates process of attachment and bonding, and allows parents to see similarities between their infant and a normal newborn. Note: Some parents, regardless of how minor the defect is, may have difficulty accepting a baby who is not "perfect."

Promote early parent-infant interaction. Assess parents' perception of infant.

Helps couple acknowledge the reality of the situation and begin to work through appropriate psychologic tasks; determines parents' readiness for involvement in infant care tasks.

Provide privacy for parents to interact with baby.

Parents may want to talk or sing to infant but may not feel comfortable with an "audience."

Review couple's parenting experience and preparation, and previous coping skills. (Refer to ND: Family Coping, ineffective: risk for compromised.)

Provides indications of emotional readiness to adopt parenting roles and responsibilities. Such readiness varies considerably, depending on coping skills and past experiences.

Assess parents for development of attachment behaviors while in the hospital (e.g., talking to, holding, and naming infant; asking appropriate questions regarding infant's condition and needs).

Indicates development of positive parent-infant ties, which help foster optimal growth and development of infant.

Note parental cues indicating readiness for involvement in infant's care and future planning. Encourage parental involvement in planning care and making decisions.

Readiness for parental involvement indicates that client/couple is attaching emotionally to infant, is becoming increasingly concerned for the infant's welfare, and is feeling emotionally able to begin to assume responsibility for infant's care. Parental involvement may enhance feelings of control, promote self-esteem, and reduce anxiety.

Demonstrate special infant care techniques, positions for holding and feeding infant, and ways of talking to infant. Assess parents' need to have staff remain with them or to be left alone with infant.

The nurse acts as a role model in caring for the infant at a time when the parents are acutely aware of others' responses and identify with those responses. Anxiety associated with a new parenting role may be minimized by participation in newborn care.

Encourage appropriate parental participation in infant care.

Reduces anxiety, improves parental self-esteem, and facilitates development of positive parent-infant attachment, which helps to assure appropriate continuity of physical and emotional care necessary for the infant's optimal development.

Identify newborn's responses and behavioral cues.

Aids parents in determining when to interact with infant, what behaviors are appropriate, and when to modify their approach based on infant's tolerance for stimulation.

Provide positive feedback as parents accomplish tasks. Inform staff of parents' capabilities.

Increases sense of self-worth and self-confidence in providing infant's care. Staff coordination provides consistency in approach and helps prevent misunderstandings.

Arrange for meeting with other parents who have faced the same or a similar problem.

May aid couple in realistically identifying infant's specific needs and abilities.

Monitor client's/couple's behaviors following client's discharge; e.g., continued visits or telephone calls, and preparation for infant's discharge, or lack of physical contact, failure to name infant or change of name from original choice, negative comments about infant, expressed concerns about adequacy in caring for infant, and failure to visit or communicate with professionals.

Involved behaviors demonstrate continued concern for child's comfort and indicate increasing strength of attachment. Although withdrawal behaviors may represent a normal response to prevent attachment to an infant who may not survive, they may also indicate potential problems, including high-risk parenting (emotional or physical abuse) following discharge, so that further evaluation and/or interventions may be needed. (Refer to CPs: Infant of an Addicted Mother; and The Infant of an HIV-Positive Mother.)

Evaluate appropriateness of discharge planning/preparation.

Realistic preparation indicates client's readiness for parenting following infant's discharge.

421

Discuss alternatives to taking baby home (e.g., foster care, institutionalization, adoption), as indicated. Be supportive of final decision; assist parents in evaluating long-term implications of decision.

Parents who choose not (or are unable) to cope with the long-term commitment of raising a child with special needs will need to seek alternative care.

Collaborative

Schedule team conference. Identify acute care and community resources for infant and parents (e.g., public health nurse, home care agencies, charitable organizations [such as Easter Seals], and support groups).

Coordinated multidisciplinary planning for discharge can ease the transition from hospital to home and reduce anxiety associated with increased parental responsibilities following discharge.

Refer for counseling or parenting classes, as indicated.

May be necessary if attachment behaviors are incomplete or absent.

NURSING DIAGNOSIS:	FAMILY COPING, ineffective: risk for compromised
Risk Factors May Include:	Situational crises, temporary preoccupation by a significant person who is trying to manage emotional conflicts and personal suffering and is unable to perceive or act effectively in regard to client's needs, temporary family disorganization/role changes
Possibly Evidenced By:	[Not applicable; presence of signs/symptoms establishes an *actual* diagnosis]
DESIRED OUTCOMES/EVALUATION CRITERIA—FAMILY WILL:	Participate in problem solving and use resources appropriately.
	Demonstrate integration of infant into family unit.

ACTIONS/INTERVENTIONS

RATIONALE

Independent

Evaluate usual family coping mechanisms and relationships among family members. Note history of high-risk behaviors (e.g., substance abuse) or presence of chronic illness.

Helps in identifying strengths and weaknesses and availability of support systems. Individual issues/limitations may overtax family's ability to be involved with client or care for infant.

Identify cultural influences relative to support systems/family involvement, including family spokesperson.

Different family members may assume leadership roles (e.g., family spokesperson/intermediary between healthcare providers and parents based on cultural dictates). For example, in Vietnamese and Iranian cultures, the father is consulted first, whereas in Puerto Rican and Russian cultures the client (mother) is consulted first. The maternal grandmother is the intermediary in Haitian families, whereas the paternal grandmother may take this role in the Hmong culture.

Provide calm, supportive environment and role modeling for parents.

External stressors may interfere with incorporation of therapeutic interventions by parents. Psychosocial needs of parents may be met through positive role modeling by healthcare providers.

Provide emotional support by allowing time, privacy, and opportunity for open discussion.

Helps client/couple to identify and clarify fears and concerns, and to correct misconceptions.

Provide information honestly; keep client/ couple informed regarding infant's condition.

Determine parental concerns, emotions, and degree of anxiety. Review past experiences with stress and past coping mechanisms and support systems.

Past experience with stress or crisis influences current stress response and management, resulting in either functional or dysfunctional behavior.

Encourage verbalization of fears, and initiate discussion of opportunities.

Parents may be hesitant to share concerns with staff. Fears may go unaddressed unless staff conscientiously creates opportunities for discussion during their client/infant care activities.

Provide parents with realistic responses and reinforcement, giving consideration to their capacity to process information and their knowledge of the situation.

Lack of knowledge contributes to increased anxiety, which interferes with the ability to cope. However, anxiety needs to be minimized for parents to process information. Repetition of explanations enhances understanding.

Encourage parents to express their own dependency needs and to focus on themselves and their own discomfort.

Both parents may need to devote time and energy to understanding and dealing with their own feelings prior to directing their concern to the infant.

Assess individual and collective responses of family members to infant's condition/appearance. Encourage family to verbalize their perceptions of the impact of the infant's illness or condition on the family.

Parental feelings toward the infant are critical, because feelings that are related to physical appearance and capabilities are internalized in the infant as development occurs.

Use role-playing techniques or play therapy with siblings. Demonstrate these techniques for parents to use. Provide information about age-appropriate discussions with siblings.

Helps young children express feelings about infant. Using words and expressions appropriate to the age of the other children helps the parents in talking with them about the new baby.

Evaluate and help parents recognize signs of ineffective coping in siblings (e.g., interpersonal problems, excessive quarreling, psychosomatic illnesses, school problems, regressive behaviors).

Early recognition allows the family to take steps to correct these problems and to seek professional help if necessary.

Encourage client/couple to arrange sibling visits and to allow older siblings the opportunity to participate in infant care, if possible.

Helps siblings to realize that they are an important part of infant care, which may eliminate feelings of abandonment and increase feelings of self-worth.

Place family photos in isolette or crib; encourage siblings to talk to infant, to make tape recordings, or to give gifts (e.g., pick out a small toy, draw a picture).

Provides sense of family unity and includes siblings in activities.

Recommend that client/couple spend special time alone with siblings.

Caring for an infant with special needs is so time-consuming that little time is left for siblings, who may feel abandoned, replaced, ignored, angry, and jealous.

Offer opportunity for contact with couples facing similar problems.

Provides peer support helpful in nurturing the couple; promotes positive behaviors and provides opportunity for sharing ideas and interventions that have been successful.

Provide 24-hr contact phone number. Initiate follow-up phone calls and/or home visits.

Provides continuity of care and a continued source of emotional support.

Be supportive of couple's decision to take infant home or to use institutional help or assistance. Help couple look at long-term effects of decision. Note cultural meaning of condition/birth anomaly.

Such decisions are difficult and may have cultural implications. To avoid increasing their guilt and confusion, make the parents aware of options, give support for their decision without judgment, and let them know that they may change their minds.

423

Encourage parents to maintain or re-establish good communication between themselves and to take time out from child care for time alone together. Encourage use of resources, such as respite care.

Facilitates rapport between parents, helps maintain healthy relationship, and fosters coping and family growth.

Encourage each partner to allow time for herself or himself, apart from the other.

Helps foster individual coping mechanisms, which can ultimately foster a stronger family.

Collaborative

Refer to community or social services, as appropriate. Identify available respite services. Provide additional referrals, including parent support groups, clergy, and psychiatric services, as indicated.

A coordinated and consistent network of multidisciplinary support enhances management of parental anxiety and assists in development of effective coping skills required by the short- and long-term complications related to the child's special needs.

Encourage couple to seek genetic counseling if appropriate. (Refer to CP: Genetic Counseling.)

Thorough evaluation of genetic factors may provide answers to some of the couple's questions.

Suggest that couple attend marital support group or seek marital counseling, as indicated.

May help couple cope with a crisis that can potentially strengthen or destroy the relationship. Family disintegration is often a consequence of the birth of an infant with a disorder or anomaly. Such disintegration is a direct response to the intense emotional and physical demands created by the infant's long-term health problems, which have a cumulative effect with preexisting stressors.

Support client/family involvement in rehabilitation programs (e.g., Alcoholics/Narcotics Anonymous; Alanon).

May not be able to adequately assume responsibility for newborn until preexisting problems impacting family are dealt with/resolved.

NURSING DIAGNOSIS:	**KNOWLEDGE deficit [LEARNING NEED], regarding infant care**
May Be Related To:	Lack of/unfamiliarity with information resources, misinterpretation, lack of recall
Possibly Evidenced By:	Verbalization of problems, concerns, misconceptions, inaccurate follow-through of instructions, hesitancy or inadequate performance of activities, inappropriate/aggravated behaviors (e.g., agitated, apathetic)
DESIRED OUTCOMES/EVALUATION CRITERIA—CLIENT/COUPLE WILL:	Verbalize understanding of infant's behaviors, physical status, and care needs.
	Participate in infant's care.
	Demonstrate mastery of infant care/treatment activities.
	Plan appropriately for discharge, home management, and use of available resources.

ACTIONS/INTERVENTIONS	RATIONALE

Independent

Keep parents informed about changes in infant's physiological status.

Helps parents to acknowledge possible positive or negative outcomes regarding infant's potential for survival and growth.

Explain plan of care for infant, including rationale for associated tests, procedures, and treatment. Discuss infant's response to treatment. Let parents know when tests are to be performed.	Promotes understanding, clarifies misconceptions, and reduces anxiety. Parents may choose not to visit infant when testing is scheduled or may desire to provide comfort following procedures.
Review normal behavior for infant's gestational age based on Dubowitz or Ballard evaluation.	Provides information to promote understanding of behaviors and motor characteristics typical for gestational age.
Discuss infant's personality traits and individual differences noted from comparison with other infants of same gestational age. Provide information about appropriate stimulation for infant.	Allows couple to gain skill in recognizing responses of infant, acknowledging individual differences, and developing methods for dealing with them.
Introduce client/couple to parent of a baby (in the nursery if possible) with the same or similar special need.	Sharing concerns with another parent can foster acceptance of the situation.
Encourage optimal participation in infant care. Reinforce the idea that infant belongs to the parents, not the nursery. Talk about the infant by name, noting attractive features and other attributes.	Fosters attachment process. Allows parents to demonstrate newly learned behaviors, increasing comfort in handling and caring for the infant. Reminds parents that child is a living being, not a disease or condition.
Encourage questions, provide answers clearly and concisely, and reinforce information as needed. Assess parents' readiness to receive information. Encourage parents to verbalize concerns.	Helps identify learning needs and clarify misconceptions. Denial used initially as a coping mechanism may interfere with learning. Repetition enhances comprehension. Verbalization of concerns promotes atmosphere of trust and is conducive to learning.
Set short-term, measurable goals with parents.	Learning to adjust to problems step by step, one day at a time, helps parents see that progress is being made and reduces the overwhelming stress of the total situation.
Provide encouragement for each task accomplished.	Increases parents' self-confidence in their ability to care for infant.
Review assessment of gestational age, expected potential, immediate and long-term prognosis, and discharge of infant. Be realistic, but positive. Keep parents informed, be honest, and let parents know whether answers are available.	Parents need to know the expectations they can have of their child. Infant may be at risk for neuromuscular disorders, developmental delays, behavior problems, or learning disabilities that may be directly associated with gestational age at birth. Honesty maintains trust between nurse and parents and promotes realistic hope.
Discuss results of ophthalmologic examination when performed prior to infant discharge. Provide information to parents about importance of scheduling reevaluations.	In the preterm infant, retinal scar tissue formation may persist for as long as 5 mo, resulting in varying degrees of visual impairment.
Review results of other routine tests, such as hearing testing and B-mode ultrasonography of the head.	These tests are performed for early identification of significant problems (presence and extent of hearing loss, intraventricular hemorrhage) and for provision of appropriate interventions.
Provide information related to home care of infant. Encourage family to read available literature.	Helps parents gain competence and comfort in caring for infant after discharge.
Discuss purpose and availability of early intervention programs and community resources.	Provides guidance for long-term planning to optimize affective, cognitive, and social development of infant.
Encourage other members of family to learn to care for infant.	Eases the parents' burden of caring for infant and promotes a sense of family unity.

Recommend parents contact other parents of children with similar needs (e.g., Down syndrome, muscular dystrophy, or cerebral palsy groups; or Parents Encouraging Parents).

Provides support and promotes the realization that parents are not alone in their struggle.

Refer to social service agencies or community resources, including national foundations (e.g., Easter Seal centers, Shriners for orthopedic defects), public assistance groups, and Medicaid, as appropriate. Discuss need to notify insurance company immediately after birth.

Couple may be unaware of available financial assistance or free services and may be overwhelmed by incurred or future expenses. Referrals help ensure continuation of support from healthcare agencies. Clarification of available insurance coverage may affect choice of treatment options. Note: Infant may not be covered by insurance if notification is not made within time period specified by third-party payor.

Provide 24-hr contact phone number, schedule follow-up phone calls and/or home visits.

Aids in adjustment of care for home environment. Lets couple know that someone cares and is available should difficulties arise.

NURSING DIAGNOSIS:	SOCIAL ISOLATION, risk for
Risk Factors May Include:	Perceived situational crisis, assuming sole/full-time responsibility for infant's care, lack of resources or inappropriate use of resources
Possibly Evidenced By:	[Not applicable; presence of signs/symptoms establishes an *actual* diagnosis]
DESIRED OUTCOMES/EVALUATION CRITERIA—CLIENT/COUPLE WILL:	Verbalize awareness of potential problems. Identify resources available for assistance. Develop plans to resume social activities.

ACTIONS/INTERVENTIONS

RATIONALE

Independent

Discuss situation with couple and determine their perceptions of how they will manage care.

Identifies problem areas and helps with planning interventions for appropriate care. After discharge, the parents quickly become consumed, both emotionally and physically, in child's care, and they may withdraw from usual social interactions and activities.

Listen to parents' expressions of feelings of inadequacy or guilt that may accompany the birth of a child with special needs. Help the couple cope with feelings that are expressed. (Refer to ND: Family Coping, ineffective: risk for compromised.)

Parents may withdraw from society or social interaction because of feelings of shame or a sense of failure as parents. They may also have fears that the child will die or will receive substandard care from others. Unresolved guilt may be responsible for overindulgent behaviors and unwillingness to let others care for the child. Resolution of guilt may promote development of effective parenting skills.

Assist couple with plans for responsible, skilled adults to care for child. Such adults may be relatives, friends, or trained caregivers, such as "mother's helpers."

The couple needs time away from child's constant demands to maintain their own relationship and to keep the situation in perspective. Reduces risk of developing impaired ability to perform family caregiver role.

Discuss plans for resumption of activities engaged

Returning to normal routines fosters self-esteem

in before the birth (e.g., hobbies, employment), if possible.

Prepare parents for/role-play responses to possible reactions by the public.

Encourage parents to plan family outings such as trips to beach, picnics, walks, and movies.

Collaborative

Provide social service and public health referrals before discharge.

Assist couple in contacting appropriate support groups.

and sense of self-worth; however, child's condition may significantly alter the family's previous patterns so that reduction or elimination of outside work or some leisure activities may be necessary. Note: Support from parents sharing similar situation provides opportunity for creative problem solving and continuation of activities.

Preparation helps couple identify possible actions or ways of managing uncomfortable social situations and eliminates the need for isolating themselves from social contacts as a protective mechanism.

Helps meet individual and collective needs for social experiences.

Maintains continuity of support network from the hospital to the home.

A support group serves as a social outlet, provides role models, and may be a resource for sharing child care.

PERINATAL LOSS

Perinatal loss may occur anytime during gestation or the neonatal period. Usually when pregnancy culminates in the death of a fetus or neonate, the loss is both unexpected and devastating for the client/couple. The loss of a child that is wanted can be as traumatic (or even more traumatic) as the loss of a close adult family member or friend. This plan of care focuses on the emotional needs of the postpartal client who must cope with the death of a child.

(To be used in conjunction with routine postpartal plans of care).

CLIENT ASSESSMENT DATA BASE

Circulation

History of essential hypertension, vascular disease

Ego Integrity

Emotionally labile; anxiety, fear, shock, disbelief, depression

Elimination

Chronic nephritis

Food/Fluid

Poor maternal nutritional status

Safety

Exposure to toxic/teratogenic agents
History of traumatic event(s)
Presence of pelvic inflammatory disease, sexually transmitted diseases (STDs), or exposure to
     contagious diseases, such as rubella, cytomegalovirus, active herpes
Premature rupture of membranes
Abnormalities of placenta/cord noted at delivery
ABO incompatibility

Sexuality

Bicornate or septate uterus, uterine fibroid tumors (leiomyoma), or other abnormalities of the
     maternal reproductive organs
Occurrence of traumatic delivery; intrapartal complications

Teaching/Learning

May report medication, drug (including alcohol) use or abuse
Family history of genetic conditions

DIAGNOSTIC STUDIES

(Refer to CP: Genetic Counseling.)

NURSING PRIORITIES

1. Facilitate the grieving process.
2. Provide information regarding events surrounding the loss and future implications.

DISCHARGE GOALS

1. Supports identified and in place
2. Plans made for disposition of infant's body
3. Demonstrated progress in dealing with grief at own pace

NURSING DIAGNOSIS:	GRIEVING [expected]
Related To:	Death of fetus/infant
Possibly Evidenced By:	Verbal expression of distress, anger, loss, guilt; crying; alteration in eating habits or sleep pattern
DESIRED OUTCOMES/EVALUATION CRITERIA—CLIENT/COUPLE WILL:	Identify and express feelings (e.g., sadness, guilt, fear) freely.
	Acknowledge impact/effect of the grieving process (e.g., physical problems of eating, sleeping) and seek appropriate help.
	Participate in self-care activities of daily living (ADLs), as able.
	Look toward/plan for future, one day at a time.

ACTIONS/INTERVENTIONS

Independent

Code patient's chart, room door, and/or head of bed, as indicated.

Provide a private room if client desires it, with frequent contact by care providers. Encourage unlimited visiting by family and friends.

Support free flow of emotional expression. Only limit behavior that is dangerous to well-being of client/couple (e.g., pulling out IV, using fists to pound on abdomen).

Include partner in planning care. Provide opportunity for partner to be seen individually. Encourage discussion of concerns.

Assess client's/couple's knowledge and interpretation of events surrounding the death of the fetus/infant. Provide information and correct misconceptions based on couple's readiness and ability to listen effectively.

Determine significance of the loss for both members of the couple. Note how strongly couple desired this pregnancy.

Identify stage of grief being expressed, e.g., denial, anger, bargaining, depression, acceptance. Use therapeutic communication skills (e.g., Active-

RATIONALE

Alerts hospital staff and volunteers so they are aware of patient's loss.

A place where family and friends can talk or cry without restriction promotes ventilation of feelings and family sharing. Note: Client may prefer carefully screened roommate(s), who can provide contact and comfort when family and friends are not available.

Expression of grief is impacted by cultural/religious beliefs and expectations running the gamut from stoic silence to screaming and pounding one's chest/throwing objects, etc. While expression of loss is cathartic, extended stoicism may impede mourning process.

Participation in planning and decision making acknowledges that partner has also lost a child and may need time to express feelings of loss and receive support without having to be supportive of client and others.

Often, after the death of a child, parents respond with shock, denial, or disbelief. These emotional reactions may hinder the couple's ability to process information and interpret the significance of events. Concrete thinking patterns (literal interpretation) may be the only available means of coping with information at this time.

The significance of the loss is a factor (e.g., whether pregnancy was planned, whether couple has lost other pregnancies, length of time associated with trying to conceive) in the extent and duration of the grief response. In addition, parents may feel the loss throughout their lives, mourning for the child they will never know or watch grow up.

When a child dies in utero, is stillborn, or dies after birth, grief is felt regardless of whether the child was wanted or unwanted. If the work of grieving

429

listening, acknowledgment), respecting client's desire/request not to talk.

is not completed, grief may become dysfunctional, resulting in behaviors that are detrimental to personal safety and to the future of the family and marriage/relationship.

Discuss the individual nature of movement through the stages of grief; tell client/couple that delays in the grief process or relapses of grief are normal.

The process of grieving is not usually a fluid progression through the stages to resolution; it is rather a fluctuation between stages and possibly involves skipping of stages. Understanding that grieving is individual helps the couple let each other grieve at his or her own pace. Note: There is no set time limitations for resolution of grief and it is not unusual for the family to be actively dealing with the loss 1–2 yr later.

Note communication patterns between members of the couple and support systems.

In many cases, parents show anger and blame toward one another. Anger may stem from fear of losing another child or threat to self-esteem.

Encourage family's expression of feelings and listen (remaining silent or commenting as appropriate). Note body language. Promote relaxed atmosphere.

Verbal and nonverbal cues provide information about family's degree of sadness, guilt, and fear. Grieving families need repeated opportunities to verbalize their experience. Time is needed to develop a therapeutic milieu. Active-listening conveys caring, which communicates an awareness of the unique meaning of the loss to the client.

Acknowledge what has happened as often as necessary, reinforcing the reality of the situation and encouraging discussion by the client.

Many families have no previous experience of coping with the death of a young person and have few role models to whom they can refer. The nurse can act as an educator and facilitator regarding ways to act and talk about the event and can clarify misconceptions.

Take pictures of the child wrapped in newborn attire. Encourage couple to see or hold the child, if appropriate. Offer the couple footprints, hospital bracelets, or lock of hair, if desired.

Pictures and touching or holding infant can be helpful and may initiate acceptance of the reality of the loss. Note: Couple may not be ready to cope with the loss. Remembrances of the infant, if not taken by the parents, should be filed with the chart, so that they are available if couple requests them at a later time.

Note client's activity level, sleep pattern, appetite, and personal hygiene.

These areas may be neglected because of the process of grieving and associated depression. Sleep patterns may be disrupted, leading to fatigue and further inability to cope with distress. Client may need assistance in meeting physical needs and may need assurance that it is acceptable to continue with usual activities.

Provide physical care (e.g., bath, back rub, nourishment) as needed. Encourage client to participate at level of ability.

Demonstrates caring and nurturing and helps client conserve energy needed to meet the demands of the grieving process. Involvement in self-care maintains self-esteem and sense of competence.

Discuss anticipated physical and emotional responses to loss. Evaluate coping skills. Note religious beliefs and ethnic background.

Helps couple recognize normalcy of their initial and subsequent responses. Grieving is individual, and the extent and nature of the response is influenced by personality traits, past coping skills, religious beliefs, and ethnic background.

Review role changes and plans to deal with loss. Note presence of siblings.

Most families anticipate a healthy pregnancy and positive outcome and are not prepared to focus on funeral arrangements, what to do with the nursery,

Discuss ways for parents to talk with siblings. Stress importance of words that are used, such as when the word "sleep" is substituted for "death." Encourage parents to give simple, honest explanations, using correct words, at the level of the child's understanding.

how to carry on their lives, and how to plan for the care of the other children.

Provides parents with ideas for handling difficult new experience. Siblings' sleeping patterns may be disturbed by their belief that they may also die. Siblings may feel guilt or responsibility for the death, especially if they had negative thoughts about the pregnancy or infant.

Assess severity of depression.

Client/couple may isolate themselves and have difficulty making decisions.

Review the client's/couple's verbal cues regularly. Note signs of developing or increasing somatic complaints, preoccupation with the death, loss of normal behavior patterns, overactivity with no apparent sense of loss, excessive hostility, or agitated depression.

May indicate change in client's/couple's manner of coping with the situation. Guilt, failure, and depression may be more pronounced in couples who have had previous child loss(es). Other signs may suggest dysfunctional grieving.

Collaborative

Refer to, or contact, clergy, according to family's wishes.

The family may want to speak to a minister or spiritual advisor to provide baptism, last rites, cultural rituals, and/or counseling. Note: Baptism is not acceptable in some religions (e.g., Jehovah's Witness, Seventh Day Adventist).

Assist with making requests and obtaining signatures for performance of autopsy if appropriate. Review benefits and limitations of autopsy.

Families may want or need explanation of cause of death, which may not be possible.

Provide information about disposition of infant's body. Contact mortician of family's choice if assistance is required.

Bodies of children, like those of adults, must be removed from hospitals to mortuary facilities or other disposition, usually within 24 hr of death. While burial may be delayed in most instances, Jewish tradition requires burial within 24 hr, which may further complicate client's grieving process if she is not able to attend ceremony.

Refer to, or contact, social services, if necessary.

Family may need assistance in planning for cost of funeral and other necessities.

Schedule follow-up meetings or phone calls, as appropriate. Refer to community resources/ support groups (e.g., visiting nurse services, Compassionate Friends, AMEND, SHARE).

Provides client/couple with opportunity for discussion and asking questions. Assists client/couple at critical moments in the grief process, providing role models and opportunity to discuss loss with others who share similar experience.

Refer for counseling or psychiatric therapy, if necessary.

Severe grief response may be noted in older women and those with longer-term pregnancies. In addition, carrying the fetus for 1 or more days after death increases risk. In cases of pathological grief, ongoing counseling may be necessary to help individual(s) identify possible causes of the abnormal reaction and to achieve resolution of the grieving process. Note: Risk of major depression episode is highest during the 1st month following the loss, whereas women without other children or who have had a prior depressive episode remain at increased risk for 6 months.

431

NURSING DIAGNOSIS:	**FAMILY PROCESSES/ROLE PERFORMANCE, risk for altered**
Risk Factors May Include:	Situational crisis (death of child)
Possibly Evidenced By:	[Not applicable; presence of signs/symptoms establishes an *actual* diagnosis]
DESIRED OUTCOMES/EVALUATION CRITERIA—FAMILY WILL:	Express feelings freely and appropriately.
	Demonstrate individual involvement in problem-solving process directed at resolution of crisis.
	Verbalize understanding of role expectations/obligations.
	Identify needs and resources to nurture roles/family ties.

ACTIONS/INTERVENTIONS	RATIONALE
Independent	
Evaluate current family situation and psychosocial status (e.g., other children, extended family, support systems).	Family members may provide support for one another. However, disbelief, anger, and denial may temporarily impair parenting skills, and other children may be ignored or treated differently from the way they had been treated before the death of the infant.
Review family's strengths, resources, and past coping skills.	Family members may be depressed, may feel totally inadequate, and may need to review what has happened and what their purpose in life may be.
Encourage discussion of feelings and listen for verbal cues indicating feelings of failure, guilt, or anger. Discuss normalcy of feelings.	Verbalization of feelings may trigger recognition of their causes and can be used to verify the acceptability of these feelings. Parents may be afraid to describe negative feelings that they consider abnormal. Realization that feelings of grief, guilt, and anger are normal may help alleviate the parents' sense of failure.
Discuss situation in terms of activities that need to be completed or continued and the available resources.	In many cases, grief causes immobilization, resulting in dysfunctional parental patterns to the point that normal household routines are disrupted and outside assistance is required.
Identify expected role changes required by the loss.	Anticipated changes include period of disorientation or breakdown in normal patterns of conduct, followed by a period of reorganization, in which energy is appropriately invested in new people and activities.
Provide information and assist parent(s) in dealing with the situation, balancing self-care, grief needs, and parenting responsibilities.	Death of a child requires unanticipated changes in parental roles. With death of a first child, the only parental function that occurs is grief. If there are other children, however, parents may express concern about their parenting abilities. Feelings of failure or guilt may lead to a sense of ultimate inadequacy.
Offer client simple choices of activities, with the opportunity to do more as she progresses.	The client needs to receive the message that she is seen as a functional, capable person, even though she may not feel competent.

Collaborative

Refer to resources such as social services, visiting nurse services, and other agencies.

May be necessary to assist family members or to replace them when they are not available to help (because of distance and/or their own lack of coping skills). Fosters growth and individuation of family members.

Refer to parent support groups (e.g., Compassionate Friends, SHARE).

Reviewing the situation with others who have gone through the same process can reaffirm normalcy of parents' feelings and responses. Note: Referral is best made when the client/couple is experiencing depression and shock. It is more difficult to refer the client/couple during the stages of denial and anger.

Refer for psychiatric counseling or psychotherapy, if indicated.

Additional support in coping with grief may be needed. Psychotherapy may be helpful in cases of pathological grief or overprotectiveness, which can negatively affect normal parenting and integration of loss into usual activities.

Administer medications judiciously, as needed (e.g., sedatives, antianxiety agents/antidepressants).

May help client obtain sleep/rest (e.g., following difficult or exhausting delivery or cesarean birth). Note: Inappropriate use of medications can cloud emotional responses and inhibit the grieving process.

NURSING DIAGNOSIS:	SELF ESTEEM, situational low
May Be Related To:	Perceived failure at a life event
Possibly Evidenced By:	Negative self-appraisal in response to life event in a person with a previous positive self-evaluation, verbalization of negative feelings about the self (helplessness, uselessness), difficulty making decisions
DESIRED OUTCOMES/EVALUATION CRITERIA—CLIENT/COUPLE WILL:	Identify strengths and resources available. Express positive self-appraisal. Demonstrate adaptation to death of infant and integration of loss into daily life by planning for the future.

ACTIONS/INTERVENTIONS

RATIONALE

Independent

Determine couple's self-perceptions as individuals and parents. Evaluate family's response to loss, noting blame placed by family members.

Giving birth provides opportunities for giving love, being loved, building self-esteem, feeling proud and accomplished, establishing a reason for living, and creating a bridge to the future. Loss of the pregnancy and newborn is, therefore, frequently associated with feelings of inadequacy, powerlessness, and inferiority, directly affecting sense of self and possibly shattering one's self-esteem as a parent. Expression of anger or blame by other family members may further reduce self-esteem. Note: Sense of loss/failure may be exacerbated in cases of repeated miscarriages or serial fetal/neonatal deaths.

Discuss with parent(s) what has occurred and ascertain how they perceive the death.

Discuss destructive behaviors, differentiating the responses of others from self-elicited responses (e.g., expressions of blame and/or guilt).

Provide opportunity for verbalization, venting of emotions, and crying.

Discuss parenting needs of other children, as appropriate.

Provide positive reinforcement for expressing needs and identifying concerns.

Collaborative

Provide referrals for counseling and assist with coordination of appointments (e.g., with social services or support groups).

Anger among family members may be transferred to client/couple, resulting in a distortion of actual events.

Destructive behaviors may be apparent during the phases of anger, isolation, and depression. Denial may be used as protection against loss of self-esteem. Guilt may be verbalized, especially if the loss is related to a genetic problem, uterine trauma (e.g., car accident or fall), or teratogens from environmental exposure or drug ingestion.

Sharing of loss provides opportunity for needed acceptance, helps parents sort through feelings, and validates parents' normal feelings of powerlessness and inadequacy.

Continuing to care and to feel needed assists in preserving client's/couple's identify as worthwhile parent(s).

Aids in coping with sadness of situation. Helps parents accept themselves as worthy human beings.

Client's/couple's ability to coordinate and perform tasks may be compromised. Referrals help provide support and assistance, which can facilitate integration of loss into daily life and enhance self-esteem.

NURSING DIAGNOSIS:	SPIRITUAL DISTRESS (distress of the human spirit), risk for
Risk Factors May Include:	Need to adhere to personal religious beliefs/practices; blame for loss directed at self or God
Possibly Evidenced By:	[Not applicable; presence of signs/symptoms establishes an *actual* diagnosis]
DESIRED OUTCOMES/EVALUATION CRITERIA—CLIENT/COUPLE WILL:	Discuss beliefs/values about spiritual issues.
	Verbalize acceptance of situation and hope for the future.
	Demonstrate ability to help self and/or participate in usual activities.

ACTIONS/INTERVENTIONS

RATIONALE

Independent

Discuss the loss with client/couple. (Refer to ND: Knowledge deficit [Learning Need]).

Grieving and trying to make sense out of the loss and to find meaning in life without the baby may cause the couple to question their religious beliefs and to feel cheated or angry. Discussion of objective findings can help the client/couple begin to cope appropriately with feelings of distress.

434

Identify supportive relationships and resources to use after discharge (e.g., extended family, friends, or religious affiliations).

Use of a support system is a constructive means of coping with grief and maintaining perspective.

Encourage discussion of perceptions of unfairness. Identify such perceptions as part of grief process. Maintain a nonjudgmental attitude while providing opportunity for client/couple to express anger.

Families suffering perinatal loss often question their religious beliefs and are concerned about the purpose of life and death. Anger related to powerlessness may result in placing blame on oneself or someone else, or at God for "selecting them to suffer."

Collaborative

Refer to hospital chaplain, rabbi, or appropriate spiritual advisor. Work with mortician, as appropriate, in assisting family with plans for funeral.

Specialists in spiritual beliefs and ritual may be needed to help in making decisions related to burial and loss. Symbolism and ritual can provide comfort and connect family members with their spiritual beliefs.

NURSING DIAGNOSIS:	KNOWLEDGE deficit [LEARNING NEED], regarding perinatal loss, future expectations
May Be Related To:	Lack of exposure to, or unfamiliarity with, information resources, misinterpretation of information
Possibly Evidenced By:	Request for information, statement of misconception
DESIRED OUTCOMES/EVALUATION CRITERIA—CLIENT WILL:	Differentiate between causes of death that are controllable and those that are uncontrollable.
	Verbalize understanding of reasons for loss, when known.
	Discuss possible short- and long-term effects of the loss.

ACTIONS/INTERVENTIONS

RATIONALE

Independent

Assess family's readiness and ability to understand and retain information.

Emotional responses may interfere with the ability to hear and process information. The stage of denial is not the best time for the individual to attempt to process information, and repetition of information may be needed because of the individual's uncertainty about, and lack of control of, the situation. Simple reinforcement of reality may be all that family members are receptive to at the moment.

Provide information about possible short- and long-term physical and emotional effects of grief, including somatic symptoms, sleeplessness, nightmares, dreams of the infant or the pregnancy, emptiness, fatigue, altered sexual response, and loss of appetite.

In many cases, parents do not know why their child died and may have a fear of future pregnancies. Causes of intrauterine death, still-birth, or perinatal death are sometimes uncertain even after autopsy, and families may feel guilty about the cause of death. Providing information about these factors can be helpful in resolving the grief of these individuals. Helps prepare couple for normal changes and difficulties associated with usual

435

	activities of daily living, and helps couple recognize extent of loss.
Review sequence of events and diagnostic tests performed, using pictures if available and appropriate.	During the severe stress that follows the loss, the client/couple understands and retains information more easily if it is presented in a concrete manner. Symbols such as footprints or pictures of the infant may be important.
Identify family's priorities when providing information.	Families have different needs for information, depending on the stage of family development and on whether death was intrauterine or caused by external factors or genetic problems.
Allow client to introduce the subject of another pregnancy.	Individuals determine their own readiness to think about and discuss this possibility. The usual recommendation is to avoid considering pregnancy until grief has been resolved, or until at least 6 mo after the loss.
Identify client's/couple's perceptions of events, and correct misunderstandings, as indicated.	Inaccurate perceptions need to be assessed on a continual basis and valid information reiterated.
Prepare parents for reactions of friends and family; role-play responses.	Family members and friends often do not appreciate the intensity of the parents' grief. Role playing can prepare parents for varied responses from friends and relatives, who may avoid talking about the loss, mistakenly believing that avoiding the topic is therapeutic/less painful for parent(s).
Refer to chaplain and community support groups. (Refer to ND: Spiritual Distress, risk for.)	In many cases, the parents do not trust information until they have heard it from multiple sources.
Review information provided by referral agencies/groups.	Support groups provide information and assistance from people who have experienced similar losses and provide reassurance of normalcy of physical and emotional responses.
Discuss appropriateness of genetic counseling as indicated.	Genetic counseling may be suggested if the parents fear reoccurrence of the problem, even if the problem is not thought to be genetic. The terms "congenital," "teratogenic," and "trauma" should be defined and differentiated so that parents can comprehend risk factors.

CHAPTER 7

NEWBORN CONCEPTS
Neonatal Assessment Tool

As in the maternal assessment tools, the neonatal assessment tool has been constructed using a nursing focus instead of the familiar "head-to-toe" or medical approach of "review of systems." The physical examination component may be done 1–24 hr after birth. The neurological examination is not valid until the neonate has successfully adapted to extrauterine life, usually after 24 hr. The information recorded here is objectively obtained from the physical assessment of the newborn and review of maternal prenatal, intrapartal, and delivery records. (The infant's health is intimately entwined with the health of the mother.) Assessment components may be deleted or added, depending on the individual practitioner's capabilities and hospital policies. On occasion, information may be recorded more than once when it has implications for multiple diagnostic divisions. In addition, some tests (e.g., the Brazelton Neonatal Assessment Scale) may not be completed initially because of the length of time they require and because of shortened hospital stays. These tests should be performed or completed during follow-up examinations or home visits, as appropriate. Whenever material is added to the data base, it is essential to note neonate age, because the assessment is an ongoing process.

Although the divisions are alphabetized for ease of presentation, they can be prioritized or rearranged to meet individual needs.

NEONATAL ASSESSMENT TOOL

Name: _____ Sex: _____ Race: _____

Mother's name: _____ Father's name: _____

Birth date: _____ Time: _____ Apgar scores: _____

Time of examination: _____ Infant age: _____ Gestational age: _____

Activity/Rest

Spontaneous activity: _____ Waking states noted: Drowsy: _____

Active alert: _____ Quiet alert: _____ Crying: _____

Sleep states noted: Deep sleep: _____ Light sleep (REM): _____

Circulation

BP _____ Apical pulse: _____ PMI: _____

Heart sounds: _____ Murmur: _____ Location: _____ Loudness: _____

Intensity: _____

Pulse: Brachial: _____ Femoral: _____ Dorsalis pedis: _____

Skin color: Ruddy: _____ Mottled: _____ Harlequin: _____ Gray: _____

Cyanosis: Location: _____ Effect of crying: _____

Hb: _____ Hct: _____

Ego Integrity

Brazelton Neonatal Assessment Scale: (general areas of concern):

  Attention to stimuli: Visual: _____   Auditory: _____

  Habituation to stimuli: _____

  Social behaviors/willingness to be cuddled: _____   Consolability: _____

  Self-consolation: _____

Elimination

Bowel sounds: Present: _____   Character: _____

Abdomen: Intact: _____   Soft: _____   Mass: _____   Protuberant: _____

  Distended: _____   Scaphoid: _____   Liver palpable: _____

  Spleen palpable: _____   Kidney palpable: R _____   L _____

  Absence of musculature: _____

Anus: Patent: _____   Fissures: _____   Pilonidal cyst: _____

Meconium passed: _____   Time: _____

Bladder: Palpable: _____   Urine: Time of first voiding: _____

  Amount/frequency (24 hr): _____   Color: _____   Urates present: _____

Male meatal opening: Normal: _____   Hypospadias: _____   Phimosis: _____

  Epispadias: _____   Circumcision: _____

Food/Fluid

Feeding: Breast: _____   Bottle: _____

Birth weight: _____   Current weight: _____   Length: _____

Skin: Moist/dry: _____   Turgor: _____   Edema: General: _____

  Localized: _____   Resolved: _____

Fontanels: Normal: _____   Depressed: _____

Mouth: Symmetrical movement of lips and mouth: _____

  Lip/palate intact: _____   Labial tubercle: _____   Sucking pads: _____

  Esptein's pearls: _____   Thrush: _____

  Tongue: Size: _____   Moves freely: _____   Midline: _____

  Mucus: Amount: _____   Character: _____

  Teeth present: _____

  Micrognathia: _____

  Drooling: _____   Character: _____

Strength of reflexes: Rooting: _____   Sucking: _____   Swallowing: _____

  Gag: _____   Feeding vigor: _____

Regurgitation: Amount: _____   Frequency: _____

Vomiting: Character: _____   Projectile: _____

Behavior: Irritable: _____   Jittery: _____

Hb: _____   Hct: _____

Hygiene

Infant is unable to care for self and is totally dependent (level 4).

Neurosensory

Level of consciousness: _____ Response to stimuli: _____ Spontaneous
alertness: _____

Cry: Strength: _____ Character: _____

Head: Appearance: _____ Circumference: _____ cm

Overriding of sutures: _____ Molding: _____

Caput succedaneum: _____ Craniotabes: _____ Cephalhematoma: _____

Fontanels (anterior/posterior): Palpable: _____ Depressed: _____ Bulging: _____

Hair texture: _____ Body distribution: _____

Facial appearance: _____ Movement: Symmetrical: _____ Paralysis: _____

Eyes: Parallel plane: _____ Hypertelorism: _____ Agenesia: _____

Color: _____ Brushfield spots: _____

Blink response: _____ Nystagmus: _____ Strabismus: Transient: _____

Constant: _____

Subconjunctival hemorrhage: R: _____ L: _____ Conjunctivitis: Chemical: _____

Infectious: _____

Tears: Present: _____ Stagnant: _____

Eyelids: Edema: _____ Inflammation: _____ Setting sun: _____ Ptosis: _____

Epicanthic folds: _____

Pupil: Size: R: _____ L: _____ Red reflex: _____ Reaction to light: R: _____

L: _____

Cornea: Clear: _____ Hazy: _____ Cloudy: _____ Reflex present: _____

Sclera color: _____

Visual response: Gazes at object: _____ Follows object: _____

Ears: Amount of cartilage: _____ Tympanic membrane: _____ Preauricular skin
tabs: _____

Position on plane with angle of eye: _____ Low-set: _____

Hearing: Response to sound: _____

Nose: Appearance: _____ Septum intact: _____

Neck/head moves freely: _____ Rigidity/torticollis: _____

Muscle tone: Strong flexor: _____ Hypotonicity: _____ Hypertonicity: _____

Comparative movement: Arms: _____ Legs: _____

Posture: Symmetrical: _____

Reflexes: Ciliary: _____ Doll's eyes: _____ Rooting: _____ Sucking: _____

Moro: Bilateral: _____ Unilateral: _____ Palmar grasp: _____

Plantar grasp: _____

Babinski's: _____ Tonic neck: _____ Traction: _____ Stepping: _____

Prone crawl: _____ Trunk incurvation: _____

Muscle tremors: Fine/rapid: _____ Coarse with activity: _____ At rest: _____

Stiffening/rigidity: _____ Deviation of eyes: _____

Pain/Discomfort

Observe (not test for) response to painful stimuli: Restlessness: _____

Irritability: _____ Constant cry: _____ Withdrawal: _____

Respiration

Apgar score: 1 min: _____   5 min: _____

Resuscitative measures/oxygen: _____   Time: _____   Narcan: _____

   Amount: _____

Respiratory rate: _____   Apnea (duration): _____

   Response to stimulation: _____

Chest: Appearance: _____   Circumference: _____cm

Chest-abdominal movement: Symmetrical: _____   Synchronized: _____

   Inspiratory lag: _____   Paradoxical breathing: _____   Diaphragmatic
      respirations: _____

Chest: Hyperexpansion: _____   Hypoexpansion: _____

Retractions: Intercostal: _____   Subcostal: _____   Substernal: _____

Air passage through both nares: _____   Flaring of nostrils (mild/marked): _____

Grunting: _____

Breath sounds: _____   Crackles: _____   Rhonchi: _____

Percussion: _____

Tracheal position: _____

Cyanosis: Location: _____   Effect of crying: _____

Mucus: Amount: _____   Character: _____

Hb: _____   ABGs: _____

Safety

Type of delivery: _____

Temperature: Rectal: _____   Axillary/skin: _____

Skin: Texture: _____   Moist/dry: _____   Color: _____   Vernix caseosa: _____

   Lanugo: _____

   Contusions: _____   Lacerations: _____   Abrasions: _____

   Milia: _____   Petechiae: _____   Erythema toxicum neonatorum: _____

   Impetigo: _____   Moles: _____   Meconium staining: _____

Pigment: Café au lait spots: _____   Mongolian spots: _____

   Telangiectatic nevi: _____   Nevus flammeus (port-wine stain): _____

   Nevus vascularis (strawberry hemangioma:) _____   Cavernous hemangioma: _____

Umbilical cord: Number of vessels: _____   Color: _____   Bleeding: _____

   Exudate: _____

   Hernia: _____   Cutis navel: _____   Granulation tissue present: _____

Clavicle: Intact: _____   Knot/crepitus/location: _____

Extremities: Comparative use: Arms: _____   Legs: _____

   Equal length: Arms: _____   Legs: _____

   Number of fingers: _____   Number of toes: _____   Syndactylism: _____

   Simian crease: _____   Sole creases: _____

   Gluteal folds: Equal: _____   Ortolani's maneuver: _____

   Talipes equinovarus (clubfoot): _____   Talipes calcaneus: _____

Spine: Straight: _____ Curved: _____

   Vertebrae present: _____

Dermal sinus: _____   Nevus pilosus: _____

Coombs' test: _____   WBC count: _____

Maternal group B beta-hemolytic streptococcus (GBS) status: _____   Hepatitis B: _____

Immunity: _____

Sexuality

Breasts: Distance between: _____ cm   Areolar diameter: _____ cm

Enlargement: _____   Discharge: _____   Supernumerary nipples: _____

Female genitalia:

Labia majora larger than labia minora (Y/N): _____   Reddened: _____

Swollen: _____

Vaginal/hymenal tag: _____   Vaginal discharge: _____   Smegma: _____

Bleeding (amount): _____

Male genitalia:

Scrotum: Rugae present: _____   Swelling: _____

Testicles descended/size: R: _____ cm   L: _____ cm   Hydrocele: _____

Ambiguous genitalia: _____

Social Interactions

Parent-infant interaction: Maternal/paternal (M/P) response:

Facial expression: _____   Use of infant's name: _____

Verbal response: To infant: _____   To spouse/significant other(s): _____

Behaviors: Eye contact: _____   Touching: _____   Examining: _____

Kissing: _____   Cuddling: _____

Identifying familial characteristics: _____   Other: _____

Interaction with other family members/siblings: _____

Pregnancy planned: _____   Prenatal care (date begun): _____

Infant care classes: _____

Teaching/Learning

Gestational age: _____   Tool used (e.g., Dubowitz, Ballard, Brazelton,

Lubchenco): _____

DISCHARGE PLAN CONSIDERATIONS

Date/time information obtained: _____   Anticipated date/time of discharge: _____

Resources available: Persons: _____   Approved car seat: _____   Fitting/trial (infant

5 lb or less): _____

Special needs: _____

Referrals made: _____

THE FIRST HOUR OF LIFE

The primary focus at this time is the transition from intrauterine to extrauterine life, with an introduction to family members as the neonate's condition warrants.

NEONATAL ASSESSMENT DATA BASE (FULL-TERM)

Circulation

Apical pulse may fluctuate from 110–180 beats per minute (bpm).
Blood pressure 60–80 mm Hg (systolic), 40–45 mm Hg (diastolic).
Heart Sounds: Located in mediastinum with point of maximal intensity just to the left of the midsternum at third or fourth intercostal space.
Murmurs common during the first few hours of life.
Umbilical cord white and gelatinous; contains two arteries and one vein.

Elimination

May void at birth
May have passed meconium at birth

Food/Fluid

Weight: 2500–4000 g (5 lb 8 oz–8 lb 13 oz)
Length: 44–55 cm (18–22 in)
Skin turgor elastic (varies according to gestational age)

Neurosensory

Muscle Tone: Hypertonic flexion of all extremities.
Awake and active, demonstrates sucking reflex for first 30 min following birth (first period of reactivity).
Asymmetrical appearance (molding, edema, hematoma).
Cry strong, lusty, medium pitch (high-pitched cry suggests genetic abnormality, hypoglycemia, or prolonged narcotic effect).

Respiration

Apgar Score: 1/5 optimal score 7–10
Rate ranges from 30–60/min; periodic pattern may be noted
Breath sounds bilateral; occasional crackles common initially
Thorax cylindrical; prominent xiphoid cartilage common

Safety

Temperature ranges from 97.7°F–99.4°F (36.5°C–37.5°C).
Some vernix present (amount and distribution dependent on gestational age).
Skin: Smooth, flexible; peeling of hands/feet may be noted; pink-tinged or ruddy color; may be mottled, display minor bruising (e.g., forceps delivery), or harlequin color changes; petechiae on head/face (may reflect increased pressure associated with delivery or nuchal cord); port-wine stains, telangiectatic nevi (eyelids, between brows, or on occiput), or mongolian spots (primarily lower back and buttocks) may be noted.
Scalp abrasion may be present (internal electrode placement).

DIAGNOSTIC STUDIES

Cord pH: Levels of 7.20–7.24 reflect a preacidotic state; lower levels indicate significant asphyxia.
Hb/Hct: Hb level of 15–20 g and Hct of 43%–61%.
Direct Coombs' Test on Cord Blood: Determines presence of antigen-antibody complexes on red blood cell (RBC) membrane, reflecting hemolytic condition.

NURSING PRIORITIES

1. Promote effective cardiopulmonary effort.
2. Provide a thermoneutral environment, and maintain body temperature.
3. Prevent injury or complications.
4. Promote parent-infant attachment.

NURSING DIAGNOSIS:	GAS EXCHANGE, risk for impaired
Risk Factors May Include:	Prenatal intrapartal stressors, excess production of mucus, and cold stress
Possibly Evidenced By:	[Not applicable; presence of signs/symptoms establishes an *actual* diagnosis]
DESIRED OUTCOMES/EVALUATION CRITERIA—NEONATE WILL:	Maintain patent airway with respiratory and heart rates within normal limits (WNL); generalized cyanosis absent.
	Be free of signs of respiratory distress.

ACTIONS/INTERVENTIONS	RATIONALE

Independent

Measure Apgar score at 1 and 5 min following delivery.	Helps determine need for immediate intervention (e.g., suctioning, oxygen). A total score of 0–3 represents severe asphyxia or possible dysfunction in neurological and/or chemical control of respiration. Scores of 4–6 signify moderate difficulty adapting to extrauterine life. Scores of 7–10 indicate no difficulty adapting to extrauterine life.
Identify prenatal complications affecting placental and/or fetal status (e.g., cardiac or kidney disorders, pregnancy-induced hypertension [PIH], or diabetes).	Such complications may result in chronic hypoxia and acidosis, increasing risk of central nervous system (CNS) damage and requiring correction after delivery.
Review intrapartal fetal status, including fetal heart rate (FHR), periodic changes in FHR, beat-to-beat variability, scalp pH level (if done), and color and amount of amniotic fluid.	As in prenatal complications, intrapartal events may create fetal distress and hypoxia that persist into the immediate postdelivery period, resulting in depressed or ineffective respiratory effort. Fetus with scalp pH level <7.20, prolonged, variable, or late decelerations, and reduced FHR variability; oligohydramnios, or meconium-stained amniotic fluid will require greater efforts to achieve stabilization following birth than fetus with no signs of hypoxia or distress.
Determine duration of labor and type of delivery.	Thoracic compression during passage through the birth canal aids in clearing the lungs of approximately 80–110 ml of fluid. An infant delivered following precipitous labor (less than 3 hr) or delivered by cesarean section has excessive mucus because of inadequate thoracic compression.
Note times at which medications (e.g., magnesium sulfate or meperidine hydrochloride [Demerol]) were administered to mother.	Medications may depress newborn's respiratory efforts and reduce the newborn's ability to oxygenate tissues.
Assess initial respiratory rate and effort.	The first breath, which is the most difficult,

443

establishes a functional residual capacity (FRC), so that 30%–40% of lung tissue remains fully expanded, provided that adequate surfactant levels are present. Failure to achieve an FRC makes each subsequent breath as tiring and difficult as the initial breath. Tachypnea (respiratory rate >60/min) is usually associated with normal anticipated changes in the first period of reactivity (30 min following birth), but may also represent an attempt to eliminate excess carbon dioxide.

Note presence of nasal flaring, chest retractions, expiratory grunting, crackles, or rhonchi.

These signs are normal and transient in the first period of reactivity, but may indicate respiratory distress if they persist. Crackles may be heard until fluid is reabsorbed from lungs. Rhonchi indicate aspiration of oral secretions.

Clear airway; gently suction nasopharynx, as needed, using a bulb syringe or DeLee mucus-trap catheter (preferably while neonate's head is on maternal perineum if meconium-stained amniotic fluid is present). Monitor apical pulse during suctioning.

Helps remove accumulated fluid, facilitates respiratory effort, and helps prevent aspiration. Suctioning of the oropharynx causes vagal stimulation leading to bradycardia.

Dry infant with warm blankets, place stockinette cap on head, and place either in parent's arms or in prewarmed heating unit.

Reduces effects of cold stress (i.e., increased oxygen needs) and associated hypoxia, which can further depress respiratory efforts and result in acidosis as neonate resorts to anaerobic metabolism with lactic acid end products. (Refer to ND: Body Temperature, risk for altered.)

Place newborn in modified Trendelenburg position at a 10-degree angle.

Facilitates drainage of mucus from nasopharynx and trachea by means of gravity.

Note pitch and intensity of cry.

Initially, a lusty, strong cry increases alveolar PO_2 and produces the necessary chemical changes to convert fetal to neonatal circulation, so that the heart rate increases to 175–180 bpm and then usually returns to normal within the next 4–6 hr.

Auscultate/evaluate apical pulse.

A heart rate less than 100 bpm indicates severe asphyxia and the need for immediate resuscitation. Tachycardia (heart rate >160 bpm) may indicate recent asphyxia or a normal response associated with the first period of reactivity.

Provide appropriate tactile and sensory stimulation.

Stimulates respiratory effort and may increase inspired oxygen.

Note presence of wide-eyed stare.

Indicates chronic intrauterine hypoxia, which is possibly associated with acidosis and requires resuscitative measures.

Observe skin color for location and extent of cyanosis. Assess muscle tone.

Acrocyanosis, suggesting sluggish peripheral circulation, occurs normally in 85% of newborns during the 1st hr; however, generalized cyanosis and flaccidity indicate inadequate tissue oxygenation.

Suction gastric contents if amniotic fluid was meconium-stained.

Helps reduce incidence of aspiration pneumonia in early neonatal period.

Collaborative

Assist with intubation at birth in presence of frank meconium in amniotic fluid.

Prevents neonate taking first breath before airway is cleared, reducing risk of meconium aspiration and subsequent pneumonia.

Administer warmed oxygen via mask at 4–7 L/min, if indicated.

Provides additional oxygen and supports respiratory effort, if marked pallor or generalized cyanosis is present. In cases of prolonged hypoxia, fetal circulation may persist, because elevated PO_2 levels are necessary to reduce pulmonary vascular resistance, enhance blood flow to the lungs, and increase pressure on the left side of the heart, which closes the ductus arteriosus and the foramen ovale.

Assist with drawing of cord blood.

If there is indication of respiratory distress in the newborn, a cord pH level may be obtained to confirm presence and duration of prenatal asphyxia.

Perform deep suctioning if newborn shows evidence of respiratory depression that does not respond to gentle suction or to gentle tactile stimulation.

Promotes patent airway. Note: If meconium staining is present, deep suctioning, in conjunction with suctioning while infant's head is on perineum, is necessary to prevent meconium aspiration.

Administer medications, as indicated (e.g., Naloxone [Narcan], administered intravenously or through umbilical vessel catheter).

Narcan is a fast-acting narcotic antagonist that counteracts respiratory depression caused by exposure to maternal anesthetics or narcotics.

Provide resuscitative measures, and prepare for transfer of newborn to a neonatal intensive care unit (NICU) or level III/IV facility, as indicated.

Infants requiring extensive resuscitative efforts must be observed and cared for by personnel who have been specifically trained to care for sick newborns.

NURSING DIAGNOSIS: BODY TEMPERATURE, risk for altered

Risk Factors May Include: Extreme of age (inability to shiver, large body surface in relation to mass, limited amounts of insulating subcutaneous fat, nonrenewable sources of brown fat and few white fat stores, thin epidermis with close proximity of blood vessels to the skin)

Possibly Evidenced By: [Not applicable; presence of signs/symptoms establishes an actual diagnosis]

DESIRED OUTCOMES/EVALUATION CRITERIA—NEONATE WILL: Maintain core, skin, and axillary temperature and vital signs WNL.

Be free of signs of respiratory distress and cold stress.

ACTIONS/INTERVENTIONS
RATIONALE

Independent

Ascertain medications mother received during prenatal and intrapartal periods. Note presence of fetal distress or hypoxia.

Fetal hypoxia or maternal use of meperidine (Demerol) alters fetal metabolism of brown fat, often causing significant drop in neonate's temperature. Magnesium sulfate can cause vasodilation and interfere with infant's ability to retain heat.

Dry newborn's head and body, place stockinette cap on head, and wrap in warm blankets.

Reduces evaporative and conductive heat loss, protects moist infant from drafts or cooling air currents, and limits stress of movement from a warm uterine environment to a much cooler environment (possibly 15°F [9.4°C] lower than intrauterine temperatures). Note: Because of the relatively large surface area of the newborn head in relation to that of

445

Place newborn in prewarmed environment or in parent's arms. Warm objects coming in contact with infant (e.g., scales, stethoscopes, examination tables, and hands.)

the body, an infant may experience dramatic heat loss from a moist, uncovered head; however, research suggests that in healthy neonates of normal weight, a cap may not be necessary if the head is dried well.

Prevents heat loss by conduction, whereby heat is transferred from the newborn to objects or surfaces cooler than the newborn. Being held close to the parent's body and skin-to-skin contact reduce the newborn's heat loss.

Note environmental temperature. Eliminate drafts and minimize use of air conditioners; warm oxygen if it is administered via mask.

A decrease in the environmental temperature of 3.6°F (2°C) is sufficient to double the oxygen consumption of a term neonate. Heat loss by convection occurs when infant loses heat to cooler air currents. Loss by radiation occurs when heat is transferred from the newborn to objects or surfaces not in direct contact with newborn (e.g., incubator sides or walls).

Assess neonate's core temperature, monitor skin temperature continually with skin probe as appropriate.

Skin temperature should be maintained close to 97.6°F (36.5°C). Core temperature (rectal) is usually 0.9°F (0.5°C) higher than skin temperature, yet continuous transfer from core to skin occurs, so that the greater the difference between core and skin temperature, the more rapid the transfer and the faster the core temperature cools.

Provide gradual warming for cold-stressed infant, keeping air temperature 2.7°F (1.5°C) warmer than body temperature.

Too-rapid increase in temperature may result in apnea in cold-stressed Infant.

Observe newborn for signs of cold stress (e.g., drop in skin temperature, increased activity, flexion of extremities, pallor and/or mottling, and cool skin, hands, and feet).

When the environmental temperature falls below the thermoneutral zone (89.6°F–96.8°F [32°C–34°C]) the neonate increases activity levels (increasing metabolic rate and oxygen consumption), flexes extremities to reduce amount of body surface exposed, and releases adrenal catecholamines, which promote heat release from stored brown fat and cause vasoconstriction, further cooling the skin.

Note signs of respiratory distress (e.g., apnea, generalized cyanosis, bradycardia, and severe grunting, retraction of respiratory muscles, and nasal flaring). Provide support as needed.

These signs indicate negative effects of prolonged cold stress, which necessitate close monitoring. Peripheral vasoconstriction leads to metabolic acidosis; pulmonary vasoconstriction results in respiratory compromise and persistence of fetal circulation with failure of ductus arteriosus and foramen ovale to close.

Collaborative

Provide metabolic support (glucose or buffer), as indicated.

Side effects of prolonged hypothermia (cold stress) may include increased oxygen consumption, leading to hypoxia, acidosis, and respiratory compromise; increased metabolic rate and glucose consumption, resulting in hypoglycemia; as well as release of free fatty acids in the bloodstream, which compete with bilirubin binding sites on albumin, therefore increasing the risk of jaundice and kernicterus. Administration of glucose or bicarbonate can correct hypoglycemia, acidosis, and/or asphyxia.

Consider admission to special care nursery (SCN) or neonatal intensive care unit (NICU).

Permits close observation and use of aggressive care methods in cases of severe neonatal cold stress with secondary symptoms.

NURSING DIAGNOSIS:	FAMILY PROCESSES, altered [bonding process]
May Be Related To:	Developmental transition and/or gain of a family member
Possibly Evidenced By:	Hesitance of parent(s) to hold/interact with infant, verbalization of concerns
DESIRED OUTCOMES/EVALUATION CRITERIA—PARENT(S) WILL:	Initiate attachment process in ways that are meaningful to family members.
	Properly identify infant to assure correct family association.

ACTIONS/INTERVENTIONS	RATIONALE

Independent

Inform parents of neonate's immediate needs and of care being provided.	Alleviates parents' anxiety regarding condition of their newborn. Helps parents to understand rationale for interventions in initial newborn period.
Place newborn in mother's/father's arms as soon as neonatal condition permits.	The 1st hr of life is an especially significant time for family interaction in that it can promote initial attachment between parents and infant and acceptance of the newborn as a new family member.
Encourage parent(s) to stroke and speak to newborn; encourage mother to breastfeed infant, if desired.	Provides opportunity for parents and newborn to initiate acquaintance and attachment process.
Share information gained from initial physical assessment of newborn.	Helps parents to view infant as a separate person with unique physical characteristics.
Discuss neonate's capabilities for interaction. (Refer to CP: Stage IV [First 4 Hours Following Delivery of the Placenta]; ND: Family Processes, altered [bonding process].)	Helps clarify expectations and facilitate parent-infant interaction.
Using legally acceptable identification system, place arm or leg bands on infant and one wrist band on mother. Take infant's footprints and mother's fingerprint (index finger).	Establishes family unit and prevents confusion regarding identification of infant. A more accurate method of identification, DNA fingerprinting, is being used and may eventually supplant traditional footprinting and fingerprinting.
Provide appropriate information in the event of unanticipated complications or the need for transfer to SCN/NICU.	Keeping parents informed about infant's change in status, and actual or potential actions to be instituted, helps to assure them that everything possible is being done to care for infant and promotes parental cooperation with emergency measures.

NURSING DIAGNOSIS:	INJURY, risk for
Risk Factors May Include:	Undetected or untreated congenital anomalies, exposure to infectious agents
Possibly Evidenced By:	[Not applicable; presence of signs/symptoms establishes an *actual* diagnosis]
DESIRED OUTCOMES/EVALUATION CRITERIA—NEONATE WILL:	Be free of injury/complications.

Independent

Perform routine physical assessment of newborn, noting number of cord vessels and presence of anomalies.	Helps detect abnormalities and neurological defects, establishes gestational age, and identifies the need for closer monitoring and more intensive care. Cord should contain three vessels. Presence of only one artery is associated with genitourinary abnormalities.
Bathe newborn immediately after delivery if exposure to infectious agents has occurred.	Prevents newborn from contracting hepatitis B virus or from becoming a chronic carrier when exposed to maternal serum blood products at delivery.
Describe to parents the appropriate rationale for actions taken to prevent injury (e.g., prophylactic administration of eye ointment and vitamin K).	Reduces parental anxiety created by a lack of understanding of the need to protect neonate against eye infection and hemorrhagic disease.

Collaborative

Clamp umbilical cord approximately ½–1 in from newborn's abdomen within 30 sec after birth, while neonate is at the level of the mother's introitus.	Holding newborn below the level of the introitus or delaying cord clamping accounts for transfer of 50–100 ml of blood from the placenta, possibly contributing to polycythemia and hyperbilirubinemia in the neonatal period.
Administer eye prophylaxis in the form of erythromycin ointment (Ilotycin) approximately 1 hr after birth (after period of parent-infant interaction).	Helps prevent ophthalmia neonatorum, caused by *Neisseria gonorrhoeae*, which may be present in the mother's birth canal. Erythromycin effectively eradicates both gonorrheal and chlamydial organisms. Note: Eye prophylaxis clouds newborn's vision, reducing infant's ability to interact with parents.
Administer Vitamin K (AquaMEPHYTON]) IM, within 2 hr after birth.	Prevents hemorrhagic disease in the newborn.
Administer hepatitis B immune globulin (HBIG) and hepatitis B vaccine if mother's serum contains hepatitis B surface antigen (HB_sAG), hepatitis B core antigen (HB_cAg), or $_e$ antigen (HB_eAg).	Provides passive immunity for newborn in presence of viral infection. First dose is administered at birth for infants of HB_sAg-positive mothers.

THE NEONATE AT 2 HOURS TO 2 DAYS OF AGE

NEONATAL ASSESSMENT DATA BASE (FULL-TERM)

(Refer to CP: The First Hour of Life.)

Activity/Rest

Wakeful state may be as little as 2–3 hr first several days.
Infant appears semicomatose while in deep sleep; grimacing or smiling is evident in rapid eye movement (REM) sleep; averages 20 hr of sleep per day.

Circulation

Apical pulse averages 120–160 bpm (115 bpm at 4–6 hr, rising to 120 bpm at 12–24 hr after birth); may fluctuate from 80–100 bpm (sleeping) to 180 bpm (crying).
Peripheral pulses may be weak (bounding pulses suggest patent ductus arteriosus [PDA]); brachial and radial pulses are more easily palpated than femoral pulses (absence of femoral and dorsalis pedis pulses suggests coarctation of the aorta).
Heart murmur often present during transition periods.
Blood pressure (BP) ranges from 60–80 mm Hg (systolic)/40–45 mm Hg (diastolic), average resting pressure approximately 74/46 mm Hg; BP lowest at 3 hr of age.
Umbilical cord clamped securely with no oozing of blood noted; shows signs of drying within 1–2 hr of birth, shriveled and blackened by day 2 or 3.

Elimination

Abdomen soft without distension; active bowel sounds present several hours after birth
Urine colorless or pale yellow, with 6–10 wet diapers per 24 hr
Passage of meconium stool within 24–48 hr of birth

Food/Fluid

Mean weight 2500–4000 g (5 lb 8 oz to 8 lb 13 oz); <2500 g suggests small for gestational age (SGA) (e.g., prematurity, rubella syndrome, or multiple gestation), greater than 4000 g suggests large for gestational age (LGA) (e.g., maternal diabetes; or may be associated with heredity). (Refer to CPs: The Preterm Infant; Newborn: Deviations in Growth Patterns).
Weight loss 5%–10% initially.
Mouth: Scant saliva; Epstein's pearls (epithelial cysts) and sucking blisters are normal on hard palate/gum margins, precocious teeth may be present.

Neurosensory

Head circumference 32–37 cm; anterior and posterior fontanels are soft and flat.
Caput succedaneum and/or molding may persist for 3–4 days; overriding of cranial sutures may be noted, slightly obliterating anterior fontanel (2–3 cm in width) and posterior fontanel (0.5–1.0 cm in width).
Eyes and eyelids may be edematous; subconjunctival or retinal hemorrhage may be noted; chemical conjunctivitis lasting 1–2 days may develop following instillation of therapeutic ophthalmic drops.
Strabismus and doll's eye phenomenon often present.
Top of ear aligns with inner and outer canthi of eye (low-set ears suggest genetic or kidney abnormalities).
Neurological Examination: Presence of Moro, plantar, palmar grasp, and Babinski's reflexes; reflex responses are bilateral/equal (unilateral Moro reflex may indicate fractured clavicle or brachial plexus injury); transient crawling movements may be seen.
Absence of jitteriness, lethargy, hypotonia, and paresis.

Respiration

Transient tachypnea may be noted, especially following cesarean or breech birth.
Breathing Pattern: Diaphragmatic and abdominal breathing with synchronous movement of

chest and abdomen (inspiratory lag or alternating seesaw movements of the chest and abdomen reflects respiratory distress); slight or occasional nasal flaring may be noted; marked nasal flaring, expiratory grunting, or marked retraction of intercostal, substernal, or subcostal muscles indicates respiratory distress; inspiratory crackles may persist for first few hours after birth (rhonchi on inspiration or expiration may indicate aspiration).

Chest circumference approximately 30–35 cm (1–2 cm smaller than circumference of head).

Safety

Skin Temperature: 96.8°F–97.7°F (36°C–36.5°C), rectal 97.8°F–99°F (36.6°C–37.2°C).

Skin Color: Acrocyanosis may be present for several days during transition period (general ruddiness may indicate polycythemia); reddened or ecchymotic areas may appear over cheeks or on lower jaw or parietal areas as a result of forceps application at delivery; facial bruising may be noted following precipitous delivery.

Cephalhematoma may appear day after delivery, increasing in size by 2–3 days of age, then be reabsorbed slowly over 1–6 mo.

Extremities: Normal range of motion in all; mild degree of bowing or medial rotation of lower extremities; good muscle tone.

Sexuality

Female Genitalia: Vaginal labia may be slightly reddened or edematous, vaginal/hymenal tag may be noted; white mucous discharge (smegma) or slight bloody discharge (pseudomenstruation) may be present.

Male Genitalia: Testes descended, scrotum covered with rugae, phimosis common (opening of prepuce narrowed, preventing retraction of foreskin over the glans).

Teaching/Learning

Gestational age between 38 and 42 wk based on Dubowitz criteria

Diagnostic Studies

White Blood Cell (WBC) Count: 18,000/mm^3, neutrophils increase to 23,000–24,000/mm^3 the 1st day after birth (decline occurs in sepsis).

Hb: 15–20 g/dl (lower levels associated with anemia or excessive hemolysis).

Hct: 43%–61% (elevation to 65% or over indicates polycythemia; decreased levels reflect anemia or prenatal/perinatal hemorrhage).

Guthrie Inhibition Assay: Tests for presence of phenylalanine metabolites, indicating phenylketonuria (PKU).

Total Bilirubin: 6 mg/dl on 1st day of life, 8 mg/dl at 1–2 days, and 12 mg/dl at 3–5 days.

Dextrostix: Initial glucose drop during first 4–6 hr after birth averages 40–50 mg/dl, raising to 60–70 mg/dl by day 3.

NURSING PRIORITIES

1. Facilitate adaptation to extrauterine life.
2. Maintain thermoneutrality.
3. Prevent complications.
4. Promote parent-infant attachment.
5. Provide information and anticipatory guidance to parent(s).

DISCHARGE GOALS

1. Newborn adapting effectively to extrauterine life.
2. Free of complications.
3. Parent-infant attachment is initiated and progressing satisfactorily.
4. Parent(s) express confidence regarding infant care.

NURSING DIAGNOSIS:	BODY TEMPERATURE, risk for altered
Risk Factors May Include:	Extreme of age (inability to shiver, larger body surface in relation to mass, limited amounts of insulating subcutaneous fat, nonrenewable sources of brown fat and few white fat stores, thin epidermis with close proximity of blood vessels to the skin)
Possibly Evidenced By:	[Not applicable; presence of signs/symptoms establishes an *actual* diagnosis]
DESIRED OUTCOMES/EVALUATION CRITERIA—NEONATE WILL:	Maintain temperature WNL. Be free of signs of cold stress or hyperthermia.

ACTIONS/INTERVENTIONS

Independent

Maintain ambient temperature within established thermoneutral zone (TNZ) considering neonate's weight, gestational age, and usual clothing provided.

Monitor neonate's axillary, skin (abdominal), or tympanic and environmental temperature at least every 30–60 min during stabilization period, or more frequently, per protocol.

Assess respiratory rate; note tachypnea (rate greater than 60/min).

Postpone initial bath until body temperature is stable and reaches 97.7°F (36.5°C).

RATIONALE

In response to lower environmental temperature, full-term infants increase their body temperature by crying or increasing motor activity, thereby possibly consuming more energy (stored glucose) and increasing their oxygen needs. Conversely, failure to maintain the environmental temperature within the upper limits of the TNZ may result in increased oxygen consumption, dehydration, hypotension, seizures, and apnea associated with hyperthermia.

Temperature stabilization may not occur until 8–12 hr following birth. Rates of oxygen consumption and metabolism are minimal when skin temperature (a reliable indicator of energy exchanges between infant and environment) is maintained above 97.7°F (36.5°C). Skin temperature measured over the abdomen (away from bony area) is an earlier, more reliable indicator of cold stress, because it drops in response to peripheral vasoconstriction. Axillary temperature readings may be misleading, because friction in the armpit, where brown fat stores are located, can cause false elevations. Core body temperature, as assessed by rectal temperatures, may remain misleadingly high, especially in the cold-stressed newborn, as a result of vasoconstriction and metabolism of brown fat stores. Core temperature may fall only after the newborn has exhausted compensatory mechanisms and has markedly increased oxygen consumption. Note: Rectal perforation may occur with insertion of rectal thermometer, and its occurrence is associated with 70% mortality.

Infant becomes tachypneic in response to increased oxygen needs associated with cold stress and attempts to eliminate excess carbon dioxide to reduce respiratory acidosis.

Helps prevent further heat losses caused by evaporation. Larger appropriate-for-gestational age (AGA) infants tend to maintain body temperature more easily than the SGA infant.

451

Bathe neonate, working rapidly, exposing only a portion of the body at a time, and drying each part immediately. Ensure that environment is free of drafts.	Reduces possible heat loss through evaporation and convection; helps conserve energy.
Note secondary signs of cold stress (e.g., irritability, pallor, mottling, respiratory distress, tremors, jitteriness, lethargy, and cool skin).	Hypothermia, which increases the utilization rate of oxygen and glucose, is often accompanied by hypoglycemia and respiratory distress. Cooling also results in peripheral vasoconstriction, with a drop in skin temperature observed as pallor or mottling. Irritability and apnea may be associated with hypoxia. Untreated or undetected cold stress may progress to metabolic acidosis, associated with anaerobic glycolysis; pulmonary vasoconstriction or persistent fetal circulation; inhibition of lecithin formation and increased severity of respiratory distress; and release of fatty acids into bloodstream, where they compete for bilirubin-binding sites on albumin molecules.
Maintain thermoneutral environment through use of automatically controlled or manually adjustable heating equipment. Maintain controlled heat source at 98.6°F (37°C). Position crib or incubator away from heat sources such as sunlight, heaters, or bilirubin lights. Promote gradual warming of infant as needed (approximately 1.2°F [1°C] per hr). Adjust clothing as indicated.	Prevents heat imbalance or losses. Gradual warming of hypothermic infant helps avoid possible apneic spells, hypotension, seizures, or dehydration associated with too-rapid warming and hyperthermia.
Assess for behavioral signs associated with hyperthermia (e.g., increased restlessness, perspiration that begins on head or face and proceeds to chest, apnea, seizure, and hypotension activity).	Heat dissipation occurs through peripheral vasodilation and through augmentation of cooling by evaporation and by increase in insensible water loss. Apnea, seizures, and hypotension may be related to peripheral vasodilation, which causes increased evaporative water losses, cerebral ischemia, and dehydration.
Note signs of dehydration (e.g., poor skin turgor, delayed voiding, dry mucous membranes, elevated temperature, sunken fontanels).	Axillary temperature >99.5°F (37.5°C) is considered hyperthermic and suggests overheated infant. Dehydration may develop in relation to a threefold to fourfold increase in insensible water loss.
Initiate early oral feeding.	For every 1.8°F (1°C) increase in body temperature, metabolism and fluid needs increase approximately 10%. Failure to replace fluid losses further contributes to dehydrated state.
Assess infant for other disease processes, such as infection, if temperature deviates more than 1.8°F (1°C) from one reading to next.	Temperature instability or subnormal temperature may indicate infection. (Refer to ND: Infection, risk for.) In addition, CNS disorders and dehydration may cause hyperthermia.

Collaborative

Make arrangements for transfer to NICU, if indicated.	If temperature remains low regardless of appropriate intervention related to thermoregulation, transfer of neonate may be necessary for closer observation and treatment.
Administer seizure-control medication (e.g., phenobarbital), as needed.	Acts directly on cerebrum to quiet excessive motor activity, which can cause hyperthermia.

NURSING DIAGNOSIS:	GAS EXCHANGE, risk for impaired
Risk Factors May Include:	Prenatal/intrapartal stressors, excess production of mucus, and fluctuations of body temperature
Possibly Evidenced By:	[Not applicable; presence of signs/symptoms establishes an *actual* diagnosis]
DESIRED OUTCOMES/EVALUATION CRITERIA—NEONATE WILL:	Maintain patent airway with respiratory rate WNL (between 30 and 60/min).
	Be free of signs of respiratory distress.

ACTIONS/INTERVENTIONS	RATIONALE

Independent

Estimate gestational age using Dubowitz criteria.	Surfactant system develops as gestation progresses. Once fetus reaches 35 weeks' gestation, the presence of phosphatidyl glycerol (a component of the surfactant complex, which indicates fetal lung maturity) markedly decreases the incidence of respiratory distress syndrome (RDS). Infants of diabetic mothers who have been exposed to prolonged hyperinsulinemia in response to maternal hyperglycemia may have depressed surfactant production and greater respiratory distress even though they are beyond 35 weeks' gestation at birth.
Review prenatal and intrapartal events, noting risk factors that could have contributed to excess lung fluid or aspiration of amniotic fluid (e.g., maternal diabetes, cesarean birth or breech delivery, maternal bleeding, intrapartal asphyxia, maternal oversedation).	Such events contribute to the neonate's inability to clear airway of excess fluid, mucus, and aspirated material, and to the collection of excess fluid in lungs, resulting in type II RDS, which usually resolves within 6 hr.
Assess respiratory rate and effort. Differentiate periodic breathing patterns from apneic episodes.	Normal respiratory rate is 30–60/min. Periodic breathing that is of no physiological significance is manifested by apneic periods lasting 5–15 sec occurring during REM sleep and periods of motor activity. It is easily converted to a normal breathing pattern by increasing inspired oxygen through tactile and sensory stimulation. Apneic episodes last longer than 20–30 sec, may be associated with changes in heart rate and skin color, and require further assessment and intervention.
Suction nasopharynx, as needed. Note color, amount, and character of regurgitated mucus.	Ensures clearance of airway, which is critical to neonate, who is an obligatory nose breather and may not learn to open the mouth in response to nasal obstruction until 3–4 wk of age. Regurgitation of mucus associated with an episode of gagging often occurs in the second period of reactivity (2–6 hr after delivery).
Position newborn on side with rolled towel for support at back.	Facilitates drainage of mucus.
Auscultate breath sounds and record equality and clarity. Note presence of crackles or rhonchi.	Breath sounds should be equal bilaterally. Inspiratory crackles may be present in the first few hours following delivery until lung fluid is absorbed from distal bronchioles. Persistent crackles may

453

Review delivery records for presence of meconium at birth or meconium-stained amniotic fluid; determine whether appropriate suctioning of oropharynx was performed while infant's head was still on perineum.	indicate RDS or pneumonia. Rhonchi heard on inspiration or expiration, caused by air moving through passages that have been narrowed by secretions or swelling, may indicate retained secretions/aspiration. When thick meconium is present, deep suctioning should take place before the initial breath is taken to avoid development of meconium-aspiration pneumonia.
Observe and record signs of respiratory distress (e.g., grunting, retraction of respiratory muscles, nasal flaring, and tachypnea).	These signs represent compensatory mechanisms to overcome hypoxia. Expiratory grunting occurs as an attempt to maintain alveolar expansion and to retain air. Retraction of respiratory muscles increases tidal volume, nasal flaring increases the diameter of the nares, and tachypnea occurs in an attempt to eliminate excess carbon dioxide.
Assess newborn for presence, location, and degree of cyanosis and its relationship to activity.	Peripheral cyanosis (acrocyanosis) associated with vasomotor instability, hypothermia, or local venous or arterial obstruction may persist through the transition period. Mild cyanosis and mottling may occur in second period of reactivity in association with fluctuations in cardiac and respiratory rates. Cyanosis that worsens with crying suggests cardiac problems (unresolved PDA or congenital anomalies) rather than respiratory problems, in which cyanosis is usually improved with crying.
Compare neonate's skin temperature and ambient air temperature.	Oxygen consumption is minimal when the difference between skin temperature and ambient air temperature is <2.7°F (1.5°C).
Monitor newborn for signs of hypothermia or hyperthermia. (Refer to ND: Body Temperature, risk for altered.)	Hypothermia and hyperthermia increase metabolic rate and oxygen consumption, causing a possible cycle of metabolic acidosis and hypoxia that perpetuates fetal circulation, reduces surfactant levels, and increases respiratory distress. A drop in skin temperature to 96.6°F (35.9°C) increases oxygen consumption by 10%. Too-rapid warming of neonate may lead to hyperthermia, which increases oxygen consumption by 6%.
Note symmetry of chest movement.	Asymmetry may indicate pneumothorax associated with previous resuscitative measures.
Auscultate heart sounds; note presence of murmurs.	Transient cardiac murmurs (usually systolic) may exist in the early newborn period because of persistence or reopening of fetal structures in response to hypoxia and crying. PDA often occurs with hypoxia, pulmonary vasoconstriction, right-to-left shunting, and congestive heart failure (CHF), or more significantly with prenatal or birth asphyxia, hyperviscosity, polycythemia, aspiration syndrome, and hypoglycemia. Foramen ovale normally closes at 1–2 hr following delivery; ductus arteriosus closes at 3–4 days of age. Inadequate lung perfusion and poorly ventilated lung tissue promote airway constriction and respiratory compromise.

Collaborative

Administer supplemental oxygen, as indicated by newborn's condition.	Persistent uninterrupted oxygen depletion increases hypoxic state, resulting in metabolic acidosis secondary to anaerobic metabolism.

454

Record use and results of mechanical monitoring of supplemental oxygen.	Unmonitored use of oxygen therapy can result in oxygen toxicity. Transcutaneous (pulse oximetry) monitoring helps prevent hypoxic states and evaluates therapeutic effectiveness.
Assess Hb and Hct levels. Note results of Kleihauer-Betke test.	The neonate whose Hb level is lower than normal has reduced oxygen-carrying capacity and possibly severe hypoxia. Hb levels <15 g/dl may be caused by blood loss, hemolysis, or decreased RBC production. Clinical signs of cyanosis may not appear until Hb levels are decreased by slightly more than 3 g/dl in central arterial blood or 4–6 g/dl in capillary blood. Kleihauer-Betke test identifies fetal bleeding in utero.
Monitor arterial blood gases (ABGs), if done.	Provides accurate measurement of acid-base balance to clarify respiratory versus metabolic deficits.
Determine Rh factor and ABO blood group of newborn and mother; note results of Coombs' test. (Refer to CP: Newborn: Hyperbilirubinemia.)	Identifies possible antigen-antibody reaction to Rh or ABO incompatibility, which contributes to lowered Hb levels and oxygen-carrying capacity.
Review chest x-ray.	May be necessary to diagnose pneumothorax.

NURSING DIAGNOSIS:	NUTRITION: altered, risk for less than body requirements
Risk Factors May Include:	Increased metabolic rate, high caloric requirement, fatigue, minimal nutritional stores
Possibly Evidenced By:	[Not applicable; presence of signs/symptoms establishes an *actual* diagnosis]
DESIRED OUTCOMES/EVALUATION CRITERIA—NEONATE WILL:	Be free of signs of hypoglycemia, with blood glucose level WNL.
	Display weight loss ≤5%–10% of birth weight by time of discharge.

ACTIONS/INTERVENTIONS	RATIONALE

Independent

| Review mother's prenatal history for possible stressors impacting on neonatal glucose stores, such as diabetes, PIH, or cardiac or renal disorders. Note results of tests related to fetal growth and placental/fetal well-being. | Full-term neonates who are especially susceptible to hypoglycemia are those who are chronically stressed in utero, are exposed to high glucose levels in utero, are SGA or LGA, or are acutely ill. The newborn has unique nutritional needs related to a rapid metabolic rate, high caloric requirement, potential loss of fluid and electrolytes caused by increased insensible water losses through pulmonary and cutaneous routes, and a potential for inadequate or depleted glucose stores. |
| Review intrapartal records for Apgar scores, condition at birth, type/timing of infant feeding. Note initial temperature on admission to the nursery. | Birth stressors and cold stress increase metabolic rate and rapidly deplete glucose stores, possibly using as many as 200 cal/kg/min in the delivery room prior to admission to the nursery. First feeding may occur in delivery room for clients choosing to breastfeed; bottle-fed infants usually have their first feeding during the second period of reactivity. Note: |

455

For client receiving mother-infant care (i.e., rooming in), neonate may be admitted briefly to nursery for purpose of assessment/medical clearance.

Reduce physical stressors such as cold stress, physical exertion, and excessive exposure to radiant warmers.

Hypothermia increases energy consumption and use of nonrenewable brown fat stores. Respiratory distress and/or ambient temperatures above TNZ increase metabolic rate and activity level as well as insensible water losses. For every 1.2°F (1°C) increase in body temperature, metabolism and fluid needs increase approximately 10%.

Weigh newborn on admission to nursery and daily thereafter. Note presence of postmaturity syndrome or wasting.

Establishes caloric and fluid needs according to baseline weight, which normally drops by 5%–10% within the first 3–4 days of life because of limited oral intake and loss of excess extracellular fluid. Infant with postmaturity syndrome has increased metabolic and caloric needs in early newborn period.

Screen for hypoglycemia using Dextrostix at 1 hr of age, and more frequently as indicated for high-risk or symptomatic infant.

Newborns may maintain maternal glucose level for up to 1 hr following birth, but after this time, glucose consumption may exceed intake and production, resulting in hypoglycemia. A history of intrauterine or postdelivery stress or hypoxia markedly increases the risk of hypoglycemia.

Observe newborn for tremors, irritability, tachypnea, diaphoresis, cyanosis, pallor, and seizure activity.

Indicates hypoglycemia associated with blood glucose levels <45 mg/dl.

Monitor newborn for ruddiness; note elevated Hb/Hct levels (Hb >20 g/dl, Hct greater than 60%).

RBCs are high consumers of glucose, predisposing the polycythemic neonate to hypoglycemia.

Auscultate bowel sounds. Note absence of abdominal distension, presence of lusty cry that quiets when oral stimulus is provided, and rooting/sucking behaviors.

Indicators showing that neonate is hungry/ready for feeding.

Initiate early oral feeding with 5–15 ml of sterile water, then dextrose and water, according to hospital protocol, progressing to formula for bottle-fed infants.

Initial feeding for breastfed infants usually occurs in the delivery room. Otherwise, water may be offered in the nursery to assess effectiveness of sucking, swallowing, gag reflexes, and patency of esophagus. If aspirated, sterile water is easily absorbed by pulmonary tissues. Early feedings help meet caloric and fluid needs, especially in an infant whose metabolic rate uses 100–120 cal/kg of body weight every 24 hr. Human milk or formula has a greater sustained effect on glucose levels and reduces risk of rebound hypoglycemia associated with bolus feeding of D_5W and $D_{10}W$.

Note frequency and amount/length of feedings. Encourage demand feedings instead of "scheduled" feedings. Note frequency, amount, and appearance of regurgitation. (Refer to ND: Knowledge Deficit [Learning Need]; and CP: The Client at 4 Hours to 2 Days Postpartum, ND: Breastfeeding [specify].)

Hunger and length of time between feedings vary from feeding to feeding. Six feedings of approximately 3 oz (an average of 17 oz of formula in 24 hr) usually meet nutritional and fluid requirements of a 6-lb neonate. Excessive regurgitation contributes to fluid loss and dehydration, increasing replacement needs.

Evaluate neonate/maternal satisfaction following feedings.

Provides opportunity to answer client questions, offer encouragement for efforts, identify needs, and problem-solve solutions.

Monitor color, concentration, and frequency of voidings.

Fluid requirements range from 140–160 ml/kg per 24 hr because the newborn has proportionately less fluid reserve and higher water needs than the older

Observe newborn for indications of feeding problems (e.g., recurrent or bile-colored regurgitation, abdominal distension, abnormal stools, excessive mucus production, choking, or refusal to feed).

child or adult. Loss of fluid and lack of oral intake rapidly deplete extracellular fluid and result in reduced urine output.

These problems may indicate intestinal obstruction, cystic fibrosis, or tracheoesophageal fistula.

Collaborative

Obtain immediate blood glucose if Dextrostix level is <45 mg/dl.

Blood glucose measurement confirms Dextrostix findings and the need for intervention.

Administer glucose immediately, orally or intravenously.

May need supplemental glucose to raise significantly low serum levels.

Follow up glucose administration with Dextrostix every 30 min–2 hr, based on severity of hypoglycemia, newborn's symptoms, and hospital protocol.

Enhances the finding and facilitates the treatment of rebound hypoglycemia. Rebound hypoglycemia is especially common following bolus feedings or bolus infusions of glucose or glucagon that are not followed by continuous glucose infusions.

Avoid oral feedings for distressed neonates, those with polycythemia and hyperviscosity, or infants with gastrointestinal (GI) anomalies. Institute IV therapy of $D_{10}W$, with infusion rate of 80–120 ml/kg/day.

Polycythemia and hyperviscosity potentially diminish circulation and availability of oxygen to digestive structures, so that introducing feedings may predispose neonate to development of necrotizing enterocolitis.

Administer glucagon or hydrocortisone if IV $D_{10}W$ therapy is not effective in resolving hypoglycemia.

Glucagon stimulates liver to break down stored glycogen. Steroids stimulate gluconeogenesis in the liver, thereby increasing blood glucose level.

NURSING DIAGNOSIS:	INFECTION, risk for
Risk Factors May Include:	Broken skin, traumatized tissue, environmental exposure, inadequate acquired immunity
Possibly Evidenced By:	[Not applicable; presence of signs/symptoms establishes an *actual* diagnosis]
DESIRED OUTCOMES/EVALUATION CRITERIA—NEONATE WILL:	Be free from signs of infection.
	Display timely healing of cord stump and circumcision site, free of drainage or erythema.

ACTIONS/INTERVENTIONS	RATIONALE

Independent

Review maternal risk factors that predispose infant to infection, which may be acquired transplacentally, via the ascending route, or at delivery. (Refer to CPs: Prenatal Infection; Puerperal Infection.)

Maternal fever during the week prior to birth, prolonged rupture of membranes (>24 hr), prolonged labor, foul-smelling amniotic fluid, and presence of infectious disease, such as gonorrhea, chlamydial infection, group B streptococcal infection, or TORCH group of viruses (toxoplasmosis, other viruses, rubella, cytomegalovirus, and herpes simplex viruses), all predispose infant to infection. Note: Use of epidural anesthesia has been correlated with increased frequency of fever in mother postpartum

457

Independent	
	(temperature of 100.4°F or more) without actual infection. This could result in neonate receiving unwarranted prophylactic antibiotics.
Determine newborn's gestational age.	Transfer of immunoglobulin E and G (IgE and IgG) antibodies via the placenta increases significantly in the last trimester, providing passive immunity to gram-positive cocci (pneumococci, streptococci, and meningococci), *Haemophilus influenzae,* viruses, and toxins (diphtheria and tetanus bacilli). However, the newborn is normally deficient in immunoglobulin M (IgM), which is stimulated by infectious agents (antibodies to blood group antigens, gram-negative enteroorganisms, and some viruses), and lacking in immunoglobulin A (IgA), which possibly provides protection on the secretory surfaces of the respiratory, urinary, and gastrointestinal tracts.
Monitor vital signs including skin temperature, as appropriate.	Aids in recognizing developing infection.
Scrub hands and arms with iodophor preparation prior to entering nursery/neonate's room, after contact with contaminated material, and after handling infant. Teach parents and siblings proper hand washing technique to use before handling infant.	Proper hand washing is the most important single factor in protecting newborns from infection. Iodophor preparation is effective against both gram-positive and gram-negative organisms.
Monitor (and instruct client to monitor) personnel, parents, and visitors for infectious illnesses, skin lesions, fever, or herpes. Limit contact with newborn appropriately.	Helps prevent spread of infection to newborn.
Maintain individual equipment and supplies for each newborn.	Prevents cross-contamination of neonate through direct contact or droplet infection.
Instruct parent(s) to inspect skin daily for rashes or interruptions in skin integrity. Recommend use of mild soaps, and gently patting skin dry after bathing; avoiding excessive rubbing.	Skin is a nonspecific immunity barrier preventing invasion of pathogens. The likelihood of infection is increased by a significant number of potential portals of entry for infectious organisms, such as umbilical vessels, site of circumcision, and skin breaks associated with forceps or internal scalp electrode application. Chemicals and perfumes in soaps may predispose skin to rashes and irritation; vigorous rubbing may traumatize delicate skin. Note: In the uncircumcised male, it is not necessary to retract the foreskin for cleaning; rather, daily external washing and rinsing is sufficient.
Suggest applying Eucerin Creme to identified dry areas, especially at ankles and wrists.	Helps prevent skin cracking and breakdown, especially in neonate with dry skin caused by excessive weight loss, dysmaturity, or prolonged exposure to phototherapy or radiant heat.
Encourage early breastfeeding, as appropriate.	Colostrum and breast milk contain high amounts of secretory IgA, which provides a form of passive immunity as well as macrophages and lymphocytes that foster local inflammatory response.
Assess cord and skin area at base of cord daily for redness, odor, or discharge. Facilitate drying through exposure to air by folding diaper below, and T-shirt above, the cord stump.	Promotes drying and healing, enhances normal necrosis and sloughing, and eliminates moist medium for bacterial growth.
Inspect newborn's mouth for white plaque on oral mucosa, gums, and tongue. Distinguish between white patches of thrush and milk curds.	White patches that cannot be removed and that tend to bleed when touched are caused by *Candida albicans,* resulting from direct contact with

458

Note presence of lethargy, poor weight gain, restlessness, lowered temperature, jaundice, respiratory symptoms, or visible lesions. Isolate newborn, as indicated; notify physician.

contaminated birth canal, hands, or breast. Note: Use of improperly cleaned nipple/breast shields or breast pump may result in colonization of the breasts.

These signs indicate possible infection. Transplacentally acquired infections tend to affect liver and CNS function; ascending route infections, in many cases, result in bacteremia or pneumonia.

Collaborative

Administer recombinant hepatitis B vaccine per state/agency policy.

Reduces risk of newborn's contracting hepatitis B or becoming a chronic carrier. First dose usually administered within 12 hr of birth. Note: The Centers for Disease Control and Prevention (CDC) and the American Academy of Pediatrics recommend immunization for all infants, regardless of mother's antigen status.

Monitor laboratory studies, as indicated:
  WBC count;

Deficiency of neutrophils, which participate in the early phagocytic response, and deficiencies of specific immunoglobulins predispose the full-term infant to infection, particularly in the first 4–6 wk of life. Normal WBC count of 18,000/mm^3 does not increase in the newborn in response to infection, and it often drops during sepsis.

  Serum levels of IgE, IgM, and IgA;

Elevated IgM levels at birth may occur in response to an infectious organism in utero. IgE levels are increased in the third trimester and provide neonate with passive immunity to some organisms. IgA is found in colostrum and provides some passive immunity until the newborn begins to produce IgA at approximately 4 wk of age.

  Cultures of lesions, pustules, or drainage, when present (distinguish between possible infectious rashes and erythema toxicum neonatorum);

Identifies possible pathogens. Vesicles or lesions of erythema toxicum neonatorum (thought to be a local inflammatory response) contain eosinophils and are of no clinical significance.

  Blood cultures.

Diagnoses presence of bacteremia or sepsis and identifies causative agents.

Administer topical, oral, or parenteral antibiotics as indicated.

Eradicates pathogenic organisms.

Apply nystatin (Mycostatin) to mouth; swab over oral mucosa, gums, and tongue. Wash mouth with sterile water prior to application.

Eradicates *Candida albicans,* the causative organism for thrush and mycotic stomatitis.

NURSING DIAGNOSIS:	INJURY, risk for
Risk Factors May Include:	Birth trauma, aspiration, abnormal blood profile, congenital anomalies, drug effects
Possibly Evidenced By:	[Not applicable; presence of signs/symptoms establishes an *actual* diagnosis]
DESIRED OUTCOMES/EVALUATION CRITERIA—NEONATE WILL	Be free of injury or aspiration.
	Display bilirubin levels below 15 mg/dL.
PARENT(S) WILL:	Identify individual risks.
	Demonstrate behaviors to protect newborn from environmental injury.

459

ACTIONS/INTERVENTIONS	RATIONALE

Independent

Perform thorough newborn assessment for possible abnormal findings. Note crepitus, interruption in clavicle, abnormal Moro reflex, skull depression, or absence of movement of extremities.

Helps detect possible birth injuries, such as fractures of the clavicle, skull, or extremities.

Assess newborn for congenital anomalies, especially cleft lip or palate, spina bifida, club foot, congenital hip dislocation, hypospadias, or epispadias.

Identifies conditions requiring immediate intervention. Note: Extra gluteal folds, unequal extremities, resistance to abduction, and Ortolani's sign (audible click on rotation) indicate congenital hip dislocation.

Position newborn on abdomen initially, or on side with rolled blanket at back. Monitor infant for difficulty in handling mucus.

Helps prevent aspiration, especially for neonates with gastric reflux or upper airway anomalies. During second period of reactivity, increased mucus production and gagging may predispose infant to airway obstruction, which can lead to asphyxia and death if it is undetected or untreated. Otherwise, research suggests positioning on back or side reduces risk of sudden infant death syndrome (SIDS).

Observe newborn frequently.

Necessary to detect possible regurgitation or position changes, which may compromise respiratory effort.

Never leave newborn on unenclosed surface.

Reduces risk of injury caused by falls.

Assess newborn for evidence of jaundice; note progression on body, color of skin/sclera/oral mucosa and stool, behavior changes, and CNS signs associated with kernicterus. (Refer to CP: Newborn: Hyperbilirubinemia.)

Increasing jaundice may indicate Rh or ABO incompatibility or breast milk–induced jaundice, with possible outcome of kernicterus if condition is left untreated. Up to 50% of full-term neonates display some degree of jaundice on day 2 or 3.

Assess newborn for CNS, gastric, vasomotor, and respiratory signs of drug effect/withdrawal. (Refer to CP: The Infant of an Addicted Mother.)

Onset of withdrawal often occurs 24 hr after delivery. Note: As many as one third of neonates who have withdrawal signs can be managed without additional medical treatment.

Collaborative

Administer vitamin K (AquaMEPHYTON) intramuscularly.

Because the newborn's intestinal tract is sterile at birth, and because feedings may be delayed, infant does not have the intestinal flora needed to promote coagulation by activation of factors II, VII, IX, and X.

Obtain/monitor direct and indirect bilirubin levels, as appropriate.

Helpful in determining need for/degree of therapeutic intervention based on specific serum bilirubin levels.

Schedule heel-stick testing for PKU, preferably within 72 hr after initiating intake of normal amounts of protein.

Identifies elevated serum levels of phenylpyruvic acid, which occur when phenylalanine is not converted to tyrosine because of absence of the liver enzyme phenylalanine hydroxylase. Excessive levels of the acid can result in CNS involvement, mental retardation, seizure activity, growth retardation, and absence of melanin.

Monitor x-ray studies; assist with diagnostic testing, as indicated.

Confirms presence of congenital abnormalities, such as hip dysplasia.

NURSING DIAGNOSIS:	FLUID VOLUME, risk for deficit
Risk Factors May Include:	Delayed feedings, limited oral intake, excessive regurgitation, increased insensible water losses
Possibly Evidenced By:	[Not applicable; presence of signs/symptoms establishes an *actual* diagnosis]
DESIRED OUTCOMES/EVALUATION CRITERIA—NEONATE WILL:	Void 2–6 times daily with output of 15–60 ml/kg/day by the second day of life.
	Produce urine free of uric acid crystals and urates.

ACTIONS/INTERVENTIONS	RATIONALE

Independent

ACTIONS/INTERVENTIONS	RATIONALE
Record initial and subsequent voidings.	Following birth, vascular resistance within renal vessels lessens and blood flow increases, but normal functioning may not be established until 24 hr following delivery. Urine output is usually limited and voiding scanty until fluid intake is adequate. During the first 2 days of life, the newborn usually voids 2–6 times daily. Thereafter, newborn usually voids 6–10 times daily, with output of 15–60 ml/kg per 24 hr.
Initiate oral feedings; note amount ingested and regurgitated.	Oral fluid requirements range from 140–160 ml/kg/day by the 3rd to 4th day of life (average is 105 ml/kg/day, or 5 oz/kg/day). Appropriate fluid ingestion helps promote hydration and offset kidney's inability to concentrate urine and to conserve fluid during periods of high insensible losses and fluid and electrolytic stress.
Monitor fluid intake and output. Note color and concentration of urine and the presence of peach-colored crystals on diaper.	Bladder usually empties when it contains between 15 and 40 ml of urine. Excessive drooling and mucus production, regurgitation, and poor fluid intake contribute to dehydration and scanty urine output. Urates and uric acid crystals reflect the need for prompt increase in fluid intake.
Note presence of blood in urine.	Bloody urine usually suggests pseudomenstruation in female infant or circumcision-related problems in male infant, but may also indicate renal injury, possibly associated with birth asphyxia, renal vein thrombosis, or infection.
Note presence of edema; assess hydration level (e.g., indicated by skin turgor and presence of mucus).	Edematous or well-hydrated neonate voids earlier after birth than dehydrated neonate and has increased urine output.
Reduce cold stressors; optimize respiratory effort and thermoregulation.	Limited tubular reabsorption and low renal threshold reduce reabsorption of bicarbonate (HCO_3), predisposing infant to metabolic acidosis associated with reduced buffering capacity to offset respiratory imbalances.
Palpate for bladder distension, restlessness, discomfort, or bladder pressure if infant fails to void within 24 hr after birth.	Helps in determining presence of urine; may suggest problem related to bladder or anomalies of urethra that may prevent voiding.

461

Collaborative

Assist with suprapubic bladder aspiration if indicated.

May be used to ascertain the presence or absence of urine, if voiding has not occurred.

NURSING DIAGNOSIS:	CONSTIPATION, risk for
Risk Factors May Include:	Inadequate fluid intake, intestinal obstruction
Possibly Evidenced By:	[Not applicable; presence of signs/symptoms establishes an *actual* diagnosis]
DESIRED OUTCOMES/EVALUATION CRITERIA—NEONATE WILL:	Pass meconium stool within 48 hr after birth.

ACTIONS/INTERVENTIONS	RATIONALE

Independent

Review intrapartal record for indications of passage of meconium.	Relaxation of anal sphincter may occur in response to vagal stimulation related to hypoxia, causing meconium passage in utero or at delivery.
Note maternal complications negatively affecting meconium passage.	Stressors such as cesarean delivery or PIH delay initial meconium passage and possibly contribute to development of hyperbilirubinemia.
Auscultate bowel sounds.	Air ingestion into the GI tract normally stimulates onset of bowel sounds within 1–2 hr after delivery.
Take rectal temperature or insert soft rubber catheter into anus with caution.	Easy passage indicates patency of anus (rules out imperforate anus).
Monitor frequency and amount/length of feeding, frequency of voiding, skin turgor and status of fontanels, and weight. Encourage early feeding; provide extra water as indicated. (Refer to ND: Fluid Volume, risk for deficit).	Inadequate oral intake, as evidenced by decreased urine output, changes in skin turgor, sunken fontanels, and excessive weight loss, can lead to constipation.
Note passage of first meconium:	Once the newborn wakens and the first feeding is initiated, passage of meconium usually follows, establishing patency of lower GI tract. Approximately 6% of healthy newborns do not defecate by 24 hr after birth. Failure to pass stool by 48 hr usually indicates intestinal obstruction.
Record frequency, color, consistency, and odor of stools; Note deviations from normal stool cycle (meconium stools for 3–4 days; they will be followed by transitional stools, which are greenish-brown and may last for 3–6 days, followed by formed or loose-yellow stools).	Number, consistency, and color of stools vary, depending on ingestion of breast milk or formula. Thick, puttylike meconium suggests meconium ileus or possible cystic fibrosis; a small, puttylike stool may indicate bowel stenosis or atresia. Loose green or diarrheal stool may indicate infection or gastroenteritis, or may be a normal result of high bilirubin content associated with phototherapy.
Assess abdomen for constant or intermittent distension. Note persistent vomiting and presence of bile in vomitus.	Abdominal distension and persistent vomiting suggest obstruction. Obstruction that is high or complete is associated with vomiting soon after birth; more distal lesions are associated with later vomiting. Bile-stained gastric contents suggest duodenal obstruction. Paralytic ileus or partial obstruction is characterized by intermittent distension. Intestinal

462

Observe for motility disturbance associated with constipation, vomiting, and fluid and electrolytic imbalances.

obstruction is the most frequent GI emergency requiring surgery in the neonatal period.

These signs may indicate aganglionic megacolon (Hirschsprung's disease), whereby absence of parasympathetic nerve cells in both the muscles and submucosa of the rectosigmoid colon inhibits passage of fecal material.

Note cluster of GI signs such as abdominal distension and tenderness, poor feeding, vomiting, presenceof blood in stool (positive result on Hematest), or presence of reducing substances in blood.

These signs may indicate necrotizing enterocolitis, the onset of which ranges from the 1st day to the 1st mo of life. Necrotizing enterocolitis is associated with ischemia of intestines precipitated by hypoxia and systemic shock.

Collaborative

Assist with diagnostic studies (e.g., abdominal x-rays, contrast studies, and upper GI barium series or enema).

Helps in determining degree and location of obstruction and in diagnosing possible malrotation.

Transfer infant to acute care setting (NICU), if indicated.

May be needed for intermittent gastric suctioning, surgical repair, or initiation of total parenteral nutrition.

NURSING DIAGNOSIS:	KNOWLEDGE deficit [Learning Need], regarding growth/development and infant care
May Be Related To:	Lack of exposure, misinterpretation, unfamiliarity with information resources
Possibly Evidenced By:	Verbalization of questions/misconceptions, hesitancy to perform care activities, inaccurate follow-through of instructions
DESIRED OUTCOMES/EVALUATION CRITERIA—PARENT(S) WILL:	Verbalize understanding of newborn's individual needs.
	Demonstrate appropriate behaviors to meet physiological and emotional needs of newborn.
	Identify signs/symptoms requiring medical intervention.
	Demonstrate proper technique for obtaining infant temperature, administering oral medication.

ACTIONS/INTERVENTIONS	RATIONALE

Independent

Appraise level of parent's understanding of infant's physiological needs and adaptation to extrauterine life associated with maintenance of body temperature, nutrition, respiratory needs, and bowel and bladder functioning.

Identifies areas of concern/need requiring additional information and/or demonstration of care activities.

Provide information and correct misconceptions, as appropriate; encourage discussion and questions.

Promotes understanding of newborn behaviors, need for specific actions/interventions.

Discuss newborn behaviors after the first and during the second periods of reactivity.	After first period of reactivity, newborn usually falls into a deep sleep, followed by the second period of reactivity, which involves wakefulness, mucus regurgitation, gagging, and often passage of first meconium stool.
Perform newborn physical assessment in presence of parent(s) as appropriate. Provide information about normal variations and characteristics, such as pseudomenstruation, breast enlargement, physiological jaundice, caput succedaneum, cephalhematoma, and milia.	Helps parents to recognize normal variations, and may reduce anxiety.
Discuss and demonstrate normal newborn reflexes; review ages at which each reflex disappears.	Encourages early detection of CNS abnormalities associated with prolonged presence of reflexes.
Provide information about newborn interactional capabilities, states of consciousness, and means of stimulating cognitive development. (Refer to CP: The Client at 4 Hours to 2 Days Postpartum; ND: Parent/Infant Attachment; Parenting, risk for altered.)	Helps parents recognize and respond to infant cues during interactional process; fosters optimal interaction, attachment behaviors, and cognitive development in infant. The state of consciousness can be divided into the sleep and wake states, involving separate and predictable behavioral characteristics.
Discuss different types of cries that the neonate may use in communication and the means to assess significance of each. Demonstrate consoling measures.	Crying does not necessarily indicate hunger. Other causes include the need to be held, burped, or changed, or just a need to express irritability, because all babies tend to have a particular part of the day (often suppertime) when irritability increases. Parents' success or failure at consoling the newborn has a tremendous impact on their feelings of competence. Crying episodes usually vary in length from 3–7 min after initiation of consoling measures.
Provide information related to thermoregulatory mechanisms of the newborn, types of heat loss, and ways to minimize or prevent excessive heat loss or overheating.	Reduces risk of possible complications associated with hypothermia and hyperthermia.
Discuss newborn's usual sleep patterns and ways of promoting sleep.	Usually requires at least 17 hr of sleep per day for normal growth.
Demonstrate and supervise infant care activities related to feeding and holding; bathing, diapering, and clothing; care of circumcised male infant; and care of umbilical cord stump. Provide written/ pictorial information for parents to refer to after discharge.	Promotes understanding of principles and techniques of newborn care; fosters parents' skills as caregivers.
Discuss infant's nutritional needs, variability in infant appetite from one feeding to the next, and means of assessing adequate hydration and nutrition.	Alleviates potential concern that may result if intake varies from feeding to feeding. Helps to ensure adequate nutritional and fluid intake.
Discuss infant feeding methods, types of formula preparations available, economics of formula use versus breastfeeding, and necessary preparation and storage of formula/expressed breast milk.	Clarifies options, helps ensure appropriateness and safety of infant feeding.
Identify dangers associated with bottle propping.	Bottle propping robs infant of needed skin-to-skin contact with parents and may cause blockage of air passage if nipple lodges against back of infant's throat, or aspiration if infant regurgitates. Bottle propping may also cause otitis media associated with drainage of nasal mucus or occlusion of duct when eustachian tube orifice opens during swallowing.

Instruct parents regarding positioning of newborn after feedings and demonstrate use of bulb syringe. Note infant's gag reflex.

Weak gag reflex predisposes newborn to aspiration. Positioning newborn on the abdomen or side with rolled towel at back allows external drainage of mucus or vomitus, reducing risk of aspiration. When infant is placed on back in carrier seat or carriage, head should be elevated 30–45 degrees. Syringe removes secretions from nasopharynx, clearing air passages.

Instruct parents regarding special care of diapers. Discuss use of cloth versus disposable diapers, recognition of rashes, and appropriate treatment.

Promotes good hygiene, reduces risk/severity of diaper rash.

Discuss nail care in newborn, including peeling of soft nails or nail trimming with manicure scissors or special infant nail scissors during infant's sound sleep.

Prevents infant's scratching with long nails and injury associated with movement during the cutting process.

Reinforce necessity of not leaving infant unattended unless in crib with siderails up.

Initially, neonate is at risk for regurgitation or aspiration. Over time, as infant matures, new concerns are associated with increasing mobility and dexterity (e.g., rolling off surface, falling down stairs, inserting inappropriate objects into mouth, which may be aspirated/swallowed, getting head caught).

Discuss requirement of federally approved car seat tailored to infant's size. Have family bring care seat to unit and demonstrate proper positioning, of infant in seat, and how seat is to be placed in car.

Accidents are the leading cause of childhood mortality, with auto accidents causing the most deaths. All states require use of approved restraint systems to protect children while passengers in automobiles. Note: There is currently ongoing discussion as to whether this requirement should be extended to include travel on airplanes.

Emphasize newborn's need for follow-up evaluation by healthcare provider and need for timely immunizations.

Ongoing evaluation is important for monitoring growth and development. Immunizations are necessary to protect the infant from childhood diseases with associated serious complications. Note: Most day-care and school systems require completed immunizations, including hepatitis B series, before enrolling.

Provide information about routine laboratory testing, as indicated.

Increases likelihood of parents following through with urine and blood testing for genetic disorders, such as PKU and congenital hypothyroidism, which if undetected can cause mental and physical retardation.

Identify signs of jaundice and when healthcare provider should be contacted.

If newborn develops yellow coloring in the face, trunk, sclera that progresses to groin, arm/legs, evaluation and treatment are indicated to prevent serious complications. Note: If neonate feeds poorly or is lethargic, prompt intervention is required.

Discuss manifestations of illness and infection and the times at which a healthcare provider should be contacted. Demonstrate proper technique for taking temperature and administering oral medications as required.

Early recognition of illness and prompt use of healthcare facilitate treatment and positive outcome. To obtain an axillary temperature appropriately, thermometer should be held in place in the center of the axilla. Use of a rectal/tympanic thermometer is not recommended until infant is older. Improper administration of medication increases risk of aspiration and ineffective treatment.

THE NEONATE AT 24 TO 48 HOURS FOLLOWING EARLY DISCHARGE

This plan of care focuses on the infant who is discharged within 30 hr of birth. It is intended to be used in conjunction with the CP: The Neonate at Two Hours to Two Days of Age. Although early discharge may be detrimental to a few infants, newborn health appears to hinge more on the parent(s) level of knowledge and support at home. The home assessment at 24–48 hr following discharge involves evaluation of the newborn's ability to adapt positively to extrauterine life.

NEONATAL ASSESSMENT DATA BASE

To meet the stringent criteria for early discharge, the newborn must be a normal, healthy infant as determined by thorough physical examination: Gestational age, 38–42 wk; birth weight, 2500–4000 g; vital signs and temperature stable; Apgar score greater than 7 at 1 and 5 min; normal elimination pattern; and successful feeding.

DIAGNOSTIC STUDIES

Hct: 40%–61%
Coombs' Test: Negative
Screening tests, including PKU and thyroid tests, dependent on individual risk factors and agency policy

NURSING PRIORITIES

1. Support transition of newborn to extrauterine life.
2. Promote positive parent-infant interaction.
3. Provide support and information regarding home care of infant.

NURSING DIAGNOSIS:	NUTRITION: altered, less than body requirements
May Be Related To:	Inability to ingest adequate nutrients (because of fatigue, excessive oropharyngeal secretions)
Possibly Evidenced By:	Weight loss, decreased urine output, dry mucous membranes, poor skin turgor, sunken fontanels
DESIRED OUTCOMES/EVALUATION CRITERIA—NEONATE WILL:	Be adequately hydrated with normal urine output.
	Display weight loss less than 10% of birth weight.

ACTIONS/INTERVENTIONS	RATIONALE
Independent	
Weigh newborn. Compare weight with birth weight and discharge weight.	Nutrient needs are based on body weight. Weight gains or losses indicate adequacy of intake. Neonates need 100–120 kcal/kg (54 cal/lb) each day. Only breast milk or formula should be given. Feedings should be provided approximately every 3 hr (6–8 times a day) or on demand. Average fluid requirements are 5 oz/kg per 24 hr.
Determine condition of fontanels, skin turgor,	Depressed fontanels, poor skin turgor, and dry

amount of mucus production. Observe newborn for jitteriness or lethargy.

Note frequency, amount, and appearance of stool and urine. Palpate abdomen for softness.

Observe newborn for possible signs of regurgitation. Encourage parents to establish relaxed mood during feedings and to place infant on right side after feeding.

Review parents' feeding practices and knowledge, noting how often baby is nursing or feeding, how many minutes newborn nurses on each breast, and whether newborn takes additional water or formula during a 24-hr period. If possible, observe parents and infant during feeding.

Assess reflexes associated with feeding, and note presence of oropharyngeal secretions.

Determine neonate's current sleep-wake pattern.

mucous membranes suggest dehydration. Jitteriness may indicate hypoglycemia.

Evaluates adequacy of oral intake. Neonates should void at least twice in the first 24 hr after discharge, advancing to approximately 7 times per 24 hr. Presence of urates in urine indicates need for additional fluid intake. The neonate may pass stool 2–7 times per 24 hr. Stool is initially meconium and changes in accordance with diet.

During the transitional period, neonates may normally regurgitate feedings. Calmness and self-assurance of parents helps neonate relax during feeding; proper positioning facilitates gastric emptying into intestines.

Knowledgeable parents are better prepared to alter schedules and respond to feeding needs and changes. Anticipatory guidance increases their self-confidence and helps avoid problems. Excessive parental anxiety may interfere with mother's let-down reflex, increase neonate's anxiety, and result in poor oral intake. Note: In addition, milk supply is usually not yet well established for specific needs of neonate.

Poor sucking and swallowing reflexes or excessive secretions may negatively affect intake.

At 24 hr of age, a healthy neonate has not yet established a sleep-wake pattern and may be excessively tired as a result of birth stress. During the first 2–3 days, the neonate may sleep almost continuously (except for feeding), progressing to a schedule of approximately 12–16 hr/day.

Collaborative

Review Dextrostix results. If newborn appears jittery or lethargic, provide feeding of dextrose solution and continue to observe.

Normal glucose levels are between 45 and 130 mg/dl; levels <45 mg/dl indicate hypoglycemia. Administration of dextrose solution should correct hypoglycemia.

NURSING DIAGNOSIS:	BODY TEMPERATURE, risk for altered
Risk Factors May Include:	Extreme of age (immature regulatory mechanisms [hypothalamus], ineffective shivering mechanism, reduced subcutaneous fat, proximity of blood vessels to the skin surface, and large ratio of body surface to mass)
Possibly Evidenced By:	[Not applicable; presence of signs/symptoms establishes an *actual* diagnosis]
DESIRED OUTCOMES/EVALUATION CRITERIA—NEONATE WILL:	Maintain axillary temperature between 97°F and 98°F (36.2°C and 36.8°C) when in an open crib with one blanket.
PARENT(S) WILL:	Identify/use individually appropriate measures to protect neonate.

467

ACTIONS/INTERVENTIONS	RATIONALE

Independent

Review importance of thermoregulation in the newborn and possible negative effects of excess chilling.

A thermoneutral home environment is needed to assist the infant's own thermoregulatory ability. Temperature fluctuations in the newborn require use of calories to regain balance at the cost of growth. In addition, chilling increases the risk of newborn jaundice because the affinity of serum albumin for bilirubin is diminished.

Demonstrate proper technique for assessing axillary temperature.

Improper technique may lead to inaccurate results.

Note signs of increased irritability, pallor, mottling, or lethargy; note restlessness and perspiration on head or face.

Indicates hypothermia or hyperthermia necessitating intervention.

Evaluate environment for thermal loss through conduction, convection, radiation, or evaporation (e.g., cool or drafty room, inadequate clothing on infant, or absence of head covering) or for thermal excess (e.g., crib in sunlight or near heaters).

Body temperature of newborn fluctuates quickly as the environmental temperature changes. Note: Cultural dictates may require bundling of neonate in excess of environmental needs necessitating sensitivity and additional discussion of temperature regulation and infant safety concerns.

Discuss appropriate actions to maintain newborn's temperature, such as appropriately bundling infant and covering head if axillary temperature is lower than 97°F (36.1°C) and rechecking temperature 1 hr later.

Information helps parents create an optimal environment. Wrapping neonate and putting cap on head helps retain body heat. Axillary temperature evaluates effectiveness of the interventions. Note: Informing parents that newborn's hands may remain cool even though body temperature is WNL reduces anxiety and inappropriate response.

NURSING DIAGNOSIS:	**INJURY, risk for CNS damage**
Risk Factors May Include:	Biochemical or regulatory function (inability to break down RBCs quickly enough during the transition period, leading to kernicterus associated with deposition of unconjugated bilirubin in the basal ganglia of the brain)
Possibly Evidenced By:	[Not applicable; presence of signs/symptoms establishes an *actual* diagnosis]
DESIRED OUTCOMES/EVALUATION CRITERIA—NEONATE WILL:	Maintain bilirubin level WNL.
PARENT(S) WILL:	Identify signs of increasing jaundice.
	Verbalize understanding of treatment needs.

ACTIONS/INTERVENTIONS	RATIONALE

Independent

Inspect neonate's buccal membranes, sclera, and skin for jaundice. Instruct parents to observe infant for passage of meconium stool.

Yellowing sclera is the first sign of jaundice and is followed by yellowed skin tone on blanching; jaundice progresses in a cephalocaudal direction.

Meconium stool may be delayed; loose/greenish-brown stools may indicate passage of bilirubin. Note: Upward of 80% of neonates develop physiological jaundice between days 2–9.

Review proper care of jaundiced neonate, providing anticipatory guidance. Refer to CP: Newborn: Hyperbilirubinemia.

Information is essential for parents to manage care appropriately and to identify changes in condition that warrant further assessment and treatment.

Collaborative

Obtain blood specimen, as indicated, if jaundice is noted.

Determines bilirubin level in presence of jaundice. Decisions regarding treatment are based on serial serum bilirubin levels. Physiological jaundice becomes pathological at level above 12.8 mg/dl.

Arrange for medical follow-up regarding hyperbilirubinemia.

Prompt, responsible follow-up and treatment are necessary to avert serious complications and reduce need for hospital readmission.

NURSING DIAGNOSIS:	PARENTING, risk for altered
Risk Factors May Include:	Lack of support between/from significant other(s), lack of knowledge, ineffective or no available role model, unrealistic expectations for self/infant/partner, unmet social/emotional maturation needs of client/partner, presence of stressor (e.g., financial, housing)
Possibly Evidenced By:	[Not applicable; presence of signs/symptoms establishes an *actual* diagnosis]
DESIRED OUTCOMES/EVALUATION CRITERIA—PARENT(S) WILL:	Verbalize realistic expectations of infant's needs.
	Identify individual methods and resources for meeting infant needs.

ACTIONS/INTERVENTIONS

RATIONALE

Independent

Reassess risk factors that may have been identified during prenatal or intrapartal periods (e.g., unwanted pregnancy, previous abortion, or lack of support systems).

Follow-up of risk factors is important to evaluate progress or areas of need. Early discharge is ideal for many families, but some clients who are at high risk for child abuse may also be included within the early discharge population.

Observe parent-infant interaction. Talk with parents about their perceptions of, and feelings toward, the newborn. Reinforce positive bonding efforts.

Because of their dependent state, infants are vulnerable to negative parental behaviors, inadequate nurturing, and abuse. The "taking-in" phase, during which the mother is still trying to assimilate the details of labor and delivery, lasts 2–3 days. Stress and inadequate help in the home during this early period may negatively affect transition to the childrearing phase, interfering with proper nurturing, with possible failure of the newborn to thrive or to develop a sense of trust during infancy.

Assist parents to identify the resources available

Enables parents to anticipate availability and

to them, e.g., community or support services, home health aide, or mother's helper.

Make arrangements for follow-up phone calls or visits as appropriate.

Provide parents with a contact phone number. Encourage them to call to ask questions, discuss concerns, or seek assistance.

Collaborative

Refer for professional mental health counseling if indicated.

appropriateness of resources. Mother normally needs additional assistance to meet the needs of her newborn, her family, and herself and to cope with unanticipated stress during the initial postpartal period.

Provides support and the opportunity to note progress. Frequency of calls or visits depends on needs of the individual situation; three visits in the 1st wk is desirable but is often dependent on financial resources/access to community programs.

Knowing that someone is available to help if needed may lessen parents' stress.

Postpartal stress may trigger depression, which is more likely to resolve quickly and not progress to more severe depression if the mother obtains help from skilled professionals.

NURSING DIAGNOSIS:	GAS EXCHANGE, risk for impaired
Risk Factors May Include:	Excessive production of mucus and/or amniotic fluid remaining in the lungs; decreased hemoglobin levels
Possibly Evidenced By:	[Not applicable; presence of signs/symptoms establishes an *actual* diagnosis]
DESIRED OUTCOMES/EVALUATION CRITERIA—NEONATE WILL:	Maintain patent airway with unlabored breathing and respirations at 30–60/min.
	Be free of signs of respiratory distress.
PARENT(S) WILL:	List signs reflecting respiratory distress and appropriate actions.

ACTIONS/INTERVENTIONS

RATIONALE

Independent

Auscultate breath sounds bilaterally to note respiratory rate and quality.

Encourage parent(s) to position neonate on abdomen or right side; demonstrate clearing of nares, as needed, with bulb syringe and possible elevation of the head of the crib mattress by 30 degrees using a rolled blanket under the mattress, as appropriate.

Assist parent(s) in learning signs of neonatal distress (e.g., grunting, retractions, nasal flaring, or tachypnea), noting when they should contact healthcare provider.

Neonate should breathe 30–60 times per minute without signs and symptoms of respiratory distress or congestion. Absence of lung sounds or persistence of crackles or rhonchi indicates possible aspiration of amniotic fluid or persistent fluid in lung tissue.

Enhances air movement and reduces risk of aspiration. Promotes drainage of mucus and relieves pressure of diaphragm on lungs. Note: Recommended position for sleep is supine (on back) or side to reduce risk of SIDS, unless neonate has difficulty handling mucus when prone or side position is preferred.

Reduces anxiety and provides guidelines for parents so they know the appropriate times at which to seek help.

Collaborative

Obtain heel-stick Hct, as indicated.

May be required routinely or if respiratory distress is noted. Hct below the normal range of 43%–61% reduces oxygen-carrying capacity and may compromise respiratory function.

Provide healthcare referral if respiratory rate is not within normal range.

Immediate care may be needed to prevent development of serious respiratory problems.

NURSING DIAGNOSIS:	KNOWLEDGE deficit [Learning Need], regarding infant care
May Be Related To:	Lack of recall and/or incomplete information presented; misinterpretation
Possibly Evidenced By:	Verbalizations of concerns/misconceptions; hesitancy in/or inadequate performance of activities
DESIRED OUTCOMES/EVALUATION CRITERIA—PARENT(S) WILL:	Carry out infant care tasks appropriately.
	Assume responsibility for own learning.
	Verbalize the rationale for specific actions.

ACTIONS/INTERVENTIONS

RATIONALE

Independent

Encourage parents to voice concerns. Provide explanations and answer questions while physical assessment is performed.

Helps determine parents' ability to care appropriately for newborn. The first 48-hr period after delivery is one of great transition for parents, especially for mothers, who must now recall and apply information related to newborn care as learned in prenatal classes or during the brief hospital stay. New, unexpected areas of needed information may arise as parents actually assume their caregiving roles.

Provide oral and written/pictorial information, as needed, about home management and care of the neonate, and indications for notifying healthcare provider.

Decreases anxiety, increases self-confidence, and promotes quality care for the neonate; helps ensure prompt treatment of problems. Note: Hospital readmissions during the 1st wk of life are usually because of jaundice, dehydration, or sepsis.

Evaluate home environment for presence of heat, running water, cleanliness, electricity; number of persons in household; size of home, and facilities, crib, and clothing for the baby.

Identifies necessary items that are lacking or conditions that present safety/health concerns. Promotes problem-solving activities.

Provide appropriate information related to infant safety. (Refer to CP: The Neonate at 2 Hours to 2 Days of Age; ND: Injury, risk for.)

Helps reduce incidence of accidental injury or trauma.

Ascertain parents' understanding of nutritional needs, feeding behaviors, and techniques.

Provides opportunity to reinforce knowledge and clarify misconceptions.

Discuss plans for follow-up appointments for tests, such as PKU or thyroid screening tests, as indicated.

Determines parent's awareness of the need for further testing. PKU testing is performed after milk stool is noted in breastfed neonates, or within 72 hr after bottle feeding is begun.

Assist parents in scheduling first appointment with healthcare provider.	Establishes importance of checkup for the infant and provides parents with opportunity to have their questions answered. Note: Based on cultural practices, some clients may be reluctant to leave home with newborn for 20–40 days following delivery.
Refer to other healthcare providers, community agencies, e.g., social services; Women, Infants, and Children (WIC) program; or support groups (e.g., La Leche League).	Helps to promote high-level wellness and family independence. Parents are more likely to use services that are familiar or recommended to them.

NURSING DIAGNOSIS:	**INFECTION, risk for**
Risk Factors May Include:	Thin, permeable skin and extra portals of entry (umbilical cord, circumcision); immature immunologic system; lack of normal intestinal flora
Possibly Evidenced By:	[Not applicable; presence of signs/symptoms establishes an *actual* diagnosis]
DESIRED OUTCOMES/EVALUATION CRITERIA—NEONATE WILL:	Be free of signs of infection.
PARENT(S) WILL:	Identify individual risk factors and appropriate actions.

ACTIONS/INTERVENTIONS	RATIONALE

Independent

Wash hands, and instruct parents to do so before handling infant.	Minimizes introduction of bacteria and spread of infection.
Observe newborn for skin abnormalities (e.g., blisters, petechiae, pustules, plethora, or pallor).	These abnormalities may be signs of infection. (Refer to CP: The Neonate at 2 Hours to 2 Days of Age; ND: Infection, risk for.)
Discuss skin care, including bathing every other day, or less often, as indicated, and using mild antibacterial soap. Recommend sponge bathing until umbilical cord detaches.	Guidelines for parents help them protect fragile skin of newborn from excessive drying or damage. Note: Foreskin of uncircumcised penis should not be retracted for cleaning; rather, external washing and rinsing are sufficient.
Inspect umbilical cord.	The umbilical cord is an open site susceptible to infection. It should show evidence of beginning dryness, and no bleeding, exudate, odor, or oozing should be present by the 2nd day of life.
Review appropriate cord care. Ensure that clothes and diaper do not cover stump. Provide information regarding the normal progression of cord resolution.	Reduces likelihood of infection; promotes drying. Cord should fall off by the 2nd wk of life. Note: Knowing it does not hurt the baby when the cord detaches provides reassurance to parents.
Inspect site of circumcision, if performed. Note undue bleeding, oozing, or swelling. (Refer to CP: Circumcision.)	Complete healing of circumcision does not occur until 7–10 days after the procedure.
Observe for/discuss signs of infection. Assess axillary temperature as indicated.	Infection in the neonate may be manifested by pallor, irritability, lethargy, poor feeding, vomiting, diarrhea, loose stools, oliguria, or temperature

Recommend avoiding contact with family members or visitors who have infections or have recently been exposed to infectious processes.

instability. Parental awareness promotes early recognition and increases likelihood of prompt medical attention.

Because the neonate is more susceptible when exposed to some infections, visitors should be screened. Note: Communicability is usually highest during the incubation period of many diseases.

THE NEONATE AT 1 WEEK FOLLOWING DISCHARGE

At 1 wk of age, the newborn continues to adapt to extrauterine life, both physiologically and behaviorally. Within this adaptation period are many normal variations. Review prior assessments for risk factors or deviations from expected norms.

NEONATAL ASSESSMENT DATA BASE

Activity/Rest

May be wakeful/fussy between feedings
May sleep more or less than the customary 17 hr/day

Circulation

Heart rate ranges from 110–160 bpm; is strong and regular.

Ego Integrity (Parents)

May verbalize unrealistic expectations of themselves and of neonate
May express feelings of ineptness or inadequate knowledge

Elimination

Urine pale and straw-colored, with output of 6–10 wet diapers per day.
Abdomen soft with bowel sounds in all four quadrants.
Defecation pattern varies; stool formed, yellow/brown, and passed 2–3 times per day in neonate fed cow's-milk formula; mustard-colored, loose, and passed initially with each feeding, then possibly every few days, in breastfed neonate.

Food/Fluid

May have difficulty adjusting to breast or bottle feeding; oral intake may be inadequate or on occasion, excessive.
Weight gain averaging 1 oz/day.

Neurosensory

Facial expression symmetrical
Reflexes associated with feeding (sucking, swallowing, gag, and rooting) present and strong
Moro, grasp, and stepping reflexes present with strong, symmetrical response
Uncoordinated motor and reflex activity present (continued development of the neurological system)
Muscle tone good; head lag present

Pain/Discomfort

Irritability, crying associated with colic may occur.

Respiration

Respiratory rate 30–60/min with no signs of difficulty (e.g., grunting, retraction, or nasal flaring).
Normal alternation between rapid and slow rate occurs in response to stimuli.
Cry strong, lusty, demanding, and purposeful.
Lungs bilaterally clear; breath sounds equal.

Safety

Skin pink and warm to the touch, with good skin turgor; free of rashes; transitory color change or mottling may appear in response to cold.

Skin may appear slightly dry or peeling in folds.
Slight jaundice involving only upper body or upper extremities may be present, peaking at day 4 or 5, subsiding within 7 days of onset.
Temperature stable; axillary/pacifier, 97.6°F–98.6°F (36.5°C–37°C); rectal, 97.8°F–99°F (36.6°C–37.2°C).
Umbilical cord stump drying, with no evidence of inflammation; slight bleeding may be noted with detachment 7–14 days after birth.

Sexuality

Circumcised penis well-healed and free of exudate

DIAGNOSTIC STUDIES

Tests dependent on individual findings/concerns
Screening repeated at 7–14 days of age to detect inborn errors of metabolism

NURSING PRIORITIES

1. Facilitate newborn's continued physiological and behavioral adaptation to extrauterine life.
2. Promote adequate fluid and nutritional intake.
3. Provide information to parent(s) about newborn's safety, developmental needs, and interactional capabilities.
4. Encourage parental use of support systems.

NURSING DIAGNOSIS:	NUTRITION: altered, risk for less than body requirements
Risk Factors May Include:	Inability to ingest/digest adequate nutrients (fatigue, increased metabolic rate, formula allergy)
Possibly Evidenced By:	[Not applicable; presence of signs/symptoms establishes an *actual* diagnosis]
DESIRED OUTCOMES/EVALUATION CRITERIA—NEONATE WILL:	Gain approximately 1 oz/day after initial weight loss.
	Remain well hydrated as evidenced by adequate urine output (6–8 wet diapers/day), good skin turgor, moist mucous membranes.
PARENT(S) WILL:	Demonstrate proper handling and comfort with infant feeding techniques.

ACTIONS/INTERVENTIONS	RATIONALE

Independent

Weigh newborn. Compare current weight with birth weight. Note weight lost and regained.	Growth is individual, but most full-term AGA infants regain birth weight within 10–14 days of birth. Large infants lose proportionately more weight than small infants. Insufficient gains indicate nutritional risks or possible malnutrition.
Emphasize importance of weighing breastfed newborn at 2 wk of age.	Evaluation at this age is critical to detect possible failure to thrive or slow weight gains.
Assess hydration level (e.g., status of fontanels, skin turgor, mucous membranes, and urine output).	Sunken fontanels, poor skin turgor, decreased production of mucus, and decreased urine output

Determine parents' knowledge of newborn's feeding needs. Observe feeding, evaluating parents' technique (e.g., positioning, burping, and length of feeding). Discuss importance of alternating infant's position (e.g., alternating right and left for bottle-fed baby to simulate breastfeeding).

Discuss emotional needs of newborn in relation to feedings (e.g., the need for holding and cuddling and for a quiet, nondistracting environment).

Observe newborn during feeding, noting presence or development of feeding reflexes (i.e., rooting, sucking, swallowing, and gag).

Note frequency and amounts of feeding.

Ascertain number of voidings per day and color of urine.

Review newborn's sleeping and waking habits.

Identify cues suggesting newborn fatigue (e.g., loss of eye contact [turning away from or closing of eyes], decreased muscle tone, and reduced activity of extremities/neck).

Determine mother's perception of her success or failure related to infant feedings.

Auscultate bowel sounds. Note color, consistency, and odor of stools.

Assess infant's temperature and pulse. (Refer to ND: Infection, risk for.)

---

indicate inadequate fluid intake. Well-hydrated tissue may indicate adequate nutrition and fluid balance.

Normal feeding should take 20–30 min. Improper positioning of infant at the breast, or improper technique of holding the bottle, may contribute to inadequate compression of maternal milk ducts or excessive air ingestion. Alternating bottle-fed infant's position provides stimulation and assists in development of eye muscles.

Skin-to-skin contact allows neonate to focus on feeding, fosters optimal emotional interaction between parents and infant, and provides tactile stimulation, which is critical to the total process of acquiring newborn's trust. Delayed gratification of hunger needs may lead to mistrust and lack of synchrony needed for the mutual gratification of mother and infant.

A deviation in any of the feeding reflexes may lead to inadequate intake of nutrients.

Breastfed neonate may initially want to nurse every 1½–3 hr with one or two night feedings, because breast milk is rapidly digested. Formula-fed infant is usually satisfied with feedings provided every 3–4 hr. Intake is considered adequate for formula-fed newborn if 6–10 feedings of approximately 2–3 oz each are ingested in a 24-hr period.

Infant is adequately hydrated if voidings occur 6–8 times per day and urine is pale or straw-colored.

Nutritional satisfaction is indicated if neonate sleeps soundly between feedings and wakes every 2–5 hr for feedings, and if feedings cause infant to stop crying.

Recognition of these cues may promote intervention to prevent undue fatigue and associated complications. Excessive handling/overstimulation can elevate newborn's metabolic rate and thereby increase caloric use in place of promoting growth.

Feelings of success or failure regarding feedings influence the mother's self-confidence. Negative self-esteem associated with the newborn's poor oral intake may establish a vicious cycle whereby mother's anxiety increases at mealtime and newborn becomes anxious in response to maternal anxiety and feeds poorly. Negative patterns at mealtime may persist throughout infancy and childhood, affecting mother-child interactions.

Hyperactivity or hypoactivity of the gastrointestinal tract leads to inadequate utilization of food. Elimination pattern is individual and is influenced by therapy (e.g., bilirubin phototherapy) and by amount and type of feedings (e.g., breast or bottle). Green or loose stool may indicate infection or passage of excess bilirubin. Constipated stool may indicate dehydration.

Infection interferes with weight gain by increasing metabolic rate and negatively affecting oral intake.

Using 24-hr diet recall, evaluate adequacy of nutritional intake in mothers who breastfeed. Note amount of calories and fluids, and the use of a variety of foods from all the basic food groups.

Good nutrition in the mother enhances the nutrition of the breastfed newborn and helps mother maintain adequate energy level.

Assess adequacy of and ways to increase milk supply and promote the let-down reflex. Review effects of smoking.

Maternal milk production may not be adequate to meet newborn's growth needs. Maternal caloric intake should be 500–800 kcal more than the level during pregnancy, with 2–3 qt of fluid consumed per 24 hr. Adequate rest is necessary for milk production. Using relaxation techniques or drinking several ounces of dark beer each day may reduce anxiety and facilitate the let-down reflex. Note: Smoking interferes with the let-down reflex, and nicotine is passed through breast milk to the infant.

Review the preparation, sterilization, and availability of different types of formula.

Enhances proper use of commercially prepared formula. Dilution of ready-to-feed formula has been linked to failures of infant growth (height and weight).

Measure specific gravity of urine.

Increased specific gravity (above 1.008) in the absence of other complications may indicate the need for additional fluid intake.

Test stool for glucose (reducing imbalance).

Increased glucose in stool may indicate an intolerance to formula or an error in metabolism.

Reinforce instructions regarding the need to obtain urine from diaper for PKU screening between 2 and 4 wk after birth, or to bring child to laboratory for Guthrie test or heel-stick method of PKU testing.

Helps ensure that newborn is screened for PKU, an autosomal recessive disorder in which absence of a liver enzyme inhibits the conversion of phenylalanine to tyrosine, with a resultant increase in phenylpyruvic acid and possible development of mental retardation.

Collaborative

Refer to community agency, visiting nurse services, or WIC program.

Nutritional problems identified in the newborn may necessitate close or frequent monitoring and financial support.

Refer lactating mother to local lactation consultant or support groups such as La Leche League International, Lact-Aid.

May be necessary to identify and meet specific nutritional needs with consideration of individual health status and resources. Can provide role model, clarify misconceptions, assist with problem solving related to breastfeeding.

Obtain consultation for breastfeeding mother as indicated.

NURSING DIAGNOSIS:	KNOWLEDGE deficit [Learning Need], regarding newborn needs/care
May Be Related To:	Lack of recall/incomplete information presented; misinterpretation
Possibly Evidenced By:	Verbalizations of concerns/misconceptions; hesitancy in, or inadequate performance of, activities; development of preventable complications
DESIRED OUTCOMES/EVALUATION CRITERIA—PARENT(S) WILL:	Verbalize understanding of infant's needs. Adopt safe child-care practices.

Independent

Assess parents' comfort and skill with infant care tasks (e.g., bathing, feeding, diapering, and recognizing infant's nutritional and physiological needs). Demonstrate, supervise, and/or reinforce skills, as needed.

Determines ability to provide appropriate care and identifies individual needs. Recognition of strengths and efforts enhances parents' sense of competence.

Review proper technique for preparation, sterilization, and storage of formula and bottles.

Faulty technique in formula preparation may lead to enteric infection. Bacterial growth can be controlled by discarding unfinished formula or by refrigerating prepared formula and discarding any unused portion after 24 hr (or per instructions on the container). Unopened commercially prepared formula may be stored at room temperature. Overdilution of formula can lead to alterations in electrolyte balance and to inadequate caloric intake. Underdilution of formula can increase renal solute load, causing dehydration.

Discuss normal patterns of newborn growth and development, behaviors, and physical and social capabilities. Provide information about newborn's temperament and about appropriate parental responses to personality. Share with parents the Brazelton assessment process.

Assists parents in monitoring neonate's physical and cognitive growth and optimizing neonate's developmental potential. By observing and understanding newborn's personality traits, parents learn to respond appropriately to individual needs of their newborn. Parents need to realize that newborn's behaviors are individually determined and not entirely a reflection of their parenting abilities.

Note stress in home environment/family relationships and discuss ways to resolve/minimize.

Research indicates that brain development is negatively affected by stress and violence in the home. Understanding of this information may help families to change behavior patterns that affect not only the infant's development but also all members of the family.

Discuss newborn's ability to become habituated to stimuli.

The ability of newborn infants to lessen their responses to repeated stimuli allows them to sleep while family members carry out normal household activities. Some newborns may not become habituated to stimuli as easily as others and need a quiet environment for sleeping.

Note family history of possible neurological or sensory deficits.

Family history of such problems may identify a genetic disorder related to seizure activity, deafness, blindness, retardation, cerebral palsy, or muscular weakness. Information may heighten parents' awareness of the need for further assessment or follow-up to determine the presence/extent of the problem and the appropriate treatment.

Provide information about home management of the common cold in infant. Discuss recognition of signs such as nasal congestion, coughing, sneezing, low-grade fever, and swallowing difficulty (indicating sore throat).

Promotes parental comfort in managing mild illnesses at home.

Recommend offering extra sterile water, reducing feeding amounts, using upright position for feeding and sleeping (elevating mattress to a 30-degree angle), nasal/oral suctioning, using a cool-mist

Promotes comfort. Smaller feedings help prevent overtiring of infant. Extra fluids and use of humidifier help liquefy secretions; upright positioning of head and chest promotes optimal humidifier, and medicating infant only with physician's orders.

Identify signs of illness necessitating medical attention, and inform parents of availability of community agencies. Provide list of emergency numbers for posting in a prominent place (e.g., next to telephone, on refrigerator).

Discuss plans for follow-up appointments for tests, such as PKU screening.

lung expansion. Note: Prone position also allows better lung expansion when infant is having difficulty handling mucus.

Prepares parents to seek prompt medical attention and to act quickly in an emergency.

Screening tests are usually repeated in 1–2 wk.

NURSING DIAGNOSIS:	**INJURY, risk for**
Risk Factors May Include:	Physical (hyperbilirubinemia), environmental (inadequate safety precautions), chemical (drugs in breast milk), psychological (inappropriate parental stimulation or interaction), cardiopulmonary (respiratory tract obstruction)
Possibly Evidenced By:	[Not applicable; presence of signs/symptoms establishes an *actual* diagnosis]
DESIRED OUTCOMES/EVALUATION CRITERIA—NEONATE WILL:	Be free of injury.
PARENT(S) WILL:	Identify individual risk factors/concerns.
	Adopt behaviors that provide safe growth-promoting environment.

ACTIONS/INTERVENTIONS	RATIONALE

Independent

Evaluate skin color from head to toe and color return on blanching of sternum. Note behavior changes (e.g., lethargy, reduced Moro's reflex, poor feeding, and listlessness). (Refer to CP: Newborn: Hyperbilirubinemia.)

Hyperbilirubinemia caused by elevated levels of unconjugated bilirubin can result in kernicterus, which is associated with deposition of excess bile pigments in the basal ganglia of the brain.

Note presence/resolution of cephalhematoma.

Large cephalhematoma may contribute to increased bilirubin levels during reabsorption of blood.

Investigate reports of cyanosis with crying, feeding, or activity.

May indicate cardiopulmonary compromise (e.g., unresolved PDA, infection) requiring prompt evaluation/intervention.

Determine parental knowledge of infant safety (e.g., use of car seats, proper restraints, and protected surfaces; proper assessment of temperature of bath water and formula).

Most common injuries in the newborn are related to accidental falls from unprotected surfaces. Bath water or formula should be comfortably warm to the inside of the wrist. Infant needs to be in federally approved car seat at all times when riding in any vehicle, with car seat positioned according to guidelines relative to infant's size/age.

Ascertain mother's use of drugs (prescription/over-the-counter/street), especially if she is breastfeeding. Discuss potentially harmful effects of specific and commonly ingested drugs, and the

Many drugs are passed to infant through breast milk. Nicotine, caffeine, alcohol, cocaine, marijuana, and other drugs tend to reach levels in newborn that are directly related to maternal

479

need to avoid taking medication until after discussion with healthcare provider.

intake. Caffeine (equivalent to more than 1 or 2 cups of coffee/tea per day) may cause restlessness, sleeplessness, and significant diuresis in infant. Excessive alcohol may increase circulating cortisol levels. Insulin, aspirin, most antibiotics, epinephrine, and antidiarrheal agents are usually viewed as safe, if used in moderation.

Collaborative

Refer to visiting nurse service as appropriate.

May benefit from additional home visits/follow-up to monitor potential complications.

Report family to social service or to protective services if potential for abuse, or possible safety or risk factors, are identified.

May be necessary for further evaluation of newborn's well-being and parents' child-care practices.

NURSING DIAGNOSIS:	BODY TEMPERATURE, risk for altered
Risk Factors May Include:	Extreme of age (immaturity of the hypothalamus, inability to shiver or perspire adequately)
Possibly Evidenced By:	[Not applicable; presence of signs/symptoms establishes an *actual* diagnosis]
DESIRED OUTCOMES/EVALUATION CRITERIA—NEONATE WILL:	Maintain temperature WNL.
PARENT(S) WILL:	Verbalize understanding of the influence of heat, cold, and dehydration on the newborn's temperature.
	Demonstrate appropriate regulation of newborn's environment and clothing.

ACTIONS/INTERVENTIONS

RATIONALE

Independent

Assess newborn's temperature. Note diaphoresis (overheating) or pallor, cyanosis, or coolness associated with hypothermia.

Detects deviations from normal range: rectal, 97.8°F–99.0°F (36.6°C–37.2°C); axillary/pacifier, 97.6°F–98.6°F (36.5°C–37.0°C). Thin skin and the proximity of blood vessels to skin surface result in rapid circulatory changes with cooling.

Review thermoregulatory needs of newborn.

Assist parents in recognizing importance of heat regulation; helps protect newborn from harm caused by temperature extremes. Note: Body temperature fluctuations require expenditure of calories to regain balance, decreasing reserves available for growth. In addition, chilling increases the risk of newborn jaundice as the affinity of serum albumin for bilirubin is diminished.

Assess environmental temperature and neonate's dress and coverings in relation to parental attire. Provide guidelines for dressing and bundling newborn, controlling environmental temperature, and evaluating infant for overheating or underheating.

Newborn is usually comfortable when dressed in the same number of clothing layers as parents. Overdressing in warm temperatures causes discomfort and prickly heat. Underdressing in cold temperatures results in discomfort and possible frostbite of cheeks, fingers, and toes.

Suggest use of appropriate hat in all temperatures.

Determine how parents check temperature of bath water. Provide guidance, as appropriate.

Informed parents can lessen the risks of such complications. Note: Cultural dictates may require bundling of newborn in excess of environmental needs, necessitating sensitivity and additional discussion of infant needs.

Protects infant's scalp from sunburn and shades eyes in summer; minimizes heat loss in cool environment.

Water temperature should feel warm to inside of wrist or elbow to avoid chilling or scalding newborn.

NURSING DIAGNOSIS:	CONSTIPATION/DIARRHEA, risk for
Risk Factors May Include:	Type and amount of oral intake; medications or dietary intake of the lactating mother; presence of allergies, infection
Possibly Evidenced By:	[Not applicable; presence of signs/symptoms establishes an *actual* diagnosis]
DESIRED OUTCOMES/EVALUATION CRITERIA—NEONATE WILL:	Evacuate with ease stool that is yellow-brown or golden-yellow and soft, with frequency appropriate for type of feeding.
PARENT(S) WILL:	Adjust specific contributing factors to promote optimal bowel pattern.

ACTIONS/INTERVENTIONS	RATIONALE

Independent

Determine frequency, amount, character, and odor of stool.

Newborn's elimination pattern is individual. Stool of newborns fed on cow's milk is pale yellow and formed, and is usually passed 1–2 times per day. Stool of newborns who are breastfed is golden or mustard-colored, and initially may be passed every few days. Diarrhea may be caused by overfeeding or enteric infection; constipation may be caused by dehydration or inappropriate lactating diet.

Ascertain total fluid intake (ounces of formula or frequency and length of feeding in breastfed infant) and number of wet diapers over 24-hr period. Determine skin turgor, observe mucous membranes. Obtain urinary specific gravity and Labstix results.

Alterations in hydration status may be associated with or cause altered bowel function. Less than five voidings per day, concentrated urine, poor skin turgor, dry mucous membranes indicate the need for increased fluid intake.

Auscultate bowel sounds.

An area of absent or diminished bowel sounds may signify blockage at a proximal segment of the bowel. Hyperactive bowel sounds indicate irritability.

Palpate for abdominal distension or tenderness.

Gas accumulation is associated with constipation or enteric infection and can cause varying degrees of discomfort.

Inspect perianal area for irritation, discharge, or rectal fissures. (Refer to ND: Skin Integrity, risk for impaired.)

Improper technique in formula preparation may result in bacterial growth, diarrhea, and resultant skin irritation.

Encourage positioning of newborn on right side after feedings.

Allows swallowed air to rise above fluid and exit through esophagus, and permits ingested formula or breast milk to flow toward pyloric sphincter.

481

Review fluid intake and diet of lactating mother, using 24-hr recall. Encourage client to increase frequency of feedings, and provide water to newborn between feedings as appropriate. Determine newborn's behavior in response to mother's ingested foods; counsel mother to avoid problem foods.

Inadequate fluid intake promotes constipation. Supplemental water may be beneficial during hot weather/in presence of constipation. In addition, certain foods ingested by lactating mother can alter newborn's elimination pattern and result in excess gas accumulation and constipation or diarrhea. Avoidance of these foods usually eliminates the problem.

Assess drug use in lactating client.

Use of cathartics may cause loose stools in infant.

Collaborative

Instruct parent(s) in proper technique of administering glycerin suppository.

Glycerin suppository aids in the passage of hard stool. Promotes parental management of infant's needs.

Refer parent(s) to healthcare provider for severe or protracted problems, or for suspected enteric infections.

May be necessary to determine exact cause of problem and to bring about resolution. Antispasmodics or antidiarrheal medications may be necessary.

NURSING DIAGNOSIS:	SKIN INTEGRITY, risk for impaired
Risk Factors May Include:	Excretions (ammonia formation from urea), chemical irritation from laundry detergent or diapering material, mechanical factors (e.g., long fingernails)
Possibly Evidenced By:	[Not applicable; presence of signs/symptoms establishes an *actual* diagnosis]
DESIRED OUTCOMES/EVALUATION CRITERIA—NEONATE WILL:	Be free of diaper dermatitis/dermal injury.
PARENT(S) WILL:	Identify and adopt measures to maintain skin integrity.

ACTIONS/INTERVENTIONS

RATIONALE

Independent

Stress need to assess diaper area for presence of rash that may be eroded, tender, indurated, or encrusted.

Early diagnosis and intervention may prevent spread of dermatitis to entire buttock area.

Recommend diaper changes, thorough cleaning and drying of area after each voiding and stool, exposure of area to air or monitored heat source, and application of a thin coat of petroleum jelly or A and D Ointment over the diaper area. Stress importance of not applying ointments before exposure to heat source, or use of cornstarch/powders.

Prevention of diaper rash maintains perineal skin integrity. Exposure to heat aids in drying and healing. Use of 25-W bulb placed 24 in (61 cm) from affected area is preferable to use of sunlight through window, which may cause sunburn. Infant may need to be gently restrained to prevent possible contact with heat source and should not be left unattended. Petroleum jelly or A and D Ointment acts as a barrier to protect the skin, but may intensify effects of heat, resulting in a burn. Powders tend to cake with urine and irritate buttocks; use of cornstarch may lead to a fungal infection.

Encourage parents to change brand of detergent and fabric softener or diaper (e.g., brand of

Eliminates possible causes of rash.

disposable diaper, or cloth versus disposable) if rash develops or fails to clear.

Review proper/safe nail-cutting techniques, e.g., cutting nails straight across with blunt-ended infant scissors/clippers while newborn sleeps.

At about 1 wk of age, the tips of the newborn's nails separate from the underlying skin. Uncoordinated activity of the upper extremities creates the risk of dermal trauma.

Collaborative

Recommend contacting healthcare provider for severe or persistent diaper rash.

May need additional help and further treatment or stronger therapeutic agents.

Demonstrate application of medicated topical creams, and explain treatment schedule.

Eradicates organisms causing dermatitis and aids in healing process.

NURSING DIAGNOSIS:	INFECTION, risk for
Risk Factors May Include:	Thin, permeable skin, extra portals of entry (umbilical cord, circumcision), and immature immunologic response
Possibly Evidenced By:	[Not applicable, presence of signs/symptoms establishes an *actual* diagnosis]
DESIRED OUTCOMES/EVALUATION CRITERIA—NEONATE WILL:	Be free of signs of infection.
PARENT(S) WILL:	Identify individual risk factors and appropriate actions.

ACTIONS/INTERVENTIONS	RATIONALE

Independent

Demonstrate proper hand-washing technique prior to handling infant. Ensure that only clean objects come in contact with newborn.

Prevents spread of infection. Hand washing is especially important following maternal perineal pad changes and following contact with vaginal lochia, because some organisms, such as listerial or streptococcal organisms, may be present in the lochia for as long as 10 days following delivery.

Instruct parents to keep newborn away from crowds and from people with known contagious illnesses until newborn is at least 1 mo of age.

Shields newborn from direct contact with infected persons, reducing cross-contamination.

Assess healing of umbilical cord stump; reinforce measures to promote healing and drying of stump through exposure to air and the use of astringents.

Stump usually heals and detaches by the 10th day of life. Small beads of blood may be present when infant strains while crying or passing stool.

Inspect penis of newborn who has been circumcised.

Penis should be well healed by 7 days following circumcision.

Discuss home management of upper respiratory infections, including the use and cleaning of cool-mist humidifiers, vaporizers, and bulb syringes; upright positioning; and increasing fluid intake. Identify possible sequelae associated with otitis media, feeding problems, breathing difficulty, and coughing. (Refer to CP: Four Weeks Following Birth; ND: Infection, risk for.)

Enhances client's ability to meet neonate's needs and promote health. Note: Water reservoirs in humidifiers and vaporizers may harbor bacteria and require special care to prevent secondary health problems.

483

Stress importance of refraining from medicating infant without first consulting healthcare provider; stress importance of using acetaminophen in place of aspirin products.

In general, safety of medications has not been determined/tested in the newborn population. The use of aspirin-containing products in presence of viral infection has been linked to Reye's syndrome.

Inspect skin for vesicular lesions surrounded by erythema (may be encrusted if ruptured).

May indicate impetigo caused by various strains of group A or B hemolytic streptococci, or by coagulase-positive *Staphylococcus aureus*.

Review signs of generalized infection (e.g., pulmonary congestion, cough, and retractions; more than one episode of forceful vomiting; refusal of two feedings in a row) or sepsis (e.g., temperature instability, lethargy, restlessness, irritability, frequent vomiting over a 6-hr period; two consecutive green, watery stools; fewer than six wet diapers per day). Discuss when to notify healthcare provider.

Studies show that neonatal infections with late onset of signs, appearing from 2–12 wk of age, are most frequently caused by cytomegalovirus and by organisms of *Chlamydia* and *Ureaplasma*.

Demonstrate proper technique for obtaining neonate's temperature.

In presence of suspected illness, healthcare provider may prefer rectal temperature readings, because core temperature is a more accurate indicator for febrile state.

Discuss advantages of breast milk for newborn.

Human milk contains iron-binding protein, which exerts a bacteriostatic effect on *Escherichia coli*; macrophages and lymphocytes, which promote a local inflammatory response; and passive transfer of maternal immunity to common mucosal pathogens, such as respiratory syncytial virus.

Inspect buccal cavity for white, curdy patches on tongue, palate, and inner aspects of cheeks; check for presence of fever and/or gastric distress.

Newborn may have been contaminated by *Candida albicans* during descent through birth canal, or as a result of poor hand-washing technique or contaminated bottles or nipples. Thrush typically causes gastrointestinal inflammation in addition to the "local" response.

Collaborative

Obtain/review complete blood count (CBC) results and cultures, as indicated.

May be necessary if temperature is elevated or presence of lesions/drainage warrants further evaluation to clarify diagnosis.

Demonstrate proper administration of local systemic antibiotics or fungicides.

Eradicates invading pathogen or infectious process. A fungicide such as nystatin (Mycostatin) applied after feedings to surfaces of oral cavity is usually effective against *Candida albicans* infections.

NURSING DIAGNOSIS:	**PAIN [acute], risk for**
Risk Factors May Include:	Accumulation of gas in a confined space, with cramping of intestinal musculature
Possibly Evidenced By:	[Not applicable; presence of signs/symptoms establishes an *actual* diagnosis]
DESIRED OUTCOMES/EVALUATION CRITERIA—NEONATE WILL:	Be free of, or display less frequent, crying spells and episodes of colic.
PARENT(S) WILL:	Report parent-infant tension is relieved or easing.

ACTIONS/INTERVENTIONS	RATIONALE

Independent

Evaluate neonate's behavior.

Colicky infant typically cries loudly, draws legs up to abdomen in pain, clenches fists, and sucks vigorously.

Obtain thorough, detailed history of normal daily events, household activity pattern, time of day in which attacks occur, and relationship of attacks to feeding.

Typically, attacks occur at a specific time of day. By determining the circumstances that possibly contribute to onset of attack and by manipulating those circumstances or environmental conditions, parents may be able to reduce overstimulation and tension that usually precipitate the attack.

Obtain 24-hr dietary recall when mother is breastfeeding. Suggest adoption of a milk-free diet for 5 days. Stress importance of reading food product labels; e.g., nondairy creamers may contain calcium caseinate, a cow's milk protein.

Gas-forming vegetables, spices, and chocolate may cause discomfort. Sensitivity to cow's milk products may precipitate colic attacks when milk products pass through the breast milk.

Observe feeding procedure. Analyze and discuss technique and behaviors with parents. Encourage burping infant in upright overshoulder position before and after feedings. Recommend smaller, more frequent feedings and placing infant in upright position after feeding. Use slow bicycling of legs from extension to knee-chest position.

Excess air ingestion from too-rapid or improper bottle position and/or inadequate burping may result in gas accumulation. Overfeeding or excess carbohydrate ingestion may lead to excess fermentation and gas production. Upright position and bicycling maneuver promote gas expulsion.

Encourage parents to administer 1–2 oz of warm, diluted tea, then to place newborn in prone position over heated towel or protected heating pad and to change infant's position frequently.

Helps stimulate peristalsis to relieve abdominal cramping.

Suggest use of collapsible bags in feeding bottles.

Reduces air ingestion.

Discuss neonate's physical condition and well-being.

Gastric acidity reduces within first week of life, affecting digestion and/or development of colic, which usually resolves within 2–3 mo. Despite colic attacks, infant normally thrives, gains weight, and tolerates feedings. However, the relationships between the parents/other family members may suffer the stressful effects of a crying, irritable infant; this may have a negative impact on the bonding process.

Assess parental response to colic attacks, methods used to relieve crying, and coping strategies. Initiate creative problem solving to diminish impact of attacks.

Parental responses of anxiety and increased tension are transmitted to the newborn, escalating tension, irritability, and crying. Adoption of different strategies may stimulate a different response in the newborn.

Encourage parents to share feelings of frustration, anger, helplessness, and insecurity. Recommend that parents spend time in diversionary activities away from the house and the newborn.

Helps support parents through crisis of colic.

Collaborative

Provide information and demonstrate insertion of glycerin suppository using a well-lubricated finger.

Stimulates passage of flatus and feces.

Discuss and demonstrate technique for administering sedatives (phenobarbital elixir), anticholinergics (atropine), antispasmodics, and antiflatulents, if used.

Medications may be needed to reduce gastrointestinal motility and provide relief.

THE INFANT AT 4 WEEKS FOLLOWING BIRTH

INFANT ASSESSMENT DATA BASE

Review prior assessments for identified risk factors.

Activity/Rest

Infant sleep pattern well-established

Circulation

Heart rate ranges from 80–150 bpm at rest, with average rate of 120 bpm.
BP obtained by using flush technique at wrist ranges from 48–90 mm Hg, with a mean of 67 mm Hg; at ankle, 38–56 mm Hg, with a mean of 61 mm Hg.

Ego Integrity

Regards faces, especially parents' faces, intently; may demonstrate beginning of social smile

Elimination

Urine pale or straw-colored, with output of 6–10 wet diapers per day
Abdomen soft, nondistended with bowel sounds present
Individual bowel elimination pattern established, dependent on type of feeding

Food/Fluid

Makes comfort noises during feeding, or may make small, throaty noises
Feeding generally 5–8 times per 24-hr period
Height gain 2.5 cm (1 in) monthly for first 6 mo
Weight gain of 3–5 oz/wk for first 6 mo
Drooling absent until 2–3 mo of age, when salivary glands begin to function

Neurosensory

Beginning to differentiate cry in relation to pain, discomfort, or hunger; uses cry to signal needs; quiets when picked up.
Head circumference increases 1.5 cm (½ in) monthly for first 6 mo.
Fontanels palpable and soft; posterior fontanel closes at 6 wk of age.
Tears present, with tear glands beginning to function at 2–4 wk of age.
Primitive reflexes present with strong, bilaterally equal responses.
Doll's eye and dance reflexes fading.
Crawling movements when prone.
Lifts head momentarily from bed while on abdomen, turns head from side to side when prone.
Demonstrates tonic neck reflex when supine.
Marked head lag when pulled from lying to sitting position (back is uniformly rounded); absence of head control in sitting position.
Strong grasp reflex: Hand closes on contact with object.
Responds to environmental stimuli: Bright objects (which are best viewed 8–12 in from face), sound, and touch.

Pain/Discomfort

Continuation of pain and cramping associated with colic may be reported.

Respiration

Signs of aspiration (continued regurgitation associated with reverse peristalsis and immature or relaxed cardiac sphincter)

Safety

Axillary temperature stable between 97.7°F–98.6°F (36.5°C–37.0°C)
Perineal area clean and free of rashes

DIAGNOSTIC STUDIES

Testing dependent on individual findings, risk factors.
Urine Specific Gravity: 1.008.

NURSING PRIORITIES

1. Promote infant's growth and development.
2. Provide information appropriate to parents' learning needs.
3. Enhance home environment to promote infant's safety, stimulation, and rest.

DISCHARGE GOALS

1. Various indicators of growth and development show progression WNL.
2. Parent(s) understand individual needs of infant.
3. Parent(s) demonstrate proficiency in infant care activities.
4. Plan in place to meet ongoing health monitoring/wellness needs.

NURSING DIAGNOSIS:	NUTRITION: altered, risk for less than body requirements
Risk Factors May Include:	Failure to ingest/digest/absorb adequate calories; e.g., biologic (insufficient intake, malabsorption, congenital problem, or neglect [failure to thrive]) or psychological factors (emotional abuse)
Possibly Evidenced By:	[Not applicable; presence of signs/symptoms establishes an *actual* diagnosis]
DESIRED OUTCOMES/EVALUATION CRITERIA—NEONATE WILL:	Display physical growth and weight gain appropriate for age and developmental stage.

ACTIONS/INTERVENTIONS	RATIONALE

Independent

Measure infant's height and weight, and compare with measurements at birth and at 1 wk of age. Review growth history.	Nutrients for infants are based on body weight. Most full-term, AGA infants regain birth weight within 10–14 days following birth. Weight gain should be 3–5 oz/wk for first 6 mo and may be as much as 1 oz/day in bottle-fed infant. Gains of less than 3–5 oz/wk may result in lifelong nutritional risks with potentially negative effects on infant development.
Assess infant for possible failure to thrive (FTT).	A breastfed infant who continues to lose weight after 10 days of life does not regain the weight by 3 wk of age, or gains weight at rate below 10th percentile after 1 mo is probably an FTT infant and requires prompt evaluation relative to issues of lactation and infant capabilities. In the bottle-fed infant, formula preparation and appropriateness (tolerance) are evaluated. Finally, concerns regarding possible neglect must be addressed. Timely intervention and resolution may prevent permanent deficits.
Determine amount, type, and frequency of oral intake over last 24 hr.	Infants require about 115 kcal/kg for first 6 mo of life, or 54 kcal/lb. Fluid needs are approximately 530 ml/day. One-third of energy is used for growth.

487

Intervention	Rationale
	Inadequate caloric and fluid intake results in nutritional inadequacies and poor weight gains. Note: Adequate protein intake is critically important to provide brain growth during the hyperplasia and hypertrophy phase in the first 6 mo of life. Inadequate protein ingestion during this phase can result in developmental delays.
Note status of fontanels, production of mucus, skin turgor, and number of wet diapers per day.	Inadequate fluid intake results in dehydration, manifested by depressed fontanels, reduced urine output, poor skin turgor, and dryness of mucous membranes. Note: Cases of hypernatremic dehydration have been associated with use of cow's milk feedings.
Obtain 24-hr dietary recall in lactating mother. Note presence of illness, infection, or dietary inadequacies. Provide dietary teaching, as appropriate, noting cultural/religious practices. Identify adequate sources of calcium and protein; suggest supplementing maternal diet with brewer's yeast as appropriate.	Illness, infection, or marginal diet may affect mother's ability to nourish the infant adequately. Factual information may help correct myths/faulty beliefs resulting in inadvertent or deliberate food restrictions. Supplementing diet with brewer's yeast improves milk production significantly more than simply adding similar nutrients.
Evaluate lactating mother' sleep and rest, noting excess fatigue, family demands, and work or social commitments. Discuss individual needs and options to meet these needs.	Inadequate sleep, resulting in excess fatigue, is most common cause of inadequate milk supply, especially during 1st mo, when milk supply is being established.
Evaluate effectiveness of let-down reflex in lacating mother. If mother smokes, suggest that she refrain or light cigarette after infant is sucking vigorously, rather than prior to feeding. Assist mother in evaluating stressors and using creative problem solving.	Smoking and psychological stress may inhibit let-down reflex. While abstinence is preferred, the reality is that cessation of smoking may not occur and achievable goals, such as reduction in frequency/number of cigarettes may still be beneficial.
Review techniques used in formula preparation and storage. Confirm that parents follow instructions for making powdered or concentrated formulas. Discourage home preparations of evaporated milk formula.	Many infant nutritional inadequacies are related to overdilution of commercial formulas, which results in inadequate calories, nutrients, and FTT. Use of home-prepared evaporated milk formulas has been linked to problems associated with improper measurement and bacterial contamination.
Encourage continued use of formula for first 12 mo of life. Discourage substitution of skim or whole cow's milk.	Skim milk contains about half the number of calories in breast or commercial formulas; may not meet the infant's energy needs; and may cause deficiencies in iron, vitamin C, and fatty acids. Use of whole milk in the first 12 mo may place the infant at risk for iron, vitamin C, and copper deficiencies.
Inspect infant for lesions; note swollen parotid glands.	May indicate poor nutritional state, affect oral intake.
Determine color, frequency, consistency, and odor of stool.	Altered elimination pattern may suggest problem with digestion and absorption. Foul-smelling stool suggests parasitic infection. Diarrhea may reflect milk intolerance or ingestion of cathartics in lactating mother.
Auscultate bowel sounds; palpate abdomen. Note presence of loose stools, cramping, crying, reports of vomiting, or chronic blood loss in GI tract.	Abdominal distension and gas accumulation may be associated with ingestion of gas-producing foods in lactating mother or with milk intolerance. Immaturity of the intestinal tract increases permeability to inadequately catabolized proteins, which produces an allergic response or milk intolerance in 1%–2% of infants.

Assess infant's color, gestational age, and weight at birth, and current weight gains.

Iron stores are usually adequate until infant weight increases by $2^1/_2$ times. Pallor and inadequate weight gain, however, may indicate anemia.

Auscultate apical pulse and count respirations as indicated.

Persistent tachycardia >160–200 bpm associated with increased respiratory rate suggests anemia.

Note excessive or forceful vomiting of nonbilious, possibly blood-tinged emesis; visible gastric waves moving right to left across epigastrium; and palpable olive-shaped mass in epigastric region.

May indicate hypertrophic pyloric stenosis, especially if infant appears alert and hungry, fails to gain weight, and has a history of recurrent vomiting.

Collaborative

Provide information as needed about prescribed alternatives to milk, such as soy milk formulas or hydrolyzed protein and amino acid mixtures.

Alternative formulas relieve symptoms associated with cow's milk intolerance.

Refer to social services or WIC program, as indicated.

Additional assistance may be needed to meet infant/maternal nutritional needs if financial resources are limited.

Instruct in addition to human milk fortifiers (HMF), as indicated, to breast milk, which is pumped and stored for feedings.

FTT infants who are breastfed may benefit from having the mother bottlefeed breast milk supplemented with extra calories until the infant is gaining weight appropriately on a consistent basis. Note: The morning and evening feeding may be from the breast in order to support the maternal breastfeeding experience.

Refer parents to pediatric nurse for assistance with surgical preparation and care if pyloric stenosis is confirmed.

Surgical management or pyloromyotomy is the standard treatment for hypertrophic pyloric stenosis; prognosis is excellent, and mortality is low.

NURSING DIAGNOSIS:	NUTRITION: altered, risk for more than body requirements
Risk Factors May Include:	Obesity in one or both parents, rapid transition across growth percentiles in infant
Possibly Evidenced By:	[Not applicable; presence of signs/symptoms establishes an *actual* diagnosis]
DESIRED OUTCOMES/EVALUATION CRITERIA—PARENT(S) WILL:	Identify and adopt appropriate infant feeding practices.
	Explain factors that promote excess weight gains and eating problems.

ACTIONS/INTERVENTIONS

RATIONALE

Independent

Assess measurement of infant's weight/height for age and sex. Determine anthropometric assessment.

Weight greater than the 85th percentile in relation to height, age, sex, and body build is considered obese. Although anthropometric assessment is most accurate, serial weight and height measurements in relation to age are fairly good predictors of obesity or excess weight gain.

Review parental weight history.

Heredity and family feeding practices contribute to obesity. There is an 80% probability that if parents

Note type of infant feeding (i.e., breast or bottle).	are obese, the child will also be obese. If parents are not obese, this probability is only 7%.
	Breastfed infants are less likely to be obese than bottlefed infants, because the breastfed infant regulates the feeding based on hunger needs. In a desire to empty the bottle, parents may overfeed the bottle-fed infant by continuing to feed even after satiation has been reached.
Determine amount and frequency of infant feedings.	Feedings in excess of infant caloric needs relative to energy expenditures result in excess weight gains, possibly leading to obesity.
Provide information about infant's energy requirements; encourage mother to let infant regulate intake based on hunger needs.	Reduces likelihood of overeating.
Encourage mother to avoid introduction of solid foods until infant is at least 4–6 mo of age.	Early addition of solid foods contributes to development of poor eating habits, excess food consumption, and infantile obesity. Mother may mistakenly think that addition of solids enhances infant's chances of sleeping through the night, but such practices have been found to have no effect on infant sleep patterns.
Encourage mother to restrict the use of infant seat during waking hours and to allow infant to spend time on mat on floor.	Enhances activity and energy expenditure.
Discuss mother's feeding of infant for emotional upsets or distress signals.	Inappropriate use of food in response to newborn's distress encourages infant to associate food with emotional gratification rather than with hunger.
Discourage substitution of skim or whole milk for commercially prepared formula for first 12 mo of life.	Such substitution may increase renal solute load as a result of excess protein and mineral ingestion. Use of whole milk may result in increased plasma osmolality, hyperphosphatemia, and hypernatremia.
Discuss possible lifelong risks associated with overeating.	Overeating increases risk of health problems related to cardiovascular system, hypertension, and diabetes.
Review family eating patterns.	Healthy eating habits and selection of appropriate amounts and types of foods can ultimately affect nutrition of the growing child.

NURSING DIAGNOSIS:	**KNOWLEDGE deficit [Learning Need], regarding infant care**
May Be Related To:	Lack of exposure/recall, misinterpretation, unfamiliarity with resources
Possibly Evidenced By:	Verbalization of problem/concern or misconceptions, inaccurate follow-through of instructions, development of preventable complications
DESIRED OUTCOMES/EVALUATION CRITERIA—PARENT(S) WILL:	Provide appropriate nutritional intake.
	Create safe, stimulating/restful infant environment.
	Identify signs/symptoms requiring medical follow-up.
	Use healthcare system appropriately.
	Plan for short- and long-term child care.

ACTIONS/INTERVENTIONS	RATIONALE

Independent

Reinforce or provide appropriate information about infant's nutritional needs for next few months.

Provide information about role of iron in body and the need for supplementation.

Discuss role of fluoride in body and in tooth development. Encourage parents to obtain fluoride supplements if appropriate.

Review information for lactating mother, as needed, including increased infant appetite and caloric needs during growth spurts at about 6 wk and 3 mo of age.

Determine how long mother plans to breast-feed. Discuss techniques of weaning from breast when desired and the process of introducing solids between 4 and 6 mo of age. (Refer to NDs: Nutrition: altered, risk for less than body requirements; Nutrition: altered, risk for more than body requirements.)

Review signs of milk sensitivities, especially if lactating mother plans to wean infant to a bottle when she returns to work.

Discuss mother's plans for possible return to work and plans for child care and feeding practices. Provide anticipatory guidance for lactating mother to allow her to continue with breastfeeding and to maintain milk supply.

Identify factors to be considered and resources available when choosing child care. Stress importance of ongoing monitoring of care provided.

Provide oral or written anticipatory guidance related to infant safety, including discussion of

Helps ensure normal growth patterns in height and weight, and may prevent overfeeding through too early introduction of solid foods.

American Academy of Pediatrics recommends 1 mg of iron per kg of body weight per day for full-term infants, starting no later than 4 mo of age. Iron-fortified commercial formula for bottle-fed infant offers most constant and predictable iron ingestion. By 4–6 mo of age, breastfed infant should have supplemental iron in form of iron-fortified cereal or oral iron drops.

Fluoride helps reduce incidence of tooth decay and improves quality of tooth enamel, making it more resistant to caries, if fluoride is ingested before eruption of teeth. Breastfed infants consume little or no water and should receive 0.25 mg of fluoride per 24 hr for 1st yr of life. Although commercial formulas have minimal amounts of fluoride, supplementation is not necessary if home/bottled water supply used in formula preparation contains 0.3 parts per million (ppm) fluoride.

The "reward period" for the breastfeeding mother may not occur until 6 wk after delivery, and she may need further encouragement and information to continue. Note: Infant may need to nurse more frequently during periods of rapid growth.

Anticipatory guidance related to the individual situation provides for anticipatory problem solving and enhances optimal outcome.

If milk sensitivity is present, infant may require use of soy or other formulas. (Refer to ND: Nutrition: altered, risk for less than body requirements.)

Allows mother to anticipate and plan for problems that may arise. Breastfeeding can be continued with adequate planning and management. Note: Some employers have an area where breastfeeding/breast pumping can be done.

Placing infant in care of others can be difficult for parents relative to issues of trust and child well-being. Informed choice and vigilance enhance parent(s) level of comfort and promote optimal outcomes.

Helps parent(s) to recognize potential safety hazards and reduce risk of injury. Crawling reflex potential accidental injury caused by suffocation, falls, burns, motor vehicle accidents, or bodily trauma. (Refer to NDs: Suffocation/Trauma, risk for.)

(which propels infant forward), rolling over, increasing eye-hand coordination, and voluntary grasp reflex increase risk of accidents in first 4 mo of life.

Provide information about importance of recommended primary schedule for immunization.

Immunizations begin in infancy to reduce incidence of infectious disease (diphtheria, tetanus, pertussis, polio, measles, mumps, rubella, and hepatitis B). Although recommendations are to begin immunizations at 2 mo of age, current discussion varies as to whether immunizations should begin at birth or after the 1st yr to avoid possible untoward responses.

Discuss timing and importance of infant's regularly scheduled well-baby visits to physician or nurse practitioner.

Helps detect any deviations from normal growth and development and ensure early intervention if deviations are identified.

Discuss infant's physical, emotional, and developmental needs. Provide oral or written/pictorial information about anticipated monthly progression of physical (gross and fine motor) development, sensory development, and vocalization and socialization.

Allows parents to monitor infant's growth and development during infancy. May help reduce parental anxiety relative to individual infant variations.

Evaluate environment for its ability to provide appropriate infant stimulation and rest. Assist parents as needed in planning for and providing appropriate visual, auditory, tactile, and kinetic stimulation as well as quiet ideas for sleep. Discuss changing needs of infant play as development progresses during the 1st yr. (Refer to ND: Sensory/Perceptual alterations, risk for.)

Helps parents recognize the balance between play and rest and to provide optimal environment for infant play, rest, and development. At 1 mo of age, placing bright hanging objects 8–12 inches from infant's face or looking at infant from close range provides visual stimulation. Talking to or singing to infant, or playing music box or radio, provides auditory stimulation. Holding, cuddling, and providing warmth offer tactile stimulation. Rocking infant in chair or cradle and using carriage provide kinetic stimulation.

Review infant's sleep-wake patterns. Suggest ways to promote sleep through provision of warm, nonstimulating environment, position changes, and sleeping arrangements separate from parents' room.

Rest periods/naps, usually after meals, are essential for continued growth. Intervals of sleep at night range from 4–10 hr with frequent naps and increased periods of wakefulness without crying. By 3 mo of age most infants have developed a nocturnal pattern.

Reassess parent-infant interaction. Discuss methods to foster mutually satisfying interactions and development of infant's trust.

Ongoing quality of emotional care is an important aspect in promoting optimal infant growth and development. Mutually satisfying parent-infant relationship fosters development of a sense of trust in newborn.

Encourage parents to pay attention to infant cues and to provide gratification soon after need is identified.

Allowing infant to feel physically comfortable, warm, emotionally loved, and secure aids in development of mutual trust and fosters development of healthy ego in the infant. Delayed gratification and/or meeting needs before infant signals them can lead to development of a sense of mistrust.

Offer anticipatory guidance, as appropriate, regarding teething, shoes, use of pacifiers, thumb sucking, and so forth.

During 1st yr of infant's life, both new and experienced parents may have concerns or questions, which if addressed early can foster positive coping, reduce anxiety, and increase problem-solving skills.

NURSING DIAGNOSIS:	INFECTION, risk for
Risk Factors May Include:	Immature immunologic response, increased environmental exposure
Possibly Evidenced By:	[Not applicable; presence of signs/symptoms establishes an *actual* diagnosis]
DESIRED OUTCOMES/EVALUATION CRITERIA—NEONATE WILL:	Be free of infection.
PARENT(S) WILL:	Identify individual risk factors and appropriate interventions.
	List signs requiring medical intervention.

ACTIONS/INTERVENTIONS	RATIONALE
Independent	
Discuss newborn development and individual risk factors.	By 4 wk of age, the infant is usually out in public more often or may even be cared for outside the home. The infant is particularly susceptible to coryza, or the common cold, which is most frequently caused by a rhinovirus and an immature immunologic response. Because the infant has been an obligatory nose breather and is only beginning to learn to open the mouth in response to an increase in mucus production and edema of nasal mucosa, respiratory problems and an increase in airway resistance may result. Possible complications such as otitis media, sinusitis, or lower respiratory tract infection may also develop.
Review signs of upper respiratory infection (e.g., poor feeding, breathing difficulty, cough, and nasal congestion) with parents.	Reinforces parental learning to assist them in identification of infant's respiratory problems.
Suggest elevating infant's head/shoulders by raising crib mattress to 30-degree angle when infant has trouble breathing.	Increases vertical chest capacity and lung expansion with descent of diaphragm. Facilitates drainage of mucus into stomach.
Recommend observing stool for passage of mucus.	Because infant cannot blow nose, excess mucus is excreted through the GI tract with the stool.
Observe parent(s) technique for using bulb suction to clear mouth/nose of excess mucus.	Bulb suctioning of mouth first, then nose second avoids introduction of microorganisms colonized in nose into oral cavity/pharynx.
Review proper handling/cleaning of syringe.	Bulb should be cleaned with hot water and allowed to dry after each use.
Encourage giving infant sterile warm water between regular feedings twice a day, as appropriate.	Promotes hydration to help liquefy secretions.
Provide information about benefits of humidified air.	Liquefies secretions and provides moisture for mucous membranes, reducing risk of excessive dryness/cracking.
Show parents how to inspect pharynx and to distinguish between viral and bacterial causative agent if area is reddened or inflamed. Discuss appropriate response.	Enlarged lymphoidal tissue and appearance of erythema (suggesting viral cause) or white exudate (indicating bacterial or streptococcal cause) characterize pharyngitis and tonsillitis. Viral infections may resolve with only palliative measures, whereas bacterial infections usually require medication.

493

Review methods for monitoring temperature.	Digital pacifier or rectal are both acceptable techniques for obtaining infant's temperature with rectal result approximately 0.5°F (0.28°C) higher. Note: Some healthcare providers prefer rectal measurements.
Discuss signs indicating a deterioration in newborn's status and necessitating evaluation by healthcare provider, such as pulling at ear (as child gets older), croupy cough, elevated temperature, cyanosis, and wheezing.	Involvement of lower respiratory structures or respiratory compromise requires further evaluation and treatment. Infant is prone to development of otitis media because of short, distensible eustachian tubes, which open inappropriately; an immature humoral defense system; and pooling of fluid in pharyngeal cavity when infant is in recumbent position.
Instruct parents not to medicate infant without discussing such action with healthcare provider.	Information about administration of medications, when to use them and when not to use them, helps parents know when to ask for assistance.
Demonstrate medication administration (e.g., antibiotics, ear or nose drops).	Enables parents to provide optimal care for infant's individual needs. For example, saline nose drops instilled 15 min before feedings may improve oral intake at mealtime. Note: Use of nose drops in newborn is somewhat controversial, because drops may lead to aspiration if they are improperly administered.

Collaborative

Provide referral for laboratory studies (e.g., complete blood count with differential [CBCD], throat culture) if needed.	Helps confirm infectious process and identify pathogens, especially when causative organism may be beta-hemolytic streptococci.

NURSING DIAGNOSIS:	**SUFFOCATION/TRAUMA, risk for**
Risk Factors May Include:	Lack of ability to protect self (infant), lack of awareness of hazards (caregivers)
Possibly Evidenced By:	[Not applicable; presence of signs/symptoms establishes an *actual* diagnosis]
DESIRED OUTCOMES/EVALUATION CRITERIA—NEONATE WILL:	Be free of injury.
PARENT(S) WILL:	Institute appropriate environmental adaptations or precautions to prevent accidental injury.
	Demonstrate concern for infant's well-being by responding to crying with soothing techniques, reacting appropriately during interactions with infant, and raising appropriate questions and concerns.

ACTIONS/INTERVENTIONS	RATIONALE

Independent

Provide oral or written/pictorial information about infant's motor development between 1 and 4 mo of age, its effect on mobility, and the increased risk of injury.	Allows parents to focus on age-appropriate safety measures. The major developmental changes that occur between birth and 4 mo of age are increased eye-hand coordination, development of voluntary grasp, ability to roll over, and increased possibility of movement associated with crawling and with Moro's reflex.

494

Review environmental factors that place infant at risk for suffocation.

Improper storage and use of plastic bags, loose-fitting sheets or soft mattress/pillows, opportunities for drowning, and strings around pacifiers/bibs (especially if they are worn at nap time or at night) place infant at risk for suffocation.

Discuss dangers associated with aspiration and proper use and storage of baby powder.

Aspiration dangers at 1 mo are most often related to baby powder container, which because of its shape may be held like a bottle, thereby creating risk of inhalation, aspiration, and possibly fatal asphyxiation.

Provide anticipatory guidance regarding necessity of burping infant before placing in bed, proper positioning, keeping small objects out of infant's reach, avoiding use of clothing with buttons, avoiding balloons or toys with removable parts.

Regurgitation associated with reverse peristalsis and immature or relaxed cardiac sphincter increases risk of aspiration. As infant's coordination and strength increase, potential exists for infant's pulling toys and decorations apart and putting small pieces in mouth.

Reassess and discuss other home safety factors, including precautions for home layout and furniture used for infant care, cigarettes and second-hand smoke, hot liquids, and motor vehicles.

Reminds parents of situations that may present danger for their infant; provides opportunity for problem-solving individual needs.

Reevaluate parents' understanding and practices related to the potential for bodily harm to infant. Provide information as needed.

Keeping diaper pins closed and out of infant's reach and carefully putting away scissors, knives, and razors reduce risks associated with bodily injury from sharp or jagged-edged objects as infant matures and becomes more active.

Assess emotional tone and quality of parent-infant interaction. Note response to infant's crying and nature of adjectives used to describe infant.

Failure of parent to have fun, talk, and make eye contact with infant; anger or frustration in response to crying episodes; and repeated use of negative adjectives to describe infant indicate a negative emotional bond with infant, which may lead to emotional or physical abuse.

Evaluate infant for physical evidence of abuse.

Excessive bruising, pinch marks, handprints, lacerations, abrasions, malnutrition, FTT, or lack of subcutaneous fat indicates possible child abuse/neglect.

Collaborative

Make appropriate referrals to healthcare provider, community agencies, and support groups.

May be necessary to help parents develop positive parenting skills and reduce possibility of physical or emotional harm to infant.

Report suspected abuse to physician and appropriate social or child-care agency.

Suspected child abuse may warrant further investigation before permanent injury or death occurs. Note: Most states have statutory guidelines requiring reporting of suspected child abuse/neglect.

NURSING DIAGNOSIS:	**PAIN [acute], risk for**
Risk Factors May Include:	Accumulation of gas in a confined space with cramping of intestinal musculature
Possibly Evidenced By:	[Not applicable; presence of signs/symptoms establishes an *actual* diagnosis]
DESIRED OUTCOMES/EVALUATION CRITERIA—NEONATE WILL:	Be free of, or display less frequent, crying spells and episodes of colic.
PARENT(S) WILL:	Identify/demonstrate appropriate techniques to relieve newborn anxiety and tension.

ACTIONS/INTERVENTIONS	RATIONALE

Independent

Evaluate infant's behavior.	Helps differentiate cause of problem. For example, colicky infant typically cries loudly, draws legs up to abdomen in pain, clenches fists, and sucks vigorously. Infant with otitis media may pull at affected ear.
Determine what parents have done previously and success of those interventions.	Assists in determining interventions that may be helpful at this time.
Reassess diet of lactating mother and infant feeding/formula preparation procedures.	Helps identify specific foods or errors in feeding process that may be causing discomfort.
Discuss physical condition and infant's well-being.	Gastric acidity reduces within 1st wk of life, affecting digestion and development of colic, which often resolves within 2–3 mo. Despite colic attacks, infant normally thrives, gains weight, and tolerates feedings.
For additional interventions, refer to CP: One Week Following Discharge; ND: Pain [acute], risk for.	

NURSING DIAGNOSIS:	SENSORY/PERCEPTUAL, risk for alterations
Risk Factors May Include:	Immature development of sensory organs, inappropriate/inadequate environmental stimuli; effects of disease, trauma, drugs
Possibly Evidenced By:	[Not applicable; presence of signs/symptoms establishes an actual diagnosis.]
DESIRED OUTCOMES/EVALUATION CRITERIA—PARENT(S) WILL:	Provide adequate/age-appropriate stimulation.
	Identify impairments.
	Initiate appropriate interventions.

ACTIONS/INTERVENTIONS	RATIONALE

Independent

Repeat the Brazelton Neonatal Assessment Scale as appropriate, and compare with previous testing.	Measures cerebral and neurological functioning and assesses interactive behavior. Although testing is usually done at 3 days of age, prolonged effects of intrapartal events/birth stress may affect initial results. Reevaluation provides opportunity for comparison and to verify appropriateness and progression of responses.
Observe responses to visual, auditory, or tactile stimuli; note motor function and reflexes.	The adequacy of sensory modes (e.g., visual, auditory, and tactile) in a 4-wk-old infant is determined by eliciting responses and evaluating the age-specific response. Causes of deviations in sensory perception may be related to vascular or traumatic injury that develops over a period of hours; toxic, infectious, or electrolyte imbalances that peak in

Determine occurrence of recent illnesses of infant or family members, prenatal or intrapartal complications and postnatal course.

several days; or congenital or degenerative injuries that develop or worsen insidiously over days, weeks, and months.
Helps detect environmental infection and illness; may rule out mechanical causes of alteration.

Assess parents' behaviors and responses to infant using such measures as Cropley's Critical Attachment Tasks, Maternal Tasks, Mother-Infant Screening Tool (MIST), and Reiser Fathering Assessment Tool.

Helps identify possible inadequacies in parent-infant interaction and establishes them as causative factors in infant's unresponsiveness to surroundings.

Encourage parents to stroke infant gently from head to toe with hand, washcloth, or cotton, and to hold, caress, cuddle, and swaddle infant.

Stimulates sense of touch; conveys feelings of warmth and protection.

Suggest parents place mobiles or bright, shiny objects within 8–12 in of infant's face, to look at infant en face (face-to-face) at close range, and to decrease intensity of light and move objects slowly.

Stimulates visual development. At 4 wk of age, infant can see shadows and outlines, showing preference for circular shapes, intricate patterns, and human faces.

Discuss placing ticking clock or radio playing soft music near infant, playing tape of parent reading a story, talking or singing to infant, and playing music box.

Provides auditory stimulation and may be soothing to infant; e.g., clock may stimulate human heartbeat.

Encourage parents to rock infant, place infant in swing, gently cradle infant in arms, and take infant for walks in carriage or in backpack placed close to back or chest.

Provides kinetic stimulation.

Assess strength of muscles, finger grasp, limb recoil, and stretching. Institute age-appropriate exercises.

Provides parents with information about the infant's ability for reciprocal behavior. Specific exercises stimulate sensory development.

Collaborative

Refer to other resources (e.g., physician, nurse practitioner, physical therapy clinic, parenting classes and support groups) as indicated.

May be necessary for follow-up care and evaluation of identified problems. (Provides role models, facilitates role transition and skill acquisition.)

THE PRETERM INFANT

Any infant born prior to completing 37 weeks' gestation is identified as premature. Thus, the level of development and maturity, and often the degree of complications, varies within this group, dependent on the length of gestation.

NEONATAL ASSESSMENT DATA BASE

Circulation

Apical pulse may be rapid and/or irregular within a normal range (120–160 bpm).
Audible heart murmur may indicate PDA.

Food/Fluid

Weight less than 2500 g (5 lb 8 oz).
Body long, thin, limp with a slight potbelly.
Suck/swallow reflex may be absent/uncoordinated (impacts feeding choices).

Neurosensory

Head size large in relation to body; sutures may be easily movable; fontanels may be large or
    wide open.
May demonstrate twitching or eye rolling.
Edema of eyelids common; eyes may be fused shut (depends on gestational age).
Reflexes depend on gestational age; rooting well established by 32 weeks' gestation; coordinated
    reflexes for sucking, swallowing, and breathing usually established by 32 wk; first
    component of Moro's reflex (lateral extension of upper extremities with opening of hands)
    appears at 28 wk; second two components (anterior flexion and audible cry) appear at 32
    wk.
Dubowitz examination indicates gestational age between 24 and 37 wk.

Respiration

Apgar scores may be low.
Respirations may be shallow, irregular; diaphragmatic with intermittent or periodic breathing
    (40–60/min).
Grunting, nasal flaring, suprasternal or substernal retractions, or varying degrees of cyanosis
    may be present.
Auscultatory presence of "sandpaper" sound indicates RDS.

Safety

Temperature fluctuates easily.
Cry may be weak.
Face may be bruised; caput succedaneum may be present; labor or delivery may have been
    precipitous.
Skin reddened or translucent; color may be pink/ruddy, acrocyanotic, or cyanotic/pale.
Lanugo widely distributed over entire body.
Extremities may appear edematous.
Sole creases may or may not be present on all or part of the foot.
Nails may be short.

Sexuality

Female labia minora may be larger than labia majora, with prominent clitoris.
Male testes may not be descended; rugae may be scant or absent on scrotum.

Teaching/Learning

Maternal history may reveal factors that contributed to preterm labor, such as young age; low
    socioeconomic background; closely spaced pregnancies; multiple gestation; poor nutrition;

previous preterm birth; obstetric complication such as abruptio placentae, premature rupture of membranes (PROM), premature dilation of cervix, presence of infection; blood incompatibility associated with erythroblastosis fetalis; or use of prescription, over-the-counter, or street drugs.

DIAGNOSTIC STUDIES

Choice of tests and the expected results depend on presenting problems and secondary complications.

Amniotic Fluid Studies: For lecithin-to-sphingomyelin (L/S) ratio, fetal lung profile, and phosphatidyl glycerol/phosphatidyl inositol may have been performed during pregnancy to assess fetal maturity.

CBC: Decreases in Hb/Hct may be associated with anemia or blood loss. WBC count may be $<10,000/mm^3$ with a shift to the left (excess early neutrophils and bands), which is usually associated with severe bacterial disease.

Dextrostix: Reveals hypoglycemia. Serum glucose test may be required if Dextrostix result is <45 mg/ml.

Serum Calcium: May be low.

Electrolytes (Na^+, K^+, Cl^-): Usually within normal limits initially, but susceptible to critical fluctuations.

Blood Type: May reveal potential for ABO incompatibility.

Rh and Direct Coombs' Determination (if mother is Rh-negative and father is Rh-positive): Determines incompatibilities.

ABGs: Po_2 may be low; Pco_2 may be elevated and reflect mild/moderate acidosis, sepsis, or prolonged respiratory difficulties.

Erythrocyte Sedimentation Rate (ESR): Elevation indicates an acute inflammatory response. Diminishing ESR indicates resolution of inflammation.

C-reactive Protein (a beta globulin): Present in serum in proportion to severity of infectious or noninfectious inflammatory process.

Platelet Count: Thrombocytopenia may accompany sepsis.

Fibrinogen Levels: May decrease during disseminated intravascular coagulation (DIC) or become elevated during injury or inflammation.

Fibrin Split Products: Present with DIC.

Blood Cultures: Identify causative organisms associated with sepsis.

Urinalysis (on second voided specimen): Detects abnormalities, renal injury.

Urine-Specific Gravity: Ranges between 1.006 and 1.013; elevated with dehydration.

Clinitest/Clinistix: Identifies presence of sugar in urine.

Hematest: Examines stools for blood; positive results suggest necrotizing enterocolitis.

Shake Test on Gastric Aspirate: Determines presence or absence of surfactant. (Intermediate results if blood or meconium is present.)

Chest X-Ray (posteroanterior [PA] and lateral) with Air Bronchogram: May have ground-glass appearance (RDS).

Serial Cranial Ultrasonography: Detects presence and severity of intraventricular hemorrhage (IVH).

Lumbar Puncture: May be performed to rule out meningitis.

Maternal GBS Status: Determines potential for meningitis/infections.

NURSING PRIORITIES

1. Promote optimal respiratory functioning.
2. Maintain neutral thermal environment.
3. Prevent or reduce risk of potential complications.
4. Maintain homeostasis.
5. Foster development of healthy family unit.

DISCHARGE GOALS

1. Maintaining physiological and behavioral homeostasis with minimal external support.
2. Weight 4½ lb or greater appropriate to age/condition.
3. Complications prevented/resolving or independently managed.

4. Family identifying and using resources appropriately.
5. Family demonstrates ability to manage infant care.
6. Plan in place to meet needs after discharge.

NURSING DIAGNOSIS:	GAS EXCHANGE, impaired
May Be Related To:	Ventilation perfusion imbalances, inadequate surfactant levels, immaturity of pulmonary arteriole musculature, immaturity of CNS and neuromuscular system, airway congestion, anemia, and cold stress
Possibly Evidenced By:	Hypercapnia, hypoxia, tachypnea, cyanosis
DESIRED OUTCOMES/EVALUATION CRITERIA—NEONATE WILL:	Maintain Po_2/Pco_2 levels WNL.
	Suffer minimal RDS, with reduced work of breathing and no morbidity.
	Be free of bronchopulmonary dysplasia.

ACTIONS/INTERVENTIONS	RATIONALE

Independent

Review information related to infant's condition, such as length of labor, type of delivery, Apgar score, need for resuscitative measures at delivery, and maternal medications taken during pregnancy or delivery, including betamethasone.	Prolonged labor increases risk of hypoxia, and respiratory depression may follow maternal drug administration or usage. In addition, infants who required resuscitative measures at birth, or those with low Apgar scores, may require more intense interventions to stabilize blood gases and may have suffered CNS injury with damage to the hypothalamus, which controls respiratory functioning. Note: Administration of corticosteroids to mother within 1 wk of delivery fosters the infant's lung maturity and surfactant production.
Note gestational age, weight, and sex.	Neonates born before 30 weeks' gestation and/or weighing less than 1500 g are at higher risk for developing RDS. In addition, males are twice as susceptible as females. Note: The majority of deaths related to RDS occur in infants weighing less than 1500 g.
Assess respiratory status, noting signs of respiratory distress (e.g., tachypnea, nasal flaring, grunting, retractions, rhonchi, or crackles).	Tachypnea indicates respiratory distress, especially when respirations are >75/min after the first 5 hr of life. Expiratory grunting represents an attempt to maintain alveolar expansion; nasal flaring is a compensatory mechanism to increase diameter of nares and increase oxygen intake. Crackles/rhonchi may indicate pulmonary vasocongestion associated with PDA, hypoxemia, acidemia, or immaturity of muscles in arterioles, which fail to constrict in response to increased oxygen levels.
Apply transcutaneous oxygen monitor or pulse oximeter. Record levels hourly. Change site of probe every 3–4 hr.	Provides constant noninvasive monitoring of oxygen levels. Note: Pulmonary insufficiency usually worsens during the first 24–48 hr, then reaches a plateau.
Suction nares and oropharynx carefully, as needed.	May be necessary to maintain airway patency,

Limit time of airway obstruction by catheter to 5–10 sec. Observe transcutaneous oxygen monitor or pulse oximeter before and during suctioning. Provide "bag" ventilation following suctioning.

especially in infant receiving controlled ventilation. Preterm infant does not develop the coordinated reflex for sucking, swallowing, and breathing until 32–34 weeks' gestation. Cilia may not be fully developed or may be damaged from use of endotracheal tube. Exudate phase associated with RDS at about 48 hr postpartum may contribute to infant's difficulty in handling secretions. Suctioning may stimulate vagus nerve, causing bradycardia, hypoxemia, or bronchospasm. Bag ventilation promotes rapid restoration of oxygen levels.

Maintain thermal neutrality with body temperature at 97.7°F (± 0.5°F). (Refer to ND: Thermoregulation, ineffective.)

Cold stress increases infant's oxygen consumption, may promote acidosis, and may further impair surfactant production.

Monitor fluid intake and output; weigh infant as indicated by protocol.

Dehydration impairs ability to clear airways because mucus becomes thickened. Overhydration may contribute to alveolar infiltrates/pulmonary edema. Weight loss and increased urine output may indicate diuretic phase of RDS, usually beginning at 72–96 hr and preceding resolution of condition.

Promote rest; minimize stimulation and energy expenditure.

Reduces metabolic rate and oxygen consumption.

Position infant on abdomen if possible. Provide "rocker" mattress, as indicated.

Prone position compensates for weak chest and abdominal muscles, decreasing the amount of respiratory effort required to expand chest, thus allowing optimal chest expansion and enhancing inhalation of air. Stimulates respirations and ventricular growth. Positioning infant on abdomen or side reduces risk of aspiration of mucus/regurgitated formula.

Observe for evidence and location of cyanosis.

Cyanosis is a late sign of low PaO_2 and does not appear until there are slightly more than 3 g/dl of reduced Hb in central arterial blood, or 4–6 g/dl in capillary blood, or until oxygen saturation is only 75%–85%, with PO_2 levels of 32–41 mm Hg. Therefore, prompt intervention is crucial.

Investigate sudden deterioration in condition associated with cyanosis, diminished or absent breath sounds, shift of point of maximal impact (PMI), bulging of chest wall, hypotension, or cardiac dysrhythmias.

Sudden or unexplained deterioration of respiratory function may indicate onset of pneumothorax.

Monitor for signs of necrotizing enterocolitis. (Refer to ND: Constipation/Diarrhea, risk for.)

Hypoxia may cause shunting of blood to brain, thereby reducing circulation to the intestines, with resultant intestinal cell damage and invasion by gas-forming bacteria.

Collaborative

Monitor laboratory/diagnostic studies, as appropriate:

Graph serial ABGs;

Hypoxemia, hypercapnia, and acidosis reduce surfactant production. PaO_2 levels should be 50–70 mm Hg or higher, $PaCO_2$ levels should be 35–45 mm Hg, and oxygen saturation should be 92%–94%. Decreased iron stores at birth, repeated blood sampling, rapid growth, and hemorrhagic episodes increase the likelihood that preterm infant will be

Hb/Hct;

Serial chest x-rays.	anemic, thereby reducing the oxygen-carrying capacity of the blood. Note: Administration of packed cells may be necessary to replace blood drawn for laboratory studies. Atelectasis, congestion, or air bronchogram suggests developing RDS.
Administer supplemental oxygen, as needed, by mask, hood, endotracheal tube, or mechanical ventilation using constant positive airway pressure (CPAP) and intermittent mandatory ventilation (IMV), or intermittent positive-pressure breathing (IPPB) and positive end-expiratory pressure (PEEP).	Hypoxemia and acidemia may further decrease surfactant production, increase pulmonary vascular resistance and vasoconstriction, and cause ductus arteriosus to remain open. Immaturity of the hypothalamus may necessitate ventilatory assistance to maintain respirations. Use of PEEP may reduce airway collapse, enhancing gas exchange and reducing the need for high levels of oxygen.
Monitor oxygen therapy closely. Record fraction of oxygen in inspired air (FIO_2) every hour. Adjust level and/or limit duration of administration as appropriate.	Amount of oxygen administered, expressed as FIO_2, is determined individually, based on transcutaneous monitoring or capillary blood samples. Prolonged high levels of serum oxygen combined with prolonged high pressures resulting from IPPB and PEEP (barotrauma) may predispose infant to bronchopulmonary dysplasia and retinal damage. Note: The retina has an immature vascular system that is susceptible to damage, leading to vaso-obliteration. New vessels that are developing may rupture, creating retinal and vitreous hemorrhage, leading to formation of scar tissue.
Initiate postural drainage, chest physiotherapy, or lobe vibration every 2 hr, as indicated, noting infant's tolerance of procedure.	Facilitates removal of secretions. Length of time allotted to each lobe is related to infant's tolerance. (Infant usually cannot tolerate a full treatment regimen each time.)
Aspirate gastric contents for shake test.	Provides immediate information about presence of surfactant. Surfactant, which is necessary to promote normal expansion and elasticity of alveoli, is usually not present in sufficient quantities until 32–33 weeks' gestation.
Provide feedings by nasogastric or orogastric tube instead of nipple feedings, as appropriate.	Reduces oxygen needs, promotes rest, conserves energy, and reduces risk of aspiration caused by poorly developed gag reflex.
Administer medications as indicated:	
Sodium bicarbonate;	If measures to increase respiratory rate or improve ventilation are not sufficient to correct acidosis, cautious use of sodium bicarbonate may help return pH to normal range. Note: Adequate circulation (HR >100) must be established.
Surfactant (artificial or exogenous).	May be given at birth or after diagnosis of RDS to decrease severity of condition and associated complications. Effect may last up to 72 hr.
Assist with procedures as needed:	
Needle aspiration, thoracentesis, or chest tube insertion;	Reinflates lung enough through removal of trapped air or fluid, reestablishing negative pressure and enhancing gas exchange.
Indirect ophthalmoscopic fundal exam;	Recommended for all infants less than 36 weeks' gestation or under 2000 g and receiving oxygen therapy. Usually done between 4 and 8 wk of age and

Laser therapy or cryotherapy.

repeated as indicated to diagnose/monitor progression of retinopathy of prematurity and determine therapy needs.

May be useful in limiting adverse effects associated with acute stages of retinopathy of prematurity by obliterating newly forming vessels, reducing traction on the retina and subsequent detachment, and limiting creation of new vessels.

NURSING DIAGNOSIS:	BREATHING PATTERN, ineffective
May Be Related To:	Immaturity of the respiratory center, limited muscular development, decreased energy/fatigue, drug-related depression, and metabolic imbalances
Possibly Evidenced By:	Dyspnea, tachypnea, periods of apnea, nasal flaring, use of accessory muscles, cyanosis, abnormal ABGs, tachycardia
DESIRED OUTCOMES/EVALUATION CRITERIA—NEONATE WILL:	Maintain periodic breathing pattern (apneic periods last 5–10 sec, followed by short periods of rapid ventilation), with mucous membranes pink, and heart rate 110–160/respiratory rate 24–60.

ACTIONS/INTERVENTIONS	RATIONALE

Independent

Assess respiratory rate and breathing pattern. Note presence of apnea and changes in heart rate, muscle tone, and skin color associated with procedures or care. Institute continuous respiratory and cardiac monitoring.

Helps in distinguishing normal cyclic periodic breathing pattern from true apneic spells, which are particularly common prior to 30 weeks' gestation.

Suction airway as needed.

Removes mucus obstructing the airway to maximize respiratory effort.

Review maternal history for drugs that might contribute to respiratory depression in the infant.

Magnesium sulfate and narcotics depress respiratory center and CNS activity.

Position infant on abdomen or in supine position with rolled diaper beneath shoulders to produce slight hyperextension.

Such positioning may facilitate respiration and reduce apneic episodes, especially in the presence of hypoxia, metabolic acidosis, or hypercapnia.

Maintain optimal body temperature. (Refer to ND: Thermoregulation, risk for ineffective.)

Even a slight increase or decrease in environmental temperature can lead to apnea.

Provide prompt tactile stimulation (e.g., rub infant's back) if apnea occurs. Note presence of cyanosis, bradycardia, or hypotonia. Encourage parental contact.

Stimulates CNS to promote body movement and spontaneous return of respirations. Sometimes, infants experience fewer or no episodes of apnea or bradycardia if parents touch and talk to them.

Place infant on neowave mattress.

Movement provides stimulation, which may reduce apneic episodes.

Collaborative

Monitor laboratory studies (e.g., ABGs, serum glucose, electrolytes, cultures, and drug levels) as indicated.

Hypoxia, metabolic acidosis, hypercapnia, hypoglycemia, hypocalcemia, and sepsis may contribute to apneic spells. Drug toxicity, which

503

Administer supplemental oxygen, as indicated. (Refer to ND: Gas Exchange, impaired.)

Administer medications, as indicated:

   Sodium bicarbonate;

   Antibiotics;
   Calcium gluconate;
   Aminophylline;

   Pancuronium bromide (Pavulon);

   Glucose solutions.

depresses respiratory function, may occur because of limited excretion and prolonged drug half-life.

Correction of oxygen and carbon dioxide levels may improve respiratory function.

Judicious use may be required to help correct acidosis, especially after hypoxic episodes, because bicarbonate is excreted at lower serum levels and immature kidneys are slower to excrete lactic acid. Treat respiratory infection or sepsis.
Hypocalcemia predisposes infant to apnea.
May increase activity of respiratory center and lower sensitivity to carbon dioxide, reducing frequency of apnea.
Induces skeletal muscle relaxation, which may be necessary if infant is to be mechanically ventilated.
Prevent hypoglycemia. (Refer to ND: Nutrition: altered, risk for less than body requirements.)

NURSING DIAGNOSIS:	THERMOREGULATION, ineffective
May Be Related To:	Immature CNS development (temperature regulation center), decreased ratio of body mass to surface area, decreased subcutaneous fat, limited brown fat stores, an inability to shiver or sweat, limited/inability to flex extremities, poor metabolic reserves (limited glycogen stores), thinner skin, muted response to hypothermia, and frequent medical/nursing manipulations and interventions
Possibly Evidenced By:	Fluctuation of body temperature below/above normal range
	Tachypnea/apnea, generalized cyanosis, bradycardia, lethargy (cold stress)
	Tachycardia, flushed color, lethargy, apnea (hyperthermia)
DESIRED OUTCOMES/EVALUATION CRITERIA—NEONATE WILL:	Maintain skin/axillary temperature within 97.7°F–99.1°F (36.5°C–37.3°C).
	Be free of signs of cold stress.

ACTIONS/INTERVENTIONS

RATIONALE

Independent

Assess temperature frequently. Check rectal temperature initially; thereafter, check axillary temperature or use thermostat probe with open bed and radiant warmer. Repeat every 15 min during rewarming.

Hypothermia predisposes infant to cold stress, utilization of nonrenewable brown fat stores if present, and reduced sensitivity to increased levels of carbon dioxide (hypercapnia) or decreased oxygen levels (hypoxia). Note: Too rapid rewarming is associated with apneic states. This causes further respiratory depression instead of increased respiratory rate, leading to apnea and reduced oxygen uptake.

Ascertain medications mother received during prenatal and intrapartal periods. Note presence of fetal distress or hypoxia.

Fetal hypoxia or maternal use of meperidine (Demerol) alters fetal metabolism of brown fat, often causing significant drop in neonate's temperature. Magnesium sulfate can cause vasodilation and interfere with infant's ability to retain heat.

Place infant in warmer, Isolette, incubator, open bed with radiant warmer, or open crib with appropriate clothing for larger or older infants. Use heating pad under infant as necessary, in conjunction with Isolette or open bed.

Maintains thermoneutral environment, helps prevent cold stress.

Use heat lamps during procedures. Warm objects coming in contact with infant's body, such as stethoscopes, linens, and clothing. Use blanket/diaper to pad cold surfaces such as scale, examination table, x-ray plate, and hands. Surround infant with warmed receiving blankets. Cover radiant warmers with plastic wrap, if appropriate. Warm blood products, if administered.

Decreases loss of heat to the cooler environment of the room/treatment surfaces, or by infusion of chilled blood.

Reduce exposure to drafts; avoid unnecessary opening of portholes in Isolette.

Reduces heat losses due to convection/conduction. Limits heat losses from radiation.

Change clothing or bed linens when wet. Keep infant's head covered.

Decreases evaporative losses.

Note environmental temperature/monitor temperature-regulating system, radiant warmers, or incubators. (Maintain upper limit at 98.6°F [37°C], depending on infant's size or age.)

Hyperthermia with resultant increases in metabolic rate, oxygen and glucose needs, and insensible water losses can occur when controlled environmental temperatures are too high. Conversely, a decrease in the environmental temperature of 3.6°F (2°C) also results in significant increase of oxygen consumption and glucose needs.

Maintain relative humidity of 50%–80%. Warm humidified oxygen to 88°F–93°F (31°C–34°C).

Prevents excessive evaporation, reducing insensible fluid losses.

Note presence of tachypnea or apnea; generalized cyanosis, acrocyanosis, or mottled skin; bradycardia, poor cry, or lethargy. Evaluate degree and location of jaundice. (Refer to CP: Newborn: Hyperbilirubinemia.)

These signs indicate cold stress, which increases oxygen and caloric consumption and predisposes infant to acidosis associated with anaerobic metabolism. Hypothermia increases risk of kernicterus, as fatty acids released with brown fat metabolism compete with bilirubin for binding sites on albumin. Note: Skin color may be bright red peripherally, with cyanosis noted centrally as a result of failure of dissociation of oxyhemoglobin.

Provide gradual warming for infant with cold stress.

Rapid increase in body temperature may cause excessive oxygen consumption and apnea.

Measure urine output and specific gravity.

Reduced urine output and increased specific gravity of urine are related to reduced kidney perfusion during periods of cold stress. Note: Use of radiant heat for warming, for longer than a few hours, potentiates water loss decreasing circulating volume and renal perfusion.

Monitor serial weight gain. If weight gain is inadequate, increase environmental temperature as indicated.

Inadequate weight gain despite sufficient caloric intake may indicate that calories are being used to maintain body temperature, necessitating increased environmental temperature. Note: Excessive warming also increases metabolic demands as infant attempts to cool down.

Note frequency and amount of food intake. Monitor Dextrostix. Assess infant for vomiting, abdominal distension, or apathy.

Poor feeding is common in infants with thermal instability; in addition, cold stress increases consumption of metabolic reserves. Dextrostix levels <45 mg/dl indicate hypoglycemia, necessitating prompt intervention.

Assess infant's progressive ability to adapt to lowered temperatures in incubator or Isolette, or to room temperature, while demonstrating appropriate weight gains.

Bassinet may be used when infant can maintain stable body temperature of 97.7°F (36.5°C) in room air and still gain weight.

Monitor infant's temperature when out of warmed environment. Provide parents with information about thermoregulation.

Out-of-bed contact, especially with parents, may need to be brief, if allowed at all, to prevent cold stress. Note: Hyperthermia can also occur when infant is held by parents.

Note development of tachycardia, flushed color, diaphoresis, lethargy, apnea, coma, or seizure activity.

These signs of hyperthermia (body temperature >99°F [37.2°C]) can progress to brain damage, if untreated.

Evaluate external sources of heat (e.g., phototherapy, heat lamp, or sunlight), limit clothing, and provide tepid sponge bath, as appropriate. Verify proper positioning of temperature probe, if used.

These measures are generally successful in correcting hyperthermia. Note: If hyperthermia persists after assuring proper position and functioning of temperature probe, the possibility of a hypermetabolic state such as sepsis or narcotic withdrawal should be considered.

Collaborative

Monitor pulse oximetry, laboratory studies, as indicated (e.g., ABGs, serum glucose, electrolytes, and bilirubin levels). (Refer to ND: Gas Exchange, impaired.)

Cold stress increases the needs for glucose and oxygen and may result in acid-base problems if infant resorts to anaerobic metabolism when sufficient oxygen levels are not available. Elevated indirect bilirubin levels may occur because of the release of fatty acids from brown fat metabolism, with fatty acids competing with bilirubin for binding sites on albumin. Metabolic acidosis may also occur with hyperthermia.

Administer $D_{10}W$ and volume expanders IV, as needed.

Administration of dextrose may be necessary to correct hypoglycemia. Hypotension caused by peripheral vasodilation may require treatment in heat-stressed infant. Hyperthermia may cause a threefold to fourfold increase in dehydration.

Provide supplemental oxygen as indicated.

If oxygen is not readily available to meet increased metabolic needs associated with efforts to increase body temperature, the infant will use anaerobic metabolism, resulting in acidosis caused by lactic acid buildup. Hypothermia reduces the preterm infant's response to hypoxia and hypercapnia, which causes further respiratory depression instead of increased respiratory rate, leading to apnea and reduced oxygen uptake. Hyperthermia caused by too rapid/excessive warming is associated with apneic states, increased insensible water losses, and increased metabolic rates with increased demands for oxygen and glucose.

Administer medications, as indicated:

Phenobarbital;

Helps prevent seizures associated with CNS irritation caused by hyperthermia.

Sodium bicarbonate.

Corrects acidosis, which may occur with both hypothermia and hyperthermia.

NURSING DIAGNOSIS:	FLUID VOLUME, risk for deficit
Risk Factors May Include:	Extremes of age and weight (premature, under 2500 g), excessive fluid losses (thin skin, lack of insulating fat, increased environmental temperature, immature kidney/failure to concentrate urine)
Possibly Evidenced By:	[Not applicable; presence of signs/symptoms establishes an *actual* diagnosis]
DESIRED OUTCOMES/EVALUATION CRITERIA—NEONATE WILL:	Be free of signs of dehydration or glycosuria with fluid intake approximating output and pH, Hct, and urine specific gravity WNL. Display weight gain of 20–30 g/day.

ACTIONS/INTERVENTIONS

Independent

Obtain daily serial weights using same scale at same time of day.

Calculate fluid balance (total intake minus total output) each shift and cumulative balance each 24-hr period. Maintain hourly records of infusing IV fluids/feedings. Determine output through measuring urine from collecting bag or through weighing/counting diapers. Also record amount of blood taken for laboratory testing.

Measure urine specific gravity after each voiding, or every 2–4 hr, by aspirating urine from diaper if infant cannot tolerate adhesive or urine collecting bag.

Test urine with Dextrostix per protocol.

Minimize insensible fluid losses through use of clothing, thermoneutral temperatures, and warm or humidified oxygen.

Monitor BP, pulse, and mean arterial pressure (MAP).

RATIONALE

Weight is the most sensitive indicator of fluid balance. Weight loss should not exceed 15% of total body weight or 1%–2% of total body weight per day. Inadequate weight gain may be related to water imbalance or inadequate caloric intake.

Output should be 1–3 ml/kg/hr, while fluid therapy needs are approximately 80–100 ml/kg/day on the 1st day of life, increasing to 120–140 ml/kg/day by the 3rd day after delivery. Lower gestational age has a negative impact on the glomerular filtration rate (GFR) and is further limited by conditions that impair renal blood flow or oxygen content (e.g., dehydration, respiratory distress), often resulting in oliguria/anuria. Positive fluid balance and corresponding weight gain in excess of 20–30 g/day suggest fluid excess.

Although renal immaturity and inability to concentrate urine usually result in low specific gravity in the preterm infant (normal range is 1.006–1.013), urine specific gravity may vary, providing an indication of the level of hydration. Low levels indicate excessive fluid volume; levels >1.013 indicate insufficient fluid intake and dehydration.

Even in cases of hypoglycemia, glycosuria occurs as immature kidneys begin excreting glucose, which may lead to osmotic diuresis, increasing risk of dehydration.

Preterm infant loses large amounts of water through skin, because blood vessels are close to surface and insulating fat levels are decreased or absent. Phototherapy or use of radiant warmer may increase insensible losses by 50%, necessitating increased intake to as much as 200 ml/kg/day. Note: Infants weighing <1500 g (3 lb 5 oz) are most susceptible to insensible fluid losses.

A loss of 25% of blood volume results in shock, with MAP of less than 25 mm Hg indicating hypotension.

507

Evaluate skin turgor, mucous membranes, and status of anterior fontanel.

Note lethargy, high-pitched cry, abdominal distension, increased apnea, twitching, hypotonia, or seizure activity.

Assess IV site every hour. Note edema or failure of fluid infusion. Do not check needle position by lowering fluid below needle level.

Monitor infusion rate closely and use pumps to administer fluids.

Institute measures to prevent infection. (Refer to ND: Infection, risk for.)

Collaborative

Monitor laboratory studies as indicated:

Hct;

Serum calcium and serum magnesium;

Serum potassium;

Blood urea nitrogen (BUN), creatinine, and uric acid levels.

Administer parenteral infusions in amounts >180 ml/kg, especially in PDA, bronchopulmonary dysplasia (BPD), or necrotizing enterocolitis (NEC).

Administer potassium chloride, 10% calcium gluconate, and 50% magnesium sulfate, as indicated. Monitor infant for potential bradycardia via cardiac monitor; observe infusion site for signs of irritation or edema.

Note: BP is related to weight, that is, the smaller the baby, the lower the MAP.

Fluid reserves are limited in the preterm infant. Minimal fluid losses/shifts can quickly lead to dehydration, as noted by poor skin turgor, dry mucous membranes, and depressed (sunken) fontanels.

These signs reflect hypocalcemia, which is most likely to occur during the first 10 days of life.

Swelling may indicate that infiltration of fluid is occurring or that tape is too tight. Back-up of blood caused by lowering fluid may clog needle.

Verifies accuracy of infusion rate to meet individual needs of infant and to prevent excess intake. Note: Limited ability of kidneys to excrete excess fluid increases risks of overhydration with cardiac or respiratory involvement as noted by presence of crackles, rhonchi, dyspnea, tachypnea, and/or peripheral edema.

Infection places increased demands on an already-compromised renal system.

Dehydration increases Hct level beyond the normal reading of 45%–53%. Removal of blood for testing causes reduction in Hb/Hct levels.

Preterm infant is susceptible to hypocalcemia (calcium level <7 mg/dl) because of low stores, depressed parathyroid stimulation, and stress caused by hypoxia, sepsis, or hypoglycemia. Hypomagnesemia often accompanies hypocalcemia. Hypokalemia may occur because of losses through nasogastric tube, diarrhea, or vomiting. Excessive levels of potassium (hyperkalemia) can result from replacement errors, potassium shifts from intracellular to extracellular compartments, acidosis, or renal failure.

Assesses adequacy of kidney function.

Fluid replacement expands blood volume; helps reverse vasoconstriction associated with hypoxia, acidosis, and right-to-left shunting through PDA; and has been helpful in reducing complications of NEC and BPD.

Correction of electrolyte imbalances is necessary to maintain or achieve homeostasis. Calcium administered through umbilical venous catheter may cause liver necrosis; if administered through umbilical artery, it may contribute to NEC. Early recognition and prompt intervention may limit untoward effects of infiltration of medication, such as sloughing, calcification, and necrosis. Note: Calcium replacement is ineffective in presence of magnesium deficit.

Administer blood transfusions.	May be necessary to maintain optimal Hb/Hct levels and replace blood losses.
Administer dopamine hydrochloride, as indicated.	May be used to counteract drops in blood pressure, especially when related to administration of pancuronium (Pavulon).

NURSING DIAGNOSIS:	**NUTRITION: altered, risk for less than body requirements**
Risk Factors May Include:	Immaturity of enzymatic production; reduced production of hydrochloric acid (reduces absorption of fat and fat-soluble vitamins); immaturity of the cardiac sphincter; lax abdominal muscles; small stomach capacity; weak, absent, or unsynchronized reflexes associated with feeding; inadequate levels of stored nutrients
Possibly Evidenced By:	[Not applicable; presence of signs/symptoms establishes an *actual* diagnosis]
DESIRED OUTCOMES/EVALUATION CRITERIA—NEONATE WILL:	Maintain growth and weight gain in a normal curve, with steady weight gain of at least 20–30 g/day.
	Maintain serum glucose WNL and positive nitrogen balance.

ACTIONS/INTERVENTIONS	RATIONALE

Independent

Assess maturity of reflexes associated with feeding (ie., sucking, swallowing, gag, and coughing).	Determines appropriate feeding method for infant.
Auscultate for presence of bowel sounds. Assess physical state and respiratory status.	The first feeding in a stable infant with peristalsis can begin 3–6 hr following birth. If respiratory distress is present, parenteral fluids are indicated, and oral fluids should be withheld.
Initiate intermittent or tube feedings, as indicated.	Gavage feedings may be necessary to provide adequate nutrition in infant who has a poorly coordinated suck-and-swallow reflex or who becomes fatigued during oral feedings. Note: Transition to oral feeding is significantly delayed if apneic episodes are experienced.
Assess infant for proper placement of feeding tube; use appropriate clamping procedures to prevent entry of air into stomach.	Improper placement of tube in trachea can compromise respiratory function. When 1 ml or less is aspirated from the stomach, this sum should be subtracted from the feeding and reinstilled in tube. When more than 2 ml is aspirated, feeding schedule may need to be altered.
Instill breast milk/formula slowly over 20 min at a rate of 1 ml/min.	Too-rapid entry of feeding into stomach may cause rapid rebound response with regurgitation, increased risk of aspiration, and abdominal distension, all of which compromise respiratory status.
Assess energy level and expenditure, degree of fatigability, respiratory rate, and length of time needed for feedings.	Excessive expenditure of energy during feedings reduces calories available for normal growth and development. Total or intermittent use of tube feedings

509

Minimize social interaction stimuli other than those directly related to feeding if infant displays signs of sensory overload. Reduce stimuli prior to feedings.

may be necessary to reduce fatigue. Oral feedings are not appropriate if respiratory rate is >70/min.

Excessive stimulation may interfere with feeding, so that the necessary stimuli must be provided between feedings. Overstimulation prior to feedings may negatively affect sucking and GI motility and may cause vomiting or regurgitation.

Provide pacifier during tube feedings. (If baby is going to be breastfed eventually, mother may rub pacifier on breast, moistening it with a dab of breast milk to scent it. She may also hold the baby during feedings.)

Accommodates infant's need for sucking. Provides oral satisfaction so that infant associates self-gratification in sucking with comfort of filling stomach.

Position infant on right side or prone, with head of mattress elevated 30 degrees.

Facilitates gastric emptying and prevents reflux.

Postpone postural drainage for at least 1 hr after feeding.

Allows optimal ingestion and absorption of feeding; helps prevent regurgitation associated with increased handling.

Note presence of diarrhea, vomiting, regurgitation, excessive gastric residual, or positive result of guaiac test. (Refer to ND: Constipation/Diarrhea, risk for.)

Indicates impaired gastric function. Gastric residual greater than 2 ml (aspirated via gavage tube before feedings) suggests a need to reduce amount of feedings and may indicate poor absorption or NEC.

Monitor Dextrostix levels and urine Clinitest per protocol.

Because the immature liver does not store or release glycogen well, risk of hypoglycemia is increased. Hypoglycemia can be diagnosed by a Dextrostix level <45 mg/dl. Note: Infant may be asymptomatic, even when Dextrostix results are as low as 20 mg/dl.

Maintain thermoneutral environment and appropriate oxygenation of tissues. Disturb infant as little as possible.

Cold stress, hypoxia, and excessive handling increase infant's metabolic rate and caloric needs, possibly sacrificing growth and weight gains.

Monitor infant for local or systemic reactions to parenteral feeding (e.g., increased temperature, dyspnea, vomiting, cyanosis, or blood vessel thrombosis).

About 50% of complications associated with total parenteral nutrition (TPN) are caused by sepsis, usually *Candida* septicemia. Other complications include fluid overload and obstruction or dislodgement of catheter.

Record growth by plotting daily weight and weekly measurements of body length and head circumference.

Growth and weight gain are criteria for establishing caloric requirements, for adjusting formula, and for determining frequency of feedings. Growth spurts increase caloric requirements and protein needs.

Encourage/support mother's efforts to pump and collect own breast milk. Identify additional resources.

Breast milk is easy to digest (reduces potential for NEC), and research suggests it boosts infant immunities and is associated with reduced occurrence of allergic food reactions, fewer ear infections, lower rate of childhood cancer. Note: There are seven breast-milk banks that can be contacted through the Human Milk Banking Association of North America (Fax 1-860-232-0113) to obtain supplements for infant, educational material, or to refer mother as potential donor if infant is not able to use breast milk presently and mother wishes to maintain lactation.

Collaborative

Start feedings of sterile water, glucose, and breast milk or formula, as appropriate.

Early feedings prevent depletion of reserves.

Feed as frequently as indicated based on infant's weight and estimated stomach capacity.

Infants <1250 g (2 lb 12 oz) are usually fed every 2 hr; infants between 1500 and 1800 g (3 lb 8 oz to 4 lb) are fed every 3 hr.

Use concentrated formula to provide 120–150 cal/kg/day or more, with 3–4 g/kg/day of protein. Add human milk fortifiers (HMF) to breast milk for gavage feeding, as needed.

Calorie intake must be sufficient to prevent catabolism. Concentrated formulas/fortified breast milk supply more calories in less volume, which is necessary because of reduced gastric capacity and emptying, and the danger of stressing immature kidneys. Note: Sick infants may require half-strength formula initially with volume/concentration advanced over 1–10 days, as infant tolerates.

Administer supplemental vitamins and minerals, especially vitamins A, C, D, and E, and iron, as indicated.

Replaces low nutrient stores to promote adequate nutrition and reduce risk of infection. Vitamin C may reduce susceptibility to hemolytic anemia and alleviate BPD and retrolental fibroplasia. Vitamin D facilitates retention of calcium and increased bone density. Vitamin E helps prevent RBC hemolysis and corrects deficiencies associated with use of iron-fortified formulas and diet high in polyunsaturated fats.

Maintain patency; assist with change of indwelling feeding tube (transpyloric, nasojejunal, nasoduodenal tubes).

Provides continuous infusion of formula in very small preterm infants who meet specific criteria; e.g., tachypnea, chronic lung disease, respirator dependence, recurrent aspiration, or repeated elevated gastric residuals with other feeding approaches. Note: Potential risks accompanying use of these indwelling tubes (e.g., gastric/intestinal perforation) must be weighed against benefits.

Administer TPN feedings via infusion pump using indwelling catheter into vena cava or peripheral line. Infuse fat emulsions (Intralipid) through peripheral line.

TPN infusion of protein hydrolysate, glucose, electrolytes, minerals, and vitamins may be necessary for infant with chronic diarrhea; malabsorption syndrome; surgical repair of GI anomalies, obstruction, or NEC; or extreme prematurity. Intralipid infusion provides essential fatty acids to infant receiving TPN. Note: Benefits of using Intralipid must be weighed against possible risk of fat accumulation in the lungs.

Monitor laboratory studies, e.g., serum glucose, electrolytes, total protein, prealbumin.

Measures necessity for and effectiveness of TPN administration.

NURSING DIAGNOSIS:	**INFANT BEHAVIOR, risk for disorganized**
Risk Factors May Include:	Prematurity (immaturity of CNS system, hypoxia), environmental overstimulation, invasive/painful procedures and therapies, separation from parent(s)
Possibly Evidenced By:	[Not applicable; presence of signs/symptoms establishes an *actual* diagnosis]
DESIRED OUTCOMES/EVALUATION CRITERIA—NEONATE WILL:	Exhibit organized behaviors that allow the achievement of optimal potential for growth and development as evidenced by modulation of physiological, motor, state, and attentional-interactive functioning.

ACTIONS/INTERVENTIONS	RATIONALE

Independent

ACTIONS/INTERVENTIONS	RATIONALE
Determine infant's chronological and developmental age; note length of gestation. Assess individual behaviors using appropriate tool (e.g., assessment of Preterm Infant Behavior Scale).	Useful in choosing interventions to meet specific needs of infant and reduce detrimental environmental stimuli. The APIB scale measures five areas of developmental behaviors, autonomic, motor control, state differentiation, attention maintenance and social interaction, self-regulation.
Provide a primary nurse for each shift. (Assign one primary nurse per baby to provide information to parents.)	Promotes continuity of care and follow-through with developmental program. Enhances recognition of subtle changes in infant's behavior and condition. Consistent and predictable care enables infant to develop trust in caregiver, environment, and self and facilitates coping. Multiple caretakers confuse the infant, increase distress during feeding, cause irritability, and upset usual attention. Note: Having one nurse responsible for giving information helps to reduce instances of parents' being uninformed or misunderstanding.
Create womblike atmosphere whenever possible by covering Isolette for extended periods, playing recorded placental or maternal heart sounds, and surrounding infant with rolled blankets or manufactured "nesting" device.	Providing dark, quiet environment reduces stress, promotes adaptation, and has been found to correlate positively with weight gain, early weaning from oxygen or ventilators, and earlier discharge. Recorded maternal heart sounds tend to reduce or eliminate infant's perception of noise from the Isolette. Nesting position facilitates hand-to-mouth behavior for self-consoling.
Cover top of radiant warmer with plastic wrap, if appropriate.	Reduces environmental stress from air currents, which startle the infant as personnel move past the warmer.
Reposition infant using rolled diapers placed at the back and front, if infant is in lateral position, or at sides, if infant can tolerate a prone position.	Neuromuscular immaturity can impair infant's ability to seek a position of comfort or to relieve stress through repositioning. Rolled diapers surrounding baby provide a sense of security and have a calming effect. Prone position promotes sleep and optimal relaxation.
Change infant's position periodically (especially if infant has nasal CPAP or endotracheal tube).	Provides kinesthetic stimulation. Neuromuscularly immature infant is unable to reposition self or move about in the Isolette.
Use containment measures when handling/moving infant and avoid sudden postural changes.	Using hands to hold infant's arms and legs in flexed position close to midline of body helps stabilize infant's motor and physiological subsystems.
Provide gentle stroking and caressing, especially at feeding time, introducing textures (tongue blade, washcloth), as appropriate.	Provides tactile stimulation, which is associated with weight gains and is especially critical when infant is 40 weeks after conception or more. Note: Slow, sure movements provide stimulation while reducing motor disorganization.
Provide pacifier/enable hand-to-mouth activity after feedings.	Nonnutritive sucking provides calming effect, decreases body movement, enhances sleep, and increases weight gain.
Talk or quietly sing to infant, call infant by name, play soft music in nursery, or play a tape of parent(s) voice.	Provides auditory stimulation. Playing tape of parents' voices may enhance infant's recognition of them.

Interact with infant at face level (en face interaction), allowing eye contact. Provide colorful linens and changing designs or pictures on side of incubator, and encourage parents to make mobiles of construction paper and string once infant reaches postconception age of 40 wk.

Visual stimulation is best provided by objects placed 7–9 in from face. Black and white faces and a checkerboard design promote visual attention. Infant may become habituated to stimuli that do not change. Involving parents in creating stimuli for infant helps ensure that the process continues after discharge.

Hold infant in ventral position (e.g., baby held to shoulder to burp) when possible, uncover eyes periodically if infant is receiving phototherapy.

Enhances visual stimulation/orientation.

Encourage periodic skin-to-skin contact, as appropriate (i.e., mother holds diaper-clad infant upright between her bare breasts).

Research suggest kangaroo-care technique not only provides closeness, strengthening mother-infant attachment, but also reduces periodic breathing and promotes deep sleep.

Assess infant for physiological signs/behavioral cues indicating stress (e.g., apnea, color change, bradycardia, sneezing, yawning), irritability or apathy, change in muscle tension, disorganized motor activity and sleep-wake cycles, measured change in sensory acuity), noting causative factors and eliminating or reducing stressors when possible.

Disorganization of the autonomic system is often associated with prematurity, resulting in some infants lacking the developmental capability of dealing with more than one sensory input at a time. Familiarity with the infant's usual behavioral responses and personality traits is necessary for identifying subtle changes that indicate stress and the need for intervention to modify causative factors.

Plan activities to allow periods of sleep. Prevent loud noises, limit conversation near bedside, respond to alarms quickly; and reduce light intermittently by covering incubator with towel, shielding infant's eyes, or lowering room lighting.

Helps protect infant from overstimulation, which can negatively affect growth and physiological status; promotes infant's sense of the day-night cycle. Note: Research reveals cycled lighting lowers infant's heart rate and motor activity, promoting longer periods of quiet inactivity resembling quiet sleep, and conserving energy.

Weigh infant daily. Note feeding frequency and intake and frequency of stools.

Vagal stimulation produced by appropriate tactile and kinesthetic stimulation promotes weight gain, increases peristalsis and expulsion of waste products, reduces gastric retention, and increases feeding activity.

Note risk factors of birth weight, coexisting conditions, and associated therapies.

Retinopathy of prematurity is no longer believed to be exclusively the result of prolonged/high levels of oxygen therapy. Immaturity, presence of some congenital anomalies, and various therapies place the infant at risk. Note: Infants with birth weight <1000 g have an 88% incidence of retinopathy.

Provide parents with information about infant's behavioral cues and responses to stressors. (Refer to CP: The Parents of a Child With Special Needs; ND: Parent/Infant Attachment, risk for altered.)

Parents must gain skill in recognizing subtle infant cues indicating stress so that they can effectively intervene to minimize stress and facilitate the infant's positive adaptation to extrauterine life. Awareness that visually impaired infant may not show recognition or feelings by changes in facial expression encourages parent(s) to observe body language/other cues reflecting self-expression, thereby strengthening the attachment bond.

Collaborative

Provide rocking or water beds, if indicated.

Kinesthetic stimulation in preterm infants of <34 weeks' gestation has been shown to improve sleep, decrease heart rate, reduce frequency of state changes, and increase head size and biparietal diameter.

ACTIONS/INTERVENTIONS	RATIONALE
Independent	
Assess respiratory effort. Note presence of pallor or cyanosis.	Respiratory distress and hypoxia affect cerebral function and may damage or weaken walls of cerebral blood vessels, increasing risk of rupture. If untreated, hypoxia may result in permanent damage. (Refer to ND: Gas Exchange, impaired.)
Monitor Dextrostix levels, and observe infant for behaviors indicating hypocalcemia or hypoglycemia (such as convulsions, twitching, myoclonic jerks, or eye rolling.) (Refer to ND: Nutrition: altered, risk for less than body requirements.)	Because of its demands for glucose, the brain may suffer irreparable damage when serum glucose levels are lower than 30–40 mg/dl. Hypocalcemia (serum calcium levels <7 mg/dl) often accompanies hypoglycemia and may result in apnea and seizures.
Observe infant for alterations in CNS function, as manifested by behavior changes, lethargy, hypotonia, bulging or tense fontanel, eye rolling, or seizure activity. Investigate deteriorating status indicated by high-pitched cry, labored respirations, and cyanosis, followed by apnea, flaccid quadriparesis, unresponsiveness, hypotension, tonic posturing, and areflexia.	Birth trauma, fragile capillaries, and impaired coagulation processes place preterm infant at risk for IVH, especially those infants weighing <1500 g or under 34 weeks' gestation. Tense or bulging anterior fontanel may be first sign of IVH, hemorrhagic shock, or increased intracranial pressure (IICP), which can easily lead to death from circulatory collapse. Infant of <32 weeks' gestation may become lethargic or hypotonic and may manifest uncontrolled "roving-eye" movements and lack of visual tracking. Note: Clinical signs of developing IVH may be absent, very subtle, or sudden and life-threatening.
Measure head circumference, as indicated.	Helps detect possible IICP or hydrocephalus, which may be a sequela of subdural hemorrhage. Only 35%–50% of infants with hydrocephalus develop normally.
Assess skin color, noting evidence of increasing jaundice associated with behavior changes such as lethargy, hyperreflexia, convulsions, and opisthotonos. (Refer to CP: Newborn: Hyperbilirubinemia.)	Preterm infant is more susceptible to kernicterus at lower serum bilirubin levels than full-term infant because of increased levels of unconjugated circulating bilirubin crossing the blood-brain barrier.
Collaborative	
Monitor laboratory studies, as indicated:	
Hb/Hct; ABGs;	Lowered Hb levels or anemia reduce oxygen-carrying capacity, increasing risk of permanent CNS

Bilirubin levels.

damage associated with hypoxemia. Abrupt fall in Hct may be first indicator of IVH. Note: Pulse oximetry may be used to monitor O$_2$ level routinely with periodic ABGs to monitor other parameters of acid/base balance.
Rapidly rising levels may result in kernicterus if not treated promptly.

Provide supplemental oxygen.

Hypoxemia increases the risk of impairment or permanent CNS damage.

Assist with diagnostic or therapeutic procedures, as indicated:

Computerized tomography (CT) scanning, cranial ultrasonography;

Identifies presence/extent of hemorrhage, which is useful in predicting likelihood of long-term complications and in choice of treatment.

Lumbar puncture;

A bloody CSF specimen confirms IVH. Some hospitals carry out serial daily lumbar punctures to reduce ICP and prevent deleterious effects of hydrocephalus.

Exchange transfusion;

Elevated or rapidly rising bilirubin levels indicate the need for a double-volume exchange transfusion with O-negative blood to remove bilirubin and to prevent further hemolysis of RBCs.

Ventriculopuncture or taps;

May be used to remove excess blood from the ventricles, although studies have not indicated any corresponding improvement in outcome.

Placement of ventriculoperitoneal shunt.

Progressive ventricular dilation unresponsive to other measures may require surgical intervention to correct or prevent hydrocephalus.

Administer medications, as indicated:

Calcium, magnesium, sodium bicarbonate, and/or glucose;

Correction of imbalances helps prevent neonatal seizure activity, which may occur in response to transient metabolic imbalances.

Phenobarbital;

Helps to control acute convulsions and status epilepticus in newborn.

Phenytoin or diazepam (Valium);

May be used if other antiepileptic drugs are not successful in controlling seizure activity. Note: Dosage should be based on blood levels.

Furosemide (Lasix), acetazolamide (Diamox), or steroids;
Vitamin E;

Helps reduce intracranial pressure and treats secondary effects of bleeding.
Antioxidant property protects RBC membranes against hemolysis.

Indomethacin (Indacin).

IV administration may correct hemodynamic imbalances through closure of PDA.

Assist with fluid replacement or maintain restrictions, as appropriate.

Cerebral perfusion depends on adequate circulatory volume. Note: Fluids may need to be restricted in cases of hypertonicity, CNS damage with bleeding, or cerebral palsy.

Perform/obtain results of car-seat test prior to discharge.

Car-seat test is performed by nursing staff or occupational therapist (OT) on infant <2500 g or <37 weeks' gestation. Infant is placed in car seat for 2 hr. During that time, infant is monitored for possible apnea, bradycardia, or oxygen desaturation. Infant is surrounded by precut foam forms or rolled receiving blankets to keep the head in a neutral, upright position.

ACTIONS/INTERVENTIONS	RATIONALE

Independent

Review record of delivery to determine whether resuscitative measures were required, length of rupture of membranes, and presence of chorioamnionitis. Note maternal GBS status and/or other sexually transmitted diseases (STDs) present.	Infant who has been resuscitated and has required invasive interventions is especially prone to introduction of pathogens and infection. Maternal factors such as PROM with preterm labor and delivery possibly caused by an infectious process predispose the preterm infant to ascending infection. Early-onset sepsis (occurring within the first 2 days of life) is affected by host defenses and duration of antepartal rupture of membranes. Transplacentally acquired infections (which affect two-thirds of all infected infants) are also a threat.
Determine gestational age of fetus, using Dubowitz criteria.	Delivery prior to 28–30 weeks' gestation increases infant's susceptibility to infection, because of reduced ability of WBCs to destroy bacteria, reduced transfer of IgG (IgG is transported across the placenta primarily in the third trimester), lack of IgA if infant does not receive breast milk, and poorly keratinized skin with ineffective barrier qualities. Note: Infant who suffers from intrauterine growth retardation/restriction is at greater risk for infection.
Promote meticulous hand washing by staff, parents, and ancillary workers per protocol. Use antiseptic before assisting with surgical or invasive procedure.	Hand washing is the most important practice for preventing cross-contamination and controlling infection in the nursery.
Monitor staff and visitors for presence of skin lesions, draining wounds, acute respiratory infections, fever, gastroenteritis, active herpes simplex (oral, genital, or paronychial), and herpes zoster.	Transmission of disease to neonate by employees or visitors can occur directly or indirectly.
Provide adequate space between infants or between Isolettes or individual units. Use separate isolation rooms and isolation technique, as indicated.	Providing 4–6 ft of space between infants helps prevent spread of droplet or airborne infections.
Assess infant for signs of infection, such as temperature instability (hypothermia or hyperthermia), lethargy or behavior changes,	Useful in the diagnosis of infection; body temperature alone is an unreliable means of assessing infection in the preterm infant with

respiratory distress (apnea, cyanosis, or tachypnea), jaundice, petechiae, nasal congestion, or drainage from eyes or umbilicus.

Establish a cohort of infants, when possible, and ensure that same nurse cares for the infants grouped together.

impaired inflammatory response and WBC mobilization.

Infants who are born within the same time frame (usually 24–48 hr), or who are colonized/infected with the same pathogen, may be grouped together until discharge. Such grouping is an important measure in infection control in that it limits the amount of contact of one infant with other susceptible infants or personnel.

Perform care of umbilical cord according to hospital protocol.

Local application of alcohol, triple dye, or various antimicrobials helps prevent colonization.

Prepare site(s) of invasive procedures with alcohol (70%), tincture of iodine, or iodophor. Monitor IV infusion site(s) and sites of invasive monitoring lines per protocol.

Reduces incidence of possible phlebitis or bacteremia.

Use aseptic technique during suctioning. Date the opened solution for humidification, irrigation, or nebulization, and discard after 24 hr. Ensure routine cleaning or replacement of respiratory equipment.

Reduces opportunity for introduction of bacteria that could result in respiratory infection.

Treat arterial line, stopcocks, and catheter as sterile fields; draw all blood specimens at the same time, when possible.

Helps prevent bacteriemia associated with arterial line and its direct access to blood and deep tissues.

Monitor infant for signs of late-onset disease or infection.

Late-onset disease may occur as early as the 5th day, but usually occurs after the 1st wk of life. Signs of late-onset infection are likely to be caused by bacteria acquired from the maternal genital tract, or from human contact or contaminated equipment/supplies after birth.

Observe for signs of shock or DIC, such as bradycardia, decreasing BP, temperature instability, listlessness, edema, or erythema of abdominal wall.

DIC may occur with gram-negative septicemia.

Provide breast milk for feeding, if available.

Breast milk contains IgA, macrophages, lymphocytes, and neutrophils, which provide some protection from infection.

Collaborative

Obtain specimens as indicated (e.g., urine through suprapubic aspiration, blood, CSF, visible skin lesions, nasopharynx, or sputum, if infant is intubated).

Cultures/sensitivity tests are necessary to diagnose pathogens and identify appropriate therapy.

Monitor laboratory studies, as indicated:

Serial WBC count and differential;

Prematurity reduces the immune response to infection. WBC count in preterm infant varies from 6000 to 225,000/mm^3 and may change from day to day, limiting diagnostic reliability. A marked and sudden increase or decrease in WBCs or band cells may suggest infection.

Platelet count;

Sepsis causes platelet count to drop, but in the preterm infant, the normal platelet range may be 60,000 (in the first 3 days) to 100,000/mm^3.

Serum glucose and pH levels.

Hypoglycemia, hyperglycemia, or metabolic acidosis (with bicarbonate levels <21 mEq/L) suggests infection.

ACTIONS/INTERVENTIONS	RATIONALE
Administer antibiotics IV based on results of culture and sensitivity.	Broad-spectrum antibiotic coverage with ampicillin and an aminoglycoside is usually initiated, pending results of culture and sensitivity tests. Indiscriminate or inappropriate use of systemic antibiotics may cause undesirable side effects, foster emergence of resistant bacterial strains, and alter the newborn's normal flora.
Monitor drug levels, especially if infant is receiving gentamicin or nafcillin.	Kidney immaturity inhibits or retards drug excretion, so that in the preterm infant, toxicity can occur more quickly and at lower levels than in the full-term infant.
Assure proper amount and concentration of supplemental formula.	Human milk contains less renal solute than does cow's milk. Kidney may be unable to handle formula with excess concentration of solute.
Assist with lumbar puncture, as needed.	Helps identify organism and site of infection when meningitis is suspected.
Assist with treatment for possible conditions associated with infection, for example, hypoxemia, thermal abnormalities, electrolyte and acid-base imbalances, anemia, or shock.	Associated physiological events and sequelae may be as life-threatening to the infant as the infection itself.
Administer IV Ig as appropriate.	Research suggests IV administration of Ig may increase survival rates in septic infants. In addition, prophylactic therapy for infants weighing <1500 g may reduce incidence of late-onset nosocomial infections.

NURSING DIAGNOSIS:	**CONSTIPATION/DIARRHEA, risk for**
Risk Factors May Include:	Dietary/fluid intake, physical inactivity, weak abdominal musculature, altered gastric motility
Possibly Evidenced By:	[Not applicable; presence of signs/symptoms establishes an *actual* diagnosis]
DESIRED OUTCOMES/EVALUATION CRITERIA—NEONATE WILL:	Establish customary bowel habits, dependent on type of feeding, with abdomen soft and nondistended.
	Be free of signs of NEC and *Clostridium difficile* organism.

ACTIONS/INTERVENTIONS	RATIONALE
Independent	
Consider frequency and characteristics of stool in relation to infant's age and type of feeding. Auscultate bowel sounds. Measure abdominal girth, reporting any increase of 1 cm or more from previous measurement.	Decreased bowel functioning and GI motility result in infrequent stools and abdominal distension.
Note presence of risk factors, such as hypoxia, sepsis, or circulatory problems associated with PDA. (Refer to NDs: Gas Exchange, impaired; Infection, risk for.)	These conditions can contribute to development of NEC. Recent findings suggest that the development of NEC is related to developmental and gestational age.

Assess hydration status and fluid intake and output. (Refer to NDs: Fluid Volume risk for deficit; Nutrition: altered, risk for less than body requirements.)

Inadequate hydration may contribute to dry or constipated stool.

Monitor for signs of NEC, such as abdominal distension, rigidity, or tenderness; shiny or taut abdominal skin; visible bowel loops; excessive spitting up, bile-stained emesis; failure of gavage feedings to be absorbed or excessive gastric residual; and absence of bowel sounds. Test stools (unless bloody diarrhea is present) using Hematest or guaiac. Test gastric residual.

NEC is a potentially life threatening complication that affects 3%–8% of preterm infants, usually presenting within the first 2 wk of life.

Minimize handling of infant; provide stroking of face, hands, and feet. Talk to infant.

Avoids further abdominal trauma. Emotional and stroking needs can be met through touching extremities and head and through quiet conversation.

Monitor for signs of C. difficile. Initiate/maintain contact precautions if detected by culture (use of gloves/gown).

Increased foul-smelling stools, thick green to tan color and texture suggest the presence of C. difficile organism. Associated cramping is manifested by infant's bringing knees to abdomen and crying. Discomfort may be noted by scowl on face and mild, continuous, moaning cry.

Avoid use of diapers and rectal thermometers.

Diapers increase lower abdominal pressure and prevent or restrict observation of abdomen. Rectal thermometers may cause trauma to rectal mucosa.

Monitor infant for signs of sepsis, shock, or DIC (e.g., bradycardia, decreasing BP, temperature instability, listlessness, and edema or erythema of abdominal wall).

NEC can progress to bowel perforation with peritonitis, resulting in sepsis, shock, and DIC.

Maintain strict policy of hand washing before/after handling each infant.

Helps prevent an epidemic of NEC from occurring in the nursery.

Collaborative

Use breast milk for feedings whenever possible.

Breast milk is more easily digested, produces softer stool, and may reduce risk of enteric infections or development of NEC.

Increase dilution of supplemental formula as indicated.

Diarrhea may indicate intolerance to formula concentration.

Monitor laboratory studies, as indicated, e.g., WBC count and differential, platelet count, PT, and PTT.

Increased or decreased WBC count or a shift to the left suggests sepsis. Thrombocytopenia or prolonged clotting times may indicate developing DIC.

Review abdominal x-rays.

Presence of distended loops of bowel, thickened walls, and ascites reflects NEC.

Send initial bloody or positive Hematest stool to the laboratory.

Alum-precipitated toxoid test is required to differentiate infant from maternal blood.

Discontinue oral or gavage feedings for 7–10 days, as indicated. Provide TPN feedings.

Allows the bowel to rest, promoting tissue healing while meeting fluid and nutritional needs.

Insert orogastric or NG tube, and connect to continuous, low suction, as needed.

May be necessary for gastric decompression in cases of suspected NEC or following surgical intervention.

Administer antibiotics, such as vancomycin, as indicated.

May be given IV or PO to combat enteric infection. May promote healing of bowel.

Prepare for surgery, as appropriate.

Operative procedure may be necessary to remove segments of inflamed bowel.

NURSING DIAGNOSIS:	SKIN INTEGRITY, risk for impaired
Risk Factors May Include:	Thin skin, fragile capillaries near the skin surface, absence of subcutaneous fat over bony prominences, inability to change positions to relieve pressure points, use of restraints (protecting invasive lines/tubes), alterations in nutritional state
Possibly Evidenced By:	[Not applicable; presence of signs/symptoms establishes an *actual* diagnosis]
DESIRED OUTCOMES/EVALUATION CRITERIA—NEONATE WILL:	Maintain intact skin.
	Be free of dermal injury.

ACTIONS/INTERVENTIONS	RATIONALE
Independent	
Inspect skin, noting areas of redness or pressure.	Identifies areas of potential dermal breakdown, which can result in sepsis. (Refer to ND: Infection, risk for.)
Provide mouth care using saline or glycerin swabs. Apply petroleum jelly to lips.	Helps prevent drying and cracking of lips associated with absence of oral intake or the drying effects of oxygen therapy.
Avoid application of harsh topical agents; carefully wash off povidone-iodine solutions after procedures.	Helps prevent skin breakdown and loss of protective epidermal barrier.
Provide range-of-motion exercises, routine position changes, and fleece or flotation pad.	Helps prevent possible necrosis related to edema of dermis or lack of subcutaneous fat over bony prominences.
Minimize use of tape to secure tubes, electrodes, urine bags, IV lines, and so forth.	Removal of tape may accidentally remove epidermal layer, because cohesion is stronger between tape and stratum corneum than between dermis and epidermis.
Bathe infant using sterile water and mild soap. Wash only grossly soiled body parts. Minimize manipulation of infant's skin.	After 4 days, skin develops some bactericidal properties because of acid pH. Frequent bathing using alkaline soaps or moisturizers may raise skin pH, compromising normal flora and natural defense mechanisms that protect against invading pathogens.
Change electrodes only when necessary.	Frequent changing may contribute to skin irritation/dermal injury.
Collaborative	
Apply antibiotic ointment to nares, mouth, and lips if they are cracked or irritated.	Promotes healing of lesions associated with administration of oxygen; reduces risk of infection.

DEVIATIONS IN GROWTH PATTERNS

Deviations in intrauterine growth patterns not only increase the risk of morbidity and mortality in the early newborn period, but may also have long-term implications for altered growth and development and for altered CNS function and learning disabilities in childhood.

This general plan of care is designed to facilitate optimal nursing management of the infant with deviations in intrauterine growth and is to be used in conjunction with the CPs: The Neonate at Two Hours to Two Days of Age, and The Preterm Infant, as appropriate. Growth deviations are classified as SGA, intrauterine growth retardation/restriction (IUGR), and LGA.

SGA/IUGR: Any newborn whose birth weight falls at or below the 10th percentile on classification charts, considering local factors (e.g., ethnicity, altitude).

LGA/Macrosomic: Any newborn whose birth weight is at or above the 90th percentile on classification charts, considering local population at any week in gestation (with special attention to determining appropriate gestational age), or who at birth weighs more than 4000 g (8 lb 13 oz).

NEONATAL ASSESSMENT DATA BASE

SGA Infant

Activity/Rest

Activity level may be excessive, with vigorous cry/hungry suck attributable to chronic intrauterine hypoxia.

MATERNAL FACTORS

Excessive/strenuous exercise program

Circulation

MATERNAL FACTORS

Resides at high altitude
Heart/lung disease; bleeding, severe anemia or sickle cell anemia; chronic hypertension or PIH

Elimination

Abdomen may appear scaphoid or concave.

MATERNAL FACTORS

Pyelonephritis, chronic renal disease

Food/Fluid

All body parts may be below expected size for gestational age but in proportion/symmetrical to each other (suggests a chronic or prolonged problem throughout gestation).
Disproportionate weight as compared to length and head circumference (appears long and thin with normal head circumference) suggests episodic vascular insufficiency in third trimester.
Sunken abdomen; absence of subcutaneous tissue.
Decreased muscle mass, especially in the cheeks, buttocks, and thighs.
May demonstrate metabolic instability associated with hypoglycemia/hypocalcemia.

MATERNAL FACTORS

Small stature
Malnutrition/poor nutritional intake (chronic or during third trimester); history of eating disorders
Advanced diabetes mellitus (class D or above); PKU

Neurosensory

Skull suture and fontanels appear widened; bulging of fontanels caused by inadequate bone growth may be evident.
Small head with protruding forehead, sunken nasal bridge, short upturned nose, thin upper lip, receding chin (indicative of fetal alcohol syndrome [FAS]).

521

Muscle tone may appear tight with flexion of upper and lower extremities, minor joint/limb abnormalities, and restricted movement (suggests FAS).
Wide-eyed appearance (associated with chronic hypoxia in utero).
Chromosomal syndromes.

Respiration

Signs of respiratory distress may be present (especially in presence of meconium aspiration syndrome [MAS], polycythemia, or infection).
Mucus may be green-tinged.

MATERNAL FACTORS

Heavy smoker

Safety

Dry, cracked, and peeling skin present, with loose skin fold; sparse scalp hair.
Meconium staining may be evident with greenish stains on fingernails and at base of umbilical cord.
Umbilical cord may have single artery and/or be thin, slightly yellow, dull, dry.
Congenital anomalies/malformations or infection may be present.

MATERNAL FACTORS

Irradiation and use of medications with teratogenic side effects (e.g., antimetabolites, anticonvulsants, trimethadione)
Collagen disease; maternal infections such as rubella, syphilis, cytomegalovirus, toxoplasmosis; uterine tumors

Sexuality

Females tend to be smaller than males at birth.

MATERNAL FACTORS

Adolescent or advanced maternal age (younger than age 16 or older than age 40)
Primiparity, grand multiparity
Placenta previa/separation, insufficiency, infarction, fibrosis, thrombosis, hemangioma, abnormal cord insertion and single umbilical artery with vascular anastomoses (twin-to-twin)
Chromosomal abnormalities, chronic intrauterine infections, congenital anomalies, multifetal pregnancy, inborn errors of metabolism

Social Interaction

MATERNAL FACTORS

Low socioeconomic class
Other child(ren) at home with history of FTT
May have previous or current involvement with Department of Social Services

Teaching/Learning

May be premature (and/or member of multifetus pregnancy)

MATERNAL FACTORS

Poor/incomplete formal education
Alcoholism, drug abuse
Lack of prenatal care

LGA Infant
Activity/Rest

Difficulty maintaining quiet, alert state; slower to arouse

Circulation

Skin color ruddy (associated with polycythemia), jaundice (indicative of hyperbilirubinemia)
May have congenital anomalies such as transposition of the great vessels, Beckwith-Wiedemann syndrome, or erythroblastosis fetalis

Food/Fluid

Macrosomia; excess fat deposits and reddened complexion; increased body size proportional (except in infant of diabetic mother [IDM], whose weight may appear disproportionately large for length)

May demonstrate metabolic instability associated with hypoglycemia/hypocalcemia, may have feeding problems

Weight may be 4000 g (8 lb 13 oz) or more (dependent on gestational age)

MATERNAL FACTORS

Inappropriate/overnutrition, excessive pregravid weight and/or weight gain >35 lb

Large stature

Diabetes mellitus (class A, B, or C)

Neurosensory

Large amount of scalp hair

May display hypotonia/hypertonia; decreased reflex functioning

Respiration

Signs of respiratory distress may be present if stress of delivery has induced meconium aspiration/asphyxiation, if delivered by cesarean section, or if infection present.

Safety

Birth injury(s) may be present, e.g., bruising, caput succedaneum, cephalhematomas; facial/phrenic nerve paralysis, brachial palsy; fractured clavicles, intracranial bleeding/depressed skull fracture(s); bulging fontanel indicative of neurological problems, depressed fontanel suggestive of dehydration.

Intrapartal/delivery events may reveal fetal distress, meconium-stained amniotic fluid, oligohydramnios, late/variable decelerations, scalp pH levels <7.20, resuscitative measures.

Evidence of congenital malformations may involve the heart, CNS, kidney, lungs, GI tract.

Long, hard nails extending beyond ends of toes and fingers.

Absence of vernix caseosa/lanugo; desquamation or epidermis.

Sexuality

Higher incidence in males

MATERNAL FACTORS

Birth of previous LGA infant

Cesarean birth because of cephalopelvic disproportion or oxytocin-induced labor related to diabetes/fetal distress/prolonged pregnancy

Multiparity

Social Interactions

Slow to orient to maternal face/voice (generally improves within 48 hr)

Teaching/Learning

May be preterm/postterm by clinical assessment

May be postterm (42 wk or more) because of postconceptional bleeding, leading to a miscalculation of dates/prolonged pregnancy associated with menstrual cycle longer than 28 days.

DIAGNOSTIC STUDIES

Dextrostix Glucose Estimations: Less than 40 mg/dl in LGA infant or 25 mg/dl in SGA infant during first 3 days indicates hypoglycemia.

Serum Glucose: Verifies Dextrostix value <40 mg/dl in LGA infant, <25 mg/dl in SGA infant.

Chest X-Ray and ABGs: Help determine cause/severity of respiratory distress if present, e.g., pneumonia, MAS, RDS.

CBC: May reveal central venous Hct elevated above 65%; central venous Hb 20 g/dl associated with polycythemia/hyperviscosity.

WBC Count: May be elevated or depressed.

Platelet Count: May be depressed if mother was pre-eclamptic or if infant was born with a congenital viral infection.

Coagulation Studies (prothrombin time [PT], partial thromboplastin time [PTT], fibrinogen, fibrin split products [FSP]): May indicate DIC, especially in the presence of polycythemia or asphyxia.

Blood Type for ABO Group, Rh Factor, and Crossmatch: Plasma exchange may be necessary if Rh incompatibility exists.

Serum Electrolytes (including ionized calcium): Assesses for hypocalcemia (level 7 mg/dl [3.5 mEq/L] or less in first 3 days of life); inappropriate antidiuretic hormone secretion, and instability related to metabolic complications.

Bilirubin: May be elevated secondary to polycythemia and resorption of bleeding associated with birth injury, e.g., intracranial hemorrhage, cephalhematoma.

Urinalysis on/after Second Voided Specimen, Including Specific Gravity and Sugar/Acetone: Assesses homeostasis, renal involvement.

Bacterial and Viral Cultures: Rule out/diagnose infectious process.

Electrocardiography (ECG), Echocardiography, Ultrasonography, Angiography, and Genetic Studies: As appropriate with suspected FAS, congenital defects, and/or complications.

NURSING PRIORITIES

1. Maintain physiological homeostasis.
2. Prevent and/or treat complications.
3. Identify/minimize effects of birth trauma.
4. Provide family with appropriate information/strategies for meeting short- and long-term needs associated with growth deviation.

NURSING DIAGNOSIS:	GAS EXCHANGE, impaired
May Be Related To:	Alveolar capillary membrane changes (decreased surfactant levels, retained pulmonary fluid, meconium aspiration), altered oxygen supply (diaphragmatic paralysis/phrenic nerve paralysis, increased intracranial pressure)
Possibly Evidenced By:	Restlessness/irritability; inability to move secretions, tachypnea, cyanosis, hypoxia
DESIRED OUTCOMES/EVALUATION CRITERIA—NEONATE WILL:	Display spontaneous, unassisted regular respiratory effort with rate of 30–50/min; and ABGs WNL.
	Be free of apnea and complications of hypoxia/lung disease.

ACTIONS/INTERVENTIONS	RATIONALE

Independent

Review history for abnormal prenatal growth patterns and/or reduced amounts of amniotic fluid, as detected by ultrasonography/fundal changes.	Low-birth-weight infant or infant with IUGR suffers chronic intrauterine asphyxia, resulting in hypoxia/malnutrition. Fetal contribution to the amniotic pool is reduced in the stressed infant. Macrosomia can be related to maternal diabetes, prolonged pregnancy, heredity, and inappropriate nutrition. Macrosomia in IDM results from excess

Note type of delivery and intrapartal events indicative of hypoxia.

Note time/onset of breathing and Apgar scores. Observe ensuing respiratory patterns.

Assess respiratory rate, depth, effort. Observe and report signs and symptoms of respiratory distress, distinguishing from symptoms associated with polycythemia.

Auscultate breath sounds regularly.

Suction nasopharynx/endotracheal tube as needed, after first providing supplemental oxygen.

Auscultate apical pulse; note presence of cyanosis.

Prevent iatrogenic complications associated with cold stress, metabolic imbalance, and caloric insufficiency.

Ensure availability of resources in the event complications occur.

Collaborative

Monitor transcutaneous oxygen/pulse oximeter readings.

Monitor laboratory studies, as indicated:

Serum pH;

ABGs;

Hct.

release of growth hormone (thyroid stimulation), increasing the number of cells and/or organ size throughout the body.

Infant with chronic hypoxia will be more susceptible to acidosis/respiratory depression/persistent fetal circulation (PFC) after delivery. Cesarean birth increases risk of excess mucus because thoracic compression by the birth canal does not occur as in a vaginal delivery.

The infant with intrapartal asphyxia may present with a delayed onset of respirations and altered respiratory pattern. Apgar scores aid in evaluation of the degree of depression or asphyxia of the newborn at birth and are directly correlated with serum pH/degree of infant acidosis.

Infant with altered growth is more susceptible to respiratory distress associated with chronic asphyxia in SGA infant, inadequate surfactant levels in IDM, perinatal asphyxia, aspiration of meconium or amniotic fluid, and PFC. Diminished lung compliance may occur as a result of polycythemia.

Presence of crackles/rhonchi reflect respiratory congestion and need for intervention.

Ensures patency of airway, removes excess mucus. Supplemental oxygen reduces hypoxic effect of procedure.

Tachypnea, bradycardia, and cyanosis may occur in response to altered oxygen levels.

Such complications increase metabolic demands and oxygen needs.

Equipment for oxygenation, suction, intubation, assisted ventilation, resuscitation, and chest tube placement must be readily available in the event of severe/prolonged respiratory distress.

Identifies therapy needs/effectiveness.

Detects possible metabolic acidosis occurring from inadequate oxygen intake/respiratory acidosis and anaerobic metabolism with acid end products. Note: Normal pH values range from 7.35–7.44; HCO_3 is 19–22 mEq/L (bicarbonate reflects buffering capacity of the blood).

Indicate degree of hypoxia/hypercapnia, as well as therapy needs/effectiveness. Note: Normal newborn arterial Po_2 ranges from 50–70 mm Hg, arterial Pco_2 from 35–45 mm Hg.

Polycythemia, which occurs in 50% of SGA infants related to excess RBC production in response to chronic intrauterine hypoxia, typically increases capillary/venous Hct levels to greater than 60%, with resultant respiratory distress associated with diminished lung compliance.

ACTIONS/INTERVENTIONS	RATIONALE
Administer warm, humidified oxygen; provide assisted ventilation, as indicated.	Corrects/prevents hypoxia, hypercapnia, and respiratory acid-base imbalances.
Review chest x-rays.	May confirm meconium aspiration pneumonia, common in SGA or postterm infant, or RDS, in IDM.
Provide chest physiotherapy, as indicated.	Percussion and postural drainage promote mobilization of secretions, enhancing airway patency and gas exchange, especially in the presence of MAS. Note: Contraindicated in preterm infant.
Administer medications as indicated:	
Sodium bicarbonate;	Corrects metabolic imbalances/acidosis resulting from prolonged respiratory acidosis.
Xanthine derivatives, e.g., aminophylline, theophylline;	Sympathomimetic bronchodilators may be useful in treating apnea of prematurity.
Tolazoline HCl (Priscoline);	Potent vasodilator that relaxes smooth muscle to maximize circulatory effort/oxygenation in cases of meconium aspiration/PFC.
Dopamine.	May be required to counteract hypotensive effect of Priscoline administration.

NURSING DIAGNOSIS:	**NUTRITION: altered, less than body requirements**
May Be Related To:	Decreased nutritional stores, increased insulin production and/or hyperplasia of the pancreatic beta cells
Possibly Evidenced By:	Weight deviation from expected; decreased muscle mass/fat stores, electrolyte imbalance
DESIRED OUTCOMES/EVALUATION CRITERIA—NEONATE WILL:	Ingest and digest adequate nutrients for weight gain (or to prevent weight loss of 2% or more).
	Display serum glucose >40 mg/dl, and other associated laboratory studies WNL.
PARENT(S) WILL:	Identify/treat/prevent short- and long-term complications of malnutrition.

ACTIONS/INTERVENTIONS	RATIONALE

Independent

Compare weight in relation to gestational age and size. Document on growth chart. Weigh daily.	Identifies presence, degree, and risk of altered growth pattern. LGA infant with excess extracellular fluid experiences a postdelivery diuresis, resulting in a loss of up to 15% of birth weight. SGA infant may have already lost weight in utero or may suffer from reduced fat/glycogen stores.
Maintain thermoneutral environment, including use of incubator/radiant warmer, as indicated. Monitor heat controls, temperature of infant and environment frequently, noting hypothermia/ hyperthermia.	The SGA infant does not have adequate adipose tissue for insulation and has a large body surface area compared to body weight. Brown adipose tissue stores may be inadequate to maintain thermoregulation. Both hypothermia and hyperthermia increase metabolic demands, necessitating increased intake in an already compromised infant. Note: Thermal instability may

Initiate early and frequent feedings and advance as tolerated.

be iatrogenically induced by improperly operated heating equipment used to maintain thermogenesis in dysmature infant. (Refer to CP: The Preterm Infant; ND: Thermoregulation, ineffective.)

Assists in maintaining fluid/electrolyte balance and meeting caloric needs to support metabolic process. Helps prevent hypoglycemia associated with inadequate body stores in SGA infant or continued pancreatic secretion of insulin in IDM.

Assess tolerance to feedings. Note stool color, consistency, and frequency; presence of reducing substances; abdominal girth; vomiting, and gastric residuals.

Advances in amount and caloric composition of feedings are dependent on tolerance. Evidence of reducing substances (increased glucose) in stool suggests inability to digest formula because of obstruction and/or disease process present. Note: Poor sucking reflex and recurrent vomiting or persistent regurgitation may be seen in FAS, requiring further evaluation/intervention. (Refer to CP: The Infant of an Addicted Mother.)

Monitor intake and output. Calculate daily caloric and electrolyte consumption.

Provides information about actual intake in relation to estimated needs for use in readjustment of dietary prescription.

Assess hydration level, noting fontanels, skin turgor, urine specific gravity, condition of mucous membranes, and weight fluctuations.

Increased metabolic demands of the SGA infant may increase fluid requirements. Hyperglycemic states may produce diuresis in the infant. IV administration of fluids may be required to meet increased demands but must be conscientiously managed to avoid fluid excess.

Monitor Dextrostix levels immediately after birth and routinely until serum glucose is stabilized.

Hypoglycemia may occur after birth because of limited glucose stores in the SGA infant and from hyperplasia/continued release of insulin in the LGA infant. Symptoms in the SGA infant usually appear between 24 and 72 hr of age, but may begin as early as 3 hr or as late as 7 days; the IDM may be symptomatic within 1–3 hr of birth. Hyperglycemia may result from inappropriate infusion of solutions containing glucose.

Observe for signs of hypoglycemia, e.g., tachypnea and irregular respirations, apnea, lethargy, flaccidity, cyanosis, temperature fluctuations, diaphoresis, poor feeding, jitteriness, high-pitched cry, tremors, eye rolling, seizure activity.

Because glucose is a major source of fuel for the brain, deficits may cause permanent CNS damage. Hypoglycemia significantly increases morbidity and mortality rates, and severity of long-term effects is dependent on duration of such episodes. Untreated symptomatic infants have a higher incidence of neurological abnormalities and/or lower mean IQ later in childhood than treated infants.

Note signs of hypocalcemia, e.g., neuromuscular irritability (tremors, twitching, seizing, clonus), hypotonia, vomiting, high-pitched cry, cyanosis, apnea, and cardiac dysrhythmias with prolonged Q-T interval.

Peak incidence of early hypocalcemia is during first 48–72 hr of life and is often related to temporary abdominal distension, neonatal hypoparathyroidism in premature infant, or prenatal asphyxia in SGA infant or IDM. Late hypocalcemia (at 6–10 days) may be caused by ingestion of milk formulas containing a higher ratio of phosphorus to calcium.

Discuss long-term complications of malnutrition in SGA infant and obesity in LGA infant; review importance of protein during phase II of brain growth.

Chronic protein deficiencies in the SGA infant make child prone to learning difficulties and cerebral dysfunction, characterized by short attention span, poor fine-motor coordination, hyperactivity behavior problems, and speech defects. Excess fat cells in the LGA/macrosomic infant may create lifelong problems associated with obesity (e.g., diabetes, cardiovascular disease, stroke). Adequate protein during hyperplasia/hypertrophy phase of brain growth during the first 6 mo of life helps to overcome insults that occurred in early gestational period of brain development.

Collaborative

Monitor laboratory studies as indicated:

Serum glucose;

Hypoglycemia may occur as early as 1–3 hr after birth. In the SGA infant, glycogen reserves are quickly depleted and gluconeogenesis is inadequate because of reduced stores of muscle protein and fat, while the IDM has decreased ability to release glucagon and catecholamines needed to stimulate glucagon breakdown/facilitate release of glucose. Frequency of screening is dependent on this risk group, i.e., IDM, intrapartal asphyxia, or preterm infants. Levels <7 mg/dl require further evaluation/intervention.

Calcium;

Sodium, potassium, chloride, phosphorus, and magnesium;

Electrolyte instability may be a consequence of deviations in growth, inadequate placental transfer, or altered maternal mineral balance. Note: Hypomagnesemia/hyperphosphatemia are usually associated with hypocalcemia.

BUN, creatinine, serum/urine osmolality, urine electrolytes;

Detects altered kidney function associated with reduced nutrient stores and fluid levels resulting from acute malnutrition/asphyxia.

Triglyceride/cholesterol levels, and liver function tests.

Useful in determining nutritional deficits and therapy needs/effectiveness.

Establish intravascular access as indicated.

IV access allows for fluid and electrolyte administration. Intra-arterial access allows for ease in obtaining samples for monitoring laboratory values.

Administer glucose-containing solutions/parenteral nutrition.

The severely compromised infant with deviations in intrauterine growth may be unable to consume adequate fluids and nutrients via an enteral route. IV glucose (i.e., infusion of D_5W) may be required when serum glucose cannot be maintained at or above 40 mg/dl, or seizure activity occurs.

Provide electrolyte supplementation as indicated, e.g., 10% calcium gluconate.

Metabolic instability in the SGA/LGA infant may necessitate supplements to maintain homeostasis, especially calcium, sodium, and occasionally magnesium.

NURSING DIAGNOSIS:	TISSUE PERFUSION, risk for altered
Risk Factors May Include:	Interruption of arterial or venous blood flow (hyperviscosity associated with polycythemia)
Possibly Evidenced By:	[Not applicable; presence of signs/symptoms establishes an *actual* diagnosis]
DESIRED OUTCOMES/EVALUATION CRITERIA—NEONATE WILL:	Maintain normal vital signs, with adequate peripheral pulses and Hct WNL.
	Be free of complications associated with polycythemia.

ACTIONS/INTERVENTIONS	RATIONALE

Independent

Note risk factors for/presence of polycythemia.

Maternal fetal or infant transfusion (during gestation or at birth), twin gestation (twin-to-twin transfusion), chronic fetal distress associated with maternal PIH, placenta previa; chromosomal anomalies, endocrine disorders; and residing at altitudes over 5000 ft place the infant at risk for developing increased blood volume. Polycythemia resulting from increased erythropoietin production in response to chronic intrauterine hypoxia may occur in both the SGA/LGA infant. In many cases, infants of diabetic mothers are polycythemic. Although the pathophysiology of the hyperviscosity is not fully understood, it may be related to decreased extracellular fluid volume or increased bone marrow stimulation associated with hypoxia.

Monitor temperature, intake/output, and urine specific gravity. Note skin turgor, condition of mucous membranes, and fontanels.

Prevention or correction of dehydration decreases the risks of hyperviscosity.

Observe skin color for ruddiness or pallor. Note presence of hyperthermia, respiratory distress, hypertension or hypotension, tachycardia, decreased pulses, oliguria, hematuria, or altered neurological findings.

Helps detect/promotes prompt intervention to prevent possible complications of polycythemia, e.g., myocardial, cerebral, and renal ischemia; cardiopulmonary congestion; hyperbilirubinemia; thromboembolism, and convulsions.

Collaborative

Monitor central/peripheral Hct/Hb and bilirubin. Send blood for type, crossmatch, and Rh. (Refer to CP: Newborn: Hyperbilirubinemia.)

Indicates degree of polycythemia/hyperviscosity. Hyperbilirubinemia often results from polycythemia (central Hct is >65%; Hb is >22 g/dl) as excess RBCs break down.

Establish intravascular access, preferably through umbilical catheterization.

Provides for fluid administration to correct hyperviscosity and exchange transfusion, if necessary.

Prepare for/assist with exchange transfusion as indicated.

Fresh frozen plasma, 5% albumin or 9% saline, replaces infant's blood in equal amounts, thereby diluting infant's remaining blood volume to prevent/correct polycythemia and hyperviscosity. Usually 10% of the infant's blood volume is removed/exchanged at one time.

Monitor for complications of procedure, including transfusion reactions, overload (CHF), catheter complications, cardiac dysrhythmias, hypovolemia, anemia, and hepatitis.

Provides for early detection/intervention.

NURSING DIAGNOSIS:	**INJURY, risk for**
Risk Factors May Include:	Altered growth patterns, delayed CNS/neurological development, abnormal blood profile, immature immune response
Possibly Evidenced By:	[Not applicable; presence of signs/symptoms establishes an *actual* diagnosis]
DESIRED OUTCOMES/EVALUATION CRITERIA—NEONATE WILL:	Be free of complications.

ACTIONS/INTERVENTIONS	RATIONALE

Independent

Inspect all LGA infants for birth injuries. Note bulging/tense fontanels; muscle spasticity, twitching, or flaccidity; high-pitched, weak, constant cry; tremors or seizure activity; changes in pupil size/reaction; or asymmetrical chest movement.

Because of disproportion between fetal size and maternal pelvis, LGA infants have a high incidence of birth injuries/trauma, such as IICP/CNS damage, cervical/brachial plexus palsy, fractured clavicle/humerus, diaphragmatic paralysis, and cephalhematoma.

Observe invasive sites, urine/stool, NG drainage, and pulmonary secretions for signs of bleeding. Note petechiae/bruising, changes in responsiveness/activity level or muscle tone, nystagmus, opisthotonic posturing, or convulsions.

Early recognition promotes timely intervention. Septicemia, congenital syphilis, cytomegalic inclusion disease, and rubella may result in DIC, resulting in pulmonary, cerebral, or IVH.

Measure occipital frontal circumference, as indicated.

Hydrocephalus may develop following IVH.

Monitor vital signs. Observe peripheral capillary refill and color and temperature of skin.

Hypotension, bradycardia, apnea, hypothermia, delayed capillary refill, and pallor reflect developing shock related to blood loss, requiring prompt assessment/intervention.

Assess home situation for abusive relationships.

Maternal abuse during pregnancy is a significant risk factor for development of SGA infant. Releasing infant into potentially unsafe environment increases risk of abuse/neglect and FTT.

Monitor for signs and symptoms of infection (e.g., changes in temperature, color, muscle tone and activity, feeding tolerance, cardiopulmonary status; or presence of petechiae, rash, jaundice).

Poor resistance to infection, cracks in epidermis, and possible exposure to infectious agents in utero place the SGA/postterm infant at risk for infection, which may be life-threatening, especially if not detected in its earliest phases. (Refer to CP: The Preterm Infant; ND: Infection, risk for.)

Discuss with parents the potential of conditions that may have long-term sequelae, such as birth injury or fetal malnutrition hypoxia (significant role in late or subnormal CNS functioning), which may result in convulsions or altered reflex responses.

Enhances early identification and promotes optimal management of long-term effects of injury/condition.

Collaborative

Monitor laboratory studies as indicated:

CBC with differential;

Dropping Hct may reflect hemorrhage; a shift of the differential may suggest infection.

Coagulation studies: PTT/activated PTT (APTT), PT, fibrinogen levels, FSP, platelets; Blood type, crossmatch, and Rh factor; Bacterial viral cultures and sensitivities.

Alterations in clotting times, presence of FSP reflect developing coagulopathies.
Blood replacement may be required.
Verifies presence, etiology, severity of infectious process.

Provide supplemental oxygen, CPAP, and/or mechanical ventilation, as needed. (Refer to ND: Gas Exchange, impaired.)

Aids in correcting hypoxia, acidemia, and hypotension; reduces risk of IVH/increased ICP.

Administer blood products, albumin, and coagulants, as necessary.

Replaces losses/enhances circulating volume; may help control bleeding.

Administer anticonvulsants (e.g., phenobarbital), as indicated.

May be necessary to quiet cerebrum and reduce electrical stimuli that precipitate seizure activity.

Assist with diagnostic studies, as indicated, e.g., lumbar puncture, CT, or ultrasound scan.

Bloody spinal fluid indicates IVH. Scans are useful in identifying site/extent of cerebral hemorrhage.

Refer family to appropriate community resources/support groups.

Provides support/guidance for dealing with possible long-term effects of condition.

NURSING DIAGNOSIS:	INFANT BEHAVIOR, risk for disorganized
May Be Related To:	Functional limitations related to growth deviations (restricting neonate's opportunity to seek out, recognize, and interpret stimuli), electrolyte imbalance, and psychological stress, immaturity or CNS damage (low threshold for stress), low energy reserves, poor organizational ability, limited ability to control environment
Possibly Evidenced By:	[Not applicable; presence of signs/symptoms establishes an *actual* diagnosis]
DESIRED OUTCOMES/EVALUATION CRITERIA—NEONATE WILL:	Exhibit organized behaviors that allow the achievement of optimal potential for growth and development as evidenced by modulation of physiological, motor, state, and attentional-interactive functioning.
PARENT(S)/CAREGIVER(S) WILL:	Recognize individual infant cues.
	Identify appropriate responses (including environmental modifications) to infant cues.
	Verbalize readiness to assume caregiving independently.

ACTIONS/INTERVENTIONS	RATIONALE

Independent

Determine infant's capacity for stimulation, noting behavioral responses involving gross and fine motor movement, presence of irritability, restlessness, crying, eye contact, and facial expressions.	Allows provision of stimuli consistent with infant's capabilities and with cues reflecting sensory overload.
Provide stimuli consistent with chronological and developmental capabilities.	Size of the infant with deviations in growth may be a false indicator of capacity for stimulation.
Monitor environmental stimulation. Minimize/remove inappropriate or hazardous stimuli.	Control of stressors can reduce infant's energy demands, aiding in maintenance of homeostasis (promotes rest, weight gain).
Provide parents with information regarding the newborn's capabilities/needs.	Parents who are informed of their newborn's capabilities can provide appropriate stimulation to optimize the newborn's development.
Encourage parental involvement in identification of coping strategies/deficits of infant, including control of behavioral state and temperament.	Fosters continued support of the infant's capacities in the acute care setting and transition to home. Identifies role for parents in providing coregulation to the infant.
Promote ongoing assessment of neurodevelopmental gains/deficits. Plan future interventions accordingly.	Prevents/minimizes complications and optimizes growth and development.

531

Collaborative

Suggest/refer to early stimulation program if available/indicated.

Optimizes infant development/interactional skills (affective, cognitive, social).

Refer for long-term neurodevelopmental assessment and intervention as indicated.

Sequelae of morbidity associated with deviations in intrauterine growth may affect long-term coping.

(Refer to CP: The Preterm Infant; ND: Infant Behavior, risk for disorganized.)

NURSING DIAGNOSIS:	KNOWLEDGE deficit [Learning Need], parent(s), regarding condition, prognosis, and treatment needs
May Be Related To:	Lack of exposure, misinterpretations, unfamiliarity with resources
Possibly Evidenced By:	Verbalization of problem, misconception, request for information
DESIRED OUTCOMES/EVALUATION CRITERIA—PARENT(S) WILL:	Identify newborn's short- and long-term needs.
	List available resources.
	Participate in discharge planning.

ACTIONS/INTERVENTIONS	RATIONALE

Independent

Provide appropriate anticipatory guidance regarding implications of growth deviations.

Malnutrition in SGA infant may result in subnormal CNS/intellectual development as well as hearing/speech deficits. LGA infant is susceptible to malnutrition problems associated with obesity. (Refer to ND: Nutrition: altered, less than body requirements.)

Review short- and long-term needs for care of the SGA/LGA infant. Assist with follow-up in discharge planning.

Provides information for parents to understand need for ongoing physical, neurodevelopmental, and psychosocial assessment needed for long-term follow-up. (Refer to CP: The Parents of a Child with Special Needs; NDs: Knowledge deficit [Learning Need]; Family Coping: ineffective, risk for compromised.)

Identify community/governmental resources as appropriate.

Presence of specific needs such as feeding problems, resolving complications, or congenital anomalies require ongoing monitoring and problem solving to foster optimal growth and development.

CIRCUMCISION

Circumcision is a surgical procedure in which the prepuce (foreskin) of the penis is separated from the glans, and a portion is excised. This elective procedure is performed in the United States based on parental choice for reasons related to hygiene, religion, tradition, social norms, and culture. It is usually performed at 12–24 hr of age or when the infant is considered physically stable. Frequency of this procedure has declined in recent years to approximately 62%.

NEONATAL ASSESSMENT DATA BASE

Circulation

Vital signs WNL, no signs of cold stress
Administration of vitamin K

Food/Fluid

Weight at least 2500 g (5 lb 8 oz)

Safety

Temperature WNL
Free of congenital anomalies; no family history of bleeding disorders or history of "proud flesh" scar formation (especially in black families)

Sexuality

Infant full-term (based on Dubowitz criteria)
Genitalia normal, with no evidence of hypospadias or epispadias; testes descended, and scrotal sac free of hydrocele; prepuce, still developing at birth, normally nonretractable

DIAGNOSTIC STUDIES

CBC: Rules out presence of anemia.
Clotting Studies: Identify coagulation problems.

NURSING PRIORITIES

1. Provide parents with sufficient information to make an informed choice.
2. Promote comfort and healing.
3. Identify and minimize postoperative complications.
4. Instruct parent(s) in proper care of circumcised infant.

DISCHARGE CRITERIA

1. Void appropriately past procedure.
2. Free of complications.
3. Parent(s) understand care needs and signs/symptoms requiring further evaluation.

NURSING DIAGNOSIS:	KNOWLEDGE deficit [Learning Need], regarding surgical procedure, prognosis, and treatment
May Be Related To:	Lack of exposure, misinterpretation, unfamiliarity with information resources
Possibly Evidenced By:	Request for information, verbalization of concerns/misconceptions, inaccurate follow-through of instructions
DESIRED OUTCOMES/EVALUATION CRITERIA—PARENT(S) WILL:	Make informed decision.
	Demonstrate proper technique of care following procedure.
	Verbalize understanding of signs of complications.

ACTIONS/INTERVENTIONS	RATIONALE

Independent

Ascertain parents' understanding of the procedure. Determine cultural/religious influences.	Provides a basis for discussion and identifies need for further information. While cultural/religious beliefs may dictate circumcision be performed, some studies have shown that many women do not know the meaning of the word or whether their husbands are circumcised.
Review information about the advantages and disadvantages of circumcision.	The routine practice of circumcision has been questioned, and the position of the American Academy of Pediatrics (1989) is that there are both potential medical benefits and advantages as well as disadvantages and risks. Proponents believe that circumcision may reduce risk of cancer of the penis and prostate in men and of the cervix in women; that it has prophylactic effects against a number of diseases, including herpes; that it facilitates hygiene; and that an uncircumcised boy may feel different from his peers. Opponents believe that the cancer link is not proved by scientific studies and that hygiene is more of a factor in cancer prevention than is circumcision; that the long-term effects of pain and stress are not known; and that complications are a significant concern.
Discuss anticipated infant behaviors following procedure.	Changes in sleep patterns, fussiness, and/or refusal of feedings usually persist for 2–3 hr following procedure. However, studies indicate that elevated cortisol levels associated with stress of the procedure can interfere with the newborn's ability to regulate sleep-wake cycles for some time following circumcision.
Note any special requests made by parents.	Parents may want to be present during the procedure or may have specific religious or cultural preferences.
Provide information about the healing process and proper care (e.g., cleaning, diapering, positioning, use of petroleum gauze dressing or bacterial ointment). Discuss the need to check infant frequently to prevent gauze from drying out and sticking to site of circumcision. Suggest soaking gauze with warm, sterile water before removing it.	Prevents complications associated with infection; promotes infant's comfort. Refer to ND: Pain [acute]. Note: If plastic bell method is used to cover the glans, petroleum gauze is not needed.
Discuss potential complications, e.g., hemorrhage, infection, or other signs warranting notification of healthcare provider.	Ensures prompt identifications and treatment of problems.

NURSING DIAGNOSIS:	**PAIN [acute]**
May Be Related To:	Trauma to/edema of tender tissues
Possibly Evidenced By:	Crying, irritability, changes in sleep pattern, refusal to eat
DESIRED OUTCOMES/EVALUATION CRITERIA—NEONATE WILL:	Appear relaxed, appropriately consolable.
	Resume normal sleeping and eating patterns.

ACTIONS/INTERVENTIONS	RATIONALE

Independent

Provide pacifier (dipped in sugar, if desired), stroke lightly, and talk gently to infant during procedure. Observe infant response.

Provides distraction and sense of reassurance to soothe the infant.

Remove infant from restraints immediately following procedure. Calm infant by holding, cuddling, dressing, and talking to him. Encourage parents to feed and cuddle infant.

A sense of uneasiness occurs because of positioning and restraint. Acute pain occurs at the time of surgical procedure, because the foreskin contains numerous nerve endings. Change of position, freedom of movement, and tactile activities refocus infant's attention and comfort infant. Feeding may promote relaxation. Note: Infant's turning head away, increased restlessness, hiccuping suggest overstimulation, which may further distress the infant.

Apply petroleum jelly and gauze dressing loosely around glans, as appropriate. Leave in place for at least 24 hr.

Protects against adherence to diaper and direct contact with urine.

Position infant on side or back, not on abdomen. Loose diaper or use no diaper at all for 24–72 hr following procedure. Note continued placement of plastic rim following circumcision with plastic bell.

Prevents friction or pressure on the penis. Plastic rim remains in place for 5–7 days. Plastic bell falls off by itself when glans is healed. Note: Removal of the bell by the healthcare provider may be required.

Avoid use of soaps on penis; clean with clear water.

Soap may cause irritation, increasing discomfort, and may cause plastic bell to fall off prematurely.

Protect the surgical site from alcohol when caring for umbilicus.

Alcohol may cause stinging, adding to infant's discomfort.

Apply a small amount of bland or petroleum-based ointment on the affected area or on the dressing that may be covering the site at each diaper change or at least 4–5 times a day for 24–48 hr.

Prevents the area from sticking to diaper.

Note infant's behavior following procedure.

Acute pain following the procedure may last approximately 30 min, whereas discomfort related to trauma, edema, and irritation from clothing may last for up to 7 days until healing is completed.

Collaborative

Assist with dorsal penile nerve block with 1% lidocaine without epinephrine or chloroprocaine (Nesacine).

Although it is not used routinely, anesthesia abolishes the pain and distress manifested in the unmedicated infant by changes in hormone levels and cardiovascular system, vigorous crying, attempts to wriggle from restraints, and trembling. Nesacine has a faster onset of action. Note: Risk of nerve damage exists if injection is not carefully placed, and the risks of elevated blood levels of lidocaine are as yet unstudied.

Apply topical agents, e.g., EMLA cream (lidocaine and prilocaine) to penis.

Topical agent applied 1-2 hr before procedure may be as effective as nerve block without associated risks.

Administer acetaminophen drops as indicated.

Helps ease acute pain, enhances effects of calming behaviors.

535

NURSING DIAGNOSIS:	URINARY ELIMINATION, altered
May Be Related To:	Tissue injury/inflammation, or development of urethral fistula
Possibly Evidenced By:	Edema, difficulty voiding
DESIRED OUTCOMES/EVALUATION CRITERIA—NEONATE WILL:	Void within 6–8 hr following circumcision.
	Establish normal elimination pattern.
• PARENT(S) WILL:	Prevent/minimize edema.

ACTIONS/INTERVENTIONS	RATIONALE

Independent

Record time of first voiding following procedure. Note amount and adequacy of stream and presence of hematuria.	Trauma to the urinary meatus from the procedure may result in delayed voidings, blocked urinary passage, or interrupted stream.
Loosely diaper the newborn and position on side or back.	Reduces pressure on affected site.
Avoid placing petroleum jelly over the meatus.	Excessive amounts of petroleum jelly may block meatus, requiring greater effort to empty bladder.
Place warm, wet washcloth over the bladder area if voiding has not occurred within 6–8 hr following procedure.	Relaxes musculature and may encourage voiding.
Notify healthcare provider if infant fails to void within 12 hr following procedure.	Failure to void may indicate urethral fistula, necessitating further evaluation.

NURSING DIAGNOSIS:	INJURY, risk for hemorrhage
Risk Factors May Include:	Decrease in clotting factors immediately after birth (do not return to prebirth levels until the end of the 1st wk); previously unidentified problems with bleeding and clotting
Possibly Evidenced By:	[Not applicable; presence of signs/symptoms establishes an *actual* diagnosis]
DESIRED OUTCOMES/EVALUATION CRITERIA—NEONATE WILL:	Be free of injury; no evidence of hemorrhage.

ACTIONS/INTERVENTIONS	RATIONALE

Independent

Delay surgical procedure until at least 12–24 hr following birth.	Postponing circumcision from the time immediately following birth to 12 or more hr following birth helps prevent complications associated with physiological instability, cold stress, undetected congenital anomaly, and illness.
Observe infant every hour for first 12 hr after the procedure.	Aids in early detection of persistent bleeding. Note: Excessive blood loss may be an initial indicator

Apply gentle, direct pressure to bleeding site, using a sterile gauze pad.

of bleeding/coagulation problems, such as hemophilia.

Promotes vasoconstriction to stop bleeding.

Apply sterile petroleum gauze dressing to site immediately following procedure and with each diaper change, if plastic bell method is not used. Moisten gauze with water if it adheres to surgical site.

Acts as a pressure dressing to control bleeding and prevent surgical site from adhering to the diaper, which could cause further irritation or loss of stable clot.

Collaborative

Apply Gelfoam to bleeding areas.

Gelfoam acts as a local hemostatic agent to promote platelet adhesion and clotting.

Assist with placement of suture(s), as needed.

May be necessary to control bleeding.

NURSING DIAGNOSIS:	INFECTION, risk for
Risk Factors May Include:	Immature immune system, invasive procedure/tissue trauma, environmental exposure
Possibly Evidenced By:	[Not applicable; presence of signs/symptoms establishes and *actual* diagnosis]
DESIRED OUTCOMES/EVALUATION CRITERIA—NEONATE WILL:	Display timely healing of circumcision site within 1 wk.
	Be free of signs of infection.

ACTIONS/INTERVENTIONS

RATIONALE

Independent

Clean penis gently with warm, sterile water or dilute hydrogen peroxide, and apply fresh sterile petroleum gauze with each diaper change.

Removes urine/feces from penis; helps promote healing. Note: Excessive scrubbing may irritate the site and provide entry for bacteria.

Note appearance of whitish yellow exudate around the glans. Do not remove.

Exudate is usually noted 24–48 hr following procedure. It is a normal sign of the granulation process and eventually disappears on its own.

Observe penis for signs of infection at each diaper change, (e.g., erythema or purulent exudate). Ensure that plastic bell is still firmly attached, if used.

Early detection of infection can prevent generalized sepsis from occurring.

Collaborative

Obtain culture of exudate, if present.

Identifies pathogens, appropriate treatment choices.

Monitor results of laboratory studies, e.g., CBC.

Helps confirm presence or resolution of infectious process.

Administer local or systemic antibiotic, as indicated.

Treats infection; prevents systemic involvement.

HYPERBILIRUBINEMIA

Elevation of serum bilirubin levels is related to hemolysis of RBCs and subsequent re-absorption of unconjugated bilirubin from the small intestines. The condition may be benign or may place the neonate at risk for multiple complications/untoward effects.

NEONATAL ASSESSMENT DATA BASE

Activity/Rest

Lethargy, listlessness

Circulation

May be pale, indicating anemia
Residing at altitudes above 5000 ft
Cardiomegaly; increased bleeding tendencies (hydrops fetalis)

Elimination

Bowel sounds hypoactive.
Meconium passage may be delayed.
Stools may be loose/greenish brown during bilirubin excretion.
Urine dark, concentrated; brownish black (bronze baby syndrome).

Food/Fluid

History of delayed/poor oral feeding, poor sucking reflex.
More likely to be breastfed than bottle-fed.
Abdominal palpation may reveal enlarged spleen, liver.
Generalized edema, ascites (hydrops fetalis).

Neurosensory

Large cephalhematoma may be noted over one or both parietal bones related to birth
        trauma/vacuum extraction delivery.
Loss of Moro reflex may be noted.
Opisthotonos with rigid arching of back, bulging fontanels, shrill cry, seizure activity (crisis stage).

Respiration

History of asphyxia
Crackles, pink-tinged mucus (pleural edema, pulmonary hemorrhages)

Safety

History may be positive for infection/neonatal sepsis.
May have excessive ecchymosis, petechiae, intracranial bleeding.
May appear jaundiced initially on the face with progression to distal parts of the body; skin
        brownish black in color (bronze baby syndrome) as a side effect of phototherapy.

Sexuality

May be preterm, SGA infant, infant with IUGR, or LGA infant, such as IDM.
Birth trauma may have occurred associated with cold stress, asphyxia, hypoxia, acidosis,
        hypoglycemia, hypoproteinemia.
Occurs more often in male than female infants.

Teaching/Learning

May have congenital hypothyroidism, biliary atresia, cystic fibrosis (inspissated bile)
Family factors; e.g., ethnic descent (Asian, Greek, or Korean), history of hyperbilirubinemia in
        previous pregnancies/siblings, liver disease, cystic fibrosis, inborn errors of metabolism
        (galactosemia), blood dyscrasias (spherocytosis, glucose-6-phosphate dehydrogenase
        [G-6-PD] deficiency)

Maternal factors, such as maternal diabetes; ingestion of medications (e.g., salicylates, oral sulfonamides late in pregnancy or nitrofurantoin [Furadantin]; Rh/ABO incompatibility; infectious illness (e.g., rubella, CMV, syphilis, toxoplasmosis)

Intrapartal contributing factors, such as preterm labor, delivery by vacuum extraction, oxytocin induction, delayed clamping of umbilical cord, or traumatic delivery

DIAGNOSTIC STUDIES

Coombs' Test on Newborn Cord Blood: Positive result of indirect Coombs' test indicates the presence of Rh-positive, anti-A, or anti-B antibodies in mother's blood. Positive result of direct Coombs' test indicates presence of sensitized (Rh-positive, anti-A, or anti-B) RBCs in neonate.

Infant and Maternal Blood Type: Identifies ABO incompatibilities.

Total Bilirubin: Direct (conjugated) levels are significant if they exceed 1.0–1.5 mg/dl, which may be associated with sepsis. Indirect (unconjugated) levels should not exceed an increase of 5 mg/dl in 24 hr, or should not be >20 mg/dl in a full-term infant or 15 mg/dl in a preterm infant (dependent on weight). Cord blood bilirubin >5 mg/dl indicates severe hemolysis.

Total Serum Protein: Levels <3.0 g/dl indicate reduced binding capacity, particularly in preterm infant.

CBC: Hb may be low (<14 g/dl) because of hemolysis. Hct may be elevated (>65%) with polycythemia, decreased (<45%) with excess hemolysis and anemia. Cord-blood Hct of <40% indicates severe hemolysis.

Glucose: Dextrostix level may be <45% whole blood glucose <30 mg/dl, or serum glucose <40 mg/dl if newborn is hypoglycemic and begins to use fat stores and release fatty acids.

Carbon Dioxide (CO_2) Combining Power: Decreased level reflects hemolysis.

Transcutaneous Jaundice Meter: Identifies infants requiring serum bilirubin determination.

Reticulocyte Count: Elevation (reticulocytosis) indicates increased production of RBCs in response to hemolysis associated with RH disease.

Peripheral Blood Smear: May reveal abnormal or immature RBCs, erythroblasts in Rh disease, or spherocytes in ABO incompatibility.

Kleihauer-Betke Test: Evaluation of maternal blood smear for fetal erythrocytes.

Ultrasound: May be done prenatally in high-risk situations to diagnose hydrops fetalis before delivery, as noted by scalp edema, cardiomegaly, hepatomegaly, plural effusions, and ascites.

NURSING PRIORITIES

1. Prevent injury/progression of condition.
2. Provide support/appropriate information to family.

DISCHARGE CRITERIA:

1. Maintaining physiological homeostasis with bilirubin levels declining.
2. Complications prevented/resolving.
3. Parent(s) understand condition/prognosis and therapeutic regimen.
4. Plan in place to meet needs after discharge.

NURSING DIAGNOSIS:	INJURY, risk for CNS involvement
Risk Factors May Include:	Prematurity, hemolytic disease, asphyxia, acidosis, hypoproteinemia, and hypoglycemia
Possibly Evidenced By:	[Not applicable; presence of signs/symptoms establishes an *actual* diagnosis]
DESIRED OUTCOMES/EVALUATION CRITERIA—NEONATE WILL:	Display indirect bilirubin levels below 12 mg/dl in term infant at 3 days of age.
	Show resolution of jaundice by end of the 1st wk of life.
	Be free of CNS involvement.

ACTIONS/INTERVENTIONS	RATIONALE

Independent

Note infant/maternal blood group and blood type.

ABO incompatibilities affect 20% of all pregnancies and most commonly occur in mothers with type O blood, whose anti-A and anti-B antibodies pass into fetal circulation, causing RBC agglutination and hemolysis. Similarly, when an Rh-negative mother has previously been sensitized by Rh-positive antigens, maternal antibodies cross the placenta and attach to fetal RBCs, causing immediate or delayed hemolysis.

Review intrapartal record for specific risk factors, such as low birth weight (LBW) or IUGR, prematurity, abnormal metabolic processes, vascular injuries, abnormal circulation, sepsis, or polycythemia.

Certain clinical conditions may cause a reversal of the blood-brain barrier, allowing bound bilirubin to separate either at the level of the cell membrane or within the cell itself, increasing the risk of CNS involvement.

Note use of vacuum extractor for delivery. Assess infant for presence of cephalhematoma and excessive ecchymosis or petechiae.

Resorption of blood trapped in fetal scalp tissue and excessive hemolysis may increase the amount of bilirubin being released and cause jaundice.

Review infant's condition at birth, noting need for resuscitation or evidence of excessive ecchymosis or petechiae, cold stress, asphyxia, or acidosis.

Asphyxia and acidosis reduce affinity of bilirubin to albumin.

Keep infant warm and dry; monitor skin and core temperature frequently.

Cold stress potentiates release of fatty acids, which compete for binding sites on albumin, thereby increasing the level of freely circulating (unbound) bilirubin.

Initiate early oral feedings within 4–6 hr following birth, especially if infant is to be breastfed. Assess infant for signs of hypoglycemia. Obtain Dextrostix levels, as indicated.

Establishes proper intestinal flora necessary for reduction of bilirubin to urobilinogen; decreases enterohepatic circulation of bilirubin (bypassing liver with persistence of ductus venosus); and decreases reabsorption of bilirubin from bowel by promoting passage of meconium. Hypoglycemia necessitates use of fat stores for energy-releasing fatty acids, which compete with bilirubin for binding sites on albumin.

Evaluate maternal and prenatal nutritional levels; note possible neonatal hypoproteinemia, especially in preterm infant.

Hypoproteinemia in the newborn may result in jaundice. One gram of albumin carries 16 mg of unconjugated bilirubin. Lack of sufficient albumin increases the amount of unbound circulating (indirect) bilirubin, which may cross the blood-brain barrier.

Observe infant in natural light, noting sclera and oral mucosa, yellowing of skin immediately after blanching, and specific body parts involved. Assess oral mucosa, posterior portion of hard palate, and conjunctival sacs in dark-skinned newborns.

Detects evidence/degree of jaundice. Clinical appearance of jaundice is evident at bilirubin levels >7–8 mg/dl in full-term infant. Estimated degree of jaundice is as follows, with jaundice progressing from head to toe: face, 4–8 mg/dl; trunk, 5–12 mg/dl; groin, 8–16 mg/dl; arms/legs, 11–18 mg/dl; and hands/feet, 15–20 mg/dl. Note: Yellow underlying pigment may be normal in dark-skinned infants.

Note infant's age at onset of jaundice; differentiate type of jaundice (i.e., physiological, breast milk–induced, or pathological).

Physiological jaundice usually appears between the 2nd and 3rd days of life, as excess RBCs needed to maintain adequate oxygenation for the fetus are no longer required in the newborn and are hemolyzed, thereby releasing bilirubin, the final breakdown product of heme. Breast milk jaundice usually appears between the 4th and 6th days of life, affecting only 1%–2% of breastfed infants. The breast milk of some women is thought to contain an enzyme (pregnanediol) that inhibits glucuronyl transferase (the liver enzyme that conjugates bilirubin), or to contain several times the normal breast milk concentration of certain free fatty acids, which are also thought to inhibit the conjugation of bilirubin. Pathological jaundice appears within the first 24 hr of life and is more likely to lead to the development of kernicterus/bilirubin encephalopathy.

Apply transcutaneous jaundice meter.

Provides noninvasive screening of jaundice, quantifying skin color in relation to total serum bilirubin.

Assess infant for progression of signs and behavioral changes: Stage I involves neuro-depression (e.g., lethargy, hypotonia, or diminished/absent reflexes). Stage II involves neurohyperreflexia (e.g., twitching, convulsions, opisthotonos, or fever). Stage III is marked by absence of clinical manifestations. Stage IV involves sequelae such as cerebral palsy or mental retardation.

Excessive unconjugated bilirubin (associated with pathologic jaundice) has an affinity for extravascular tissue, including the basal ganglia of brain tissue. Behavior changes associated with kernicterus usually occur between the 3rd and 10th days of life and rarely occur prior to 36 hr of life.

Evaluate infant for pallor, edema, or hepatosplenomegaly.

These signs may be associated with hydrops fetalis, Rh incompatibility, and in utero hemolysis of fetal RBCs.

Collaborative

Monitor laboratory studies, as indicated:

Direct and indirect bilirubin;

Bilirubin appears in two forms: direct bilirubin, which is conjugated by the liver enzyme glucuronyl transferase, and indirect bilirubin, which is unconjugated and appears in a free form in the blood or bound to albumin. The infant's potential for kernicterus is best predicted by elevated levels of indirect bilirubin. Elevated indirect bilirubin levels of 18–20 mg/dl in full-term infant, or >13–15 mg/dl in preterm or sick infant, are significant. Note: Stressed or preterm infant is susceptible to deposition of bile pigments within brain tissue at far lower levels than nonstressed full-term infant.

Direct/indirect Coombs' test on cord blood;

Positive results of indirect Coombs' test indicate presence of antibodies (Rh-positive or anti-A, anti-B) in mother's and newborn's blood; positive results of direct Coombs' test indicate presence of sensitized (Rh-positive, anti-A, or anti-B) RBCs in neonate. A decrease is consistent with hemolysis.

CO_2 combining power;
Reticulocyte count and peripheral smear;

Excessive hemolysis causes reticulocyte count to increase. Smear identifies abnormal or immature RBCs.

Hb/Hct;

Elevated Hb/Hct levels (Hb >22 g/dl; Hct >65%) indicate polycythemia, possibly caused by delayed cord clamping, maternal-fetal transfusion, twin-to-twin transfusion, maternal diabetes, or chronic intrauterine stress and hypoxia, as seen in LBW infant or infant with compromised placental circulation. Hemolysis of excess RBCs causes

Total serum protein.	elevated levels of bilirubin with 1 g of Hb yielding 35 mg of bilirubin. Low Hb levels (14 mg/dl) may be associated with hydrops fetalis or with Rh incompatibility occurring in utero and causing hemolysis, edema, and pallor. Low levels of serum protein (<3.0 g/dl) indicate reduced binding capacity for bilirubin.
Calculate plasma bilirubin-albumin binding capacity.	Aids in determining risk of kernicterus and treatment needs. When total bilirubin value divided by total serum protein level is <3.7, the danger of kernicterus is very low. However, the risk of injury is dependent on degree of prematurity, presence of hypoxia or acidosis, and drug regimen (e.g., sulfonamides, chloramphenicol).
Initiate phototherapy per protocol, using fluorescent bulbs placed above the infant or bile blanket (except for newborn with Rh disease). (Refer to NDs: Injury, risk for side effects of phototherapy; Injury, risk for complications of exchange transfusions.)	Causes photo-oxidation of bilirubin in subcutaneous tissue, thereby increasing water solubility of bilirubin, which allows rapid excretion of bilirubin in stool and urine. Rate of hemolysis in Rh disease usually exceeds rate of bilirubin reduction related to phototherapy, so that an exchange transfusion is the only appropriate treatment.
Discontinue breastfeeding for 24–48 hr, as indicated. Assist mother as needed with pumping of breasts and reestablishment of breastfeeding.	Opinions vary as to whether interrupting breastfeeding is necessary when jaundice occurs. However, formula ingestion increases GI motility and excretion of stool and bile pigment, and serum bilirubin levels do begin to fall within 48 hr after discontinuation of breastfeeding.
Administer enzyme induction agent (phenobarbital, ethanol), as appropriate.	Stimulates hepatic enzymes to enhance clearance of bilirubin.
Assist with preparation and administration of exchange transfusion. Use same type of blood as infant's, but Rh-negative or type O-negative blood, if results of direct Coombs' test on cord serum are >3.5 mg/dl in the 1st wk of life, serum unconjugated bilirubin levels are >20 mg/dl in the first 48 hr of life, or Hb is <12 g/dl at birth in infants with hydrops fetalis. (Refer to ND: Injury, risk for complications of exchange transfusions.)	Exchange transfusions are necessary in cases of severe hemolytic anemia, which are usually associated with Rh incompatibility, to remove sensitized RBCs that would soon lyse; to remove serum bilirubin; to provide bilirubin-free albumin to increase binding sites for bilirubin; and to treat anemia by providing RBCs that are not susceptible to maternal antibodies.

NURSING DIAGNOSIS:	**INJURY, risk for side effects of phototherapy**
Risk Factors May Include:	Physical properties of therapeutic intervention and effects on body regulatory mechanisms
Possibly Evidenced By:	[Not applicable; presence of signs/symptoms establishes an *actual* diagnosis]
DESIRED OUTCOMES/EVALUATION CRITERIA—NEONATE WILL:	Maintain body temperature and fluid balance WNL.
	Be free of *skin/tissue* injury.
	Demonstrate expected interaction patterns.
	Display decreasing serum bilirubin levels.

ACTIONS/INTERVENTIONS	RATIONALE

Independent

Note presence/development of biliary or intestinal obstruction.

Phototherapy is contraindicated in these conditions because the photoisomers of bilirubin produced in the skin and subcutaneous tissues by exposure to light therapy cannot be readily excreted.

Measure quantity of photoenergy of fluorescent bulbs (white or blue light) using photometer.

The intensity of light striking skin surface from blue spectrum (blue lights) determines how close to the light source the infant should be placed. Photometer should register between 8 and 9 $\mu W/cm^2/nm$ of light when placed flush with infant's abdomen. Blue and special blue lights are considered more effective than white light in promoting bilirubin breakdown, but they create difficulty in evaluating the newborn for cyanosis.

Document type of fluorescent lamp, total number of hours since bulb replacement, and the measured distance between lamp surface and infant.

Light emission may decay over time. Infant should be placed approximately 18–20 in (45 cm) from light source for maximal benefit. Note: Use of fiberoptic blanket connected to an illuminator (light source) allows infant to be "wrapped" in therapeutic light without risk to corneas. In addition, infant can be held and fed without interrupting therapy.

Apply patches to closed eyes; inspect eyes every 2 hr when patches are removed for feedings. Monitor placement frequently.

Prevents possible damage to the retina and conjunctiva from high-intensity light. Improper application or slipping of patches can cause irritation, corneal abrasions, and conjunctivitis, and compromise breathing by obstructing nasal passages.

Cover testes and penis of male infant.

Prevents possible testicular damage from heat.

Place Plexiglas shield between baby and light.

Filters out ultraviolet radiation (wavelengths less than 380 nm) and protects infant if bulb breaks.

Monitor neonate's skin and core temperature every 2 hr or more frequently until stable (e.g., axillary temperature of 97.8°F (36.5°C), rectal temperature of 98.8°F (37.4°C). Regulate incubator/Isolette temperature, as appropriate.

Fluctuations in body temperature can occur in response to light exposure, radiation, and convection.

Reposition infant every 2 hr.

Allows equal exposure of skin surfaces to fluorescent light, prevents excessive exposure of individual body parts, and limits pressure areas.

Monitor fluid intake and output; weigh infant twice a day. Note signs of dehydration (e.g., reduced urine output, depressed fontanels, dry or warm skin with poor turgor, and sunken eyes). Increase oral fluid intake by at least 25%.

Increased water losses through stools and evaporation can cause dehydration. Note: Infant may sleep for longer periods in conjunction with phototherapy, increasing risk of dehydration if frequent feeding schedule is not maintained.

Note color and frequency of stools and urine.

Frequent, greenish, loose stools and greenish urine indicate effectiveness of phototherapy with breakdown and excretion of bilirubin.

Carefully wash perianal area after each passage of stool; inspect skin for possible irritation or breakdown.

Early intervention helps prevent irritation and excoriation from frequent or loose stools.

Bring infant to parents for feedings. Encourage stroking, cuddling, eye contact, and talking to infant during feedings. Encourage parents to interact with infant in nursery between feedings.

Fosters attachment process, which may be delayed if separation required by phototherapy. Visual, tactile, and auditory stimulation helps infant overcome sensory deprivation. Intermittent

543

phototherapy does not negatively affect photo-oxidation process. Note: Dependent on infant condition and policies/capabilities of hospital, phototherapy may be provided in conjunction with rooming-in.

Note behavioral changes or signs of deteriorating condition (e.g., lethargy, hypotonia, hypertonicity, or extrapyramidal signs).

Such changes may signify deposition of bile pigment in the basal ganglia and developing kernicterus.

Evaluate appearance of skin and urine, noting brownish black color.

An uncommon side effect of phototherapy involves exaggerated pigment changes (bronze baby syndrome), which may occur if conjugated bilirubin levels rise. The changes in skin color may last for 2–4 mo but are not associated with harmful sequelae.

Collaborative

Monitor laboratory studies, as indicated:

Bilirubin levels every 12 hr;

Decreases in bilirubin levels indicate effectiveness of phototherapy; continued increases suggest continued hemolysis and may indicate the need for exchange transfusion. Note: Blood sample drawn for bilirubin determination should be protected from light to prevent continued photo-oxidation.

Hb levels;

Continued hemolysis is manifested by progressive decreases in Hb level.

Platelets and WBCs.

Thrombocytopenia during phototherapy has been reported in some infants. Decrease in WBCs suggests a possible effect on peripheral lymphocytes.

Administer fluids parenterally as indicated.

May be necessary to correct or prevent severe dehydration.

NURSING DIAGNOSIS:	INJURY, risk for complications of exchange transfusions
Risk Factors May Include:	Invasive procedure, abnormal blood profile, chemical imbalances
Possibly Evidenced By:	[Not applicable; presence of signs/symptoms establishes an *actual* diagnosis]
DESIRED OUTCOMES/EVALUATION CRITERIA—NEONATE WILL:	Complete exchange transfusion without complications. Display decreasing serum bilirubin levels.

ACTIONS/INTERVENTIONS

RATIONALE

Independent

Note condition of infant's cord prior to transfusion, if umbilical vein is to be used. If cord is dry, administer saline soaks for 30–60 min prior to procedure.

Soaks may be necessary to soften cord and umbilical vein prior to transfusion for IV access and to ease passage of umbilical catheter.

Maintain NPO status for 4 hr prior to procedure, or aspirate gastric contents.

Reduces risk of possible regurgitation and aspiration during procedure.

Ensure availability of resuscitative equipment.

To provide immediate support if necessary.

544

Maintain infant's temperature prior to, during, and after procedure. Place infant under radiant warmer with servomechanism. Warm blood prior to infusion by placing in incubator, warm basin of water, or blood warmer.

Verify infant's and mother's blood type and Rh factor. Note blood type and Rh factor of blood to be exchanged. (Exchanged blood will be the same type as the baby's but will be Rh-negative or type O–negative blood that has been cross-matched with mother's blood beforehand.)

Ensure freshness of blood (not more than 2 days old), with heparinized blood preferred.

Monitor venous pressure, pulse, color, and respiratory rate/ease before, during, and after transfusion. Suction as needed.

Carefully document events during transfusion, recording amount of blood withdrawn and injected (usually 7–20 ml at a time).

Monitor for signs of electrolyte imbalance (e.g., jitteriness, seizure activity, and apnea; hyperreflexia, bradycardia, or diarrhea).

Assess infant for excessive bleeding from IV site following the transfusion.

Collaborative

Monitor laboratory studies, as indicated:

Hb/Hct levels prior to and following transfusion;

Serum bilirubin levels immediately following procedure, then every 4–8 hr;

Total serum protein;

Serum calcium and potassium;

Glucose;

Serum pH levels.

Helps prevent hypothermia and vasospasm, reduces risk of ventricular fibrillation, and decreases blood viscosity.

Exchange transfusions are most often associated with Rh incompatibility problems. Using Rh_o(D)-positive blood would only increase hemolysis and bilirubin levels, because antibodies in infant's circulation would destroy new RBCs.

Older blood is more likely to hemolyze, thereby increasing bilirubin levels. Heparinized blood is always fresh, but must be discarded if not used within 24 hr.

Establishes baseline values, identifies potentially unstable conditions (e.g., apnea or cardiac dysrhythmia/arrest), and maintains airway. Note: Bradycardia may occur if calcium is injected too rapidly.

Helps prevent errors in fluid replacement. Amount of blood exchanged is approximately 170 ml/kg of body weight. A double-volume exchange transfusion ensures that between 75% and 90% of circulating RBCs are replaced.

Hypocalcemia and hyperkalemia may develop during and following exchange transfusion.

Infusion of heparinized blood (or citrated blood without calcium replacement) alters coagulation for 4–6 hr following the exchange transfusion and may result in bleeding.

If Hct is <40% prior to transfusion, a partial exchange with packed RBCs may precede full exchange. Dropping levels following the transfusion suggest the need for a second transfusion.
Bilirubin levels may decrease by half immediately following procedure but may rise shortly thereafter, necessitating a repeat transfusion.
Multiplying level by 3.7 determines the degree of elevation of bilirubin necessitating exchange transfusion.
Donor blood containing citrate as an anticoagulant binds calcium, thereby decreasing serum calcium levels. In addition, if blood is more than 2 days old, RBC destruction releases potassium, creating a risk of hyperkalemia and cardiac arrest.
Low glucose levels may be associated with continued anaerobic glycolysis within donor RBCs. Prompt treatment is necessary to prevent untoward effects/CNS damage.
Serum pH of donor blood is typically 6.8 or less. Acidosis may result when fresh blood is not used and infant's liver cannot metabolize citrate used as an

ACTIONS/INTERVENTIONS	RATIONALE

Administer albumin prior to transfusion if indicated.

Although somewhat controversial, administration of albumin may increase the albumin available for binding of bilirubin, thereby reducing levels of freely circulating serum bilirubin. Synthetic albumin is not thought to increase available binding sites.

anticoagulant, or when donor blood continues anaerobic glycolysis, with production of acid metabolites.

Administer medications, as indicated:

  5% calcium gluconate;

From 2–4 ml of calcium gluconate may be administered after every 100 ml of blood infusion to correct hypocalcemia and minimize possible cardiac irritability. Note: Some controversy exists as to the purpose and effectiveness of this practice.

  Sodium bicarbonate;
  Protamine sulfate.

Corrects acidosis.
Counteracts anticoagulant effects of heparinized blood.

NURSING DIAGNOSIS:	KNOWLEDGE deficit [Learning Need], regarding condition, prognosis, and treatment needs
May Be Related To:	Lack of exposure, misinterpretation, unfamiliarity with information resources
Possibly Evidenced By:	Request for information, statement of problem/misconceptions, inaccurate follow-through of instructions
DESIRED OUTCOMES/EVALUATION CRITERIA—PARENT(S) WILL:	Verbalize understanding of cause, treatment, and possible outcomes of hyperbilirubinemia.
	Demonstrate appropriate care of infant.
	Identify signs/symptoms requiring prompt notification of healthcare provider.

ACTIONS/INTERVENTIONS

RATIONALE

Independent

Provide information about types of jaundice and pathophysiological factors and future implications of hyperbilirubinemia. Encourage questions; reinforce or clarify information, as needed.

Promotes understanding, corrects misconceptions, and can reduce fear and feelings of guilt. Neonatal jaundice may be physiological, breast milk–induced, or pathological, and protocol of care depends on its cause and contributing factors.

Demonstrate means of assessing infant for increasing bilirubin levels (e.g., observing blanching of skin over bony prominence or behavior changes), especially if infant is to be discharged early. Provide parents with 24-hr emergency telephone number and name of contact person, stressing importance of reporting increased jaundice.

Enables parents to recognize signs of increasing bilirubin levels and to seek timely medical evaluation/intervention.

Discuss home management of mild or moderate physiological jaundice, including increased feedings, diffused exposure to sunlight (checking

Parents' understanding helps foster their cooperation once infant is discharged. Information helps parents to carry out home management infant frequently), and follow-up serum testing program.

Provide information about maintaining milk supply through use of breast pump and about reinstating breastfeeding when jaundice necessitates interruption of breastfeeding.

Review rationale for specific hospital procedures/ therapeutic interventions (e.g., phototherapy, exchange transfusions) and changes in bilirubin levels, especially in the event that neonate must remain in hospital for treatment while mother is discharged.

Discuss need for Rh immune globulin (RhIg) within 72 hr following delivery for an Rh-negative mother who has an Rh-positive infant and who has not been previously sensitized.

Assess family situation and support systems. Provide parents with appropriate written explanation of home phototherapy, listing technique and potential problems, and safety precautions. Discuss appropriate monitoring of home therapy, e.g., periodic recording of infant's weight, feedings, intake/output, stools, temperature, and proper reporting of infant status.

Provide appropriate referral for home phototherapy program, if necessary.

Make appropriate arrangements for follow-up testing of serum bilirubin at same laboratory facility.

Discuss possible long-term effects of hyperbilirubinemia and the need for continued assessment and early intervention.

safely and appropriately and to recognize the importance of all aspects of management program. Note: Exposure to direct sunlight is contraindicated as infant's tender skin is highly susceptible to thermal injury.

Helps mother maintain adequate milk supply to meet infant's needs when breastfeeding is resumed.

Assists parents in understanding importance of therapy. Keeps parents informed about infant's status. Promotes informed decision making. Note: Some hospitals have overnight rooms that allow mother/father to remain with infant.

In Rh_o(D)-negative client with no Rh antibodies, who has given birth to an Rh_o(Du)-positive infant. Rh-Ig may reduce incidence of maternal isoimmunization in nonsensitized mother and may help to prevent erythroblastosis fetalis in subsequent pregnancies.

Home phototherapy is recommended only for full-term infants after the first 48 hr of life, whose serum bilirubin levels are between 14 and 18 mg/dl with no increase in direct reacting bilirubin concentration.

Lack of available support systems and education may necessitate use of visiting nurse to monitor home phototherapy program.

Treatment is discontinued once serum bilirubin concentrations fall below 14 mg/dl, but serum levels must be rechecked in 12–24 hr to detect possible rebound hyperbilirubinemia.

Neurological damage associated with kernicterus includes death, cerebral palsy, mental retardation, sensory difficulties, delayed speech, poor muscle coordination, learning difficulties, and enamel hypoplasia or yellowish green staining of teeth.

(Refer to CP: The Parents of a Child with Special Needs; ND: Knowledge deficit [Learning Need].)

THE INFANT OF AN ADDICTED MOTHER

Although abuse of alcohol, heroin, and marijuana has remained relatively stable, cocaine and crack use is growing dramatically, affecting approximately 1 in 10 pregnancies (higher in urban areas). In addition to alcohol and illicit drugs, abuse of prescription medications also occurs and use of multiple substances is common. From 80%–90% of infants born to addicted mothers are physiologically addicted and experience passive signs of drug withdrawal, commonly referred to as neonatal withdrawal syndrome or neonatal abstinence syndrome. It is estimated that cocaine use alone impacts 30,000–50,000 infants born annually. An additional 3000–5000 infants yearly are determined to be suffering from FAS. This plan of care is to be used in conjunction with the previous newborn plans of care. Refer also to CPs: The Preterm Infant and Deviations in Growth Patterns, as appropriate.

NEONATAL ASSESSMENT DATA BASE

Severity and time of onset of symptoms are related to substance(s) abused, duration of use, and maternal drug level at birth.

Activity/Rest

High-pitched cry, wakefulness, short or unquiet sleep patterns, yawning
Difficulty maintaining alert states

Circulation

Tachycardia
Hypertension

Ego Integrity

Poor state organization (cocaine use)

Elimination

Diarrhea
Hyperactive bowel sounds (hypermotility)

Food/Fluid

May be LBW or SGA infant; may have IUGR (maternal use of heroin, alcohol, or cocaine, or maternal malnutrition); or may be higher-birth-weight/LGA infant (maternal use of methadone)
Poor feeding with uncoordinated frantic sucking, hyperphagia, drooling, hiccups, possible cleft lip
Weight decrease or failure to gain weight
Vomiting/regurgitation
Dry mucous membranes, poor skin turgor, sunken fontanels
Abdominal distension, changes in bowel sounds, dilation of bowel (paralytic ileus, NEC)

Neurosensory

Apgar score may be low (e.g., intrauterine asphyxia or medication given to mother during intrapartal period).
Small head circumference/SGA (nicotine); microcephaly (FAS, cocaine use, toxic vapor abuse); facial abnormalities (FAS, toxic vapor abuse).
Hyperirritability (including increased startle response), hyperactivity, poor state organization; hypertonicity may be present.
Hyperacusis (abnormal sensitivity to sound), difficulty attending to/actively engaging in auditory and visual stimuli.
Tremors, persistent or rhythmic myoclonic jerks, or seizure activity may be noted.
Increased or exaggerated reflexes (e.g., gag, sucking, rooting, deep tendon, and Moro reflex) may be noted; absent or poor reflexes; poor muscle tone/limpness (perinatal infarcts).
Dilated/tortuous vessels of the iris.

Respiration

Periods of apnea (cocaine), transient tachypnea (heroin).
Increased tearing, rhinorrhea, stuffy nose, yawning, or sneezing may be present.
Signs of respiratory distress; green-tinged mucus (meconium aspiration) (heroin).
Tracheoepiglottal abnormalities (FAS).

Safety

Temperature variations.
Sweating, mottling, and flushing may be seen.
Rub marks on face and knees related to constant "mouthing/crawling" motions pressure-point abrasions.
Sclera, skin may be jaundiced.
Congenital anomalies (associated with cardiovascular or genitourinary systems) may be present.
Signs of infection or sepsis (acquired in utero), history of premature rupture of membrane, impaired immunologic mechanisms (marijuana).

Social Interaction

May exhibit poor tolerance for being held, decreased interactive behavior (difficulty responding to human voice/face, environmental stimuli), gaze aversion.

Sexuality

Female more commonly affected, ratio 2:1 (FAS)
Genital abnormalities in females (FAS)

Teaching/Learning

May be premature.
Mother may have received no prenatal care (literature suggests that 75% of women who abuse drugs during pregnancy do not seek prenatal care until the onset of labor), or may report prenatal problems associated with preterm labor, abruptio placentae, or placenta previa (placental insufficiency/fetal asphxia); infections such as pneumonia, endocarditis, STD, or hepatitis; PIH; and anemia.

Diagnostic Studies

Toxicology or Drug Screen (maternal/infant blood and urine, and fetal meconium): Identifies current substance exposure. Cocaine metabolites may persist in urine for 4–7 days after use, or even longer in infant.
Serum Electrolytes: Vomiting/diarrhea resulting in electrolyte imbalances.
Serum Glucose: May be decreased (increased metabolic rate, poor feeding, limited nutritional reserves [FAS]).
CBCD and Blood Cultures: For differential diagnosis associated with sepsis. GBS is becoming one of the most insidious and lethal infections of the newborn.
Platelet Count: May be decreased (tranquilizers or infectious process).
Serologic Tests: Determine presence of STDs, e.g., syphilis, hepatitis B, HIV.
Bilirubin Levels: Increased risk of jaundice (especially in infant of methadone user).
Electroencephalogram (EEG): May be abnormal, demonstrating cerebral irritation, in cocaine-exposed infant. Normalization of EEG noted by 3–12 mo of age.
Lumbar Puncture: Determines presence of white cells/bacteria, specific GBS antigens.

NURSING PRIORITIES

1. Facilitate and support drug withdrawal in infant.
2. Detection of infectious process.
3. Prevent injury, and reduce risk of short- and long-term complications.
4. Foster parent-infant interaction and attachment.
5. Provide information and support to parent(s) during rehabilitation process.

DISCHARGE GOALS

1. Gaining weight appropriately.
2. Free of injury, complications resolving.
3. Parent-infant interactions progressing satisfactorily.
4. Parent(s)/caregiver understand infant's present condition, prognosis, and needs.
5. Parent(s)/caregiver participate in care and use available resources.
6. Plan in place to meet ongoing needs after discharge.

NURSING DIAGNOSIS:	**INJURY, risk for CNS damage**
Risk Factors May Include:	Prematurity, hypoxia, effects of medications/substance use and/or withdrawal, possible exposure to infectious processes (perinatal/intrapartal)
Possibly Evidenced By:	[Not applicable; presence of signs/symptoms establishes an *actual* diagnosis]
DESIRED OUTCOMES/EVALUATION CRITERIA—NEONATE WILL:	Be free from injury and complications.
	Display reduced periods of hyperactivity or irritability; free of seizure activity.
	Display CNS function WNL.

ACTIONS/INTERVENTIONS

RATIONALE

Independent

ACTIONS/INTERVENTIONS	RATIONALE
Determine maternal history of addiction, noting duration, type of drug(s) used (including alcohol), and time and strength of last dose before delivery.	Degree of infant narcosis and withdrawal is related to the amount of mother's regular drug intake, the length of time mother has been addicted to drug(s), and the drug level at time of delivery. The closer the drug ingestion is to the time of delivery, the longer it takes for the infant to develop withdrawal and the more severe the manifestations may be. Note: An addicted mother frequently uses more than one substance, e.g., alcohol, cocaine, heroin, and phencyclidine (PCP).
Review prenatal/intrapartal record, and note any anesthesia or analgesia administered during intrapartal period.	The newborn is susceptible to possible long-term effects from fetal asphyxia associated with placental insufficiency, fetal drug withdrawal in utero (secondary to maternal withdrawal), and increased incidence of strokes and intracerebral hemorrhage. Medications administered to the mother during the intrapartal period, acidosis, and hypoxia associated with meconium aspiration may also contribute to temporary or permanent alterations in CNS function.
Observe infant for initial signs of acute withdrawal (e.g., tremors, restlessness, hyperactive reflexes, sneezing, high-pitched shrill cry, and hypertonicity).	Although these signs may appear soon after delivery (6–24 hr), the mean is 72 hr after birth, with delay of onset for as long as 10–14 days following delivery, especially if mother was on methadone maintenance during prenatal period. Note: Frequency of withdrawal signs is significantly less if methadone dose at time of delivery was <20 mg.
Monitor withdrawal using an evaluative tool or a seizure withdrawal chart (e.g., Neonatal Abstinence Score).	Consistent use of an objective tool provides a cumulative record that is useful in judging progress of withdrawal and/or effectiveness of

Place infant on abdomen. Provide pacifier/allow hand-to-mouth contact.

Swaddle infant in prone fetal (flexed) or side-lying position. Provide quiet, dimly lit area and scheduled periods of uninterrupted sleep.

Observe sleep patterns and degree and timing of irritability. (Refer to CP: The Preterm Infant; ND: Infant Behavior, risk for disorganized.)

Place baby in infant carrier, play soft music, and provide gentle rocking during periods of arousal.

Monitor effects of handling; decrease handling, as indicated.

Monitor vital signs and neurological status.

Observe infant for change in withdrawal signs and/or for side effects of drug therapy.

Observe infant for signs of seizure activity, such as twitching (rhythmic movements not decreased when limbs are held), rigidity, arching of back, nystagmus, and tongue thrusting or sucking motions. Institute seizure precautions.

Suction airway, and provide resuscitative measures, as indicated.

Collaborative

Monitor laboratory values, as indicated:

Glucose;

ABGs;

CBCD, sodium, calcium, and blood cultures.

---

supportive care and in determining need to institute or alter pharmacological therapy. Early identification of infants requiring medical or pharmacological intervention decreases incidence of mortality and morbidity. Subacute effects of narcotic drug withdrawal may last 4–6 mo.

Facilitates quieting and behavior organization. May reduce tension levels, decrease crying and irritability, and may actually reduce amount of drug treatment needed.

Decreases external stimuli, reducing CNS stimulation. Note: Infant may need to be positioned on side when risk of vomiting or regurgitation is present.

Excessive jitteriness and irritability interrupt sleep cycle, possibly necessitating initiation or alteration of pharmacological therapy. Withdrawal prevents adequate periods of deep sleep, but therapy promotes REM and deep sleep cycles.

Mimics intrauterine posture, helps soothe infant; provides body closeness.

Holding infant and providing close contact usually reduces hyperactivity and quiets child, although some infants become more irritable when they are held.

Early detection and treatment of potential complications such as meningitis, intracranial hemorrhage, and pyrexia reduce risk of long-term sequelae. Prematurity and liver immaturity, especially when associated with use of methadone, increase the risk of jaundice and kernicterus.

Changes in withdrawal signs may necessitate alteration in medication dosage to produce the best effect at the lowest dose without the side effects of excessive CNS depression, impaired sucking, or delayed bonding. Note: The greater the number and severity of withdrawal signs, the higher the probability of infant mortality or morbidity.

Newborns experiencing passive withdrawal from addiction are subject to convulsions associated with CNS stimulation, which increases risk of injury.

Maintains airway patency and supports vital functions.

Useful in differentiating signs of withdrawal from those of hypoglycemia. Note: Increased risk of hypoglycemia exists in FAS infants, who are often SGA with limited nutritional reserves.
Hypoxia and acidosis may develop, requiring prompt intervention.
Alterations in electrolytes and presence of sepsis or meningitis can produce signs similar to those of withdrawal.

Administer medications, as indicated:	Note: Infant experiencing cocaine withdrawal usually does not require pharmacological support.
Paregoric (administered orally);	Paregoric is the drug of choice for pharmacological management of drug withdrawal in the infant because of its sedative effect and lack of adverse effects.
Phenobarbital;	Sedatives may prevent or control seizure activity and modify hyperactive movement by depressing cerebrum, reducing CNS stimuli, and controlling irritability and insomnia.
Lorazepam (Ativan);	Often used for sedation by itself or with denatured tincture of opium (DTO). May decrease amount of DTO needed. Respiratory depression is main adverse effect, especially when used with other anticonvulsants.
Chlorpromazine (Thorazine);	While these drugs are generally not recommended, Thorazine may be used to control CNS and GI effects of withdrawal, but may be associated with prolonged excretion time and hypothermia.
Diazepam (Valium).	Valium can rapidly suppress narcotic withdrawal effects, but is poorly metabolized and excreted by infant and may require as long as 1 mo for total elimination. Parenteral administration may displace bilirubin and is contraindicated in jaundiced or premature infant.
Administer supplemental oxygen, as needed.	Corrects hypoxia and may prevent associated CNS damage.
Refer to foster care or child protection agency. (Refer to ND: Parenting, risk for altered.)	Psychosocial environment of home setting may predispose infant to neglect, addiction, or personality problems in later life. Some state laws require that all addicted mothers be reported to a child protection agency.

NURSING DIAGNOSIS:	**AIRWAY CLEARANCE, ineffective/GAS EXCHANGE, impaired**
May Be Related To:	Excess production of mucus, depression of cough reflex and respiratory center, intrauterine asphyxia
Possibly Evidenced By:	Tachypnea, tachycardia, cyanosis, nasal flaring, grunting respirations, hypoxia, acidosis
DESIRED OUTCOMES/EVALUATION CRITERIA—NEONATE WILL:	Display ABGs and respiratory rate WNL, with pink mucous membranes.
	Be free of signs of respiratory distress.

ACTIONS/INTERVENTIONS	RATIONALE

Independent

| Note respiratory rate and effort, color, heart rate, presence of cough reflex, and signs of respiratory distress. | Narcotic may depress respiratory center and cough reflex. Transient tachypnea (>60 respirations per min) secondary to excess fluid reabsorption in the lungs may occur. Tachycardia, cyanosis, nasal flaring, or grunting indicates hypoxia and respiratory failure. Mottling may occur as a vasomotor response during withdrawal and may be unrelated to peripheral oxygenation. |

Review and record fetal status during prenatal and intrapartal periods, and at delivery, for evidence of stress, hypoxia, or meconium-stained amniotic fluid.

Place infant on side or in semi-Fowler's position.

Note nasal stuffiness; suction prior to feedings, as indicated.

Monitor infant's temperature. Control environment to promote cooling if infant's temperature is elevated.

Collaborative

Monitor and graph serial ABGs.

Administer supplemental oxygen, if indicated.

Avoid use of narcotic antagonists, such as naloxone hydrochloride (Narcan) and naltrexone hydrochloride (Trexan).

Place infant on cardiopulmonary monitor and pulse oximeter. Initiate resuscitative measures, as appropriate.

Provides data about infant's respiratory status and indicates occurrence and degree of hypoxic insults.

Reduces risk of aspiration.

Increased nasal stuffiness and production of mucus interfere with breathing, especially during feedings.

Pyrexia associated with CNS stimulation increases metabolic rate and oxygen needs.

Drug withdrawal causes an increase in oxygen consumption. In addition, respiratory depression or failure may result in hypoxia and acidosis. Although narcotic-addicted infants are usually delivered prematurely, chronic intrauterine stress, especially when associated with heroin addiction, can increase surfactant production, thereby reducing risk of RDS.

Increased oxygen demands and respiratory depression are associated with withdrawal and may compromise respiratory function, causing hypoxia and respiratory acidosis and alkalosis.

These drugs are contraindicated in narcotic-addicted infants because they may precipitate acute withdrawal.

May be necessary in cases of severe respiratory interference. Note: Increased incidence of SIDS has been reported in cocaine-exposed infants, possibly because of altered neurotransmitter content and disruption of brain structures regulating respiration.

NURSING DIAGNOSIS: INFECTION, risk for

Risk Factors May Include: Maternal cultures positive for GBS or any STDs

Possibly Evidenced By: [Not applicable; presence of signs/symptoms establishes an *actual* diagnosis]

DESIRED OUTCOMES/EVALUATION CRITERIA—NEONATE WILL: Display no signs of infection as evidenced by normal CBCD, stable vital signs; afebrile, negative blood culture.

ACTIONS/INTERVENTIONS

RATIONALE

Independent

Identify maternal immune status and blood culture results; note prolonged rupture of membranes, infant's birth weight.

Monitor vital signs closely and assess respiratory status (rate and effort).

Infant may acquire STDs/GBS, either during intrapartum stage or during parturition. Transmission may also occur in the nursery. GBS is the single most common cause of fatal bacterial infection during the first 2 mo of life. It occurs most frequently in LBW infants and with prolonged rupture of membranes.

Respiratory-distress-like syndrome characterizes the infection. It then progresses to apnea, shock, and respiratory failure.

Inspect conjunctiva and eyelids.	Herpes simplex virus, gonococcal ophthalmia, and *Chlamydia* infections present with thick yellow eye discharge, accompanied by eyelid edema. These infections can progress to pneumonia and superficial corneal vascularization and blindness from scarring.
Note skin lesions, e.g., vesicles, pustules, petechiae.	Herpes simplex virus lesions appear in groups of small vesicles, which evolve into pustules with crust. Frequently found around the face, mouth, and on the scalp.

Collaborative

Review laboratory/diagnostic studies, e.g.:

CBCD, platelet count;	Development of septicemia (as evidenced by shift of differential to left, decreased platelets) is a high index of suspicion.
Gram's stain and cultures;	Identifies specific agent(s) involved to determine appropriate therapy.
Giemsa-stained smear;	Identifies herpes simplex virus (obtained from a smear from the base of a vesicular lesion), *Chlamydia* (obtained from lower conjunctival scrapings).
Lumbar puncture with CSF for bacteria, protein and glucose; cell count and differential;	CSF analysis helps to detect specific GBS antigens.
Viral culture, liver function tests (LFTs);	Optional testing for viral sepsis may be indicated if tachycardia and/or hepatosplenomegaly or liver function abnormalities are present. Viral organisms may include CMV, herpes, enteroviruses (coxsackie, echo), and rubella.
Chest x-ray.	Presentation on x-ray can vary and may include asymmetrical densities, pleural effusion, or pulmonary granularity (often associated with GBS).
Administer antibiotics as indicated, e.g.:	Dosage and schedule may vary with gestational and postnatal age.
Ampicillin;	May be indicated in early sepsis;
Vancomycin (Vancocin);	May be used.
Gentamicin (Garamycin);	May be effective in early or late sepsis. Note: Check drug levels before and after third dose and adjust accordingly.
Acyclovir (Zovirax);	Indicated in herpes exposure.
Ocular medications, such as vidarabine (Vira-A).	Prevents eye infections.

NURSING DIAGNOSIS:	**NUTRITION: altered, less than body requirements**
May Be Related To:	Inability to ingest/digest/absorb adequate nutrients to meet metabolic needs (e.g., poor/uncoordinated sucking and swallowing, frequent GI irritation with vomiting, diarrhea, and repeated regurgitation; frequent hyperactivity)
Possibly Evidenced By:	Failure to gain weight or weight loss, decreased adipose tissue
DESIRED OUTCOMES/EVALUATION CRITERIA—NEONATE WILL:	Tolerate feedings, free of aspiration. Maintain adequate nutritional intake as evidenced by normal weight gain and customary stool cycle.

ACTIONS/INTERVENTIONS	RATIONALE

Independent

Determine infant's gestational age. Note maternal prenatal nutritional state and evidence of maternal prenatal care.	IUGR and delivery of LBW infant can result from heroin use, which decreases cellular multiplication and growth hormone production in utero. Many addicted mothers are malnourished throughout the pregnancy, leading to birth of a preterm SGA/LBW infant having low protein, iron, and glucose stores. Approximately 75% of women who abuse drugs during pregnancy do not seek prenatal care until labor begins.
Monitor strength and coordination of sucking and swallowing reflexes.	CNS hyperactivity may negatively affect feeding behaviors and oral intake of nutrients.
Assess infant for nasal congestion, stuffiness, or sneezing. Use bulb suction prior to feedings as indicated.	Clears respiratory passage of excess mucus, allowing newborn to breathe more easily while eating, which may improve oral intake.
Encourage mother to feed infant, and assist her with activity as appropriate. Note effects of drugs and withdrawal syndrome on infant's feeding behaviors.	Hyperactive or sedated newborn is difficult to feed and put to the breast. In addition, FAS infants may display feeding problems and persistent vomiting for 6–7 mo and have difficulty adjusting to solid foods.
Provide small, slow, or frequent feedings. Use high-calorie formula, as appropriate. Encourage mother to avoid overfeeding.	Reduces risk of abdominal distension with resultant regurgitation. Slow feedings may allow infant to coordinate sucking and swallowing reflexes, improving intake. High-calorie formulas maximize nutrients available for energy production. In many cases, mothers overfeed, offering milk whenever the newborn cries, which may actually prolong the GI dysfunction. Note: If mother chooses to breastfeed infant, addition of HMF to pumped milk may be indicated.
Position infant on right side; do not disturb after feedings.	Facilitates emptying of stomach; promotes absorption. Disturbances may increase likelihood of regurgitation.
Monitor infant's intake and output, including frequency and consistency of stools.	Identifies imbalances, permitting early intervention. GI irritability is associated with frequent loose or watery stools, vomiting, and regurgitation, with resultant dehydration and malnutrition.
Weigh infant as indicated. Graph weight gains and losses.	Excessive or steady weight loss may indicate that caloric intake is inadequate for amount of energy being expended.
Institute a calorie count.	Inadequate weight gain may require use of higher-calorie formula and supplements, especially in LBW/SGA infant.
Note dryness of skin and mucous membranes, sunken fontanels, poor skin turgor, fever, diaphoresis, and increased urine specific gravity.	Dehydration can occur quickly in newborns because of fluid/electrolyte losses through diarrhea, vomiting, fever, and sweating.
Provide pacifier between feedings, position to facilitate hand-to-mouth activity.	Satisfies infant's need for sucking, promotes self-quieting, and may decrease metabolic demands.
Reduce external stimuli, and swaddle infant. (Refer to ND: Injury, risk for CNS damage.)	Reduces activity level, metabolic needs, and energy expenditure.

555

Test stool for presence of reducing substances.	Identifies possible lactose intolerance or poor nutritional state, necessitating use of soy-based formula.

Collaborative

Monitor laboratory studies, as indicated:	
Hb/Hct;	Identifies anemia.
WBC count with differential, blood cultures;	Infection/sepsis may be acquired in utero.
Serum glucose;	Hypoglycemia may develop as a result of poor feeding, hyperactivity with increased metabolic demands, or GI disturbances resulting in faulty utilization of formula.
Serum electrolytes.	Electrolyte imbalances may result from profuse diaphoresis, diarrhea, and inadequate fluid and nutrient intake.
Administer supplemental fluids parenterally, as appropriate.	May be necessary to prevent dehydration and to correct fluid and electrolyte imbalances associated with diarrhea, sweating, and vomiting.
Provide gavage feedings as indicated.	Conserves energy and decreases risk of regurgitation and aspiration. Gavage may be necessary if sucking and swallowing reflexes are ineffectual or uncoordinated and result in slower, difficult feedings, or if tachypnea or respiratory distress is present.
Administer antispasmodics (e.g., paregoric, tincture of opium) between feedings, as indicated.	Reduces GI irritation, controls loose or watery stools, and helps prevent dehydration.

NURSING DIAGNOSIS:	**SKIN INTEGRITY, risk for impaired**
Risk Factors May Include:	Mechanical factors (continual rubbing of face and knees against bedding, scratching of the face with hands), presence of excretions
Possibly Evidenced By:	[Not applicable; presence of signs/symptoms establishes an *actual* diagnosis]
DESIRED OUTCOMES/EVALUATION CRITERIA—NEONATE WILL:	Maintain intact skin.

ACTIONS/INTERVENTIONS	RATIONALE

Independent

Inspect skin for abrasion or excoriation, especially on face, nose, knees, elbows, and shoulders, and under buttocks.	Changes in tissue color and integrity indicate increased irritation and need for intervention.
Provide soft bedding or sheepskin; cover hands with mitts.	Decreases risk of dermal injury.
Reposition infant at least every 2 hr.	Avoids prolonged pressure on body parts.
Swaddle infant; place in infant carrier.	Provides sense of containment, decreases external stimuli, reducing activity level and risk of dermal irritation.
Provide skin care and meticulous cleansing of diaper area.	Prevents breakdown in diaper area, which is more susceptible to excoriation because of loose excretions/moisture and lack of air circulation.

Collaborative

Apply zinc oxide cream; nystatin medicated cream (Micronazole).

Forms a barrier between skin and irritants. Used to treat fungal infections of the buttocks. Note: *Candida* organisms gravitate to warm, moist areas such as buttocks or groin.

NURSING DIAGNOSIS:	PARENTING, altered
May Be Related To:	Lack of available or ineffective role model, lack of support between/from significant other(s), unmet emotional maturation needs of parent, interruption in bonding process, lack of knowledge, lack of appropriate response of child to relationship
Possibly Evidenced By:	Verbalization of role inadequacy, inability to care for infant, inattention to infant needs, inappropriate caretaking behaviors, lack of parental attachment behaviors
DESIRED OUTCOMES/EVALUATION CRITERIA—PARENT(S) WILL:	Demonstrate appropriate attachment behaviors. Verbalize realistic perception of the maternal/parental role. Verbalize insight into own dependency needs. Contact/use support resources effectively.

ACTIONS/INTERVENTIONS

RATIONALE

Independent

Evaluate mother's prenatal and current physical and emotional status. Assess family stressors. Note mother's involvement in prenatal care, childbirth classes, and drug or alcohol rehabilitation programs.

Provides data necessary to evaluate parenting capabilities and the family/home situation. Because of her own emotional state, the addicted mother is often unable to assume the overwhelming task of unselfish giving and nurturing, so that the potential for infant abuse or neglect exists.

Discuss mother's perception of herself, noting realistic and unrealistic appraisals and her desire to change. Maintain nonjudgmental attitude.

Fosters mother's desire to provide data about drug dependence, to discuss her emotional status, and to look realistically at her own ability to cope with the stress of childrearing and with the infant's withdrawal behaviors. The drug-addicted mother is usually dependent and depressed, and has low self-esteem and inadequate support systems stemming from an inability to form lasting intimate/mutually supportive relationships. Her drug dependence has resulted from her inadequate coping skills. Fear and guilt associated with her observation of infant's physiological withdrawal may reinforce her negative self-image and may negatively affect her ability to cope and care for the infant.

Encourage mother to express anxieties, fears, and anger. Discuss ways to release frustrations and manage stress (e.g., stating concern directly or use of physical exercise).

Helps mother to ventilate her concerns. Abusive behavior, guilt, and fear may reinforce feelings of incompetence.

Discuss current status of substance abuse. Initiate plans for enrollment in drug or alcohol rehabilitation program.

Mother's insight into her dependency needs and her ability to use resources to promote change may affect the decision regarding newborn placement with parent(s) or in foster care.

Ascertain maternal/paternal perceptions of parenting role and state of the family.	Provides realistic appraisal of parenting capabilities. Aids in predicting the amount of follow-up needed, and influences decisions regarding custody of newborn.
Encourage frequent visits/telephone contact as appropriate.	Minimizes separation between mother and newborn if infant is confined to the nursery, reducing interruption in bonding process. (Refer to CP: The Parents of a Child with Special Needs; ND: Parent/Infant Attachment, risk for altered.)
Recommend bringing infant to eye contact gradually while speaking slowly and softly.	May limit infant irritability and enhance interactive behavior. Note: Limited ability to tolerate visual activity may result in infant's taking a time-out by averting eyes after only 30–60 sec of interaction. Parent may erroneously interpret this as rejection by the infant.
Observe attachment behaviors and quality of parent-infant interaction.	Previous lifestyles, a potential lack of knowledge regarding child care and the needs of a growing infant, and the possibility of the infant's experiencing problems of withdrawal can interfere with the attachment process. Poor maternal interactional capabilities increase risk for a disturbed mother-child relationship. Furthermore, separation related to the infant's withdrawal, treatment, and hospitalization of the infant required after discharge of the mother may negatively affect the acquaintance process.
Assess parent's ability and desire to keep child.	Subtle cues of parental anxiety may be apparent in parents' behavior or in the expression of their concerns. The child may need to be placed in foster care if the mother/couple is unable to care for infant for a protracted period of time.
Support parents' efforts to understand and care for child.	Many parents require constant emotional support to build confidence.
Encourage performance of infant care tasks by mother and father.	Fosters positive adaptation to parenting role; facilitates the parent-newborn acquaintance process.
Provide information about the signs of acute newborn withdrawal, anticipated behaviors, and the therapeutic measures to be employed. Let parents know that these signs are usually temporary; however, infants with FAS can have subacute or long-term withdrawal effects, as well as mental retardation.	Prepares parents for management of withdrawal. Information about therapy may help relieve feelings of guilt, fear, and ambivalence. Feeding problems, excessive crying, irritability, inconsolability, and sleep disturbances may further reinforce parents' low self-esteem, may create potential negative feedback patterns (e.g., avoidance or rough handling of infant), and may interfere with or prevent positive attachment.
Provide names, phone numbers, and addresses of supportive resources providing 24-hr availability. Encourage use of these resources.	Allows parents to obtain help and information to help them to cope with stressful situations.
Schedule home visit within 7–10 days of infant's discharge from hospital.	Helps to monitor home setting and to assess the possibility of substance abuse, poor parenting, and infant neglect or abuse.

Collaborative

Refer parents to community resources, such as addiction counselor, social service, visiting nurse services, or peer/support group.	Ongoing support and assistance in a protective or therapeutic environment such as a halfway house or the use of ongoing services in the home may help parents develop appropriate parenting skills and promote well-being of the infant.

Make appropriate referral to foster care or child care agency.

Some state laws require notification of such agencies if mother is a known substance abuser. Maternal maturation may be insufficient to meet increasing demands of infant care. Note: Studies show an increased incidence of illness in the offspring of substance abusers believed to be directly related to poor parenting.

Refer mother to drug assistance program, as indicated (e.g., Narcotics Anonymous or Alcoholics Anonymous).

Mother needs to take care of herself before she can assume responsibility for another person.

NURSING DIAGNOSIS:	KNOWLEDGE deficit [Learning Need], regarding infant condition, prognosis, and care
May Be Related To:	Lack of exposure/unfamiliarity with information resources, misinterpretation, lack of recall, lack of interest in learning
Possibly Evidenced By:	Request for information, statement of misconceptions, inaccurate follow-through of instructions, inappropriate behaviors
DESIRED OUTCOMES/EVALUATION CRITERIA—PARENT(S) WILL:	List behaviors/signs associated with substance withdrawal. Verbalize/demonstrate appropriate infant care activities.

ACTIONS/INTERVENTIONS

RATIONALE

Independent

Provide information to parents about infant's behavior and physiological signs of withdrawal. Discuss rationale of treatment plan.

Fosters cooperation and understanding of interventions; promotes safety of infant. Encourages informed decision making.

Review altered responses of infant during withdrawal (increased sensitivity to auditory stimuli, depressed visual orientation and response, increased lability, and reduced alertness). Encourage mother to provide early visual input and pattern stimulation.

Information helps parent(s) understand infant's needs, optimizing infant's capabilities and interactional qualities, which can increase parents' self-esteem and provide reinforcement for efforts. Note: Long-term effects, particularly associated with cocaine, include behavior lability and inability to express strong feelings.

Identify long-term physiological effects of addiction on infant.

Although most infants are free of withdrawal signs by 10 days of age, mild patterns of irritability may persist for 3–4 mo, and sleep problems may persist for as long as 1 yr, creating stress for parents. Use of opiates, methadone, and possibly other drugs has been correlated with SIDS, feeding problems (FTT), hyperactivity, and brief attention span (which may be manifested with apparent long-term growth retardation and disturbed behavior patterns, especially in the FAS infant). In addition, smaller head size associated with cocaine use can lead to neurological impairment and difficulties with language skills as the infant matures.

559

Discuss passage of drugs (e.g., nicotine, narcotic, or alcohol) through breast milk.

Provide information about infant's needs following discharge (e.g., food, clothing, and equipment) and verify availability of resources. (Refer to CPs: The Neonate at 1 Week Following Discharge; and The Infant at 4 Weeks Following Birth; ND: Knowledge deficit [Learning Need].)

Recommend that parent(s) learn infant cardiopulmonary resuscitation (CPR).

Stress importance of continued medical monitoring and periodic reevaluation.

Alternative feeding method may need to be considered if maternal withdrawal program includes prescribed pharmacological agents. Mother needs to be aware that any drugs she takes can be passed on to the infant. Note: Cocaine may remain in breast milk for up to 60 hr following maternal use.

Helps ensure that parent(s) have necessary supplies in the home to care for the child.

Research suggests a fivefold increased incidence of SIDS in cocaine-exposed infants.

Once withdrawal is complete, infant/child may be asymptomatic until school age, at which time some limitations in general intelligence may be noted (FAS). In addition, lack of early diagnosis/timely intervention increases risk of behavioral problems.

NURSING DIAGNOSIS:	FAMILY COPING, ineffective: disabling
May Be Related To:	Significant person with chronically unexpressed feelings of guilt, anxiety, hostility, despair, and so forth; dissonant discrepancy of coping styles for dealing with adaptive tasks by/among significant person(s)
Possibly Evidenced By:	[Not applicable; presence of signs/symptoms establishes an *actual* diagnosis]
DESIRED OUTCOMES/EVALUATION CRITERIA—FAMILY WILL:	Verbalize realistic understanding and expectations of family members.
	Participate positively in care of infant, within limits of family's abilities.
	Express feelings and expectations openly and honestly, as appropriate.

ACTIONS/INTERVENTIONS

RATIONALE

Independent

Discuss parents' expectations of themselves and of infant, noting realistic and unrealistic perceptions.

Assess family stressors, history, and situation, and available support systems. Involve other family members in plan of care, if appropriate.

Observe parent-infant interaction and child care

Increases parents' awareness of common problems that may arise and helps them to have a more realistic view of parenting.

A stable relationship, the presence in the home of adults who are not substance abusers, and previous success in childrearing increase chance of positive outcome for infant. Family disorganization and disruption, with absence of strong, consistent father figure, or a history of sexual abuse of female who is addicted, may negatively affect mothering qualities.

Identifies areas of weakness or misunderstanding.

skills. Evaluate parents' level of knowledge and decision-making skills in regard to keeping and raising the infant. (Refer to ND: Parenting, risk for altered.)

Anxiety, depression, low self-esteem and self-confidence, and poor interpersonal skills typically render parents ineffective as primary caregivers and may foster intergenerational problems of child abuse or child neglect and predispose family members to substance abuse.

Ascertain long-range plans and mother's commitment to seeking assistance and making necessary lifestyle changes to achieve and maintain drug-free life.

Mother's drug problem and treatment status, together with her poor coping skills and lack of family support, may interfere with integration of infant into the family, necessitating alternative placement.

Collaborative

Provide referrals, as indicated, to meet physical, emotional, and financial needs (e.g., visiting nurse services, group homes, halfway houses, drug programs, and counseling or psychotherapy).

May be necessary to provide ongoing care, to reduce incidence of recidivism, and to foster optimal growth and development of parent(s) and infant.

THE INFANT OF AN HIV-POSITIVE MOTHER

Frequently, the newborn who is subsequently determined to be HIV-positive will be asymptomatic during the nursery stay. The CDC classifies HIV-positive newborns as indeterminate, asymptomatic, or symptomatic. Between 20% and 65% of infants born to HIV-positive mothers are themselves infected.

This plan of care is to be used in conjunction with the previous newborn plans of care.

NEONATAL ASSESSMENT DATA BASE

As a rule, the neonate is asymptomatic at birth, although a few may show signs of opportunistic infections within several days of birth. In addition, the effects of maternal substance use/abuse and/or prematurity may be present.

Circulation

Prolonged bleeding, petechiae (thrombocytopenia) noted on occasion

Elimination

Diarrhea
Enlarged liver, spleen may be noted

Food/Fluid

LBW
Feeding difficulties
Oral lesions (candidiasis)

Neurosensory

Neurological deficits
Microcephaly

Respiration

Varied degree of impairment (relative maternal drug use, cesarean birth)

Safety

Swollen glands (lymphadenopathy) noted on occasion
MATERNAL FACTORS
History of high-risk behaviors, STDs
Seropositive HIV

Sexuality

MATERNAL FACTORS
History of multiple sexual partners

Teaching/learning

Prematurity
Developmental delays
MATERNAL FACTORS
History of parental drug use (mother or partner)

DIAGNOSTIC STUDIES

CBC and Total Lymphocyte Count: Provides baseline immunologic data regarding WBC and lymphocyte counts to monitor disease progression.

Enzyme Immunoassay or Enzyme-Linked Immunosorbent Assay and Western Blot Test (EIA/ELISA): May be positive, but invalid because test does not distinguish between maternal and infant antibodies. (The infant may test negative by 9–15 mo of age.)

HIV Cultures (with peripheral blood mononuclear cells and, if available, plasma): Diagnostic for infants under 15 mo of age.

Polymerase Chain Reaction Test: Detects nucleic acid in small quantities of infected peripheral mononuclear cells.

Serum or Plasma p24 Antigen: Increased quantitative values can be indicative of progression of infection (may not be detectable during very early stages of HIV infection) in infants 30 days or older and who have had the second dose of hepatitis vaccine.

Quantitative Serum IgG, IgM, and IgA Determinations: Nondiagnostic in newborns, but provide baseline immunologic data.

Blood/Lesion/Urine Cultures: Diagnostic for opportunistic infections.

X-ray: May reveal lymphoid interstitial pneumonia.

NURSING PRIORITIES

1. Prevent/minimize infections.
2. Maximize nutritional intake.
3. Promote attachment, growth, and development.
4. Provide information to parent(s)/caregivers about disease process/prognosis and treatment needs.

DISCHARGE GOALS

1. Free of opportunistic/nosocomial infection.
2. Gaining weight appropriately.
3. Perform skills typical of age group within scope of present developmental level.
4. Parent/caregiver understands condition/prognosis and treatment needs.
5. Plan in place to meet specialized needs after discharge.

NURSING DIAGNOSIS:	INFECTION, risk for
Risk Factors May Include:	Immature immune system, inadequate acquired immunity, suppressed inflammatory response, invasive procedures, malnutrition, chronic disease (infections)
Possibly Evidenced By:	[Not applicable; presence of signs/symptoms establishes an actual diagnosis]
DESIRED OUTCOMES/EVALUATION CRITERIA—NEONATE WILL:	Be free of opportunistic infection.
PARENT/CAREGIVER WILL:	Verbalize understanding of individual risk factors.
	Identify interventions to reduce risk of infection.
	Provide safe environment for infant.

ACTIONS/INTERVENTIONS	RATIONALE

Independent

Note maternal HIV status/presence of high-risk behaviors, and prenatal/intrapartal use of zidovudine (AZT).	Affects care of neonate from time of delivery. Anti-HIV antibodies are transmitted across the placenta and are present in all infants of HIV-seropositive mothers. Between 20% and 67% of these infants will themselves eventually test positive for HIV. Note: Maternal antibodies may not be cleared from infant's system until 9–15 mo of age.

Use mechanical suction or bulb syringe in place of oral mucus extractors (e.g., DeLee trap) to clear airways. Avoid mouth-to-mouth contact for resuscitation.

Prevents exposure of healthcare provider to virus.

Wash neonate at time of delivery, or as soon as possible, using warm water and mild soap. Minimize exposure to maternal blood and body fluids.

Although maternal blood is contaminated, at birth infant may not be HIV-positive. Prompt care may help reduce risk to infant.

Provide customary physical care of neonate (e.g., skin care, eye care, vitamin K administration) the same as for all newborns, using universal precautions.

Universal precautions are routinely required for contact with body fluids/blood products to protect the healthcare provider from potential infection.

Stress need for care providers/family members washing hands before and after contact with infant. Wear gloves for contact with secretions (e.g., diapering, cord care, injections, handling of blood/blood by-products).

Reduces risk of cross-contamination and risk to care providers.

Sealed soiled tissues, paper wipes/trash, and disposable diapers in plastic bags per protocol.

Reduces risk of cross-contamination and alerts appropriate personnel/departments to exercise specific hazardous materials procedures.

Apply mittens; file infant's nails, as indicated.

Protects skin from injury that can provide additional portals of entry for infectious agents.

Monitor temperature and secretions. Auscultate breath sounds. Note behavioral changes, e.g., irritability, lethargy. Palpate lymph node chains.

HIV-seropositive infants have increased risk for developing recurrent upper respiratory infection, otitis media, thrush, cytomegalovirus, erythematous rash, and lymphadenopathy. Note: Although *Pneumocystis carinii* pneumonia (PCP) is common is both infants and adults, lymphocytic interstitial pneumonitis (LIP) is rarely seen in adults and is the second most common indicator disease for diagnosing AIDS in infants.

Prepare skin with soap and water and then alcohol prior to injections/heel-sticks. Notify laboratory of HIV status and mark specimens accordingly.

Proper preparation and handling reduces risk of cross-contamination for infant and care providers/laboratory staff.

Monitor/limit contact with care providers and family members, as appropriate.

Reduces number of pathogens presented to the infant's immune system and decreases possibility of infant's contracting a nosocomial infection. Note: Depending on specific facility policy, pregnant care providers may be excluded from caring for infant to reduce risk of HIV contamination.

Provide for complete isolation as indicated.

Presence of enteritis, congenital syphilis, CMV, or other viral infections increases risk of cross-contamination to other infants.

Investigate sudden fever, dyspnea, dry cough, hypoxia, abnormal breath sounds, or use of accessory muscles, retractions and nasal flaring.

Up to 50% of HIV-infected infants develop PCP during 1st yr of life.

Observe infant for seizure activity, neck stiffness, muscle rigidity, irritability or lethargy, or positive Kernig's sign.

Suggests meningitis or opportunistic CNS infection. Note: If symptoms develop slowly over weeks, may reflect HIV effect on CNS rather than acute infectious process.

Collaborative

Monitor laboratory studies as indicated:

Urine screening;

Increased risk of CMV in utero or during hospital stay necessitates routine microscopic evaluation.

IgG, IgM, IgA;	Note: Once infant is discharged, exposure to CMV is a risk in day-care setting as well. Elevated serum immunoglobulins are a hallmark of pediatric HIV infections and may develop before the decrease in CD4 (T-helper cells) is noted. Note: Polyclonal hypergammaglobulinemia occurs in approximately 80% of infected infants, usually in first months of life.
CD4 counts;	Decline reflects immunologic compromise and need for institution of AZT therapy. Note: CD4 counts of $3000/m^3$ or more are normal in healthy infants and gradually decline to adult levels. Counts below $1500/mm^3$ in 1st yr place infant at increased risk of developing PCP.
CBCD, liver function tests.	Establishes baseline prior to initiation of drug therapy to be compared with repeat studies at 2, 6, and 12 wk of age to monitor effects of therapy/progressions of condition.

Administer medications, as appropriate:

Zidovudine (AZT/ZVD);	Useful in preventing replication of HIV in infants older than 3 mo of age; however, side effects may limit its usefulness. Note: Recent CDC publications recommend 6 wk of combination therapy beginning within 12 hr of birth for infants born to seropositive mothers.
cidobudine (CBD); trimethoprin (TMP); sulfamethasoxazol (SMX) 2 divided doses;	Given orally immediately following birth to prevent *Pneumocystis carinii* pneumonia
didanosine (Videx);	May be used to treat HIV strains resistant to AZT.
ketoconazole (Nizoral);	Effective treatment for systemic yeast infections.
trimethoprim-sulfamethoxazole (Bactrim) prophylaxis;	Instituted for symptomatic infants or asymptomatic infants with CD4 counts below $500/mm^3$ to prevent PCP.
Triple dye, bacitracin;	Antimicrobial agents used in cord care to reduce risk of infection.
Ganciclovir (Cytovene).	Treatment of choice for CMV infection to prevent blindness/life-threatening dissemination.
Recommend/coordinate periodic ophthalmologic examinations as appropriate.	Early detection of retinitis in presence of CMV infection allows for prompt intervention.

NURSING DIAGNOSIS:	**NUTRITION: altered, risk for less than body requirements**
Risk Factors May Include:	Inability to ingest, digest, or absorb nutrients (e.g., impaired suck/swallow, GI infection, malabsorption, diarrhea)
Possibly Evidenced By:	[Not applicable; presence of signs/symptoms establishes an *actual* diagnosis]
DESIRED OUTCOMES/EVALUATION CRITERIA—NEONATE WILL:	Demonstrate progressive weight gain toward goal. Display laboratory values WNL. Be free of signs of malnutrition/FTT.
PARENT/CAREGIVER WILL:	Demonstrate understanding of feeding techniques and infant's specific needs.

ACTIONS/INTERVENTIONS	RATIONALE

Independent

Obtain baseline weight. Establish regular schedule for weighing following discharge (e.g., three times per week). Identify resources if scale is not available in home setting.	These infants are at increased risk for FTT as evidenced by weight loss or little weight gain from birth. Early recognition provides opportunity for prompt intervention. Note: If infant is eating well, but not gaining weight, evaluate for GI infection.
Observe coordination of sucking and swallowing reflexes.	Abnormal oral motor patterns may impair feeding ability.
Inspect oral cavity. Review procedure with caregivers.	Development of oral sores (e.g., thrush) impairs ability to feed, and, if untreated, can spread to the esophagus, necessitating alternative feeding techniques.
Counsel mother regarding risk of breastfeeding. Encourage alternative feeding method.	HIV is present in colostrum and breast milk and although limited, does present some risk to the infant.
Note infant tolerance of feedings.	Feeding difficulties, gastric distress, or signs of fatigue may require small, frequent feedings for optimal intake.
Hold infant during feedings.	Provides human contact/stimulation and may enhance intake.
Observe feeding techniques of caregivers. Provide assistance and encouragement.	Attention to positioning and handling may be required to normalize postural tone while feeding and to maximize sucking/swallowing efforts.
Investigate presence of diarrhea.	May indicate lactose intolerance requiring lactose-free formula or reflect GI manifestations of HIV infection (e.g., diarrhea, malabsorption, impaired gastric motility, and liver dysfunction).
Stress importance of close monitoring for infectious processes.	Infant is prone to parotitis, as well as frequent episodes of rapid-onset pneumonia, interfering with both appetite and feeding. In addition, presence of infectious process greatly increases metabolic rate and thereby nutritional needs.
Review future nutritional needs, age-appropriate diet and addition of solid foods considering developmental abilities.	Provides optimal nutrition based on individual needs following discharge.

Collaborative

Provide enteral/parenteral feedings as appropriate.	Motor impairments and/or presence of infection may necessitate alternative feeding techniques to meet dietary needs/prevent dehydration.
Obtain stool specimens, as indicated.	Stool cultures; tests for ova/parasites, *Cryptosporidium*, *C. difficile* (toxin produced by bacteria), acid-fast bacillus and Gram's stain may identify causes for gastric distress/diarrhea and weight loss or failure to gain.
Administer nystatin, as indicated.	Effective treatment for oral yeast infection.

NURSING DIAGNOSIS:	**GROWTH AND DEVELOPMENT, risk for altered**
Risk Factors May Include:	Separation from significant others, inadequate caretaking, inconsistent responsiveness/multiple caretakers, environmental and stimulation deficiencies, effects of chronic condition/disabilities
Possibly Evidenced By:	[Not applicable; presence of signs/symptoms establishes an *actual* diagnosis]
DESIRED OUTCOMES/EVALUATION CRITERIA—NEONATE WILL:	Respond to parent/caregiver interactions.
	Perform motor, social, and/or expressive skills typical of age group, within scope of present capabilities.
PARENT/CAREGIVER WILL:	Verbalize understanding of developmental status and plans for intervention.
	Demonstrate skills in handling infant needs.

ACTIONS/INTERVENTIONS	RATIONALE
Independent	
Determine individual status using Denver Developmental or similar screening tool.	Provides baseline to note future progress/changes and identify therapy needs. Cognitive impairments vary, may be present at birth, or may develop as a result of environmental deprivation or viral infections affecting the CNS. In addition, some infants may have delayed sensorimotor development, while others display abnormal muscle tone and movement patterns with delayed development of righting and equilibrium reactions. (Refer to CP: Deviations in Growth Patterns.)
Identify developmental milestones and anticipated time frames for achievement.	Reinforces belief that infant may progress with appropriate support and interventions. Note: Lack of development or regression is an indicator of need for further evaluation and may reflect effect of infectious process.
Discuss caregiver's perceptions of infant's capabilities and plan for growth.	Increased frequency of illness, prolonged/recurrent hospitalizations, neglect/overprotection by caregivers may limit sensory/movement stimuli and motivation.
Observe infant-parent/caregiver interactions.	Eye contact, reaching out of infant promotes adult response. Effect of maternal drug use, presence of illness, or developmental delays may prevent or limit infant interactions, impairing bonding/attachments.
Encourage verbalization of feelings by parent(s)/family members.	Frequently, feelings of guilt and despair may be expressed as hostility, denial, or defensiveness regarding diagnosis. Awareness of these feelings provides opportunity to work through them and develop a positive relationship with the infant.
Avoid confronting denial. Counsel without lecturing, provide information without patronizing, and support and give hope without making false promises.	Parent(s) need to progress at their own rate and denial may be very strong especially when the infant is asymptomatic. Providing information, Active-listening, and acceptance of the person in nonjudgmental ways promotes more positive

567

Encourage/support family efforts to care for infant.

Personal interactions, even after a period of abandonment, enhance the bonding process. Note: Volunteers may be required to support staff efforts in the absence of family participation or ineffective family involvement.

progression to acceptance and resolution of dealing with reality of the situation.

Discuss ways to provide a normal atmosphere (e.g., spending time outdoors, using support systems effectively).

Enhances sense of control and provides encouragement for enjoying the present and possibilities of the future.

Collaborative

Coordinate multidisciplinary team conference to include pediatrician, primary nurse, social worker, nutritional support, psychologist/psychiatrist or clinical specialist psychiatric nurse, physical/occupational therapists, and speech therapists.

Necessary to address complex issues and maximize infant's potential because all areas are interrelated to growth and development.

Stress importance of frequent screening and formal evaluations by developmental specialists.

Identifies developmental delays and effectiveness of therapy (e.g., early intervention program [EIP]).

NURSING DIAGNOSIS:	KNOWLEDGE deficit [Learning Need], regarding condition, prognosis, and treatment needs
May Be Related To:	Lack of exposure, misinterpretation, unfamiliarity with resources, lack of recall, lack of interest in learning
Possibly Evidenced By:	Request for information, statement of misconceptions, inaccurate follow-through of instructions, development of preventable complications
DESIRED OUTCOMES/EVALUATION CRITERIA—PARENT/CAREGIVER WILL:	Verbalize understanding of condition and treatment needs. Identify signs/symptoms requiring intervention. Perform necessary procedures correctly and explain reasons for the actions. Establish plan for ongoing therapy and evaluations.

ACTIONS/INTERVENTIONS

RATIONALE

Independent

Determine parent(s)'/caregivers' understanding of condition and prognosis.

Provides starting point for information and opportunity to clarify misconceptions. Incubation period of initial HIV infection to progressive encephalopathy varies from 2 mo to 5 yr. HIV directly affects CNS, cardiovascular, GI, and renal function. Median age for appearance of opportunistic infection is 9 mo. Impaired brain growth, loss of developmental milestones, and progressive motor dysfunction indicate a very poor prognosis. Note: Children rarely develop Kaposi's sarcoma,

Provide realistic, optimistic information during each contact with parent.

tuberculosis, toxoplasmosis, cryptococcosis, or histoplasmosis.

Enhances attachment process and reduces likelihood of abandonment. Many people have been exposed to media information about AIDS or have friends/lovers who have died of the disease, and parent/caregiver may be pessimistic about outcome for infant.

Note response to contact with infant by parent(s)/family, and other caregivers. Discuss individual concerns.

Interactions may be affected by fear of contamination and of personal judgments regarding suspected high-risk behaviors of parents. Note: To date, there have been no documented cases of individuals contracting AIDS from routine care of infected infants when following established CDC precautions.

Note roles of family members and availability of extended family.

HIV infection is frequently a multigenerational disease, directly affecting mothers, offspring, and other family members. Because the mother must deal with her own chronic illness, awareness of the role of the father and/or grandparents is necessary in determining family needs or necessity of alternative placement.

Review current medication/treatment options.

Research is ongoing and often openly discussed in the media, sometimes raising false hopes that must be clarified to enhance the decision-making process. Current studies suggest monthly IV immunoglobulins (IV-Ig) may reduce infections and incidence of hospitalization. In addition, trials of experimental vaccines for asymptomatic HIV-seropositive infants are presently being tried in the hope of enhancing the response of the immune system.

Discuss safe formula preparation and feeding techniques.

Reduces risk of bacterial infection and aspiration. Note: Infant should not be put to bed with formula/juice bottle because of risk of bacterial growth.

Recommend prompt diaper changing/perineal care, use of disposable gloves, and proper handling of soiled diapers/other pericare items.

Reduces risk of skin irritation providing entry of infectious agents. Protects others from exposure to HIV.

Identify ways to protect infant from exposure to common infections, diseases, or contact with recently vaccinated individuals.

Impairment of immune system reduces infant's ability to ward off disease. Depending on infant's immune status, placement in day care may be contraindicated to reduce risk of cross-contamination from other infants.

Stress importance of routine immunization as appropriate.

Provides protection from some infectious agents. Note: Infant should receive injectable (Salk) instead of oral (Sabin) polio vaccine, which contains live virus. In addition, asymptomatic infants do not require influenza vaccine.

Review side effects of therapy, e.g., AZT.

Nausea/vomiting, abnormalities of liver function, and suppression of bone marrow limit therapy/drug dosage.

Determine current living conditions, physical care needs, immune status/presence of opportunistic infections.

Mother's lifestyle/condition may preclude her providing appropriate care for infant. Other family members (e.g., grandparents, aunt/uncle) may be providing care for mother and/or other involved family members and be unable to care for infant too.

Discuss placement options as appropriate.

Chronically ill/impaired mother and extended family members who may be overtaxed with caring for ill family members may not be able to meet the needs of even a well infant. Residential or foster home may be indicated at least for a period of time until family or parent(s) are able to assume responsibility for infant. However, many foster homes refuse HIV-infected infants, and as a rule, these children are not usually available for adoption, making placement very difficult.

Stress frequency and content of follow-up care, especially with health professionals experienced in caring for HIV-seropositive women and infants.

Knowledgeable providers are better equipped to deal with the complex health issues and use newly developed treatment options to promote optimal outcomes for the infant/family.

Discuss significance of HIV and other testing.

Regular testing to age 2 is necessary to verify HIV status in absence of opportunistic infections. Viral cultures, polymerase chain reaction, IgA, IgM, p24 antigen assay, and evaluation of CD4 lymphocyte count monitor presence/progression of infection. In addition, some resources believe all infants born to HIV-risk women require vigilant pediatric follow-up for early diagnosis of true HIV infection.

Identify signs/symptoms requiring notification of healthcare provider, e.g., fever, pain, altered activity level, difficulty breathing, poor appetite, weight loss, vomiting, diarrhea, skin rashes, oral thrush, or developmental regression.

Prompt evaluation and intervention may limit process and progression to AIDS.

Encourage parents/caregivers to care for their own health and to make time to meet their own needs for rest and relaxation.

As they learn to take time for themselves, parents/caregivers can better manage long-term care of a chronically ill child.

Review individual/family coping strategies. Discuss/encourage use of effective stress management techniques, including use of medication/prayer as appropriate.

Individuals providing care for infant with complex medical regimen and emotional needs are exposed to multiple, continuous stressors that can quickly exhaust coping abilities, increasing risk for caregiver role strain.

Identify sources for family counseling, community support groups, and other resources (e.g., visiting nurse services, home care agency, social services, respite care).

Mother-infant dyads are at increased risk for impaired bonding. Physical illness, financial stressors, depression, maternal drug use, and poor support systems interfere with parenting abilities, placing infant at risk for physical and emotional neglect/abuse. In addition, family members will require assistance in coping with chronic illness and future prognosis of other family members. Note: Recent studies suggest mothers who provide primary care for their infant with HIV report lower quality of life scores as compared to alternative caregivers, reflecting need for special attention/support of this population.

Bibliography

General Reference: Articles

Sevo, M: Keeping the faith: *Jewish tradition in pregnancy and childbirth.* AWHONN Lifelines, 1(4)46, 1997.

General Reference: Books

American Academy of Pediatrics and American College of Obstetrics and Gynecology: *Guidelines for Perinatal Care,* ed 2, American Academy of Pediatrics and American College of Obstetrics and Gynecology, 1997.

The American College of Obstetricians and Gynecologists: *Guidelines for Women's Health Care,* The American College of Obstetricians and Gynecologists, 1996.

Association of Women's Health, Obstetrics, and Neonatal Nursing (AWHONN): *Core Curriculum for Neonatal Intensive Care Nursing,* WB Saunders, Philadelphia, 1993.

Berkow, R, (ed): *The Merck Manual,* ed 16, Merck & Co., Rahway, 1992.

Cella, J, and Watson, J: *Nurse's Manual of Laboratory Tests,* ed 2, FA Davis, Philadelphia, 1995.

Cox, HC, et al.: *Clinical Applications of Nursing Diagnosis,* ed 3, FA Davis, Philadelphia, 1997.

Deglin, JH, and Vallerand, AH: *Davis's Drug Guide for Nurses,* ed 5, FA Davis, Philadelphia, 1997.

Doenges, ME, and Moorhouse, MF: *Nurse's Pocket Guide: Nursing Diagnoses with Interventions,* ed 6, FA Davis, Philadelphia 1998.

Gordon, T: *PET in Action.* Wiley Pub, 1976.

Joint Program in Neonatology, Harvard Medical School, Beth Israel Hospital, Brigham & Women's Hospital, The Children's Hospital, Boston, MA,: *Manual of Neonatal Care,* ed 3, Little, Brown, & Co, Boston, 1991.

Lipson, JG, Dibble, SL, and Minarik, PA: *Culture and Nursing Care:* A Pocket Guide, UCSF Nursing Press, 1996.

Manual of the Office Management of Sexually Transmitted Diseases. Cornell postgraduate course, Reed & Carnrick Pub, Piscataway, NJ, 1988.

Mishell, D, Herbst, A, and Kirschbaum, T: *Year Book of Obstetrics and Gynecology,* Mosby, St. Louis, 1996.

National Council for Excellence in Critical Thinking. Critical Thinking: *Shaping the Mind of the 21st Century,* Sonoma State University, Center for Critical Thinking and Moral Critique: Rhonert Park, CA, 1992.

Niswander, KR, and Evans, AT: *Manual of Obstetrics,* ed 5, Little, Brown, & Company, 1996.

Olds, SB, London, ML, and Ladewig, PW: *Maternal Newborn Nursing:* A Family-Centered Approach, ed 5, Addison-Wesley, Redwood City, CA, 1996.

Rivlin, MF, and Martin, RW: *Manual of Clinical Problems in Obstetrics and Gynecology,* Little, Brown & Company 1994.

Suddarth, DS: *The Lippincott Manual of Nursing Practice,* ed 5, JB Lippincott, Philadelphia, 1991.

Chapter 1: Articles

American College of Nurse-Midwives (ACNM): *Clinical practice guideline, clinical practice committee.* Nurse Midwifery, 40(2)58, 1995.

Attenborough, R: *The Canadian health care system: Development, reform, and opportunities for nurses.* JOGNN, 26(2) 229, March/April, 1997.

Bendell, A: *Health care in the 1990s: Changes in health care delivery models for survival.* JGONN, 26(2)212, March/April, 1997.

Boucher, MA: *Delegation alert!* Am J Nurs, 98 (2)26, February, 1998.

Cox, RP: *Family health care delivery for the 21st century.* JOGNN, 26(1)109, January/February, 1997.

Fitzgerald, SM: *Advanced practice nursing: Back to the future.* JOGNN, 26(1)101, January/February, 1997.

Henry, J: *Community nursing centers: Models of nurse managed care.* JOGNN, 26(2)224, March/April, 1997.

Honn, A: *Are you ready for genetic counseling?* AWHONN Lifelines, 1(3), June, 1997.

Jones, R: *Patient satisfaction with home care.* Home Care Provider, 2(5)235, October, 1997.

Jones, SL: Genetics: *Changing health care in the 21st century.* JOGNN, 25(9)777, November/December, 1996.

Keepnews, D: *Welfare reform and health care.* Am J Nurs, 98(3)55, March, 1998.

Lea, DH, Anderson, G, and Black, R: *A multiplicity of roles for genetic nursing: Building toward holistic practice.* Holistic Nursing Practice, 12(3)77, April, 1998.

Leininger, M: *Transcultural nursing research to transform nursing education and practice: 40 years.* Image J Nurs Schol, 29(4)341, Fourth Quarter, 1997.

Loescher, L, and Ronan, J: *Toward a holistic view of genetic technology as a way of knowing.* Holistic Nursing Practice, 12(3)1, April, 1998.

Lynn, M, and Kelley, G: *Effects of case management on the nursing context: Perceived quality of care, work satisfaction, and control over practice.* Image J Nurs Schol, 29(3)237, Third Quarter, 1997.

National Council of State Boards of Nursing (1995). *Delegation: Concepts and decision-making process.* Issues, (suppl 4,) 16: 4, May/June, 1997.

Pence, M: *Patient-focused models of care.* JOGNN, 26(3)320, May/June, 1997.

Penticuff, JH: *Ethical dimensions in genetic screening: A look into the future.* JOGNN, 25(9)785, November/December, 1996.

Pesut, DJ: *The future, virtue-ethics, and Sigma Theta Tau.* Reflections, 23(3)56, Third/Fourth Quarter, 1997.

Raines, D: *From covenant to contract.* AWHONN Lifelines, 1(4)41, August, 1997.

Simpson, K: *What nurses need to know.* AWHONN Lifelines, 1(3)26, June, 1997.

Sinclair, B: *Advanced practice nurses in integrated health care systems.* JOGNN, 26(2)217, March/April, 1997.

Ventura, MJ: *NPs vs. MDs.* RN, 61(2)27, February, 1998.

Williams, LR, and Cooper, MK: *A new paradigm for postpartum care.* JOGNN, 25(9)745, November/December, 1996.

Chapter 2: Articles

Starn, J, and Neiderhauser, V: *An MCN model for nursing diagnosis to focus interventions.* Mat Child Nurs, 15:180–183, 1990.

Chapter 2: Books

Doenges, ME, Moorhouse, MF, and Geissler, AC: *Nursing Care Plans: Nursing Diagnoses in Patient Care,* ed 4, FA Davis, Philadelphia, 1997.

Doenges, ME, Townsend, MC, and Moorhouse, MF: *Psychiatric Care Plans: Guidelines for Planning and Documenting Client Care,* ed 3, FA Davis, Philadelphia, 1998.

Chapter 3: Books

Doenges, ME, and Moorhouse, MF: *Application of Nursing Process and Nursing Diagnosis: An Interactive Text,* ed 2, FA Davis, Philadelphia, 1995.

Lampe, SS: *Focus Charting,* ed 4, Creative Nursing Management, Minneapolis, 1986.

Chapter 4: Articles

Amaya, M: *Perinatal lead exposure.* Reflections, 22(3)18, Third Quarter, 1996.

Astley, S, and Little, R: *Maternal marijuana use during lactation and infant development at one year.* Neurotoxicology and Teratology, 12:161, 1990.

Bartholomew, SD: *Healthy moms, healthy babies: 1st, 2nd, 3rd Trimester.* Diabetes Forecast, 50(9)25–33, December, 1997.

Bresnahan, K, Brooks, C, and Zuckerman, B: *Prenatal cocaine use: Impact on infants and mothers.* Pediatric Nursing, 17(2)123, 1991.

Casey, K: *Malnutrition associated with HIV/AIDS, part 2: Assessment and interventions.* J Assoc Nurses AIDS Care, 8(5)39, September/October, 1997.

Chasnoff, IJ, et al: *Cocaine/polydrug use in pregnancy: Two-year follow-up.* Pediatrics, 89(2)284, 1992.

Chasnoff, IJ, et al: *Perinatal cerebral infarction and maternal cocaine use.* J Pediat, 108:456, 1986.

Clarifying the risks of delayed childbearing. Am J Nurs 96(8) 11, August, 1996.

Cohen, M: *Building a better baby.* Parenting, December/January, 1997.

Craig, DI: *The adaptation to pregnancy of spinal cord injured women.* Rehabilitation Nursing, 15(1)6, 1990.

Detecting heart defects prenatally. Science News, 152(6)89, August 9, 1997.

Dunn PA, and Feinberg, RF: *Oncofetal fibronectin: New insight into the physiology of implantation and labor.* JOGNN, 25(9)753, November/December, 1996.

Duley, L, et al: *Which anticonvulsant for women with eclampsia? Evidence from the collaborative eclampsia trial.* Lancet, 345:1455, 1995.

Forrest, F, Florey, C, and Taylor, D: *Maternal alcohol consumption and child development.* Int J Epidemiol, 21(4)S17, 1992.

Frenkel, L, et al: *Effects of Zidovudine use during pregnancy on resistance and vertical transmission of human immunodeficiency virus Type 1.* Clin Infec Dis 20:1321, 1995.

Gill, P, Smith, M, and Katz, M: *Tocolysis for preterm labor.* Tokos Medical Corp., Santa Ana, CA.

Gill, P, and Katz, M: *Let's prevent preterm birth.* Tokos Medical Corp., Santa Ana, CA.

Haddad, A: *Ethics in Action.* RN, 60(7)17, July 1997.

Hoegerman, G, and Scholl, S: *Narcotic use in pregnancy.* Clin Perinatol, 18(1)51, 1991.

Jones, SL: *Genetics: Changing health care in the 21st century.* JOGNN, 25(9)777, November/December, 1996.

Kane, A: *Herbal medicine and childbirth: Do they mix?* International Journal of Childbirth Education, 12(2)22, May/June, 1997.

Kearney, MH, Murphy, S, and Rosenbaum, M: *Mothering on crack cocaine: A grounded theory analysis.* Social Science Medicine, 18(2)351, 1994.

Kivikoski, AI, Martin, CM, and Smeltzer, JA: *Transabdominal and transvaginal ultrasonography in the diagnosis of ectopic pregnancy.* Am J Obstet Gynecol, 163:123–128, 1990.

Klebanoff, M. et al: *Outcome of the vaginal infections and prematurity study: Results of a clinical trial of erythromycin among pregnant women colonized with Group B Streptococci.* Am J Obstet Gynecol, 172:1540, 1995.

Langer, A, and Kudart, E: *Construction of a family pedigree in genetic counseling before amniocentesis.* J Reprod Med, 35:715–718, 1990.

Lucas, LS, and Jordan, ET: *Phenytoin as an alternative treatment for preeclampsia.* JOGNN, 26(3)263, May/June, 1997.

MacMullen, NJ, Dulski, LA, and Naber, SJ: *Women's reactions to monitoring of high-risk pregnancy at home or in the hospital.* Mother Baby Journal, 2(5)23, September, 1997.

Maloni, J, and Ponder, MB: *Fathers' experience of their partners' antepartum bed rest.* Image J Nurs Schol, 29(2)183, Second Quarter, 1997.

McFarlane, J, Parker, B, and Soeken, K: *Abuse during pregnancy: Associations with maternal health and infant birth weight.* Nurs Res, 45(1)37, Jan/Feb, 1996.

Ostrea, EM, et al: *Meconium analysis to assess fetal exposure to nicotine by active and passive maternal smoking.* J Pediatr, 124(3)471, 1994.

Patient guide: When diabetes develops during pregnancy. Medical Aspects of Human Sexuality, 91:45–46, 1991.

Paulson, RJ: *Conservative surgical treatment of ectopic pregnancy.* J Reprod Med, 35:22–24, 1990.

Penticuff, JH: *Ethical dimensions in genetic screening: A look into the future.* JOGNN, 25(9)785, November/December, 1996.

Pietrantoni, M, and Knuppel, R: *Alcohol use in pregnancy.* Clin Perinatol, 18(1)93, March, 1991.

Pregnancy after 35. Harvard Women's Health Watch, 4(11)2, July, 1997.

Pregnancy, smoking, and HIV. HIV Frontline, 28(7), May/June, 1997.

Prozac and pregnancy. Science News, 150(16)249, October 19, 1996.

Richardson, P: *Sleep in pregnancy.* Holist Nurs Pract, 10(4)20–26, July, 1996.

Schroeder, C: Women's experience of bed rest in high-risk pregnancy. Image J Nurs Sch 28(3)253, Fall, 1996.

Sibal, B, et al: *Aggressive versus expectant management of severe preeclampsia at 28 to 32 weeks' gestation: Randomized controlled trial.* Am J Obstet Gynecol 171:818, 1994.

Sisson, MC: *Preventing preterm labor.* AWHONN Lifelines, 1(2)42, April, 1997.

Shiono, P, et al: *The impact of cocaine and marijuana use on low birth weight and preterm birth: A multicenter study.* Am J Obstet Gynecol, 172, 1995.

Stark, M: *Psychosocial adjustment during pregnancy: The experience of mature gravidas.* JOGNN, 26(2)206, March/April, 1997.

Sternfeld, B, et al: *Exercise during pregnancy and pregnancy outcome.* Med Sci Sports Exerc 27:634, 1995.

Stevie, MM: *Pregnancy-induced hypertension: A comprehensive review.* Mother Baby Journal, 2(4)20, July 1997.

Stewart, R: *Female circumcision implications for North American nurses.* J Psychosoc Nurs Ment Health Serv, 35(4)35, April, 1997.

Stirrat, GM: *Common causes of recurrent miscarriage.* Medical Aspects of Human Sexuality, 25(7)36–44, 1991.

Teen birth rate falls again. Family Life Matters, 30:7, Winter, 1997.

Tutelian, L: *A good night's sleep, the first trimester.* Parenting, December/January, 1997.

Urbanski, P: *How does hydration affect preterm labor?* AWHONN Lifelines, 1(3)25, June, 1997.

Visser, W: *Temporising management of severe pre-eclampsia with and without the HELLP syndrome.* Br J Obstet Gynaecol, 102:111, 1995.

Wilkins-Haug, L, Gabow, Pa: *Toluene abuse during pregnancy: Obstetric complications and perinatal outcomes.* Obstet Gynecol, 77(44)504–509, 1991.

Chapter 4: Books

Flandermeyer, A: The drug-exposed neonate. In Kenner, C, Grueggemeyer, A, and Gunderson, L (eds), *Comprehensive Neonatal Nursing,* WB Saunders, Philadelphia, 1993, pp. 997–1033.

Loftus, JA: Antepartum home care. In *Community and Home Health Nursing,* Aurowich, I, and Burkhart, L (eds), Delmar Publishers, Albany, 1996.

Peragallo-Dittko, V, Godfrey, K, and Meyer, J: *A Core Curriculum for Diabetes Education,* ed 3, American Association of Diabetes Educators, Chicago, 1995.

Stovall, T: *The Use of Methotrexate for the Treatment of Ectopic Pregnancy,* Mosby-Year Book, St. Louis, 1996.

Chapter 5: Intrapartal: Articles

Acosta, YM, et al: *HIV disease and pregnancy: Antepartum and intrapartum care,* part 2. JOGNN, 21(2)97–103, 1992.

Cook, A, and Wilcox, G: *Pressuring pain.* AWHONN Lifelines 1(2)36, April, 1997.

Furst, S, and Reisner, L: *Risk of high spinal anesthesia following failed epidural block for cesarean delivery.* J Clin Anesth 7:71, 1995.

Harvey, CS: *Coming to terms: Electronic fetal monitoring update.* AWHONN Lifelines, 1(3)43, June, 1997.

Johnson, K, and Rodgers, S: *When cultural practices are*

health risks: The dilemma of female circumcision. Holist Nurs Pract, 8(2)70, January, 1994.

Jukelevics, N: *Reducing cesarean rates while improving maternal and infant outcomes.* International Journal of Childbirth Education, 12(1)30, February, 1997.

King, D: *Electronic fetal monitoring.* International Journal of Childbirth Education, 12(1)28, February, 1997.

Maier, J, and Maloni, J: *Nurse advocacy for selective versus routine episiotomy.* JOGNN, 26(2)155, March/April, 1997.

Martin, J: *The gentle truth about infant bonding.* Parenting, December, 1993.

Ment. L, et al: *Antenatal steroids, delivery mode, and intraventricular hemorrhage in preterm infants.* Am J Obstet Gynecol, 172, 1995.

Schmidt, J: *Fluid check, making the case for intrapartum amnioinfusion.* AWHONN Lifelines, 1(5)47, October, 1997.

Shorten, A: *Female circumcision: Understanding special needs.* Holistic Nursing Practice 9(2)66, January, 1995.

Stem, J: *Flirting with disaster.* AWHONN Lifelines, 1(1):31, February, 1997.

Swayze, SC: *Electronic fetal monitoring.* Nursing 98, 28(1) 20, January, 1998.

Winslow, EH, and Jacobson, AF: *Research for practice; benefits of continuous support during labor.* Am J Nurs, 98(1) 16, January, 1998.

Chapter 6: Postpartal: Articles

Acosta, YM, et al: *HIV disease and pregnancy: Antepartum and intrapartum care, part 2.* JOGNN, 21(2)97–103, 1992.

Bastin, N, et al: *HIV disease and pregnancy: Postpartum care of the HIV-positive woman and her newborn, part 3.* JOGNN, 21(2)105–111, 1992.

Eaton, AP: *Current controversies in infant feeding: Why breast is best.* Pediatric Rounds, 2(1)7–9, 1993.

Fertility and contraception: Some diabetics can use OCs safely. Medical Aspects of Human Sexuality, 25(3)16, 1991.

Gennaro, S: *Leave and employment in families of preterm low birthweight infants.* Image J Nurs Schol, 28(3)193, Fall, 1996.

Hanna, K: *Helping grieving parents explain perinatal death to children.* The Journal of Perinatal Education, 5(3)45, March, 1996.

Hoeman, SP: *A research-based transdisciplinary team model for infants with special needs and their families.* Holist Nurs Pract, 7(4)63–72, 1993.

Janssen, HJEM, et al: *A prospective study of risk factors predicting grief intensity following pregnancy loss.* Arch Gen Psychiatry, 54, January, 1997.

Jones, R: *Patient satisfaction with home care.* Home Care Provider, 2(5):235, October, 1997.

Martin, J: *The gentle truth about infant bonding.* Parenting, December, 1993.

Nagle, B: *Low molecular weight heparin.* RN, 61(4)40, April, 1998.

Neifert, M: *The working mother's guide to breastfeeding.* Parenting, December/January, 1997.

Neugebauer, R, et al: *Major depressive disorder in the 6 months after miscarriage.* JAMA, 277(5), 383, February 5, 1997.

Postoperative Epidural Analgesia: A Guide for Nurses. Astra Pharmaceutical Products, Inc, Westborough, MA, 1993.

Postpartum disorders. The Harvard Mental Health Letter, 14(3)1, September, 1997.

Probing the cause of after-baby blues. Science News, 148(6)15, July 1, 1995.

Quinn, A, and Koepsell, D: *Breastfeeding incidence after*

early discharge and factors influencing breastfeeding cessation. JOGNN, 26(3)289, May/June, 1997.

Rose, M, and Clark-Alexander, B: *Caregivers of children with HIV/AIDS: Quality of life and coping styles.* Journal of the Association of Nurses in AIDS Care, 9(1)58, January/February, 1998.

Schnare, S, and Matsuda, K: *Today's contraceptive choices.* RN, 60(12)30, December, 1997.

Smith-Stoner, M, and Frost, AL: *Coping with grief and loss.* Nursing 98, 28(2)49, 1998.

Strimike, C, Wojcik, J, and Stark, B: *Incision care that really cuts it.* RN, 60(7)22, July, 1997.

Williams, LR, and Cooper, MK: *A new paradigm for postpartum care.* JOGNN, 25(9)745, November/December, 1996.

Wolf-Gabor, S: *The individuality of grief.* AWHONN Lifelines, 1(2)72, April, 1997.

Chapter 6: Postpartal: Books

Groeschell, BJ, and Revolinski, MA: Breast feeding. In *Community and Home Health Nursing,* Anrowich & Burkhart, Delmar Publishers, Albany, 1996

Loftus, JA: Postpartum home care. In Androwich, I, and Burkhart, L (eds), *Community and Home Health Nursing,* Delmar Publishers, Albany, 1996.

Chapter 7: Articles

Anderson, J, et al: *Occupational therapy for children with perinatal HIV infection.* Am J Occup Ther, 44(3)249–55, 1990.

Bastin, N, et al: *HIV disease and pregnancy: Postpartum care of the HIV-positive woman and her newborn,* part 3. JOGNN, 21(2)105–111, 1992.

Blass, JL, Mehta, KA, and Camara, J: *Monitoring premature infants in car seats: Implementing the American Academy of Pediatrics policy in a community hospital.* Pediatrics, 91(6), June, 1993.

Bourland, J: *The circumcision decision.* Parenting, 102–106, February, 1997.

Christmas, JT: *The risks of cocaine use in pregnancy.* Medical Aspects of Human Sexuality, 26(2)36, 1992.

Dusick, AM, et al: *Risk of intracranial hemorrhage and other adverse outcomes after cocaine exposure in a cohort of 323 very low birth weight infants.* J Pediatr, 122(3)438–445, 1993.

Early hospital release not the only factor in newborn health. HealthNews, 3(11)6, August, 26, 1997.

Gallagher, MA and Klima, C: *The challenge of maternal-infant transmission of HIV.* JANAC, 7(1)47, January/February, 1996.

Gingras, JL, et al: *Cocaine and development: Mechanisms of fetal toxicity and neonatal consequences of prenatal cocaine exposure.* Early Hum Dev, 31:1–24, 1992.

Hess, DJ, and Kenner, C: *Families caring for children with fetal alcohol syndrome: The nurse's role in early identification and intervention.* Hol Nurs Pract, 12(3)47, April, 1998.

Keolahan, C, and James, EJP: *The natural history of neonatal jaundice.* Pediatrics, 74:368, 1984.

Lawrence, R: *Breastfeeding is more than just good nutrition.* International Journal of Childbirth Education, 12(1)16, February, 1997.

Lockridge, T: *Now I lay me down to sleep: SIDS and infant sleep positions.* Mother Baby Journal, 2(2)8, March, 1997.

Lutes, L: *Bedding twins/multiples together.* Neonatal Network, 15(7)61, October, 1996.

Mandich, MB, and Ritchie, SK: *Transition times to oral feeding in premature infants with and without apnea.* JOGNN, 25(9)771, November/December, 1996.

McFarlane, J, Parker, B, and Soeken, K: *Abuse during pregnancy: Associations with maternal health and infant birth weight.* Nurs Res, 45(1)37, January/February, 1996.

Noerr, B: *Keeping the newborn warm: Understanding thermoregulation.* Mother Baby Journal, 2(5)6, September, 1997.

Pasers, CL: *Pain control: Pain during circumcision.* AJN 97(10)21, October, 1997.

Peters, KL: *Bathing premature infants: Physiological and behavioral consequences.* Am J Criti Care, 7(2)90, March, 1998.

Plessinger, MA, and Woods, JR: *The cardiovascular effects of cocaine use in pregnancy.* Reprod Toxicol, 5(2)99–113, 1991.

Porcher, FK: *HIV-infected pregnant women and their infants: Primary health care implications. Nurse Practitioner.* Am J of Primary Health Care, 17(11)46, 49–50, 53–54, 1992.

Pressler, J, and Hepworth, J: *Behavior of marosomic and appropriate-for-gestational-age newborns.* JOGNN, 26(2)198, March/April, 1997.

Raine, A, et al: *Interaction between birth complications and early maternal rejection in predisposing individuals to adult violence: Specificity to serious, early-onset violence.* Am J Psychiatry, 154:1265, September, 1997.

Riordan, J, and Koehn, M: *Reliability and validity testing of three breastfeeding assessment tools.* JOGNN, 26(2)181, March/April, 1997.

Rose, M, and Clark-Alexander, B: *Caregivers of children with HIV/AIDS: Quality of life and coping styles.* JANAC, 9(1)58, January/February, 1998.

Safe transportation of premature and low birth weight infants. Pediatrics, 97(5), May, 1996.

Seppa, N: The dark side of immunizations? A controversial hypothesis suggests that vaccines may abet diabetes, asthma. Science News, 152(21)332, November 22, 1997.

Shiao, S: Fluid and electrolyte problems of infants of very low birth weight. AACN Clinical Issues in Critical Care Nursing, 3(3)698–704, 1992.

Singer, L, et al: Neurodevelopmental effects of cocaine. Clinics in Perinatology, 20(1)245–261, 1993.

Smith, J: Bringing Theresa home. Nursing 91, 21(3)94, 1991.

Sternberg, S: Pinpoint cold saves sight, not acuity. Science News, 149(16)244, April, 20, 1996.

Taking baby's temperature. HealthNews, 3(9)8, July, 15, 1997.

WHO/UNICEF issue statement on HIV and breastfeeding. Int Nurs Rev, 39(4)108, 1992.

Wilfert, CM: *HIV infection in maternal and pediatric patients.* Hosp Pract, 26(5)55–62, 65–67, 1992.

Zuckerman, B, et al: *A preliminary report of prenatal cocaine exposure and respiratory distress syndrome in premature infants.* AJDC 145:696–698, June 1991.

Chapter 7: Books

Groeschell, BJ, and Revolinski, MA: Breast feeding. In Anrowich, I and Burkhart, L (eds), *Community and Home Health Nursing,* Delmar Publishers, Albany, 1996.

Grubman, S, and Simonds, RJ: *Preventing Pneumocystis corinii pneumonia in HIV-infected children.* New Guidelines for Prophylaxis, Pediatric Infections Disease Journal, 15:165, 1996.

Kotulak, R: Inside The Brain. Andrews McMeel Pub, Kansas City, 1996.

Merenstein & Gardner: *Handbook of Neonatal Critical Care,* (ed 3), Mosby, 1997.

Index of Nursing Diagnoses